COSMETIC SURGERY AFTER MASSIVE WEIGHT LOSS

COSMETIC SURGERY AFTER MASSIVE WEIGHT LOSS

Edited by

SETH R. THALLER, MD, DMD
Chief and Professor
Division of Plastic, Aesthetic, and Reconstructive Surgery
Dewitt Daughtry Family Department of Surgery
University of Miami Health System
Miami, Florida
USA

MIMIS COHEN, MD, FACS, FAAP
Professor and Chief
Division of Plastic, Reconstructive and Cosmetic Surgery
University of Illinois
Chicago, Illinois
USA

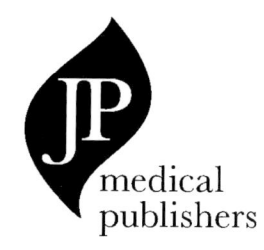

JP medical publishers

London • St Louis • Panama City • New Delhi

© 2013 JP Medical Ltd.
Published by JP Medical Ltd, 83 Victoria Street, London, SW1H 0HW, UK
Tel: +44 (0)20 3170 8910   Fax: +44 (0)20 3008 6180
Email: info@jpmedpub.com   Web: www.jpmedpub.com

The rights of Seth R. Thaller and Mimis Cohen to be identified as editors of this work have been asserted by them in accordance with the Copyright, Designs and Patents Act 1988.

All rights reserved. No part of this publication may be reproduced, stored or transmitted in any form or by any means, electronic, mechanical, photocopying, recording or otherwise, except as permitted by the UK Copyright, Designs and Patents Act 1988, without the prior permission in writing of the publishers. Permissions may be sought directly from JP Medical Ltd at the address printed above.

All brand names and product names used in this book are trade names, service marks, trademarks or registered trademarks of their respective owners. The publisher is not associated with any product or vendor mentioned in this book.

Medical knowledge and practice change constantly. This book is designed to provide accurate, authoritative information about the subject matter in question. However readers are advised to check the most current information available on procedures included and check information from the manufacturer of each product to be administered, to verify the recommended dose, formula, method and duration of administration, adverse effects and contraindications. It is the responsibility of the practitioner to take all appropriate safety precautions. Neither the publisher nor the editors assume any liability for any injury and/or damage to persons or property arising from or related to use of material in this book.

This book is sold on the understanding that the publisher is not engaged in providing professional medical services. If such advice or services are required, the services of a competent medical professional should be sought.

Every effort has been made where necessary to contact holders of copyright to obtain permission to reproduce copyright material. If any have been inadvertently overlooked, the publisher will be pleased to make the necessary arrangements at the first opportunity.

ISBN: 978-1-907816-28-4

British Library Cataloguing in Publication Data
A catalogue record for this book is available from the British Library

Library of Congress Cataloging in Publication Data
A catalog record for this book is available from the Library of Congress

JP Medical Ltd is a subsidiary of Jaypee Brothers Medical Publishers (P) Ltd, New Delhi, India.

Publisher:	Geoff Greenwood
Development Editor:	Gavin Smith
Design:	Designers Collective Ltd

Indexed, typeset printed and bound in India.

Foreword

It is an honor and great privilege to write this foreword. Seth Thaller and Mimis Cohen are both renowned educators, forward thinkers and internationally recognized leaders in plastic surgery.

Obesity is an epidemic; however, bariatric surgery has been proven to be an effective and safe option for patients afflicted with massive obesity, a condition that is resistant to traditional diet and exercise regimens. Long-term studies show that the procedures used cause significant long-term loss of weight, recovery from diabetes, improvement in cardiovascular risk factors, and a reduction in mortality.

In the past, reconstructive and cosmetic surgeons have developed new, innovative techniques in craniofacial, micro- and endoscopic surgery in order to meet the needs of patients suffering from burns, cancer and trauma. In a similar way, plastic and reconstructive surgeons have once again risen to the challenge of rapidly developing new and safe techniques to help post-bariatric patients to deal with redundant skin and fat.

The editors have assembled a group of knowledgeable experts who have contributed to this comprehensive and practical text covering all aspects of cosmetic surgery after massive weight loss. The book features contributions from numerous residents and young colleagues, as well as very experienced authors who are leaders in their fields and who have already published extensively on this challenging topic.

Among the interesting topics covered, I was particularly fascinated by the by first few chapters, which describe the surgical options, psychological evaluations, and medical management of post-bariatric patients. Subsequent chapters deal with cosmetic surgical options that improve various anatomical areas after massive weight loss. The final chapters report on new, unique approaches to tissue transfer for cancer reconstruction, techniques to avoid unfavorable results, and important medicolegal issues related specifically to cosmetic surgery for the massive weight loss patient.

Congratulations should go to the editors and the very distinguished group of authors responsible for developing this landmark contribution to plastic surgery. This book should become a key focal point for cosmetic surgeons specializing in body contouring surgery for massive weight loss patients.

Renato Saltz MD, FACS
Vice-President,
International Society of Aesthetic Plastic Surgery (ISAPS)
Founder and Chairman,
Image Reborn Foundation of Utah Saltz Plastic Surgery
Salt Lake City and Park City
Utah, USA

Preface

Due to the almost epidemic proportion of the population afflicted with morbid obesity and associated morbidity, there has been an ever expanding number of patients undergoing bariatric surgical procedures. Postbariatric body contouring surgery is centered on enhancing the overall quality of life following weight loss surgery. This focuses on the overall loss of skin tone, resultant sagging fat and skin, and concomitant functional deficiencies associated with these clinical issues. At the completion of the plastic surgical rehabilitation, the patient should enter a final stage where they are able to obtain a more natural look. Prior to embarking on this surgical endeavor, the plastic surgeon must ensure that the patient is an appropriate candidate for surgical intervention. Key considerations are that the patient's weight is stabilized, they have developed a new, healthy and fit lifestyle, they have satisfactory motivation, are medically stable, and possess reasonable goals and expectations. However, all surgical procedures and sequences must be individualized and may even require serial operative approaches. The priority must always remain patient safety.

This book has solicited experts and innovators in their field to impart their experiences with these challenging patients. The authors have shared their extensive knowledge and have covered every aspect of the comprehensive management of post-bariatric patients, from the actual options for weight loss surgery, to the psychological needs of the individual patient. The authors then describe how to approach the patient and develop an overall treatment plan. With these goals in mind, this book will serve to introduce the plastic surgeon early on in their career to how best to approach and successfully manage these patients, and importantly, avoid complications. In addition, the more seasoned plastic surgeon will be able to employ this book to review, update, and enhance their skills prior to embarking on operative treatment.

Seth R. Thaller
Mimis Cohen
August 2012

Contents

Foreword   v

Preface   vii

Contributors   xi

Chapter 1
Surgical options for weight loss   1
Michael C. Cheung, Bassan J. Allan, Veer Chahwala, Nestor F. De La Cruz

Chapter 2
Psychological evaluation of the postbariatric patient   5
Veer Chahwala, Michael C. Cheung, Bassan J. Allan, Nestor F. De La Cruz

Chapter 3
Medical management of the postbariatric patient and evaluation before body contouring procedures   7
Bassan J. Allan, Michael C. Cheung, Veer Chahwala, Nestor F. De La Cruz

Chapter 4
Preoperative evaluation of the postbariatric patient   11
Yash J. Avashia, Narayanan M. Nair, ChiChi Berhane, Zubin Jal Panthaki

Chapter 5
Anesthetic challenges encountered in the postbariatric patient   19
Gian Paparcuri, Miguel Cobas

Chapter 6
Anatomical deformities secondary to massive weight loss   25
Michele A. Shermak

Chapter 7
Outpatient lower body lift   39
Richard H. Tholen, Douglas L. Gervais

Chapter 8
Sequencing and timing of surgery of the postbariatric patient   57
Dennis J. Hurwitz

Chapter 9
Panniculectomy and abdominoplasty   73
Urmen Desai, Andrew M. Rivera, Bryan R. Wilner, Seth R. Thaller

Chapter 10
Belt lipectomy and total body lift   89
Megan C. Jack, Martin I. Newman

Chapter 11
Hernia repair in the massive weight loss patient 105
Jason W. Edens, Ergun Kocak, Carmen S. Ceron,
Liliana Camison, Christopher J. Salgado

Chapter 12
Reconstruction of abdominal wall defects after bariatric 113
surgery and simultaneous abdominal lipectomies
Mimis Cohen, Rebekah M. Zaluzec

Chapter 13
Brachioplasty 125
Michele A. Shermak

Chapter 14
Male breast surgery after massive weight loss 133
Brian D. Kubiak, Milton B. Armstrong

Chapter 15
Female breast surgery after massive weight loss 137
Ari S. Hoschander, Steven M. Henriques, Catherine Gordon,
John C. Oeltjen

Chapter 16
Gluteal contouring after massive weight loss 145
Morad Askari, Haaris S. Mir

Chapter 17
Medial and lateral thigh surgery after massive weight loss 153
Susan E. Downey

Chapter 18
Facial contouring after bariatric surgery 161
Kenneth L. Fan, Benjamin T. Lemelman, Seth R. Thaller

Chapter 19
Role of suction-assisted lipectomy 165
Joseph F. Capella

Chapter 20
Unfavorable results: identification and avoidance 179
Michael S. Golinko, Albert Losken

Chapter 21
Tissue transfer for cancer reconstruction in the massive 189
weight loss patient
Deniz Dayicioglu

Chapter 22
Medicolegal issues 203
Walter G. Sullivan

Index 211

Contributors

Bassan J. Allan, MD, MBA
General Surgery Resident
Department of Surgery
University of Miami
Miami, Florida
USA

Milton B. Armstrong, MD
Professor and Chief, Division of Plastic Surgery
Medical University of South Carolina
South Carolina
USA

Morad Askari, MD
Assistant Professor of Surgery, Assistant Professor of Orthopaedic Surgery
Departments of Surgery and Orthopaedic Surgery
University of Miami Miller School of Medicine
Miami, Florida
USA

Yash J. Avashia, BS
University of Miami
Miller School of Medicine
Miami, Florida
USA

ChiChi Berhane, MD, MBA
Plastic Surgeon
Division of Plastic Surgery
University of Miami
Miami, Florida
USA

Liliana Camison, MD
Division of Plastic Surgery
University of Miami Miller School of Medicine
Miami, Florida
USA

Joseph F. Capella, MD
Chief, Division of Post-Bariatric Body Contouring
Division of Plastic Surgery
Hackensack University Medical Center
Hackensack, New Jersey
USA

Carmen S. Ceron, BS
Division of Plastic Surgery
University of Miami Miller School of Medicine
Miami, Florida
USA

Veer Chahwala, MD
General Surgery Resident
Department of Surgery
University of Miami
Miami, Florida
USA

Michael C. Cheung, MD
Plastic Surgery Fellow
Department of Surgery
Division of Plastic, Maxillofacial, and Oral Surgery
Duke University, North Carolina
USA

Miguel Cobas, MD
Associate Professor of Anesthesiology
University of Miami Leonard M. Miller
  School of Medicine
Department of Anesthesiology, Perioperative Medicine
  and Pain Management
Miami, Florida
USA

Deniz Dayicioglu, MD
Assistant Professor,
Plastic and Reconstructive Surgery
Department of Surgery
Division of Plastic Surgery
University of South Florida
Tampa, Florida
USA

Nestor F. De La Cruz, MD, FACS, FASMBS
Associate Professor of Surgery
Chief, Division of Laparoendoscopic and
  Bariatric Surgery
Director of the Bariatric Fellowship Training Program
Co-Director, Center of Excellence in Minimally
  Invasive Surgery
Department of Surgery
University of Miami
Miami, Florida
USA

Urmen Desai, MD, MPH
Fellow in Plastic and Reconstructive Surgery
Department of Plastic and Reconstructive Surgery
University of Miami
Miller School of Medicine
Miami, Florida
USA

Susan E. Downey, MD, FACS
Clinical Associate Professor of Plastic Surgery
Keck School of Medicine
University of Southern California
Los Angeles, California
USA

Jason W. Edens, MD
Resident in Plastic Surgery
Division of Plastic Surgery
University of Miami Miller School of Medicine
Miami, Florida
USA

Kenneth L. Fan, MD
Resident in Plastic Surgery
Georgetown University Hospital
Department of Plastic Surgery
Washington, D.C.
USA

Douglas L. Gervais, MD
Minneapolis Plastic Surgery Ltd
Minneapolis, Minnesota
USA

Michael S. Golinko, MD, MA
Plastic Surgery Fellow
Department of Surgery
Division of Plastic Surgery
Emory University School of Medicine
Atlanta, Georgia
USA

Catherine Gordon, BA
University of Miami
Miller School of Medicine
Miami, Florida
USA

Steven M. Henriques, MD
Associate Professor
Department of Surgery
The University of Illinois at Peoria
Peoria, Illinois
USA

Ari S. Hoschander, MD
Resident in Plastic, Aesthetic and Reconstructive Surgery
Department of Plastic, Aesthetic and Reconstructive Surgery
University of Miami
Miami, Florida
USA

Dennis J. Hurwitz, MD
Clinical Professor of Plastic Surgery
Department of Plastic Surgery
University of Pittsburgh Medical Center
Director of the Hurwitz Center for Plastic Surgery
Pittsburgh, Pennsylvania
USA

Megan C. Jack, MD
Plastic and Reconstructive Surgeon
Sanctuary Plastic Surgery
Boca Raton, Florida
Cleveland Clinic Florida
Weston, Florida
USA

Ergun Kocak, MD, MS
Assistant Professor of Plastic Surgery
Department of Plastic Surgery
The Ohio State University Medical Center
Columbus, Ohio
USA

Brian D. Kubiak, MD
Resident in Plastic Surgery
Division of Plastic Surgery
Medical University of South Carolina
South Carolina
USA

Benjamin T. Lemelman, MD
Resident in Plastic and Reconstructive Surgery
Department of Plastic and Reconstructive Surgery
University of Chicago
Chicago, Illinois
USA

Albert Losken, MD, FACS
Professor of Surgery
Division of Plastic and Reconstructive Surgery
Emory University
Atlanta, Georgia
USA

Haaris S. Mir, MD
Assistant Professor Surgery
Department of Surgery
Division of Plastic and Reconstructive Surgery
University of Miami
Leonard M. Miller School of Medicine
Miami, Florida
USA

Narayanan M. Nair, MD
General Surgery Resident
Department of General Surgery
Cleveland Clinic Florida
Weston, Florida
USA

Martin I. Newman, MD, FACS
Director of Education
Head of Clinical Research
Associate Program Director
Department of Plastic Surgery
Cleveland Clinic Florida
Weston, Florida
USA

John C. Oeltjen, MD, PhD
Assistant Professor of Surgery
Division of Plastic and Reconstructive Surgery
Department of Surgery
University of Miami
Miami, Florida
USA

Zubin Jal Panthaki, MD, CM, FRCS(C), FACS
Associate Professor of Clinical Surgery
(Division of Plastic Surgery)
Associate Professor of Clinical Orthopaedics
University of Miami Miller School of Medicine
Chief of Plastic Surgery and Hand Surgery, Miami VA
Chief of Hand Surgery, University of Miami Hospital
Miami, Florida
USA

Gian Paparcuri, MD
Assistant Professor of Anesthesiology
University of Miami Leonard M. Miller School of Medicine
Department of Anesthesiology, Perioperative Medicine
  and Pain Management
Miami, Florida
USA

Andrew M. Rivera, MD
Resident in Otolaryngology Department of Otolaryngology
University of Miami
Miller School of Medicine
Miami, Florida
USA

Christopher J. Salgado, MD
Associate Professor of Surgery (Plastic Surgery)
Co-Director, University of Miami Center for Genital Surgery
Section Chief, University of Miami Hospital
Division of Plastic Surgery
University of Miami Miller School of Medicine
Miami, Florida
USA

Michele A. Shermak, MD, FACS
Plastic Surgeon
The Plastic Surgery Center of Maryland
Lutherville, Maryland
USA

Walter G. Sullivan, MD, JD, LLM
Health Law Attorney of Counsel
Levine, Garfinkel and Eckersley
President, Plastic Surgery Transitions Inc.
Las Vegas, Nevada
USA

Richard H. Tholen, MD
Minneapolis Plastic Surgery Ltd
Minneapolis, Minnesota
USA

Bryan R. Wilner, BS
University of Miami
Miller School of Medicine
Miami, Florida
USA

Rebekah M. Zaluzec, DO
Resident Surgeon
Department of Surgery
University of Illinois College of Medicine at
Chicago – Mount Sinai Hospital
Chicago, Illinois
USA

Dedication

A special thanks and appreciation to my wife, Pat, who has been by my side throughout the highs and lows: I couldn't manage without her support. She makes everything worthwhile. Also to my children, Cody and Lexi, who make it interesting, and my mother.

ST

To my wife Andrea and my daughter Saranna with my thanks and appreciation for their love and support.

MC

Chapter 1 Surgical options for weight loss

Michael C. Cheung, Bassan J. Allan, Veer Chahwala, Nestor F. De La Cruz

■ INTRODUCTION

Worldwide, an estimated 1.7 billion individuals are overweight or obese.[1] In the USA, approximately two-thirds of the population are overweight and about 5% are morbidly obese.[2] The increase in the prevalence of obese patients is also associated with a rise in a number of medical conditions, including type 2 diabetes, hyperlipidemia, hypertension and asthma. Moreover, obesity imposes a considerable economic burden on society, and an estimated 2.5 million deaths a year are attributed to comorbidities associated with obesity.[3]

■ PREOPERATIVE EVALUATION

Estimates suggest that close to 350 000 bariatric operations were performed worldwide in 2008.[4] However, despite the high volume of bariatric procedures performed there is no consensus about the ideal preoperative evaluation for bariatric surgical candidates.[5] Weight loss improves obesity-related comorbidities and may have a mortality effect.[6] For any given age, obesity significantly increases the risk of dying, and those with prolonged overweight/obesity exhibit the highest risk. The management of overweight patients starts with medical therapy, but moves to surgery if the degree of obesity increases, initial measures fail, or comorbidities arise. Both pharmaceutical agents and dietary restrictions have not been shown to be as effective as bariatric surgery in the treatment of weight loss in the long term.[7]

Bariatric surgery should be considered as a treatment option for patients with a body mass index (BMI) of 40 kg/m² or more who instituted but failed an adequate exercise and diet program (with or without adjunctive drug therapy), or for patients with a BMI >35 kg/m² who present with obesity-related comorbid conditions, such as hypertension, impaired glucose tolerance, diabetes mellitus, hyperlipidemia, and obstructive sleep apnea. In addition, potential bariatric surgery candidates should be well informed and have an acceptable risk to undergo surgery.

Contraindications to bariatric surgery are similar to those that apply for most elective surgical cases, with some exceptions. In general, patients with severe bleeding disorders, high cardiac risk, and severe pulmonary disease are considered poor surgical candidates. In addition, specific to bariatric surgery, patients with ongoing untreated psychiatric conditions (i.e. major depression, psychosis) and patients with active drug and/or alcohol dependence should not undergo bariatric procedures. Moreover, a rigorous preoperative evaluation must demonstrate that a patient is capable of complying with and understanding postoperative nutritional requirements.

Preoperative evaluation should be tailored based on general risks to undergo surgery. All patients should undergo a thorough physical exam, laboratory tests, chest radiograph, electrocardiogram (EKG), and both nutritional and psychological evaluations. Additional evaluations must be performed as needed for the high-risk medical patients and should start a medical consultation for clearance to surgery.

■ CHOICE OF PROCEDURE

The choice of bariatric surgery depends on a patient's preference and a surgeon's expertise. Discussion of surgical options should include the long-term side effects, such as possible need for reoperation, gallbladder disease, malabsorption, and body dysmorphic syndrome. Patients must understand the pros and cons of each bariatric procedure, as well as the lifestyle and dietary changes that they are expected to take part of.

Bariatric surgery is becoming increasingly popular due its effectiveness in weight loss control and reduction of obesity-related comorbidities.[8] Bariatric surgical options may be grouped into three main categories: malabsorptive, restrictive, and mixed procedures. Malabsorptive procedures reduce the size of the stomach, although they function primarily by creating malabsorption. They effectively decrease the length of functioning small bowel, hence reducing nutrient absorption which leads to weight loss. Restrictive procedures are those that act to reduce oral intake by limiting gastric volume, produce early satiety, and leave the alimentary canal in continuity. They tend to produce more gradual weight loss than malabsorptive procedures. Mixed bariatric procedures utilize both malabsorptive and restrictive components simultaneously. Roux-en-Y- gastric bypass (RYGB) is an example of a mixed procedures, by which reduction of the stomach to a smaller gastric pouch limits intake (restrictive component), and the anatomic reconfiguration of the small bowel reduces the length of functional intestine (malabsorptive component). This chapter covers the most common types of bariatric surgery procedures performed.

■ Biliopancreatic diversion

Biliopancreatic diversion (BPD) is a type of malabsorptive procedure. The technique involves the removal of part of the stomach. The remnant of the limited horizontal gastrectomy is a gastric pouch, larger than that of a gastric bypass. However, there is no restrictive component, so the patient may consume a free diet. The ileum is then connected to the pouch. Approximately 2% of patients experience severe malabsorption and nutritional deficiency.[9] All patients require life-long nutritional supplements. Overall, BPD is performed by fewer surgeons compared with other weight-loss surgery, in part because of the need for long-term nutritional follow-up and monitoring of BPD patients. Worldwide, it constitutes less than 2% of bariatric surgery.

BPD has been replaced with a modification known as duodenal switch (BPD/DS), which incorporates a restrictive component and reduces the risk of ulcer disease. The restrictive component of the surgery involves removing 70% of the stomach along the greater curvature whereas the malabsorptive portion of the surgery re-routes a lengthy portion of the small intestine, creating two separate pathways and one common channel. The shorter of the two pathways, the digestive loop, takes food from the stomach to the common channel. The much longer pathway, the biliopancreatic loop, carries bile from the liver to the common channel. The common channel is the portion of small intestine, usually 75–150 cm long, in which the contents of the digestive path mix with the bile from the biliopancreatic loop before emptying into the large intestine. As a result, after surgery, these patients absorb only approximately 20% of the fat they intake.

Hospital stay after BPD ranges between 2 and 7 days, with an associated operative mortality rate of 2% and perioperative morbidity rate of 10%. Common side effects include foul-smelling loose stools and stomal ulcers. The more serious complications include anastomotic leak (3–10%), anemia (3–5%), and protein malnutrition (2–4%).

Adjustable gastric band

Adjustable gastric band (AGB) is a type of restrictive bariatric procedure. A band encircles the proximal part, fundus, of the stomach and connects to a subcutaneous port/reservoir (**Fig. 1.1**). Initially, the band remains deflated and is then progressively inflated via the subcutaneous port, during subsequent postoperative outpatient visits, to achieve gastric restriction and weight loss. AGB is considered one of the safest bariatric procedures performed today with a mortality rate of 0.05%.[10] Compared with gastric bypass procedures, weight loss observed with AGB is less and not as rapid. AGB can lead to a percentage excess weight loss of 15–20% at 3 months, between 40 and 50% at 1 year, and 45–75% at 2 years.[6]

AGB is a reversible procedure. It is performed laparoscopically with a hospital stay ranging between 1 and 3 days. Complications specific to this procedure include band slippage, band erosion, band migration, reservoir leak, persistent vomiting, and failure to lose weight. Albeit a safe procedure, the reoperative rate due to band failure ranges between 20 and 30%, highlighting the importance of long-term follow-up despite a deceitfully simple case.[11]

Sleeve gastrectomy

This is another restrictive bariatric procedure. The stomach is reduced to about 15–25% of its original size, by surgical removal of a large portion its greater curvature (**Fig. 1.2**). The stomach is left shaped like a tube, or a sleeve and its size is permanently reduced. Although the stomach volume is reduced, it functions normally so that food can be consumed in small portions. This procedure also removes the portion of the stomach that produces ghrelin, the hormone responsible for hunger, hence incorporating a metabolic component for weight loss. In addition, by avoiding intestinal bypass, the chance of intestinal obstruction, anemia, osteoporosis, protein deficiency, and vitamin deficiency is significantly reduced. Evidence from one randomized controlled trial showed a laparoscopically isolated sleeve gastrectomy to be more effective than AGB with greater excess weight loss up to 3 years (66% versus 48%, respectively, $p = 0.0025$).[6] This procedure is relatively safe and has a low complication rate. Hospital stay ranges between 1 and 2 days.

Roux-en-Y gastric bypass

Roux-en-Y gastric bypass is the most commonly performed bariatric procedure and it is a type of mixed procedure. The roux-en-Y technique

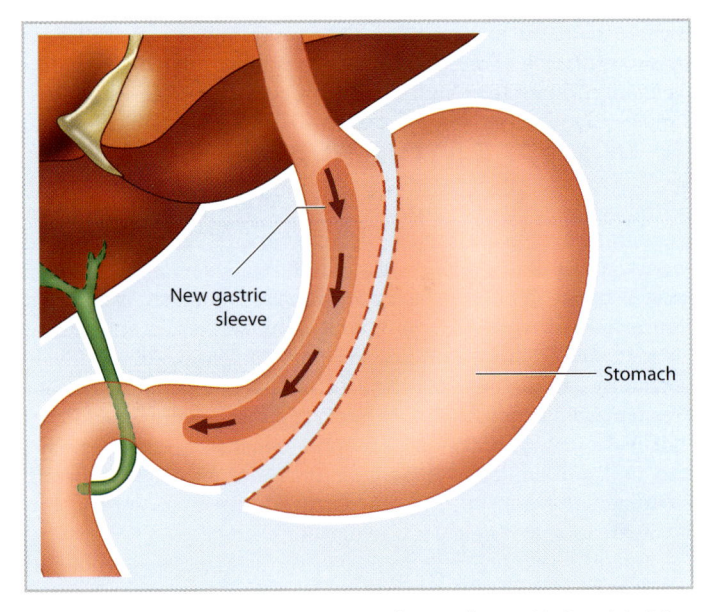

Figure 1.2 Sleeve gastrectomy. New gastric sleeve is about 15% of its original size.

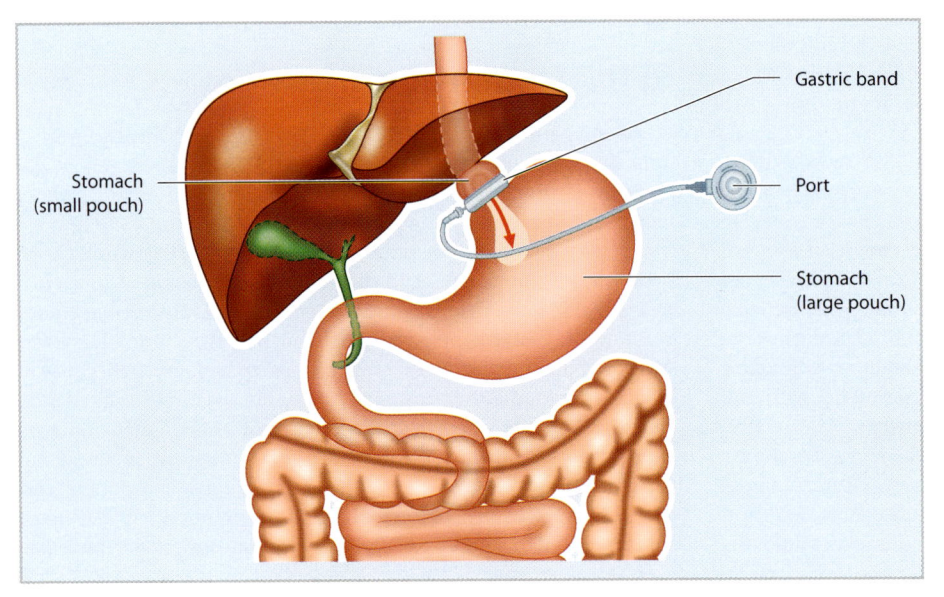

Figure 1.1 Adjustable gastric band. Subcutaneous port connects to gastric band to inflate and achieve gastric restriction.

is utilized to avoid loop gastroeneterostomy and the bile reflux that may follow. The proximal stomach is separated from the distal stomach to form a small, restrictive gastric pouch with a capacity of 15–20 ml (**Fig. 1.3**). This pouch is then connected to the mid-jejunum in a retrocolic or retrogastric fashion, forming the alimentary (roux) limb. This limb is diverted away from the biliopancreatic secretions by the biliary (biliopancreatic) limb. The 'common limb' is the length of small intestine distal to the site at which the roux limb and the biliary limb join. The common limb represents the intestinal area where biliopancreatic secretions mix with ingested food and most absorption occurs. The alimentary limb is typically 100–150 cm in length and the biliopancreatic limb 30–50 cm in length. RYGB has been known to be the most effective of the stomach-stapling procedures since the 1980s.

Postoperatively patients stay in the hospital for 1–5 days after laparoscopic RYGB, and are able to return to work 4 weeks after surgery. Dietary restrictions include a liquid diet for the first few weeks after surgery. Subsequently a diet must be composed of small meals, daily multivitamins, oral iron, and vitamin B_{12} supplementation. Multiple randomized controlled trials provide evidence that RYGB is more effective than AGB. RYGB achieves good weight loss, particularly in the short term. In the first 12 months after RYGB, a weight loss of 60–70% excess weight loss (EWL) can be expected. This effect is maintained for 12 months and then begins a gentle fade to an average of 50–60% EWL for those still attending follow-up at 5 years.

OPEN VERSUS LAPAROSCOPIC TECHNIQUES

In excess of 90% of bariatric surgery performed in the USA is via some form of minimally invasive surgery.[12] Compared with open procedures, laparoscopic bariatric surgery, in expert hands, is associated with decreased perioperative morbidity. Minimally invasive procedures are associated with a lower rate of wound infections and incisional hernias, a reduced length of hospital stay, and an earlier return to work. Specific to gastric bypass surgery, patients with open gastric bypass are more likely to experience pulmonary and cardiovascular complications, complications during the procedure, sepsis, and anastomotic leaks compared with laparoscopic gastric bypass patients.[13] Although there is a steep learning curve, the evidence supports a minimally invasive approach to bariatric surgery being more beneficial and cost-effective than an open approach.

REVISIONAL SURGERY

Patients requiring reoperative surgery are at higher risks of perioperative complications. A surgeon must make every effort to attain all medical records, including surgical reports to be able to understand the anatomy and adequately plan the revision procedure. Moreover, in addition to a general preoperative evaluation, revisional surgery patients should undergo a preoperative upper endoscopy and an upper gastrointestinal swallow test to help further delineate the rearranged gastrointestinal anatomy.

CONCLUSION

Obesity remains a major epidemic in developing countries. Currently, bariatric surgery is the only therapeutic strategy that can lead to sustained weight loss and resolution of medical comorbidities. The evidence indicates that bariatric surgery is a more effective option for weight loss than non-surgical treatments. Also, economic models suggest that bariatric surgery is more cost-effective than non-surgical interventions.[6] Obesity treatment should be personalized to each patient and factors such as sex, the degree of obesity, individual health risks, psychobehavioral and metabolic characteristics, and the outcome of previous weight loss attempts should be taken into account. Ideally, patients should be referred to high-volume accredited bariatric centers with experienced surgeons.

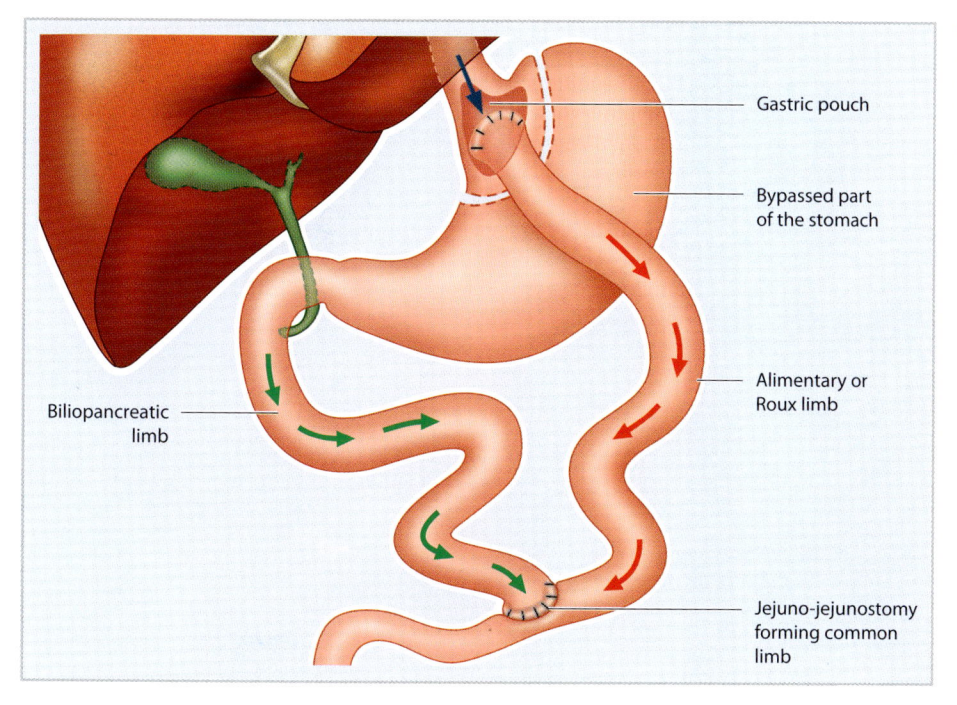

Figure 1.3 Anterocolic–anterogastric (front of colon and stomach – most common) roux-en-Y gastric bypass. Red arrows portray flow of food. Green arrows depict flow of bile and digestive juices. The junction of the alimentary and biliopancreatic limb forms the common channel.

REFERENCES

1. Deitel M. Overweight and obesity worldwide now estimated to involve 1.7 billion people. *Obes Surg* 2003;**13**:329–30.
2. Buchwald H, Avidor Y, Braunwald E, et al. Bariatric surgery: a systematic review and meta-analysis. *JAMA* 2004;**292**:1724–37.
3. Fontaine KR, Redden DT, Wang C, Westfall AO, Allison DB. Years of life lost due to obesity. *JAMA* 2003;**289**:187–93.
4. Buchwald H, Oien DM. Metabolic/bariatric surgery worldwide 2008. *Obes Surg* 2009;**19**:1605–11.
5. Eldar S, Heneghan HM, Brethauer S, Schauer PR. A focus on surgical preoperative evaluation of the bariatric patient--the Cleveland Clinic protocol and review of the literature. *Surgeon* 2011;**9**:273–7.
6. Picot J, Jones J, Colquitt JL, et al. The clinical effectiveness and cost-effectiveness of bariatric (weight loss) surgery for obesity: a systematic review and economic evaluation. *Health Technol Assess* 2009;**13**:1–190, 215–357, iii–iv.
7. NIH conference. Gastrointestinal surgery for severe obesity. Consensus Development Conference Panel. *Ann Intern Med* 1991;**115**:956–61.
8. Smith BR, Schauer P, Nguyen NT. Surgical approaches to the treatment of obesity: bariatric surgery. *Endocrinol Metab Clin North Am* 2008;**37**:943–64.
9. Crookes PF. Surgical treatment of morbid obesity. *Annu Rev Med* 2006;**57**:243–64.
10. Buchwald H, Estok R, Fahrbach K, Banel D, Sledge I. Trends in mortality in bariatric surgery: a systematic review and meta-analysis. *Surgery* 2007;**142**:621–32; discussion 32–5.
11. Suter M, Calmes JM, Paroz A, Giusti V. A 10-year experience with laparoscopic gastric banding for morbid obesity: high long-term complication and failure rates. *Obes Surg* 2006;**16**:829–35.
12. Nguyen NT, Masoomi H, Magno CP, Nguyen XM, Laugenour K, Lane J. Trends in use of bariatric surgery, 2003–2008. *J Am Coll Surg* 2011;**213**:261–6.
13. Weller WE, Rosati C. Comparing outcomes of laparoscopic versus open bariatric surgery. *Ann Surg* 2008;**248**:10–5.

Chapter 2

Psychological evaluation of the postbariatric patient

Veer Chahwala, Michael C. Cheung, Bassan J. Allan, Nestor F. De La Cruz

The psychological evaluation of a bariatric patient must begin preoperatively. Of extremely obese patients who pursue bariatric surgery 20–60% have an axis I psychiatric disorder. The risk for major depression was found to be almost five times higher in patients with a body mass index (BMI) >40 kg/m^2 compared with patients with a normal BMI (18.5–24.9 kg/m^2) in a population study of 40 000 US adults.[1] The primary care physician mostly provides patients with their psychiatric (particularly antidepressant) medications. However, the plastic surgeon should not assume that these medications are adequately controlling the patient's depressive symptoms. Rather, they should further assess and observe patients for depressive symptoms, as well as their mood, affect, and overall presentation during the body-contouring consultation. Should the patient endorse symptoms of a mood disorder, a mental health professional consultation is necessary. Preoperative psychological evaluation may also help identify who should not undergo surgery. Commonly cited contraindications for bariatric surgery include patients with active substance abuse, active psychosis, bulimia nervosa, or severe uncontrolled depression, because these features are thought to limit the capacity for informed consent and also increase the likelihood of postoperative medical complications.[1]

Gastric bypass surgery has become the gold standard among the various surgical techniques available for the management of morbid obesity. Generally, patients experience positive changes in quality of life and body image postoperatively. However, surgically assisted massive weight loss often results in loose, hanging, excessive skin which may negatively impact quality of life and body image, and may also prevent further weight loss. It is vital that patients are counseled about motivations and expectations after bariatric surgery, particularly with respect to expected weight loss, body image, and psychosocial functioning. In one study, 96% of all patients developed surplus skin after bariatric surgery. Of these, 65–75% reported a discontent with their body image and a desire for body-contouring surgery.[2] Patients' expectations after body-contouring surgery included improved appearance, self-confidence, and ability to be physically active, and reduced feelings of embarrassment. Indeed, patients who have massive weight loss may have unrealistic expectations about postoperative results. They may expect a total body transformation that makes their bodies comparable to those of people who have never experienced massive weight loss. They should be counseled about the possibility of large scars, skin irregularities, and residual deformities in body shape. Patients should not expect a 'perfect' body shape. They should also be constantly reminded of the possible need for multiple, staged procedures. It is important that expectations are framed within the context of realistic outcomes via extensive preoperative counseling by a multidisciplinary team.

As previously mentioned, postbariatric patients are particularly at risk of psychiatric disorders due to long-standing social discrimination and social isolation, leading to emotional lability. Pre- and postoperative screening for psychological disturbances should be performed by trained psychologists or psychiatrists with some expertise in the treatment of bariatric patients. The goal of bariatric surgery is not only weight reduction and associated physical comorbidities, but also improved psychosocial functioning and quality of life.[3] Although most studies report broad psychosocial improvement in terms of depression, negative body attitude, and low self-esteem, a significant minority of patients do not benefit psychosocially from surgery. Enhanced psychosocial functioning and improved quality of life can motivate postoperative patients to adhere to healthy behaviors that maintain surgically established weight loss. Psychological factors, as opposed to technical failures, are often attributed to failures of bariatric surgery. As such, a meticulous approach to the psychological functioning of postoperative bariatric patients will facilitate the development of postoperative interventions to enhance successful outcomes.

The initial assessment of the postbariatric patient should ideally be a continuation of the preoperative psychological evaluation. Before surgery, patients should receive counseling on the expected changes that the surgery will bring them and any significant psychiatric disorder should be identified. In addition, lifestyle factors, such as increase in physical activity and social support, and improvement in dietary habits, which will require significant effort by the patient, have to be continuously addressed throughout the surgical process. Many bariatric patients have poor coping mechanisms and reduced food intake post-surgery, which can place them at risk of surgical failure and development of mental health illnesses. Following patients' changes in personality, body image, eating habits, quality of life, and social functioning are critical in evaluating the mental health of postoperative bariatric patients.

Personality aspects are relevant in postoperative eating behaviors and adjustment to bariatric surgery in general. Studies have shown that most patients have improved personality features, including reduction in defensiveness, immature identity, and increased self-esteem.[4] Those patients with poor weight loss showed more personality pathology than comparison groups in borderline, avoidant, and passive–aggressive personality features. Improvements in self-esteem were highly correlated to the amount of weight loss.

Body image is also a major postbariatric psychosocial factor. Generally, weight loss after bariatric surgery leads to marked improvements in body image, attractiveness, and decreased feelings of shame. This is particularly true in the first 6 postoperative months. These improvements appear to be an underlying source of overall psychosocial improvement, because morbidly obese patients have very poor preoperative body image.[5] Patients' reporting of improved postoperative body image seems to dissipate with time. These patients often still feel overweight and exhibit discontent with increasing skinfolds. Furthermore, there have been mixed results in the literature: some studies show that patients satisfied with their appearance have less weight loss, whereas others suggest that patients who experienced more weight loss were more satisfied with their appearance.

Bariatric surgery patients may suffer from a particular dysfunction in body image – body dysmorphic disorder (BDD), or dysmorphophobia. In this syndrome, the patient is obsessed with some aspect of physical appearance that is quite normal to objective viewers. It is characterized by extreme body image dissatisfaction. As opposed to people with mild body image dissatisfaction, most BDD patients experience little change or an actual worsening in their BDD symptoms postoperatively.[6] Hence, some authorities cite BDD as an additional contraindication to plastic surgery. Patients with massive weight loss who are undergoing reconstructive procedures have neither slight nor imagined physical deformities, so it is difficult to apply the technical definition of BDD to them. However, some studies of patients undergoing other reconstructive procedures have reported symptoms consistent with BDD. Thus, patients undergoing preoperative evaluation for body-contouring procedures may well present with some form of BDD, and they should be counseled appropriately.

Postbariatric surgery eating behavior is a critical factor in determining weight loss and influencing overall outcome. Bariatric surgery reduces the physical capacity for food and reduces hunger. Compliance with dietary advice is required. Dietary changes are incompletely facilitated by the anatomic changes of bariatric surgery. Therefore, significant patient effort is required to adjust dietary habits. In general, patients report a decrease in binge eating and emotional eating and better, more flexible, control of eating behaviors. However, some patients are not as successful. They report loss of control of eating behaviors: Overeating, emotional eating, consumption of calorie-dense soft liquid foods, and binge eating. Up to a third of patients do not adhere to post-surgery treatment dietary regimens.[7] These patients generally have a less favorable outcome, including greater weight regain and postoperative complications.

Social functioning and health-related social quality of life generally improve after bariatric surgery. In particular, they become more socially active, have extended social networks, show better sexual functioning, and get more social support.[8] However, some patients experience negative outcomes. Certain studies reveal worsening sexual problems, divorce, and difficulty adjusting to the demands of increased social functioning. Generally, quality of life substantially improves, especially in the first 2 postoperative years. However, some studies do show deterioration after some years. This may be related to stabilized weight loss or regaining of weight, or the occurrence of disturbed eating patterns as previously discussed. Still other studies even demonstrate negative effects in the quality of life, which suggests that postbariatric patients need long-term evaluation.[9]

After bariatric surgery, there is a general tendency toward normalization of psychopathology.[10] However, as with the previously mentioned psychosocial aspects, there are studies that show decline in improvements over the years and even some reports of moderate-to-severe psychopathological problems after surgery. Similar patterns are seen with depressive symptoms as well. Although various studies indicate a postoperative decrease in depression to the norm, others fail to show much difference between pre- and postoperative depressive symptoms.

As described above, most studies show broad improvements in the psychosocial functioning of postoperative bariatric patients. However, there remains a significant minority of patients who do not experience these improvements, or show deterioration over the years. There are several possible explanations to these findings. One is the stabilization of weight loss, or weight regain. Patients may also be disappointed that their lives do not dramatically improve after experiencing significant weight loss. In addition, patients realize that, once their morbid obesity has resolved, other life problems arise. Patients realize that they can no longer blame negative life events on their obesity. Clearly, then, bariatric surgery and subsequent weight loss are not the universal solution for psychosocial problems of morbidly obese patients, but certainly a very important part of successful outcomes. It is imperative that postoperative bariatric patients receive a multidisciplinary approach, including continued and close follow-up care from a mental health professional.[11]

REFERENCES

1. Sarwer DB, Fabricatore AN. Psychiatric considerations of the massive weight loss patient. *Clin Plast Surg* 2008;**35**:1–10.
2. Kitzinger HB, Abayev S, Pittermann A, et al. After massive weight loss: patients' expectations of body contouring surgery. *Obes Surg* 2012;**22**:544–9.
3. van Hout GC, Boekestein P, Fortuin FA, Pelle AJ, van Heck GL. Psychosocial functioning following bariatric surgery. *Obes Surg* 2006;**16**:787–94.
4. Dymek MP, le Grange D, Neven K, Alverdy J. Quality of life and psychosocial adjustment in patients after Roux-en-Y gastric bypass: a brief report. *Obes Surg* 2001;**11**:32–9.
5. Schok M, Geenen R, van Antwerpen T, de Wit P, Brand N, van Ramshorst B. Quality of life after laparoscopic adjustable gastric banding for severe obesity: postoperative and retrospective preoperative evaluations. *Obes Surg* 2000;**10**:502–8.
6. Sarwer DB, Thompson JK, Mitchell JE, Rubin JP. Psychological considerations of the bariatric surgery patient undergoing body contouring surgery. *Plast Reconstr Surg* 2008;121:423e–34e.
7. Gentry K, Halverson JD, Heisler S. Psychologic assessment of morbidly obese patients undergoing gastric bypass: a comparison of preoperative and postoperative adjustment. *Surgery* 1984;**95**:215–20.
8. Kinzl JF, Traweger C, Trefalt E, Biebl W. Psychosocial consequences of weight loss following gastric banding for morbid obesity. *Obes Surg* 2003;**13**:105–10.
9. Shai I, Henkin Y, Weitzman S, Levi I. Determinants of long-term satisfaction after vertical banded gastroplasty. *Obes Surg* 2003;**13**:269–74.
10. Mamplekou E, Komesidou V, Bissias C, Papakonstantinou A, Melissas J. Psychological condition and quality of life in patients with morbid obesity before and after surgical weight loss. *Obes Surg* 2005;**15**:1177–84.
11. Hsu LK, Benotti PN, Dwyer J, et al. Nonsurgical factors that influence the outcome of bariatric surgery: a review. *Psychosom Med* 1998;**60**:338–46.

Chapter 3 | Medical management of the postbariatric patient and evaluation before body contouring procedures

Bassan J. Allan, Michael C. Cheung, Veer Chahwala, Nestor F. De La Cruz

INTRODUCTION

Obesity is a worldwide epidemic. About 1.1 billion adults and 10% of children are currently classified as obese.[1] These statistics reflect progressive societal dietary changes and decreasing physical activity with tremendous overconsumption of energy. Obesity has been shown to reduce life expectancy and it is directly related to the development of comorbidities, such as cardiovascular disease, diabetes mellitus (type 2), and several cancers. Approaches to control obesity include low-calorie, low-fat diets, increased physical activity, and strategies contributing to the modification of lifestyle. Pharmacological options may also facilitate weight loss and contribute to further amelioration of obesity-related health risks. Short-term weight loss in up to 6 months can be achieved easily with the aforementioned strategies. However, long-term weight management is far more difficult to achieve. Bariatric surgery is an effective strategy to treat severely obese patients. Bariatric surgery leads to a substantial improvement of comorbidities as well as a reduction in overall mortality rate by 25–50% during long-term follow-up.[2]

Over the past two decades, bariatric surgery has gained more public acceptance as an effective treatment strategy for weight loss. Postbariatric patients need close medical follow-up because many chronic conditions related to obesity may change dramatically with weight loss. Postoperative medical management after bariatric surgery should focus on healthy dietary habits, weight maintenance, medication management, and screening for complications (e.g. prolonged vomiting, dumping syndrome, obstruction).

FOLLOW UP AFTER BARIATRIC SURGERY

Medical visits

Medical visits should be as frequent as 4–6 weeks in the initial postoperative period, and extended to 6 months to a year as the patient's initial rapid weight loss subsides. Based on current recommendations, each medical visit should include a full physical exam, review of systems, review of medications and adjustment of doses based on a patient's weight, and a laboratory panel. The review of systems is an important part of the patient's history. Patients should be asked for resolution of preoperative symptoms (i.e. fatigue, musculoskeletal pain, reflux) and when indicated medications discontinued. The laboratory panel should focus on metabolic and nutritional markers; a recommended schedule for postoperative management is shown in **Table 3.1**.

An additional component to each medical visit should include a complete nutritional assessment. This group of patients is at high risk for malnutrition, either from poor food intake or from changes in the digestive track. Additional counseling by a nutritionist should be given

Table 3.1 Laboratory values recommended for postoperative management of bariatric surgery patients.

	1 month	3 months	6 months	12 months	18 months	Annually
Electrolyte panel	+	+	+	+	+	+
CBC	+	+	+	+	+	+
LFTs	+	+	+	+	+	+
Albumin/Prealbumin[a]			+	+	+	+
Iron panel[a]			+	+	+	+
Vitamin B_{12}/D or folate[a]			+	+	+	+
Intact PTH[a]			+	+	+	+

[a]Not indicated after AGB.
AGB, adjustable gastric band CBC, complete blood count; LFTs, liver function tests; PTH, parathyroid hormone.

to all postbariatric patients to minimize eating disorders and stress the importance of adequate eating patterns.

Nutrition

The dietary approach to patients after bariatric surgery is divided into stages. The early postoperative stages emphasize energy consumption that is adequate for healing after surgery. The late dietary stages after bariatric surgery highlight the development of long-term healthy habits, reduction in weight fluctuation, and prevention of metabolic/nutritional derangements.

There are a number of protocols for dietary management of obese patients after bariatric surgery. The various protocols vary with the length of each dietary stage and the type of foods allowed. However, the principles are generally the same. Dietary advancement should be based on an individual basis. Assessment of tolerance for foods, bearing in mind the rearrangements in the anatomy due to the specific bariatric procedures, should be made frequently in the early stages, and less frequently in the late stages if no complications arise. Basic general guidelines for the dietary management of patients after bariatric surgery are shown in **Table 3.2**.

Medications

Many obesity-related medical conditions may improve dramatically with postoperative weight loss seen with bariatric surgery. Bariatric procedures may also alter the manner in which medications are absorbed and metabolized; hence close follow-up is mandatory to change either the dose or a medication itself. **Table 3.3** lists the most common medical conditions related to obesity and the expected changes in medical management after bariatric surgery.

Complications

Recognition of complications is an important aspect of the medical management of postbariatric patients, as the complication rate can be as high as 40%.[3] For ease of understanding, complications can be divided into two main categories: Early and late, or long term. Although there can be some overlap, some of the early complications may have a delayed clinical presentation.[4] In addition, some complications may be specific to the type of operation performed (**Table 3.4**). This chapter focuses on complications seen after the most common bariatric surgery procedures performed (i.e. roux-en-Y gastric bypass, gastric band, and gastric sleeve).

Table 3.2 Guidelines for dietary management of bariatric surgery patients.

Stage	Recommendations
Early (postop day 1–14)	Sips of clear liquids if Gastrografin swallow test (if indicated) is negative As tolerated, advance to clear liquids and full liquids Encourage consumption of at least 1400 grams of liquids daily Discourage/restrict carbonated, high sugar/calorie options
Late (>2 weeks postop)	Advance diet to soft foods After about 1 month advance diet as tolerated to solid food Encourage a balanced diet, with emphasis on protein consumption Continue routine nutritional check-ups to ensure diet adequacy and weight loss

Table 3.3 Obesity-related medical conditions and their changes after bariatric surgery.

	Expected change	Medication
HTN	Blood pressure decreases to normal	Antihypertensives are usually reduced in dose or discontinued postoperatively
Diabetes	Decreased need for insulin	Continue metformin until patient is eating and normoglycemia is achieved. Discontinue meglitinides and oral sulfonylureas because they may lead to hypoglycemia
GERD	Decreased acid reflux	Discontinue PPIs, unless symptoms persist
Psychiatric	Variable, patient dependent	Safe to continue medications, see Chapter 2 for further details

GERD, gastroesophageal reflux disease; HTN, hypertension; PPIs, proton pump inhibitors.

Table 3.4 Common bariatric procedures and specific complications.

Roux-en-Y gastric bypass	Weight regain Marginal ulcers Cholelithiasis Gastric remnant distension Incisional hernias Internal hernias Dumping syndrome Metabolic derangements Hypoglycemia
Adjustable gastric band	Esophageal irritation Port infection/malfunction Band erosion/slippage Hiatal hernia
Gastric sleeve	Staple line disruption and leak Bleeding Stenosis

Early complications

This type of complication is generally seen during hospital admission or becomes apparent up to 4 weeks after the bariatric procedure. Most of these complications are treated by the bariatric surgeon. Depending on the complication, it will require either surgical re-exploration or medical management. The most life-threatening early complications include gastrointestinal (GI) leaks, deep venous thromboembolism/pulmonary embolus, and early intestinal obstructions. These conditions can be very serious and early recognition is imperative.

Late complications

This type of complications is usually a result of the changes in the anatomy of the GI track or dietary changes leading to nutritional deficiencies. The most common late complications include nausea/vomiting, dehydration, diarrhea, acid reflux, cholelithiasis, anemia, and vitamin/mineral deficiencies.

BODY CONTOURING AFTER MASSIVE WEIGHT LOSS

After massive weight loss, skin and soft tissue excess leads to contour deformities that can potentially affect every part of the body. This tissue excess fails to retract completely and becomes redundant, especially in areas where the fat deposits used to be in these patients. In the upper body, excess tissue can be found in the axilla as well as on the back and flank. In addition, breast deformities can be variable. In the lower body, excess tissue can be found on the abdominal wall, mons pubis, and thighs. An inclusive and illustrative classification system has been developed to help systematically assess and quantify the level of deformity in 10 areas of the body: Arms, breast, abdomen, flank, mons pubis, back, buttock, medial thigh, hips/lateral thigh, lower thighs/knee.[5] This rating scale facilitates preoperative planning and is a useful tool in determining how extensive the procedure that a patient would require.

Preoperative evaluation and screening

As with any surgical procedure, good patient selection and thorough preoperative evaluation may identify potential problems and prevent postoperative complications. The ideal time for surgery is approximately 12–18 months after the bariatric procedure. The patient's maximum and current body mass index (BMI) should be calculated[6] – approximately 3 months without weight fluctuation is recommended. Patients should be free from nausea and vomiting because these may represent mechanical problems resulting from the bariatric procedure; these patients should be referred back to the bariatric surgeon for further workup. Nutritional concerns, such as iron and vitamin B_{12} levels, are important in these patients as the GI tracts are altered. Furthermore, daily protein intake should be assessed because these patients may not be consuming enough protein for wound healing. Medical problems, such as diabetes and hypertension, should be re-evaluated and optimized by their respective specialists before surgery. A thorough physical exam should be performed by the operating surgeon. For patients who have undergone an adjustable gastric band (AGB) procedure, location of the port is important because it may have to be moved for abdominoplasty. Furthermore, incisional hernias from the bariatric procedure should be assessed and documented. Patients currently smoking should be required to quit smoking for at least a month before the surgical procedure.[7] Smoking causes small vessel constriction and is associated with higher rates of complications in patients undergoing body contouring operations.[6] Importantly, the patient must be of adequate anesthesia risk.

Combined versus staged procedures

Body contouring procedures are divided into upper and lower body procedures. It is not uncommon for patients to undergo multiple procedures, either all in one setting or staged over a period of time. The advantages of combined procedures include one anesthetic setting as well as reducing total time off work, recovery time, and total costs. On the other hand, combined procedures may result in increased postoperative pain and increased overall operative time. As a result, risk for deep vein thrombosis and pulmonary embolus is also increased. Therefore, relative contraindications to combined procedures include a history of smoking, a history of deep vein thrombosis or pulmonary embolus, a high residual BMI, or substantial medical risk factors that increase the risk of perioperative complications.[6] Taken altogether, the approach and plan for every patient must be individualized.

Upper body

Post bariatric deformities of the upper body may be most notable on the medical aspect of the upper extremities. Patients with minimal redundancy of skin may have a reasonable cosmetic result with liposuction alone. For those with excess skin and fat, a brachioplasty is the best option. This most commonly includes circumferential liposuction of the upper extremity, followed by resection of skin with minimal subdermal undermining. This is accomplished via a longitudinal incision along the bicipital groove from the elbow to the axilla, with extension onto the chest wall.

Breast changes after bariatric surgery include excess skin, ptosis, and deficient or excess breast volume. The volume loss and nipple position may be asymmetric. Removal of redundant skin and raising of the nipple areola complex through mastopexy are the mainstay of correcting deformities of the breast. This is usually accomplished using the Wise pattern or the inverted T-incision, the latter allowing for maximal skin removal while preventing retraction of remaining skin.[8,9] In patients with deficient breast volume, breast augmentation with implants or autologous tissue can be performed at the time of surgery.[8]

Lower body

Lower body deformities after bariatric surgery are more complex than those seen in the upper body. Perhaps the most common complaint is of excess skin and fat located below the umbilicus on the anterior aspect of the abdomen. Poor hygiene, constant skin-to-skin contact, and irritation of this area with constant moisture retention may lead to superficial infections. These infections must be addressed before any intervention is carried out. The procedure most commonly carried out is panniculectomy, which involves excision of the skin hanging inferior to the umbilicus. A limited undermining of the soft tissue is performed. Although this procedure addresses the superficial skin irritation issues, it fails to be completely aesthetically pleasing because it does not address other issues such as vertical and horizontal skin excess, abdominal wall laxity, and malpositioning of the umbilicus.

To some degree, abdominoplasty addresses many of these issues. More extensive tissue undermining is performed with dissection and preservation of the umbilical stalk, with the intent to relocate the umbilicus. The dissection may be carried out to the xiphoid process and costal margins.[10] This allows for more significant skin and fat resection than with a panniculectomy. The fascia of the abdominal wall is then plicated from the xiphoid process to the pubis, which helps tighten the stretched abdominal wall transversely. Although abdominoplasty addresses the anterior aspect of the abdomen, circumferential torso or truncal excess and lateral excess may also need attention.

To address these issues, a belt lipectomy (also known as a torsoplasty or circumferential lipectomy) can be performed. This procedure is started in a similar fashion as an abdominoplasty. In addition to elevation of flaps to the xiphoid process and costal margins, lateral elevation is also performed to allow for lateral resection. In the lateral decubitus position, resection from the anterior axillary line to the midline of the back is performed. This eliminates upper back and midback rolls. To correct saddlebag deformities and contour issues involving the buttock, a lower body lift can be performed. This combines circumferential abdominoplasty with a lateral thigh and buttock lift.[10] This can also be performed together with a medial thigh lift.

Ptosis of the mons pubis may also affect patients who have undergone bariatric surgery. Monsplasty consists of excisional lipectomy and liposuction for correction of this area.[11]

REFERENCES

1. Buchwald H, Williams SE. Bariatric surgery worldwide 2003. *Obes Surg* 2004;**14**:1157–64.
2. Buchwald H, Avidor Y, Braunwald E, et al. Bariatric surgery: a systematic review and meta-analysis. *JAMA* 2004;**292**:1724–37.
3. Flum DR, Belle SH, King WC, et al. Perioperative safety in the longitudinal assessment of bariatric surgery. *N Engl J Med* 2009;**361**:445–54.
4. Ukleja A, Stone RL. Medical and gastroenterologic management of the post-bariatric surgery patient. *J Clin Gastroenterol* 2004;**38**:312–21.
5. Song AY, Jean RD, Hurwitz DJ, Fernstrom MH, Scott JA, Rubin JP. A classification of contour deformities after bariatric weight loss: the Pittsburgh Rating Scale. *Plast Reconstr Surg* 2005;**116**:1535–44; discussion 45-6.
6. Rubin JP, Nguyen V, Schwentker A. Perioperative management of the post-gastric-bypass patient presenting for body contour surgery. *Clin Plast Surg* 2004;**31**:601–10, vi.
7. Gusenoff JA, Rubin JP. Plastic surgery after weight loss: current concepts in massive weight loss surgery. *Aesthet Surg J* 2008;**28**:452–5.
8. Hurwitz DJ, Golla D. Breast reshaping after massive weight loss. *Semin Plast Surg* 2004;**18**:179–87.
9. Wise RJ, Gannon JP, Hill JR. Further experience with reduction mammaplasty. *Plast Reconstr Surg* 1963;**32**:12–20.
10. Borud LJ, Warren AG. Modified vertical abdominoplasty in the massive weight loss patient. *Plast Reconstr Surg* 2007;**119**:1911–21; discussion 22–3.
11. Hurwitz DJ, Rubin JP, Risin M, Sajjadian A, Sereika S. Correcting the saddlebag deformity in the massive weight loss patient. *Plast Reconstr Surg* 2004;**114**:1313–25.

Chapter 4: Preoperative evaluation of the postbariatric patient

Yash J. Avashia, Narayanan M. Nair, ChiChi Berhane, Zubin Jal Panthaki

PREOPERATIVE EVALUATION: A HOLISTIC APPROACH

The upward trend in bariatric surgery has led to a concomitant increase in body-contouring procedures. Massive weight loss (MWL) is defined as a loss of ≥50% of excess weight, and is commonly observed with patients losing ≥100 lb (≥45 kg) after bariatric surgery. The primary goal of a plastic and reconstructive surgeon in operating on the patient who has undergone bariatric surgery with sustained MWL is to provide an improvement in form and function in the safest possible setting. Bearing in mind that patients who require surgical intervention for weight loss have failed medical therapy and typically had a body mass index (BMI) that exceeded 35–40 kg/m², residual medical problems secondary to morbid obesity often place these patients in a high-risk category for surgery.1 Cumulative postbariatric plastic surgery can reach up to 10 hours in the operating room. Proper preoperative evaluation for postbariatric plastic surgery is a necessary prerequisite to both intraoperative and postoperative success.

Plastic surgeons performing these procedures should be cognizant of the various bariatric procedures offered to patients today, and should be able to differentiate the physiological changes that follow these procedures, anticipate potential late complications, and identify associated underlying medical issues in the patient. Many patients will present for body-contouring procedures as their weight loss stabilizes between 12 and 18 months after bariatric surgery. Unfortunately, as the goal weight is approached and weight loss stabilizes, follow-up with their respective bariatric surgeon often starts to seem of lesser importance. Incidentally, a significant number of patients will be lost to follow-up by their bariatric surgeon when they first present for plastic surgery evaluation. This heightens the criticality of plastic surgeons' preoperative evaluation and its potential to identify late complications that linger in the postbariatric patient seeking massive body-contouring surgery. A comprehensive preoperative evaluation is mandatory because these procedures are often extensive, with the potential for significant morbidity and even mortality. There should be a low threshold for recommending treatment or referral to a specialist, in preparation of the patient who has undergone bariatric surgery and sustained MWL.

BARIATRIC PROCEDURES

The most radical option for weight loss is bariatric surgery, and it remains the treatment of choice for severely obese patients. Over the years, numerous modifications and novel additions have been made to the armamentarium of bariatric surgery procedures. Although patient-specific and surgeon-specific factors influence the choice of bariatric procedure, relevant factors to the plastic surgeon operating on a postbariatric patient are (1) what type of bariatric procedure was performed and (2) what the associated nutritional deficiencies are (Table 4.1).

Table 4.1 Bariatric procedures and associated nutritional deficiencies.

Procedure	Type	Mechanism	Potential nutritional deficiency
Roux-en-Y gastric bypass	Restrictive/Malabsorptive	Restricts volume of consumption, mild malabsorption, dumping syndrome	Iron, vitamin B_{12}, folate, calcium, vitamin D, copper, zinc
Biliopancreatic diversion with duodenal switch	Restrictive/Malabsorptive	Moderately restricts consumption volume, moderate malabsorption of fat	Fatty acids, protein, calcium, vitamins A, D, E, and K, iron, vitamin B_{12}, folate
Gastroplasty	Restrictive	Restricts volume by decreasing size of gastric pouch	Vitamin B_{12}, folate, vitamin B_6
Lap-band procedure	Restrictive – adjustable	Restricts volume, only procedure that is adjustable	Vitamin B_{12}, folate, vitamin B_6

At the present time, there are three main categories of bariatric procedures: Restrictive, malabsorptive, and combination restrictive–malabsorptive. Restrictive procedures produce early satiety by creating a small gastric pouch and outlet. It achieves weight loss by indirectly decreasing patient meal portions through early satiety. Procedures in this category include horizontal gastroplasty, gastric partitioning, Silastic ring gastroplasty, vertical banded gastroplasty (VBG), and laparoscopic adjustable gastric banding (LAP-BAND). Malabsorptive procedures contrast restrictive procedures by keeping the gastric pouch intact, and altering the length of absorptive surface of the small intestine. Procedures in this category include biliopancreatic diversion (BPD), jejunoileal bypass (JIB), and combination BPD with duodenal switch. With altered length and access to specific absorptive surface, long-term nutritional and metabolic complications are common, along with undesirable effects such as foul-smelling stools. Malabsorptive procedures are usually limited for patients with a BMI exceeding 50 kg/m². A hybrid of restrictive and malabsorptive bariatric procedures came about in the 1960s and eventually led to the development of the gastric bypass procedure. A major modification to this has been the creation of a roux-en-Y anastomosis to reduce the incidence of alkaline gastritis from bile reflux. This modified procedure is the roux-en-Y gastric bypass (RYGB). Restriction is achieved through a small gastric pouch with a 1-cm outlet whereas malabsorption is achieved through bypassing the fundus, duodenum, and proximal jejunum.

Today, the two most common operations are LAP-BAND and RYGB. The risk for nutritional deficiencies is significantly higher for malabsorptive procedures but does not rule out the possibility of encountering them in patients with restrictive procedures. Nutrient deficiencies in malabsorptive procedures develop from disruption of one or more steps in the physiology of nutrient absorption. Restrictive procedures are associated with nutrient deficiencies through inadequate intake secondary to improper nutrition. Restrictive procedures can alter the physiology of nutrient absorption but not as extensively as malabsorptive procedures.

PATIENT HISTORY

Weight loss history

Evaluation for body-contouring procedures after bariatric surgery typically occurs when the patient has achieved a stable weight for a period of 2 months. Past studies have calculated ideal body weight for men and women with the following formulae:[2]

Men: [48 + height (cm) − 150] = ideal body weight (kg)
Women: [45 + height (cm) − 150] = ideal body weight (kg).

Patients should be within 10–15% of their ideal goal weight, with no more than a 1- to 2-lb per month (0.45- to 0.90-kg per month) fluctuation over a 3- to 6-month period. This often corresponds to 12–18 months after gastric bypass surgery. Confirmation of weight stability provides time for metabolic and nutritional homeostasis, which also improves wound healing and reduces surgical morbidity and mortality. A number of studies point to the increased incidence of wound infections, pulmonary complications, and thrombotic events associated with surgery in obese patients. Patients with a higher BMI (>32 kg/m^2) tend to achieve suboptimal aesthetic results. Patients who have plateaued above their goal weight or those who have experienced significant weight regain should be referred back to their bariatric program. Causes for weight regain may include poor compliance with postoperative dietary and exercise regimen, underlying psychological conflict, or mechanical complication such as gastric band slippage in LAP-BAND patients.

Diet and exercise habits

The decision to undergo bariatric surgery and subsequent body-contouring plastic surgery requires a commitment from the patient. although the surgery provides a radical answer to the patient's chronic burden of morbid obesity, poor compliance with postoperative lifestyle modifications, including diet and exercise, can be a harbinger for poor prognosis and surgical results. An evaluation of the patient's diet and exercise habits and compliance with nutritional supplements is important. Exercise capacity is often a reliable indicator of the patient's level of fitness for major surgery.

Medical history

Along with weight loss after bariatric surgery comes a tremendous improvement, if not resolution, of many medical disorders associated with obesity, although not all patients experience complete resolution of obesity-related comorbidities. The plastic surgeon must be aware of this and properly screen for continued underlying medical issues that may affect surgical outcomes.[3] Depending on the severity of these issues, referral to the bariatric team may be necessary to properly manage the ongoing medical problem. It is important to inquire about residual medical issues or chronic disease states that could affect the safety of major body-contouring procedures.

Diabetes

Ample evidence has shown that insulin resistance correlates with truncal obesity and physical inactivity. Severely uncontrolled diabetes is a risk factor that may lead to secondary disease processes, including heart disease, hypertension, blindness and eye problems, kidney disease, nervous system damage, and the potential for foot amputation from severe diabetic foot infections. As you know, the value of MWL goes beyond the mere idea of fitting into a smaller dress or pant size. Immediately after gastric bypass, serum glucose levels decrease with concomitant improved glucose control. Pories et al.[4] showed that 82% of obese patients with diabetes mellitus type 2 had resolution of their disease after surgery. RYGB in people with diabetes has been shown to lead to resolution in 64–93% of cases. Patients who do not have diabetes but have impaired glucose tolerance have witnessed a 99% improvement. Although resolution is attained by most, there are still patients who do not achieve this endpoint. For the plastic surgeon during preoperative evaluation, checking serum glucose and hemoglobin A1c (HbA1c) may provide insight into the extent of diabetes resolution and glucose intolerance.

Underlying diabetes after gastric bypass surgery is an important detail to document. Patients with diabetes have a depressed immune system response and an increased susceptibility to infection, and are especially prone to streptococcal and staphylococcal skin infections. Diabetes and perioperative hyperglycemia were shown to independently increase the prevalence of these infections.[5] On the same note, risks for streptococcal and staphylococcal skin and nosocomial infections correlates with the degree of glucose elevation.

In the case of patients with poorly controlled glucose levels, intensive therapy has been shown to improve short- and long-term prevention of morbidity. Patients with HbA1c >7% should be placed on a low-carbohydrate meal and an insulin drip on admission to hospital for proper glycemic control. Goals for glycemic control should be glucose concentrations between 70 and 120 mg/dl and postprandial concentrations of <180 mg/dl. The oral hypoglycemic agents used should not be taken on the morning of surgery.

Cardiac disease

Premature morbidity and mortality in severely obese patients are related to the adverse effects of obesity on the heart and lung function, as well as related metabolic abnormalities. Increases in total body fat mass require blood flow to support the active metabolism of adipose tissue. In addition to increased cardiac output, hypertension is also associated with an increased waist:hip ratio, indicative of abdominal adiposity. This combination of hypertension and increased cardiac output, in a setting of peripheral vascular disease, directly exposes patient to the risk of developing left ventricular hypertrophy. These factors are associated with an increased risk of myocardial infarction (MI), congestive heart failure, and other cardiovascular events.

Numerous studies have shown weight reduction to reduce blood pressure in obese hypertensive patients in a linear fashion.[6] The mechanism is thought to relate to diuresis and contraction of blood volume with a concomitant decrease in sympathetic drive. In addition to improving blood pressure, surgically induced weight loss has been documented to reduce cardiovascular risk by means of lowering triglycerides and low-density lipoprotein, with associated increases in high-density lipoprotein.[7]

Although obesity-related hypertension should be resolved by the time that the postbariatric patient arrives for body-contouring evaluation, certain steps in the visit should be performed. During the preoperative evaluation, discussion about angina, exertional dyspnea, fatigue, and syncope may provide clues to underlying cardiac disease. On physical examination, hallmark signs for congestive heart failure include jugular venous distension, an additional S3 heart sound, respiratory crackles, and peripheral edema, which all need to be assessed. Assessing patient exercise tolerance provides insight into the patient's ability to withstand cardiac stress experienced during surgery. A patient with a weekly exercise routine of swimming 30 minutes four times a week is less likely to have as significant heart disease as the patient who does not exercise at all. Sedentary, inactive patients may have underlying cardiac disease that is unmasked in the operating room. Patients aged >30 should have cardiac screening with an electrocardiogram to reveal ventricular hypertrophy or any ischemic changes from prior cardiac events. Any concern indicates prompt referral to a cardiologist for further evaluation.

Pulmonary disease

Obesity is one of the strongest risk factors for obstructive sleep apnea (OSA) and obesity hypoventilation syndrome (OHS), present in >50% of obese individuals.[8] OSA is defined by the occurrence of more than five apneic episodes per hour due to repetitive collapse of the upper airways during sleep. Risks and complications of OSA include MI, sudden death from arrhythmia, and stroke during apneic episodes. The potential consequences of OSA are intractable daytime somnolence, impaired daytime function, and metabolic dysfunction, in addition to the above cardiovascular complications. First-line therapy for OSA is positive airway pressure delivered through a specific timing regimen, most commonly continuous.

Postoperative follow-up after gastric bypass surgery has demonstrated improved apnea indices in up to 93% of patients. Patients with continued OSA who use continuous positive airway pressure should have inpatient arrangements made before plastic surgery. Analgesics including opiates and sedatives may exacerbate mild apnea symptoms postoperatively. Some recommend intensive care unit monitoring for apneic episodes and associated arrhythmias during the first 24 hours after extubation.

OHS exists when obese patients (BMI >30) present with hypoventilation defined by an arterial blood gas demonstrating hypercapnia ($PaCO_2$ >45 mmHg) or hypoxemia (PaO_2 <55 mmHg). Most patients with OSH have coexisting OSA. Associated complications include pulmonary hypertension and right-sided heart failure. Resolution of pulmonary hypertension and improvements in blood gas measurements has been demonstrated after gastric bypass surgery in patients with OHS. Patients with OSH and pulmonary hypertension should have preoperative invasive hemodynamic monitoring and optimization of cardiopulmonary function. Evaluation by a pulmonologist is vital to determine surgical risk associated with elective body-contouring surgery.

Gastroesophageal reflux disease

Although weight loss is often recommended for obese patients with acid reflux, clinical studies of obesity and reflux disease have shown conflicting results. Gastroesophageal reflux disease (GERD) has a well-known constellation of symptoms and complications, with cancer being the most threatening. A multivariate analysis demonstrated a direct relationship between increased BMI and reflux symptoms.[9] Studies have shown that gastric bypass alleviates symptoms of GERD. Patients with active GERD should be stabilized on appropriate medication by their bariatric surgeon or gastroenterologist before body-contouring surgery. In addition, patients should be counseled about the potential risk of worsening symptoms if abdominal fascial plication is performed.

Deep venous thrombosis

Obesity is an independent risk factor for deep vein thrombosis (DVT) and pulmonary embolism (PE), and this risk must be taken into account when operating on patients with a high BMI. Risk for DVT also increases with age, with a linear increase after the age of 40. Type of surgery and magnitude of the procedure are additional important factors; most body-contouring procedures that occur postbariatric surgery should be considered equivalent to major general surgery operations. Prior DVT or PE is an especially notable risk. Aly et al.[10] reported a 9% incidence of PE in postbariatric patients.

Proper prophylactic treatment is a balance between efficacy and risk of bleeding complications. Body-contouring procedures create large dead spaces from tissue undermining and liposuction, increasing concern for bleeding. Patients may be stratified based on their likelihood of thromboembolic event: Low, moderate, high, and highest.

Sequential compression devices (SCDs) are an effective measure with essentially no complications. Comprehensive evidence-based guidelines published from the sixth American College of Chest Physicians Consensus Conference on Antithrombotic Therapy state that either heparin therapy or SCD is acceptable as solo therapy for general surgery patients at moderate or high risk for DVT.[11] SCD stockings are suitable for all patients who undergo procedures longer than 1 hour and should be applied preoperatively before anesthesia. The best preventive measure is early ambulation; however, if this is not possible, heparin or low-molecular-weight heparin (LMWH) should be initiated 30–60 min preoperatively or 12 h postoperatively for patients in the high- and highest-risk categories.

Psychiatric considerations

Many morbidly obese patients have impairments in quality of life and psychosocial distress. Several studies have shown the presence of psychopathology in extremely obese patients.[12] Of this patient population seeking bariatric surgery, 20–60% have been diagnosed with an axis I psychiatric disorder. Mood and anxiety disorders were most common among these, although substance abuse and personality disorders followed. A population-based study of more than 40 000 adults in the USA showed a fivefold increase in the risk for major depression in patients with a BMI >40 kg/m².

Dissatisfaction with one's body image is believed to motivate many behaviors, including weight loss, exercise, and plastic surgery. Marked body image dissatisfaction is related to lower self-esteem and increased symptoms of depression in obese individuals. When these issues drive motivation for bariatric surgery, weight loss is certainly efficacious, but risky from a psychiatric point of view. Most bariatric surgery programs in the USA require a mental health evaluation as part of the patient selection process. Despite the variability in the preoperative mental health evaluations conducted, any significant psychiatric issue is universally considered a contraindication to bariatric surgery.

Dissatisfaction with one's appearance or body image has long been believed to play a role in an individual's decision to undergo plastic surgery. Several studies have shown that the presence of binge-eating disorder (BED) predicts suboptimal surgical weight loss and late complications of weight regain within the first 2 years after bariatric surgery. BED is characterized by eating large amounts of food within a 2-hour period of time while feeling a subjective loss of control. Purging is not associated with this disorder as it is with bulimia nervosa. Patients with this disorder may also have mood, anxiety, personality, and substance-use disorders.

Psychopathology independent of the degree of obesity was postulated to inhibit one's ability and capacity to make the necessary dietary and behavioral changes to achieve a successful postoperative result. Understanding the psychological aspects of these patients likely plays an important role in preoperative assessment and postoperative management. Factors that motivate patients' decisions to seek these procedures, along with the psychosocial and physical outcomes, require attention. A preoperative psychological assessment of the MWL patient should be the central focus of the initial plastic surgery consultation.[13] Topics discussed should include, but not be limited to, patients' motivations and expectations of postbariatric plastic surgery, their body image concerns, and presence and explanation of any previous psychiatric history. It is fundamental to confirm weight stability at this time because any sign of instability or weight regain may reveal underlying psychiatric issues among other possibilities. Many patients after MWL have an unrealistic expectation of their postoperative results for plastic surgery. They often fail to understand that body-contouring surgery leaves large, visible scars, skin irregularities, and residual deformities in body shape.

A small degree of body image dissatisfaction is expected and well recognized in patients seeking bariatric and plastic surgery, and is not to be misconstrued as psychopathological. Although this judgment may be subjective, patients who report that they dwell on their appearance for more than 1 hour daily, or experience emotional disruption from thinking about their appearance, strongly indicate body image dissatisfaction suggestive of body dysmorphic disorder (BDD). Approximately 40% of postbariatric patients are involved in some form of psychiatric treatment often including antidepressant medications. Despite treatment, the plastic surgeons should assess for ongoing depressive symptoms, including observing the patient's mood, affect, and behavior. Patients should be asked whether they experience frequent crying or irritability, social isolation, feelings of emptiness, and any suicidal ideation. Affirmative answers to these questions necessitate mental health consultation. In the event of unclear answers, referral to the patient's treating mental health physician is encouraged. Previous reports have described cases in which patients dissatisfied after plastic surgery used their preoperative psychiatric history as leverage for legal action. For such cases, it may behoove the plastic surgeon to obtain written psychiatric confirmation of the patient's mental stability and capacity before plastic surgery.

■ NUTRITIONAL DEFICIENCY

Given the time frame during which postbariatric patients consider body-contouring evaluation, many of the early complications experienced with bariatric procedures have potentially subsided. Late complications are of more concern, of which nutritional deficiencies predominate. They often become evident years after bariatric surgery, and are often unidentified and remain undertreated within this patient population. Although there is significant variability in the literature for the reported incidence of macro- and micronutrient deficiencies, plastic surgeons must be diligent about unmasking them. Many patients may present as chronically malnourished if they failed to maintain compliance with diet and vitamin supplementation. Many gradually fail to continue with their regular, scheduled, postoperative follow-up appointments as their weight drops and they begin to feel better. Patients who are older, witness greater weight loss than expected, or experience dumping syndrome after their bariatric procedure are more likely to present with inadequate nutrition.

Nutritional deficits have a wide range of clinical presentations (**Table 4.2**). During the preoperative evaluation, familiarity with them supports suspicion of any clinical or subclinical micro- and macronutrient deficiency. These deficiencies do affect postoperative morbidity and even mortality. Several play an important role, adversely affecting wound healing, which is detrimental to the postoperative aesthetic result.

Table 4.2 Nutritional deficiencies and associated clinical findings.

Protein–energy	Poor growth, muscle wasting, edema, fine, sparse hair, dry, scaling, flaky skin, altered skin pigmentation, cheilosis, ridging of nails, abdominal distension, hepatomegaly
Essential fatty acids	Desquamating dermatitis, alopecia, poor growth
Vitamin A	Night blindness; xerophthalmia; follicular hyperkeratosis; corkscrew hairs
Vitamin D	Craniotabes, enlarged fontanel, epiphyseal enlargement, knock-knees or bowing of extremities, costochondral beading, tetany
Vitamin E	Hemolytic anemia, edema, ataxia, hyporeflexia, ophthalmoplegia, hypotonia
Vitamin K	Petechiae, purpura, ecchymoses, bleeding diathesis
Thiamine (vitamin B_1)	Calf tenderness, hyporeflexia, muscle weakness, ataxia, ophthalmoplegia, tachycardia, edema, apathy
Riboflavin (vitamin B_2)	Angular stomatitis, cheilosis, glossitis, seborrheic dermatitis, normocytic anemia
Niacin (vitamin B_3)	Symmetric dermatitis in light-exposed areas, cheilosis, glossitis, diarrhea, apathy
Pyridoxine (vitamin B_6)	Seborrheic dermatitis, glossitis, angular stomatitis, cheilosis, seizures, peripheral neuropathy, microcytic anemia
Cyanocobalamin (vitamin B_{12})	Megalobastic anemia, peripheral neuropathy
Folate	Megaloblastic anemia
Biotin	Seborrheic dermatitis, alopecia, glossitis, irritability, lethargy
Vitamin C	Follicular hyperkeratosis, corkscrew hairs, gingival hypertrophy and bleeding, perifollicular petechiae, ecchymoses, hemarthroses, periosteal hemorrhage, anemia, bone tenderness
Iron	Fatigue; headache; koilonychia; pallor; tachycardia; anemia
Zinc	Periorificial dermatitis, angular stomatitis, alopecia, poor wound healing, impaired taste sensation
Copper	Poor growth, depigmentation of hair, brittle hair, pallor, microcytic anemia, neutropenia, osteoporosis, fractures
Selenium	Cardiomyopathy, osteoarthropathy

■ Macronutrients

Protein is the primary macronutrient that requires close surveillance after bariatric surgery. Protein-calorie malnutrition is defined by a history of inadequate protein and energy intake, unintentional weight loss, or low body weight for height.[14] Due to inadequate protein intake, up to 25% of weight loss surgery patients are at risk of developing protein–calorie malnutrition for several months after surgery. Coughlin et al.[15] reported the gradual progression in energy intake and protein–calorie intake in the months after bariatric surgery. For the first 3 months, energy intake is < 500 kcal/day with < 20 g/day being protein. By the sixth month, numbers increase to roughly 1000 kcal/day and 38 g/day, respectively. At 1 year, although energy intake is maintained at 1000 kcal/day, protein intake generally increases to 60 g/day. After major surgery, such as massive body contouring, protein-calorie requirements may increase by up to 25%. At the time of plastic surgery evaluation, dietary sources of high-quality protein should provide a minimum of 60 g/day or 1.0–1.5 g/kg ideal body weight per day.

Protein–calorie insufficiency may result from low food intake, food intolerance, or malabsorption. During rapid weight loss, amino acid stores are mobilized toward gluconeogenesis. Patients with malabsorption from their surgery, in addition to food intolerance to high protein foods, can end up with significant protein depletion. Albumin has been shown to be a predictor for postoperative morbidity and mortality. A history of dumping syndrome after a bariatric procedure and continued change in BMI are relatively good predictors of low albumin levels. Hypoalbuminemia has been reported as high as 13% in patients who received RYGB. Low serum albumin with low phosphorus is a good diagnostic indicator for total body protein depletion. Due to its shorter half-life of 2–4 days, prealbumin is a more sensitive measure of acute protein malnutrition. In the same sense, it is the best assessment for response to protein supplementation. Compared with nonsurgical and gastric banding weight loss, patients with previous gastric bypass have lower prealbumin levels on average, at 23 g/l. Naghshineh et al.[16] showed that low daily protein intake does not significantly correlate with low serum protein measures. Therefore it is vital to obtain the three measurements for a valid nutritional workup: Albumin, prealbumin, and protein intake.

Complications for low protein nutrition can be detrimental to the successful recovery of body-contouring surgery. A decrease in serum albumin from 46 g/l to 21 g/l has been shown to increase morbidity and mortality, predominantly from sepsis and major infections. This association of severe protein–calorie malnutrition with immunosuppression increases wound complication rates after clean surgical procedures. Low caloric intake has been shown to decrease collagen synthesis, extracellular matrix protein deposition, and formation of granulation tissue. Furthermore, insufficient protein intake and low serum protein are known to cause delayed wound healing, skin and fascial wound breakdown, and ultimately wound dehiscence. In addition, any consequent edema from hypoalbuminemia will adversely affect perfusion of the healing tissues. It is crucial that protein–calorie-deficient patients are asked to increase intake to fulfill daily protein requirements. Liquid protein is an effective means that may be necessary. Any concern for abnormal protein intake should prompt further evaluation by a bariatric nutritionist and surgery should be postponed.

Micronutrients

Vitamins and minerals serve as coenzymes or factors in a multitude of metabolic pathways incorporated in carbohydrate, fat, and protein metabolism. Some function in oxidation and reduction reactions and others serve as antioxidants or even hormones. Regardless of the type of bariatric surgery, micronutrient homeostasis changes for different reasons. For patients with VBG, the small intestine remains intact and micronutrient deficiencies are considered to be rare, provided that adequate food intake is maintained, which in some cases is not easily achieved. Due to their malabsorptive mechanism, RYGB and BPD are commonly associated with micronutrient deficiencies. Miskowiak et al.[17] showed that, several months after bariatric surgery, the intake of a wide spectrum of vitamins, except for vitamin K, decreased from well above to well below the minimum recommended daily allowance (RDA).

Minerals
Iron
Iron deficiency is a persistent complication after all types of bariatric surgery. Sources for dietary iron include animal hemoglobin and myoglobin (heme iron) or plant inorganic iron. Heme iron is more rapidly absorbed compared with nonheme iron. After removal of globin by proteolytic duodenal enzymes, intestinal mucosal cells, primarily of the duodenum and upper jejunum, absorb iron. Due to the inorganic form of iron in nonheme iron, gastric hydrochloric acid is required to reduce it from the ferric to the ferrous state before absorption. Therefore, in RYGB patients, the pathophysiology behind iron deficiency arises from reduced iron intake, bypassing the acid environment of the stomach, and curtailing the absorptive surface in the small intestine.

With iron deficiency observed in both restrictive and malabsorptive procedures, the reported incidence is up to 47%, with variation depending on the type of procedure. The RDA for iron is 10 mg/day in men and 15 mg/day in nonmenstruating women. RYGB patients may only consume 6–9 mg iron daily from limited energy intake of 1000–1500 kcal/day.[18] Chronic causes of blood loss including menstruation or stomal ulceration increase risk for iron deficiency in postbariatric patients. Iron deficiency worsens with time and has shown to peak at 3–4 years postoperatively.

Iron deficiency is associated with cognitive impairment, immune dysregulation, and cellular dysfunction. More commonly, iron deficiency presents as microcytic anemia, which appears to increase with follow-up time in the postbariatric population with rates of up to 52–75%. Microcytic anemia can affect circulation in the healing tissues, increasing the risk of opportunistic infections. Severe iron deficiency impairs collagen production, which may lead to developing wound contractures. Weakness and fatigue from iron deficiency anemia promotes inactivity and immobilization in the postoperative postbariatric patient, increasing the risk for developing DVT. With an incumbent risk of significant blood loss during postbariatric body contouring, identification of iron deficiency anemia and optimization of the patient's hemoglobin and hematocrit are vital preoperatively. Any iron deficiency dictates treatment. Patients benefit rapidly from oral ferrous sulfate or gluconate supplements. The addition of vitamin C enhances intestinal absorption of iron. Patients refractory to oral iron supplementation require parental iron infusion.

Zinc
Zinc is an essential trace mineral used in cellular growth and replication. It plays a role in supporting the immune system in leukocyte function and cell-mediated immunity. It also behaves as an antioxidant and has antiatherogenic properties. Zinc deficiency impairs cellular and humoral immune functions. Deficient patients are at risk of decreased collagen synthesis and fibroblast proliferation. Wound infection and delayed wound healing are the results of this process. In postbariatric patients, zinc deficiency is often subclinical. RDA for men and women is 11 mg/day and 8 mg/day, respectively. Prior studies show a direct correlation between dietary protein and zinc intake. A well-recognized manifestation of zinc deficiency is hair thinning and loss. Incidentally, zinc deficiency is not commonly reported after bariatric surgery.

Copper
Copper is an important cofactor for enzymes vital to the functioning of the nervous system. Copper deficiency can manifest in parallel with vitamin B_{12} and other nutritional efficiencies. Deficiency is rarely reported with RDA at 0.9 mg/day for most adults. It is linked to demyelinating neuropathies and sideroblastic anemia. Neurological problems may include myelopathy, peripherally neuropathy, and optic neuropathy. Copper deficiency can be treated with either oral copper supplements or intravenous copper.

Selenium
Few studies have been published regarding selenium deficiency after weight loss surgery. Madan et al.[19] demonstrated significant deficiency of this trace element in 58% of the preoperative morbid population.

Postoperatively only 3% continued with this mineral deficiency after proper supplementation and had no other complications.

Water-soluble vitamins
Vitamin B$_{12}$
Vitamin B$_{12}$ (cobalamin) is an important coenzyme involved in amino acid metabolism, DNA synthesis, and neurological function. The RDA of cobalamin is 2.4 µg/day. Vitamin B$_{12}$ deficiency is fairly prevalent in postbariatric patients and may manifest as early as 6 months, but commonly at 12 months and thereafter. The hallmark laboratory finding for this is macrocytic anemia with increased serum methylmalonic acid. When vitamin B$_{12}$ is deficient, abnormal fatty acids accumulate and become incorporated into cell membranes, including those of the nervous system, accounting for some of the neurological manifestation of vitamin B$_{12}$ deficiency. Neurological symptoms include sensory or motor deficits and subacute combined degeneration of the spinal cord. In addition to neurological symptoms, prolonged vitamin B$_{12}$ deficiency has hematological and atherosclerotic manifestations.

Up to a third of patients with gastric bypass will develop vitamin B$_{12}$ deficiency. Absorption of vitamin B$_{12}$ is a complex process compared with other vitamins. The pathophysiology behind vitamin B$_{12}$ malabsorption involves disruption of any one of the following steps: Gastric acid release and pepsin hydrolysis, stomach parietal cell release of intrinsic factor, pancreatic enzyme release into the duodenum, and an adequate terminal ileum length.[20] After gastric bypass patients are supplemented on 500–600 µg vitamin B$_{12}$ daily. Deficient patients may need monthly intramuscular injections of 1000 µg until their liver stores have been replenished. Only a few cases of macrocytic anemia from vitamin B$_{12}$ deficiency in postbariatric patients have been published.

Folate
Folic acid is an essential water-soluble vitamin that serves as a coenzyme for DNA production. Folate deficiency is less common than vitamin B$_{12}$ and iron deficiency. Widely found in animal and plant dietary sources, absorption requires folate to be hydrolyzed by intestinal brush border conjugates. The increased intraluminal pH found in the absence of gastric hydrochloric acid inhibits these enzymes and disrupts folate absorption, 100 µg of which is excreted in the bile daily. Folate deficiency can occur up to 38% of patients after gastric bypass. Many RYGB patients with folate deficiency are asymptomatic or have subclinical disease. Severe deficiency manifests as megaloblastic anemia. Associated with folate deficiency and rapid weight loss are elevated levels of homocysteine, which are atherogenic and have a direct effect on vascular endothelium dysfunction. It is a known risk for MI, stroke, and other vaso-occlusive processes.[21] Supplementation with vitamin B$_{12}$ and folate can normalize this level. In addition to folate, vitamin B$_{12}$ and B$_6$ deficiencies can contribute to hyperhomocysteinemia. Deficiency of vitamin B$_6$, vitamin B$_{12}$, and folate in postbariatric patients can potentially contribute to a hypercoagulable state in those with hyperhomocysteinemia. Recommendations for postsurgical patients is supplementation of 400 µg folate.

Vitamin B$_1$
Thiamine (vitamin B$_1$) is a coenzyme in oxidative decarboxylation reactions and plays a central role in carbohydrate metabolism. Total body stores are approximately 30 mg, and last 3–6 weeks with a half-life of 15 days. Clinical manifestations of thiamine deficiency include peripheral neuropathy, which may present as weakness, ataxia, and numbness in the extremities. Prolonged deficiency may progress to Wernicke-Korsakoff syndrome, characterized by mental confusion, memory loss, progressive paralysis, coma, and ultimately even death. Thiamine is absorbed in the small intestine, namely the jejunum and ileum. Similar to other vitamins, its deficiency is likely to remain subclinical. Patients can develop symptoms of deficiency in less than 3 weeks of deficient intake. If patients are deficient, parental thiamine 50–200 mg/day should be started until symptoms clear. This may be followed by oral supplementation of 10–100 mg/day.[14] Administration of glucose or other carbohydrates with our thiamine replacement can be dangerous and deplete any remaining stores, further precipitating central nervous system deterioration.

Vitamin B$_2$
Riboflavin (vitamin B$_2$) is another water-soluble vitamin obtained from ingested food by small intestine absorption. It is important for energy production, enzyme function, and normal fatty acid and amino acid synthesis, and is necessary for the reproduction of glutathione, a free radical scavenger. Colonic bacteria serve as another source through colonic absorption. Increased dietary fiber promotes colonic bacteria to produce more riboflavin. A high-fiber diet is often maintained with recommendations for a protein-rich postbariatric surgery diet. Despite supplementation, riboflavin deficiency in RYGB patients has been reported at 13.6 and 7.1% at 1- and 2-year follow-ups. Riboflavin is not stored in large amounts and requires constant supply through diet. Deficiency rarely stands alone and is usually part of a multiple-nutrient deficiency. Deficiency should be treated by 6–30 mg riboflavin by mouth daily.

Vitamin B$_6$
Pyridoxine (vitamin B$_6$) is an essential cofactor in DNA synthesis and various transamination, decarboxylation, and synthesis pathways. Clements et al.[22] have reported deficiency of vitamin B$_6$ after RYGB. Deficiencies may present clinically as sideroblastic anemia and, in extreme cases, as peripheral neuropathy and convulsions. Recommendation for treatment is variable on clinical presentation.

Fat-soluble vitamins
Vitamin A
Vitamin A deficiency has been shown in 61% of patients after BPD by Dolan et al.[23] Despite multivitamin supplementation, Brolin and Leung[24] reported up to 10% of patients with distal RYGB developing vitamin A deficiency after 2 years. Studies have demonstrated vitamin A deficiency after weight loss surgery. Effects of deficiency include impaired night vision. Excessive supplementation has toxic effects including papilledema and seizures, hepatitis, and bone pain. The RDA for men is 3000 IU and for women is 2300 IU.

Vitamin D
Vitamin D (calcitriol) is a sterol with hormone-like function, involved in the maintenance of adequate plasma levels of calcium. Vitamin D increases uptake of calcium by the intestine, minimizes loss of calcium by the kidney, and stimulates resorption of bone when necessary. It can be found naturally in fatty fish, liver, and egg yolk. Unfortified milk is a poor source. Cholecalciferol (vitamin D$_3$) is a biologically inactive form of the vitamin converted in vivo to the active form of vitamin D by two sequential reactions in the liver and kidney. Cholecalciferol is synthesized in the skin after ultraviolet light (sunlight) reacts with its precursor, 7-dehydrocholesterol. Patients with insufficient sunlight exposure may need dietary preformed vitamin D. The RDA for adults is 5 µg cholecalciferol or 200 IU vitamin D. Patients with malabsorptive procedures are at higher risk of calcium and vitamin D deficiency than patients with restrictive procedures, but may present in patients with either procedure. Logically, in patients with combination malabsorptive and restrictive procedures such as RYGB, vitamin D deficiency is significantly higher.[18] Long-term manifestations of these deficiencies

include osteoporosis, osteomalacia, and secondary hyperparathyroidism. Despite supplementation with calcium and vitamin D after RYGB, Coates et al.[25] showed increased bone resorption and decreased bone mass at 3–9 months postoperatively. Patients with RYGB and BPD should be placed on supplements. Recommended ranges include 100–1500 mg/day of calcium and 8 μg/day of vitamin D.

Vitamin E

Vitamin E (tocopherol) is an essential fat-soluble nutrient that serves as an antioxidant. Its role is to prevent nonenzymatic oxidation of cell components by molecular oxygen or free radicals. Deficiency is rare after weight loss surgery. Supplementation has not shown to be clinically significant in these patients. Excess supplementation has been shown to inhibit collagen synthesis and damage tensile strength of wounds. The RDA for vitamin E is 15 IU.

Vitamin K

The main function of vitamin K is modification of various blood-clotting factors involved in the coagulation cascade. Vitamin K is produced by intestinal bacteria and its deficiency is rare. Patients with deficiency have symptoms of prolonged bleeding including ecchymosis, petechiae, and hematomas. A study of 170 patients after BPD and BPD/DS found a relatively high incidence of vitamin K deficiency by the fourth year with no clinical manifestation. It is apparent that there are inadequate data on vitamin K deficiency in weight loss surgery procedures.

LABORATORY WORKUP

During the preoperative evaluation, clinical suspicion guided by history, physical examination, and type of bariatric procedure will dictate which laboratory tests to order. Electrolyte analysis and a complete blood count with differential should be expanded to include ferritin, folate, calcium, vitamin B_{12}, prealbumin, and albumin levels.[26] Ideally, laboratory work-up should be performed several weeks before surgery to allow sufficient time for additional tests and for addressing any abnormalities before surgery.

REFERENCES

1. Brolin RE. Update: NIH Consensus Conference. Gastrointestinal surgery for severe obesity. *Nutrition* 1996;**12**:403–4.
2. Moize V, Geliebter A, Gluck ME, et al. Obese patients have inadequate protein intake related to protein intolerance up to 1 year following Roux-en-Y gastric bypass. *Obes Surg.* 2003;**13**:23–8.
3. Rubin JP, Nguyen V, Schwentker A. Perioperative management of the post-gastric-bypass patient presenting for body contour surgery. *Clin Plast Surg* 2004;**31**:601–10, vi.
4. Pories WJ, Swanson MS, MacDonald KG, et al. Whom would have thought it? An operation proves to be the most effective therapy for adult-onset diabetes mellitus. *Ann Surg* 1995;**222**:339–50.
5. The Diabetes Control and Complications Trial Research Group. The effect of intensive treatment of diabetes on the development and progression of long-term complications in insulin dependent diabetes mellitus. *N Engl J Med* 1993;**329**:977–86.
6. Carson JL, Ruddy ME, Duff AE, et al. The effect of gastric bypass surgery on hypertension in morbidly obese patients. *Arch Intern Med* 1994;**154**:193–200.
7. Foley EF, Benotti PN, Borlase BC, et al. Impact of gastric restrictive surgery on hypertension in the mobidly obese. *Am J Surg* 1992;**163**:294–7.
8. Choban PS, Flancbaum L. The impact of obesity on surgical outcomes: a review. *J Am Coll Surg* 1997;**185**:593–603.
9. Ruhl CE, Everhart JE. Oerweight, but not high dietary fat intake, increases risk of gastroesophageal reflux disease hospitalization: the NHANES I Epidemiologic Followup Study. First National Health and Nutrition Examination Survey. *Ann Epidemiol* 1999;**9**:424–35.
10. Aly AS, Cram AE, Chao M, et al. Belt lipectomy for circumferential truncal excess : the University of Iowa experience. *Plast Reconstr Surg* 2003;**111**:398–413.
11. Geerts WH, Bergqvist D, Pineo GF, et al., American College of Chest Physicians. Prevention of venous thromboembolism: American College of Chest Physicians Evidence-Based Clinical Practice Guidelines (8th Edition). *Chest* 2008;133(6 suppl):381S–453S.
12. Bocchieri LE, Meana M, Fisher BL. A review of psychosocial outcomes of surgery for morbid obesity. *J Psychosom Res* 2002;**52**:155–65.
13. Sarwer DB, Fabricatore AN. Psychiatric considerations of the massive weightloss patient. *Clin Plast Surg* 2008;**35**:1–10.
14. Sebastian JL. Bariatric surgery and work-up of the massive weight loss patient. *Clin Plast Surg* 2008;**35**:11–26.
15. Coughlin K, Bell RM, Bivins BA et al. Preoperative and postoperative assessment of nutrient intakes in patients who have undergone gastric bypass surgery. *Arch Surg* 1983;**118**:813–6.
16. Naghshineh N, O'Brien Coon D, McTigue K, Courcoulas AP, Fernstrom M, Rubin JP. Nutritional assessment of bariatric surgery patients presenting for plastic surgery: a prospective analysis. *Plast Reconstr Surg* 2010;**126**:602–10.
17. Miskowiak J, Honore K, Larsen L, et al. Food intake before and after gastroplasty for morbid obesity. *Scand J Gastroenterol* 1985;**20**:925.
18. Slater GH, Ren CJ, Siegel N, et al. Serum fat-soluble vitamin deficiency and abnormal calcium metabolism after malabsorptive bariatric surgery. *J Gastrointest Surg* 2004;**8**:48.
19. Madan AK, Orth WS, Tichansky DS, Ternovits CA. Vitamin and trace mineral levels after laparoscopic gastric bypass. *Obes Surg* 2006;**16**:603–6.
20. Agha-Mohammadi S, Hurwitz DJ. Nutritional deficiency of post-bariatric surgery body contouring patients: what every plastic surgeon should know. *Plast Reconstr Surg* 2008;**122**:604–13.
21. Welch GN, Loscalzo J. Homocysteine and atherothrombosis. *N Engl J Med* 1998;**339**:1042–50.
22. Clements R, Katasani V, Palepu R, et al. Incidence of Vitamin Deficiency after Laparoscopic Roux-en-Y Gastric Bypass in a University Hospital Setting. *Am Surgeon* 2006;**72**:1196–1204.
23. Dolan K, Hatzifotis M, Newbury L et al. A clinical and nutritional comparison of biliopancreatic diversion with and without duodenal switch. *Ann Surg* 2004;**240**:51–6.
24. Brolin RE, Leung M. Survey of vitamin and mineral supplementation after gastric bypass and biliopancreatic diversion for morbid obesity. *Obes Surg* 1999;**9**:150–4.
25. Coates PS, Fernstrom JD, Fernstrom MH, Schauer PR, Greenspan SL. Gastric bypass surgery for morbid obesity leads to an increase in bone turnover and a decrease in bone mass. *J Clin Endocrinol Metab* 2004;**89**:1061–5.
26. Rhode BM, Maclean LD. Vitamin and mineral supplementation after gastric bypass. In: Deitel M, Cowan GSM Jr (eds), *Update: Surgery for the morbidly obese patient: the field of extreme obesity including laparoscopy and allied care.* Toronto: FD Communications, 2000.

SUGGESTED READING

Agha-Mohammadi S, Hurwitz DJ. Nutritional deficiency of post-bariatric surgery body contouring patients: what every plastic surgeon should know. *Plast Reconstr Surg* 2008;**122**:604–13.

Sebastian JL. Bariatric surgery and work-up of the massive weight loss patient. *Clin Plast Surg* 2008;**35**:11–26.

Chapter 5: Anesthetic challenges encountered in the postbariatric patient

Gian Paparcuri, Miguel Cobas

As a direct result of the vastly increasing incidence of obesity and bariatric surgery, body-contouring surgery after massive weight loss (MWL) is a major growth field in plastic surgery. It has developed into a unique specialty within the specialty.

OBESITY

Obesity is a complex, multifactorial, chronic disease that has grown in severity over the past decades. It has become a major health concern worldwide.[1] In the USA, the obesity epidemic is a public health issue, and is considered a leading cause of preventable death and morbidity in all age groups,[2] with a prevalence of almost 34% according to recent national surveys.[3]

Obesity is clinically expressed in terms of the body mass index (BMI). This is derived by dividing the weight of the patient in kilograms by the square of the height in meters. Measurement of BMI provides an accurate and reproducible screening tool for obesity. The BMI-based obesity definitions of the World Health Organization and the National Institutes of Health (NIH) can be found in **Table 5.1**.

Increased BMI >25 kg/m^2 is strongly associated with cardiovascular risk. With BMI >30 kg/m^2, the risk of death from any cause increases abruptly.[4] Over the past decade, in the USA, the prevalence of BMI >30 kg/m^2 has increased twofold, that of BMI >40 kg/m^2 fourfold, and that of BMI >50 kg/m^2 fivefold.[5]

Elevated BMI is also linked to several comorbid conditions, including hypertension, coronary artery disease, diabetes, dyslipidemia, venous stasis disease, obstructive sleep apnea, pulmonary hypertension, nonalcoholic fatty liver disease, gastroesophageal reflux disease, infertility, and cancer.

Current treatment options for morbid obesity include pharmacological agents, low-calorie diets, behavioral modification, exercise, and surgery. In morbidly obese patients, most of these conventional (nonsurgical) interventions have been unable to show meaningful weight loss.[6]

Recently, bariatric surgery has become an excellent evidence-based option for obesity. It offers significant and sustainable weight reduction, and complete resolution of obesity-associated comorbidities.[7] Since its introduction in 1950, bariatric surgery has risen dramatically in recent years. Over 200 000 people now undergo bariatric surgery annually.[8]

According to the NIH, patients must meet strict criteria to qualify for bariatric surgery. Surgical treatment should be considered for patients with a BMI exceeding 40 kg/m^2 and for those between 35 kg/m^2 and 40 kg/m^2 who have life-threatening comorbidities. In addition, they must have failed nonsurgical modalities and be free of any significant psychiatric disorders.[9]

Gastroplasty procedures are generally classified according to their mechanism of action: gastric restriction, intestinal malabsorption, or a combination of the two.

Common contemporary bariatric surgical procedures, performed either open or laparoscopically, include:

- *Adjustable gastric band*: purely restrictive method that limits the size of the stomach, reducing food intake.
- *Roux-en-Y gastric bypass*: mainly a restrictive procedure with some malabsorption. Malabsorptive procedures segregate the food from digestive enzymes and bile, reducing digestive capacity.
- *Biliopancreatic diversion*: restrictive and malabsorptive.

Morbidly obese patients undergoing MWL surgery are considered a challenge for the surgical team. The following is a list of common concerns among anesthesia providers encountering obese patients:

- To the anesthesia provider, the airway is a priority. The degree of airway difficulty is directly proportional to the BMI, because fat deposits in and around the neck and face limit cervical spine mobility (flex extension) and mouth opening, as well as increasing the intrusion of the tongue into the oral pharynx.
  Prepare for the possibility of a difficult intubation. A surgeon familiar with surgical airways should always be readily available.
  Optimize head and neck positioning, in order to align oropharyngeal axes before attempting direct laryngoscopy. Use a ramp under the shoulders so that the chin is higher than the chest.
  In some cases, two anesthesiologists are necessary to maintain ventilation via a mask, one to keep the mask in position and the other to operate the bag.
- Anticipate rapid oxygen desaturation during periods of hypoventilation due to higher oxygen consumption and carbon dioxide production (excess of metabolically active fat tissue). Patients with an anticipated difficult airway should be intubated awake, sitting up, under fiberoptic guidance.
- Patients with severe, life-threatening, obesity-related comorbidities might benefit from invasive monitoring (pulmonary artery catheterization and arterial line).
- Central venous access may be required for patients with thick pannus and difficult peripheral intravenous access.

Table 5.1 Body mass index (BMI)-based obesity definitions.

	Adult BMI (kg/m^2)
Normal	18.5–24.9
Overweight	25–29.9
Obese, class I (moderate obesity)	30–34.9
Obese, class II (severe obesity)	35–39.9
Obese, class III (extreme obesity)	40–49.5
Super obese	50–59.9
Super, super obese	>60

- Arterial cannulation may be necessary, especially in those patients with poorly fitting noninvasive blood pressure cuffs encircling <75% of the upper arm's circumference. Other options include obtaining readings from the ankle or wrist with appropriately sized blood pressure cuffs.
- Obese patients can present with severe nutritional deficiencies, especially after bariatric surgery. Consider vitamin K administration to correct abnormal prothrombin time within 6–24 hours. For emergency surgery or active bleeding use fresh frozen plasma.
- Histamine H_2-receptor antagonists (ranitidine, famotidine, cimetidine), nonparticulate antacid (sodium bicitrate), and proton pump inhibitors (omeprazole, lansoprazole) will reduce gastric volume, acidity, or both. This reduces the risk of and complications arising from aspiration.
- Discuss a thromboprophylaxis regimen with the surgeon.
- Appropriate equipment and tables to accommodate extra weight should be available. A standard surgical table can safely support a 500-lb (227-kg) patient. Attention should always be paid to the manufacturer's maximum weight limit recommendations. Specially designed tables (extra width) or two regular tables joined together may be required.
- Bariatric patients are prone to slipping off the operating table during table position changes. They should be well strapped to the table or positioned on the bean bag.
- Super-obese and diabetic patients are prone to pressure ulcers. All pressure points should be checked and well padded.
- Calculate drug dosage based on lean body mass. Most anesthetic drugs are strongly lipophilic; expect an increased volume of distribution.
- Ventilate with moderate levels of positive end-expiratory pressure. Avoid a large tidal volume (no more than 10–12 ml/kg) to improve functional residual capacity and oxygenation without causing excessive barotraumas.
- Postoperative atelectasis in obese patients can be managed with noninvasive positive airway pressure ventilation. Continuous positive airway pressure (CPAP) or bilevel positive airway pressure (BiPAP) ventilation, starting in the recovery room and continuing overnight, accelerates recovery of preoperative pulmonary function without increasing the risk of pouch distension and anastomotic disruption (postbariatric surgery patients).[10]
- Other options to prevent pulmonary complications include incentive spirometry, deep breathing, and intermittent positive pressure breathing.
- Thoracic epidural analgesia is not only a safe and effective form of postoperative analgesia with few side effects, but it also prevents deep venous thrombosis (DVT) and facilitates early recovery of intestinal motility. Ultrasonography can be used to identify the location of the spinal process and dura.

The results of bariatric surgery are impressive. Approximately 80% of patients experience a 60–80% excess weight loss (body weight in excess of the ideal or BMI >25 kg/m^2) in the first year, with a longer-term stabilization at 50–60% excess weight loss.[11]

Other benefits also far exceed the commonly recognized significant and sustained weight loss. Many studies have shown improvement and sometimes resolution of most comorbid conditions, with concomitant reduction in mortality- and patient-related health costs. In a large Canadian study, surgical weight loss reduced the mortality risk eightfold among morbidly obese patients.[12]

BODY-CONTOURING SURGERY – CONSIDERATIONS FOR THE ANESTHESIOLOGIST

After MWL, patients are left with an excess of lax, overstretched skin. This causes physical discomfort and psychosocial problems. Frequently, these patients consult plastic surgeons to correct such deformities.

To complete the metamorphosis, a multidisciplinary and comprehensive approach offers the best alternative in terms of safety and efficacy to address clinical issues regarding postbariatric patients. Reconstructive procedures include:
- Abdominoplasty (belt lipectomy or mid-body lift)
- Abdominal panniculectomy
- Breast reduction
- Mastopexy (breast lift)
- Brachioplasty (upper arm lift)
- Lower body procedures (thigh and buttocks)
- Liposuction

Preoperative considerations

Body-contouring procedures are considered high-risk and complex surgery. They involve prolonged surgical times, substantial blood loss, significant fluid shifts, and greater physiological stress than even the bariatric procedure.[13]

Complete preoperative history and physical examination, proper patient selection, and medical optimization all help to minimize complications and improve safety.

Staging

During body lift surgery, attention may directed to more than one body part (arms, chest, breasts, back, abdomen, and thighs). These can be performed as a single-stage total body lift or as multiple-stage 'smaller' surgeries.

Relatively healthy patients can be operated on in one single-stage total body lift procedure by a team experienced in body-contouring surgery. This approach reduces costs, reduces time off work, and decreases the number of general anesthesia inductions.

On the other hand, performing a body lift in two or three stages exposes the patient to shorter surgical procedures (less anesthesia time) and decreases overall blood loss. Additional benefits of staging procedures may include the following:
- Areas of greater concern can be tackled first (abdomen, flanks, lower back, and buttocks).
- Skin exposure to opposing pulling vectors when correcting adjacent areas (upper and lower body lifts) is minimized.
- Any contour irregularities and skin laxity that might have occurred after previously performed procedures can be corrected.
- Stress of recovery (and length of stay) is minimized.
- Morbidity may be reduced.

Preoperative medications and NPO (nothing per os) guidelines

It is recommended that the patient's usual medications be continued until the time of surgery. Exceptions include insulin and oral hypoglycemic agents.

The American Society of Anesthesiologists (ASA) has published practice guidelines for preoperative fasting to reduce the risk of pulmonary aspiration. To increase patient comfort and satisfaction, the ASA recommends a minimum of 6 hours for light meals and 2 hours for clear liquids (water, fruit juices without pulp, carbonated beverages, clear tea, and black coffee). A typical light meal consists of toast and clear liquids. Meals that include fried or fatty foods or meat may prolong gastric emptying time.[14]

For patients with an apparent increased risk of pulmonary aspiration, the ASA recommends the use of preoperative pharmacological agents to reduce the volume and acidity of gastric contents.

Nutritional assessment

A thorough nutritional assessment is necessary to determine whether the patient will be able to tolerate the demands of a major surgical procedure. Frequently ordered laboratory tests include complete blood count, electrolytes, albumin, and prealbumin levels.

Daily protein intake and positive nitrogen balance, before and after surgery, is assessed by patient recall of a typical day's diet. Patients are encouraged to increase their protein intake (typically between 50 and 70 g/day) and to select protein sources that have low fat and low carbohydrate content.

Suboptimal protein intake may lead to postoperative complications and impaired healing. This should trigger immediate nutritional counseling and diet changes. These dietary changes could also include vitamin and mineral supplements, such as calcium, vitamin A, vitamin D, vitamin B_{12}, folate, zinc, selenium, and ferrous sulfate.

For those patients requiring additional weight loss before body-contouring surgery, customized diets and exercise plans can be added to optimize cosmetic results. It is crucial that the patient's weight be stable and close to the goal weight, for a minimum of 3 months, preferably with a BMI of ≤ 28 kg/m^2.[15] This usually occurs 12–18 months after bariatric surgery for further evaluation and management.

Finally, it is also important to assess the presence of any issues regarding the bariatric surgery such as nausea, vomiting, or dumping symptoms, because these patients might need to be referred back to their bariatric surgeon.

Anemia screening

Anemia, related to nutritional deficiencies, is very common after bariatric surgery and, as significant blood loss frequently occurs during body-contouring surgery, patients should be optimized and preoperative autologous blood donation considered.[16]

Thromboembolism prophylaxis

The American College of Chest Physicians classifies postbariatric patients as at high risk of thromboembolism. This is due to specific high-risk factors: Major surgery, age >40 years, immobility, obesity (BMI >30), varicose veins, and estrogen use.[17] In fact, the most common cause of mortality and morbidity after contouring surgery is DVT. Strategies for DVT prevention (**Table 5.2**) are initiated preoperatively and should be continued in the postoperative period.

Smoking cessation

As body lifting involves the creation of large tissue flaps and nicotine is a vasoconstrictor and a well-known cause of wound infection, flap necrosis, and wound dehiscence after plastic surgery, patients are required to have stopped taking all nicotine-containing products for a minimum of 4 weeks before surgery.

Table 5.2 Venous thromboembolism prevention strategies.

- Aggressive postoperative pain control
- Early ambulation
- Chemoprophylaxis:
  - LMWH once daily postoperatively
  - Low-dose unfractionated heparin three times a day postoperatively
- Mechanical prophylaxis (functional before induction of general anesthesia):
  - Intermittent compression (pneumatic) devices
  - Graded compression stocking
- Temporary inferior vena cava filters for high risk patients presenting before bariatric surgery for giant panniculectomy

LMWH, low-molecular-weight heparin.

Medical comorbidities

- During the preoperative examination, patients should be evaluated for residual morbidly obese-related disease. In addition, exercise tolerance can be assessed to estimate major surgery tolerance and presence of silent ischemia.
- The American College of Cardiology and the American Heart Association have established guidelines on perioperative cardiovascular evaluation for patients undergoing non-cardiac surgery.[18] Since the ASA endorsement, perioperative physicians have being encouraged to familiarize themselves with its algorithms and apply these to their clinical practice.
- Patients with a personal or a family history of thrombophilia should be referred for a hematology consult to guide perioperative anticoagulation.

Intraoperative considerations

Airway

These patients often have anatomies that can complicate ventilation and intubation. In addition, as a result of their bariatric surgery (distorted gastroesophageal junction), there are increased risks of reflux and aspiration. They should be considered to have a full stomach and at risk of aspiration.[19]

Blind insertion of foreign objects, including a nasogastric tube, is contraindicated in patients with a smaller gastric pouch secondary to bariatric surgery. Endoscopic guidance is recommended to avoid esophageal or gastric perforation.

Infection

A first-generation cephalosporin is routinely administered before incision and continued in the postoperative period. This is because of an increased risk of postoperative wound infection.

Hypothermia

Lengthy procedures exposing large areas of the body increase the risk for hypothermia and with it morbidity, blood loss, transfusion rate, surgical wound infection, seroma formation, cardiac events, and lengthened hospital stay. Many centers implement active warming devices such as forced-flow air warmers, both preoperatively in the holding area and continued throughout the case. When repositioning the patient and moving from one anatomic region to another, warming devices should be replaced to cover as much of the exposed body surface as possible.

Operating room temperature should be set to 21°C (70°F). Skin preparation should be performed with warm solutions.

All intravenous fluids should be either pre-warmed or run through a fluid warmer system, including tumescent solutions. Core temperature should be monitored at all times using an esophageal probe.

Positioning

- Careful positioning and padding of pressure points prevents injuries.
- The head and neck should remain in a neutral position and always be supported.
- Anesthesia providers should be granted access to the endotracheal tube. Care must be taken to avoid dislodgement and unplanned extubation during turning.
- Supine is the most common position. This allows access to the face, breast, abdomen, and anterior aspects of the upper and lower extremities. Placing a pillow under the knees reduces tension over the lumbar spine.
- To avoid stretching injuries of the brachial plexus, shoulder adduction should be limited to <80°. This avoids hyperextension, especially during breast surgery.
- Also during cosmetic breast procedures, it is common to move the patient from the supine position to the seated position several times. If the arms are not properly secured, they can slip off the arm board.
- To minimize ulnar nerve injuries, confirm appropriate positioning and padding of the elbow. Avoid pronation of the forearm in the abducted position and limit elbow flexion to no more than 90°.
- The prone position is frequently used for liposuction. This position is carried out by supine intubation followed by transition to the prone position.
- To minimize pressure on the chest and facilitate ventilation in the prone position, patients are elevated off the table by using parallel gel rolls. Direct pressure on the male genitalia and nipples should be avoided. Breasts should be positioned medially and genitalia should be free from any stress from urinary catheters.
- The use of headrest support systems designed for the prone position offers additional protection to the face, ears, nose. and eyes. It also allows stabilization of the head and neck in the neutral position, preventing obstructions, dissection, and even thrombosis of the vertebral arteries when a patient's heads is laid on its side.
- To decrease intraocular pressure when prone, 15° of reverse Trendelenburg can be applied.
- Lateral decubitus is facilitated by the use of a beanbag. It should be placed before the start of surgery. Use of an axillary roll (placed caudal to the axilla, not in the axilla) minimizes pressure on the neurovascular structures of the axilla. The dependent lower extremity is flexed at the hip, and the nondependent lower extremity remains straight. Pillows and extra padding are placed between the legs and under the dependent greater trochanter, fibular head, and lateral malleolus.
- During the many frequent changes in position, the anesthesiologist should remain vigilant. He or she should re-check all pressure points and joint positions. Deepening anesthesia minimizes coughing, bucking, and straining, all of which might exacerbate bleeding during these position changes.
- Eye injury is infrequent but, when it happens, the results can be devastating. Lack of lacrimation, improperly placed facemasks, or eyes left open are all risk factors for such injuries. Ocular protection strategies include the use of lubricants and artificial tears, closure of the eyelids with tape immediately after intubation, and hard goggles.

Muscle relaxants

During certain body lift procedures (e.g. mastopexy), nerve monitoring and avoiding muscle relaxation might be necessary.

Liposuction

Liposuction can complement body-contouring surgery. Administration of epinephrine-containing tumescence fluid decreases associated blood loss.

Anesthetic literature recommends a maximum lidocaine dose of 7 mg/kg. This limit is surpassed during tumescent liposuction, reaching up to 35 mg/kg. Toxic blood levels (5 mg/dl) are usually never reached because of immediate suctioning of some of the infiltrate, as well as delayed absorption of an extremely diluted lidocaine tumescent solution.

Large-volume lipoaspirates (>4–5 l) have been associated with epinephrine and lidocaine toxicity. Tinnitus and circumoral numbness are early symptoms of local anesthetic toxicity, followed by muscle twitching, seizures, coma, and cardiopulmonary collapse.

As the plasma concentration of lidocaine peaks at 8–16 h, admission and observation are recommended for large-volume liposuction (after 4 l).[20]

Other complications of large-volume liposuction include fluid overload, and pulmonary and fat embolism.

Epidural anesthesia

If regional anesthesia is planned, special attention should be exercised during catheter placement and removal if perioperative venous thromboembolism chemoprophylaxis is to be employed.

The use of subcutaneous heparin is not a risk factor for spinal hematoma and neuraxial blockage as stated by the American Society of Regional Anesthesia and Pain Medicine.[21] In cases of preoperative low-molecular-weight heparin (LMWH) chemoprophylaxis, the consensus is to delay needle placement 10–12 h after the last dose. Postoperative management is based on the dosing schedule:

- *Twice daily dosing*: This associated with an increased risk of spinal hematoma. Indwelling catheters should be removed before initiation of LMWH thromboprophylaxis (usually no earlier than 24 h postoperatively).
- *Single daily dosing*: The first postoperative LMWH dose is usually administered 6–8 h postoperatively and the second dose is given no sooner than 24 h after the first dose. Indwelling neuraxial catheters may be safely maintained. They should be removed 10–12 h after the last dose of LMWH, with subsequent dosing no earlier than 2 h after catheter removal.

Postoperative considerations

After extubation, the head of the bed should be elevated to at least 30° to facilitate ventilation and minimize the risk of aspiration.

Strategies to prevent thromboembolism (already started preoperatively) should continue in the postoperative period. Patients should be encouraged to ambulate early, starting on the day of surgery and at least three times a day thereafter. Compression boots should be worn when the patient is not ambulating.

To prevent lung atelectasis, pulmonary rehabilitation with incentive spirometry should start immediately, 10 times an hour while awake. Noninvasive positive pressure ventilation (CPAP or BiPAP) overnight should also be considered.

Aggressive pain management facilitates early ambulation and deep breathing. This helps to prevent venous thromboembolism and pneumonia.

In addition to epidural analgesia, some surgeons choose to thread catheters along the fascia in abdominal surgery for continuous administration of long-acting local anesthetics. Another option to manage acute postoperative pain is the use of intravenous patient-controlled analgesia pain pumps.

REFERENCES

1. World Health Organization. *Obesity: Preventing and managing the global epidemic*. WHO Obesity Technical Report Series 894. Geneva: WHO, 2000.
2. American Obesity Association. *Obesity in the United States*. Available at www.obesity.org (accessed February 17, 2012).
3. Flegal KM, Carroll MD, Ogden CL, et al. Prevalence and trends in obesity among US adults, 1999–2008. *JAMA* 2010;**303**:235–41.
4. Calle EE, Thun MJ, Petrelli JM, Rodriguez C, Heath CW Jr. Body mass index and mortality in a prospective cohort of US adults. *N Engl J Med* 1999;**341**:1097–105.
5. Sturm R. Increases in clinically severe obesity in the United States, 1986–2000. *Arch Intern Med* 2003;**163**:2146–8.
6. Bjorntorp P. Treatment of obesity. *Int J Obes Relat Metab Disord* 1992;**16**(suppl 3):S81–4.
7. National Institutes of Health. Gastrointestinal surgery for severe obesity. *NIH Consens Statement Online* 1991;**9**:1–20.
8. Belle SH, Berk PD, Courcoulas AP, et al. Safety and efficacy of bariatric surgery: Longitudinal assessment of bariatric surgery. *Surg Obes Relat Dis* 2007;**3**:116–26.
9. NIH conference. Consensus development conference panel. Gastrointestinal surgery for severe obesity. *Ann Intern Med* 1991;**115**:956–61.
10. Weingarten TN, Kendrick ML, Swain JM, et al. Effects of CPAP on gastric pouch pressure after bariatric surgery. *Obes Surg* 2011;**21**:1900–5.
11. Buchwald H, Avidor Y, Braunwald E, et al. Bariatric surgery: a systematic review and meta-analysis. *JAMA* 2004;**292**:1724–37.
12. Christou NV, Sampalis JS, Liberman M, et al. Surgery decreases long-term mortality, morbidity, and health care use in morbidly obese patients. *Ann Surg* 2004;**240**:416–24.
13. Colwell AS, Borud LJ. Optimization of patient safety in postbariatric body contouring: a current review. *Aesthet Surg J* 2008;**28**:437–42.
14. Practice guidelines for preoperative fasting and the use of pharmacologic agents to reduce the risk of pulmonary aspiration: application to healthy patients undergoing elective procedures. *Anesthesiology* 1999;**90**:896–905.
15. Rubin JP, Nguyen VU, Schwentker A. Perioperative management of the post-gastric bypass patient presenting for body contour surgery. *Clin Plast Surg* 2004;**31**:601–10.
16. Ellsworth WA, Basu CB, Iverson RE. Perioperative considerations for patient safety during cosmetic surgery – preventing complications. *Can J Plast Surg* 2009;**17**:9–16.
17. Geerts WH, Pineo GF, Heit JA, et al. Prevention of venous thromboembolism: The Seventh ACCP Conference of Antithrombotic and Thrombolytic Therapy. *Chest* 2004;**126**:338S–400S.
18. Fleisher LA, Beckman JA, Brown KA, et al. ACC/AHA 2007 Perioperative Guidelines. *J Am Coll Cardiol* 2007;**50**(17):e159–e241.
19. Cannon-Diehl MR. Emerging issues for the postbariatric surgical patient. *Crit Care Nurs Q* 2010;**33**:361–70.
20. Gordley KP, Basu CB. Optimal use of local anesthetics and tumescence. Optimization of patient safety in cosmetic surgery. *Semin Plast Surg* 2006;**20**:219–24.
21. Horlocker TT, Wedel DJ, Rowlingson JC, et al. Regional anesthesia in the patient receiving antithrombotic or thrombolytic therapy: American Society of Regional Anesthesia and Pain Medicine Evidence-Based Guidelines (Third Edition). *Reg Anesth Pain Med* 2010;**35**:64–101.

Chapter 6

Anatomical deformities secondary to massive weight loss

Michele A. Shermak

Although massive weight loss (MWL) improves the body mass index (BMI) and medical profile, those who sustain MWL have negative physical sequelae, including the effects of volume loss, tissue damage, and residual fat pockets. More specifically, these individuals may have significant deflation of body regions, skin excess and redundancy, rolls with fat deposits made more remarkable by adhesions, and striae. Extent of the deformity varies between and within patients. Body regions may be affected from head to toe. Some regions are impacted more than others. It is not known which patients are most affected physically by MWL. The deformity is related to degree of weight loss, mode of weight loss, and/or duration of weight loss. In addition, there are factors intrinsic to the patient's biology.

MWL of the order of 100 lb (45 kg) or more often leads to skin deflation and redundant skin from head to toe. Individuals with MWL may experience functional symptoms, composed of rashes and irritation with requirement for constant hygiene, pain, backache with exacerbation of osteoarthritis of the joints and spine, and disability with activity and exercise. They complain of difficulty with clothing. Many individuals report deflated body image after MWL. Many even state that they wished they never lost all the weight. The success of MWL is diminished with lack of completion of care. This is somewhat analogous to women who undergo mastectomy and are never offered reconstruction. Plastic surgery can provide completion to care, with improved physical and mental functioning.

The goal of postbariatric body-contouring surgery is to correct deformities that result from significant weight loss. These consist of resection of excess tissue, and repositioning and tightening of lax tissues. Analyzing the patient presentation results in an informed discussion between patient and doctor to determine an appropriate individualized surgical plan.

Standardized classification systems have been presented to describe deformities of the abdomen, chest, thigh, and other body regions. Some systems are specific to the MWL patient. Surgeons create these systems to improve academic and administrative communication and to guide surgical repair. There is, however, difficulty in adopting a universal classification system, due to the intrinsically cumbersome nature of a system that must account for enormous variability in individual presentation. The Pittsburgh Rating Scale, a 10-region, 4-point grading system, with '0' describing normal, up to '3' describing the most severe deformity, was developed to describe deformities of all body regions impacted by MWL.[1] This system has been criticized for its use of body regions that are not fixed landmarks, and for its cumbersome nature, manifested by its lack of universal adoption and its absence of use outside Pittsburgh. Iglesias et al.[2] attempted to address the Pittsburgh scale's shortcomings by using fixed anatomic structures unaltered by weight loss. This system has, however, also not been universally adopted.

Anatomic deformities sustained with MWL associated with each body region are described in this chapter.

FACE AND NECK

A youthful face is a full face. Volume loss from the facial skeleton and soft tissues, paired with skin damage from MWL, results in a more aged appearance. MWL mimics facial aging. It is associated with deflation and descent of soft tissues. The brow falls down into the orbital region, the cheek drops into the jowl, and the jawline becomes less distinct from the neck. Lost volume results in more prominent lines and folds, drooping eyebrows, thinned lips, 'marionette lines' and jowls, and skin laxity and platysmal banding in the neck (**Fig. 6.1**).

The upper face includes the forehead and periorbital region. Brow descent and loss of soft tissue result in hooding of the eye and a more hollow orbit. The lower lid may lose support, and is lengthened with cheek ptosis. Elongation of the lower lid enhances the appearance of pseudo-herniated periorbital fat, a lack of smooth transition between the lower lid and midface, and dark circles with thinned skin and more visible vasculature.

The midface includes the region between the cheek and upper lip. Fullness of the cheek deflates and descends in the face. Skeletal loss contributes to lack of fullness. Nasolabial folds, marionette lines, and jowls are also enhanced with MWL.

The lower face includes the perioral region and jawline to the neck. Changes from the midface impact the lower face with descent. The neck angle becomes more obtuse, with jowling effacing jaw angularity. Skin laxity and loss of fat result in more remarkable platysmal banding, which may also be more pronounced with loss of fat between the platysma in the neck. The lips may thin with enhancement of dynamic or static perioral rhytides. Marionette lines between the mouth and chin become deeper and more pronounced.

Plastic surgeons draw on volume enhancement with off-the-shelf fillers, such as hyaluronic acids, autogenous fat graft, suspension of lax and descended tissues, and skin tightening and repair. A full facelift may be necessary. Incisions may need to start as high as the temple, and travel as low as the earlobe and around the back of the ear, to obtain adequate suspension of the soft tissue. More conservative neck-lift techniques may be appropriate for younger patients. In these patients incisions may travel from the sideburn to the area around the ear (**Fig. 6.2**).

ARMS

The arms in MWL demonstrate varying degrees of skin laxity and focal fat deposits. This may involve only the upper arm, and extend distally to the elbow. In more severe cases of batwing deformity, excess skin

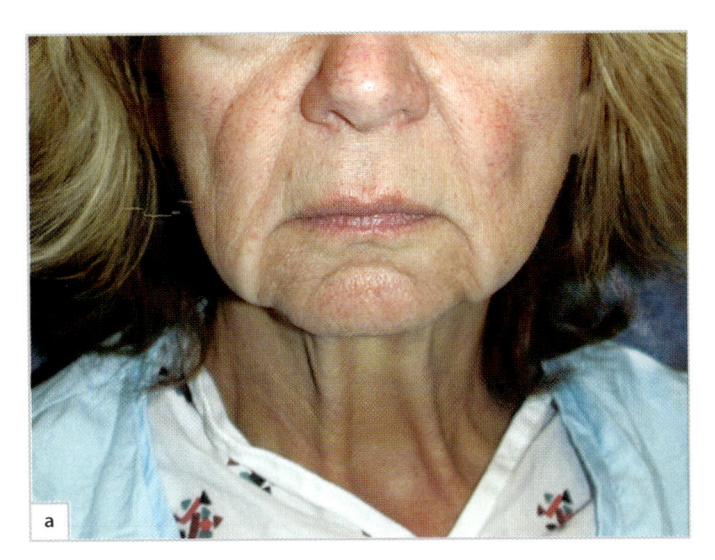

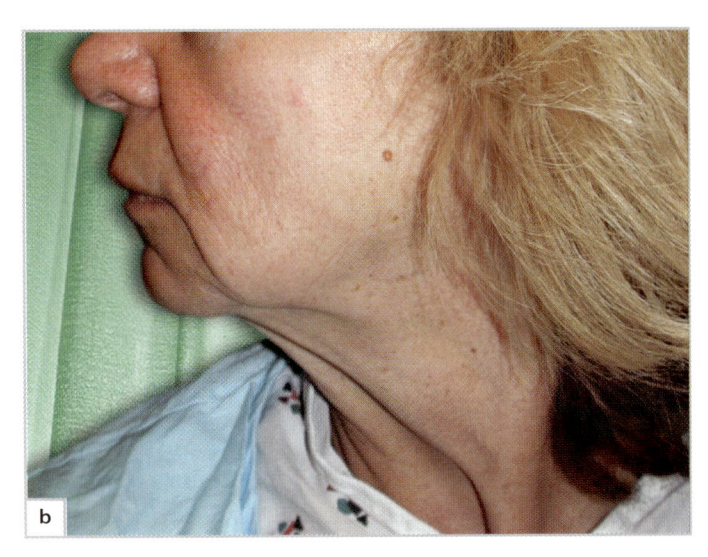

Figure 6.1 Frontal and lateral views of a 47-year-old woman who lost 140 lb (63 kg) after gastric bypass surgery. She demonstrates advanced aging throughout the face, including brow ptosis; dermatochalasis with upper lid hooding; loss of fat in the orbit with pseudo-proptosis of the globe; elongated lower lid with enhancement of pseudo-herniated orbital fat; loss of fullness in the midface; enhanced nasolabial folds and marionette lines; and an obtuse cervicomental angle with visible platysmal banding. She requires a full facelift to help suspend lax tissues and remove skin redundancy, with fat augmentation to address her deflation and folds.

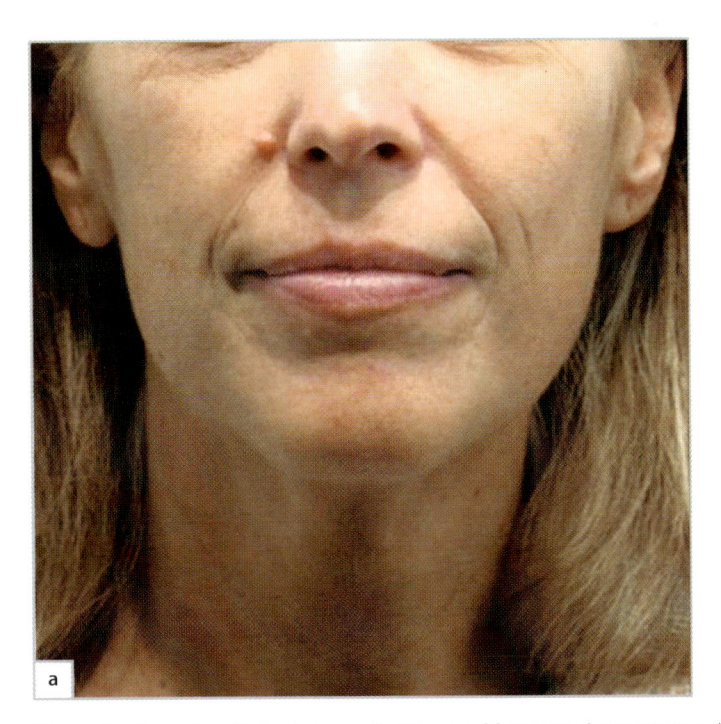

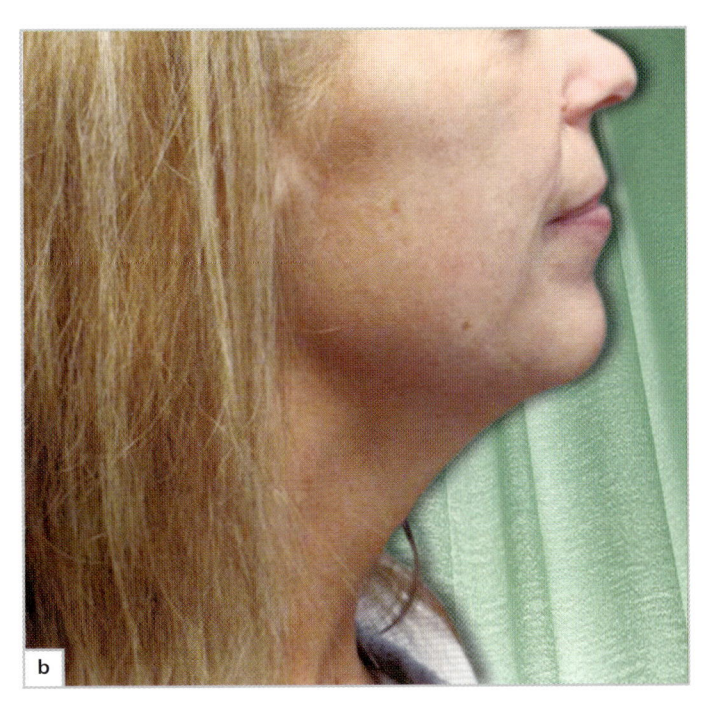

Figure 6.2 Frontal and lateral views of a 40-year-old woman, demonstrating classic enhanced aging of the mid and lower face, with descent and deflation of cheek fullness, prominent nasolabial folds, lip thinning, and remarkable platysmal banding. She will benefit from a lower facelift with platysmal repair in the midline and suspension laterally, with fat grafting to fill the folds and lips.

and fat may run from the axilla down the lateral chest wall. El Khatib et al.[3] developed a formal classification system for arm deformities from MWL, based on the amount of adipose deposits and degree of skin ptosis. This classification system is as follows: Stage 1 comprises minimal adipose, no ptosis, stage 2a moderate adipose and grade I ptosis, and stage 2b severe adipose and grade 2 ptosis; stage 3 comprises severe adipose with grade 3 ptosis; and stage 4 comprises minimal adipose and grade 3 ptosis. This classification system has not been universally adopted.

Degree of skin and fat excess and skin quality help guide surgical repair. Patients who manifest minimal adipose and localized proximal skin excess may benefit from a more proximal, limited brachioplasty, whereas more significant weight loss and skin excess merit a more comprehensive approach, including the arm to the elbow and the lateral chest wall (**Fig. 6.3**).

MALE CHEST

With MWL, men may have fullness in the chest, with skin and subcutaneous fat excess. The degree of chest deformity varies across a broad spectrum. In some cases men have pseudogynecomastia (no breast tissue with minimal to moderate skin and fat excess) or true gynecomastia (breast tissue present), with ptosis. This may extend posteriorly into the axilla and upper back. A nipple–areolar complex (NAC) may be widened or more prominent from herniation of breast tissue into it. An inframammary fold (IMF), which is not typically remarkable in the male chest, may be developed and ptotic below the transitional level between the chest and abdomen.

Classification systems of gynecomastia may be general, or describe MWL specifically. Simon et al.[4] developed one of the original generalized gynecomastia classification systems that could apply to MWL. In this system, grade 1 describes small visible breast enlargement without skin redundancy; Grade 2A describes moderate breast enlargement without skin redundancy; grade 2B describes moderate breast enlargement with skin redundancy; grade 3 describes marked breast enlargement with marked skin redundancy, such as that seen with MWL.[4] Interestingly, the authors recommended that skin resection outside of the nipple and nipple grafts are discouraged. However, these may be necessary with more extreme manifestations with NAC deformities of MWL.

Gusenoff et al.[5] described a grade 1–3 classification system for pseudogynecomastia specific to MWL. Grade 1 comprises minimal excess skin and fat, grade 2 comprises ptosis of the NAC and IMF below the ideal IMF, with a lateral chest roll and minimal upper abdominal laxity, and grade 3 comprises location of the NAC and IMF below the ideal IMF, with a lateral chest roll and upper abdominal laxity. Although the system attempts to specifically classify chest wall deformity for MWL, the presentation of gynecomastia is not as distinct as this simplified system.

Functional problems correlate with the degree of deformity manifested. As tissue redundancy and ptosis increase, symptoms experienced may include rashes from overhanging skin. Physical appearance may also impair body image and cause psychiatric distress resulting in functional disability (**Fig. 6.4**).

Surgical reconstruction ranges from liposuction, to Wise pattern skin resections with subcutaneous tissue removal. Extent of resection to the back requires removal of skin rolls. This circumferential approach defines a male upper body lift and would apply to men with marked weight loss and skin redundancy.

FEMALE BREAST

In women who sustain MWL, breast tissue loses its fullness. This is secondary to loss of fat, and results in a deflated appearance with ptosis. Breasts may be asymmetric. IMF becomes less distinct and ptotic as well and, rather than lie over the base of the pectoralis muscle origin, the IMF may descend to a level at the superior rectus abdominis muscle. NAC may be distorted, stretched, and/or medially displaced. The extent of vertical and horizontal skin laxity and ptosis, as well as breast size, varies greatly in women with a history of MWL. Many of these women have underlying skeletal deformity with a barrel chest and more bowed, angular ribs. These likely develop from the prior obese state and pulmonary requirements (**Fig. 6.5**). Physical deformity may translate into functional issues such as those experienced with macromastia, which consist of back, neck, and shoulder pain, bra grooving, and intertrigo rashes between and under the IMF. Many women had breast reduction surgery before MWL. Often this develops into an even more remarkable deformity, characterized by marked breast tissue loss, skin redundancy, and scars. A breast reduction

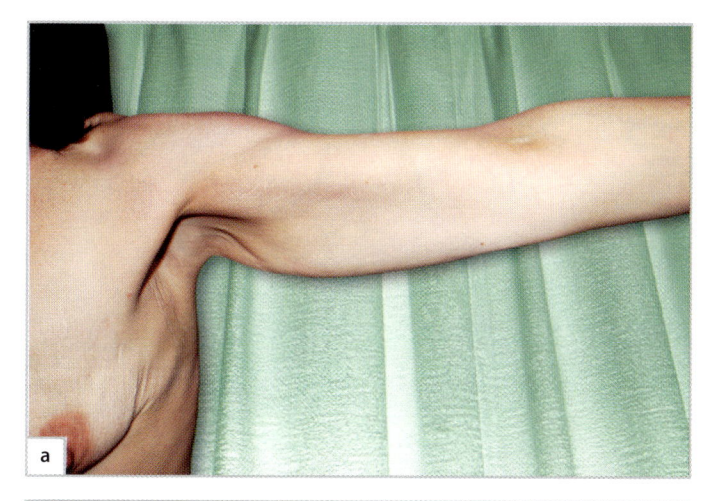

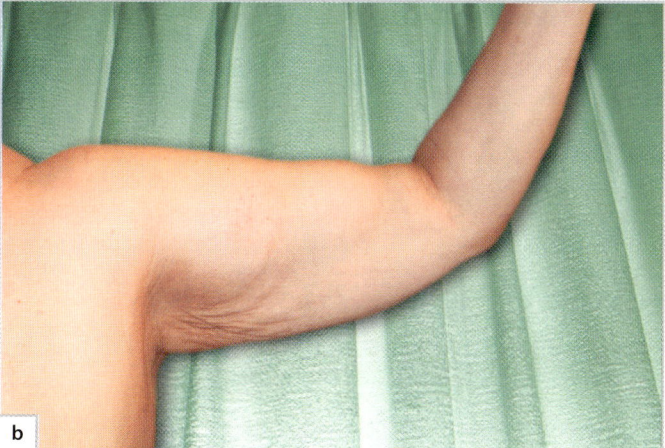

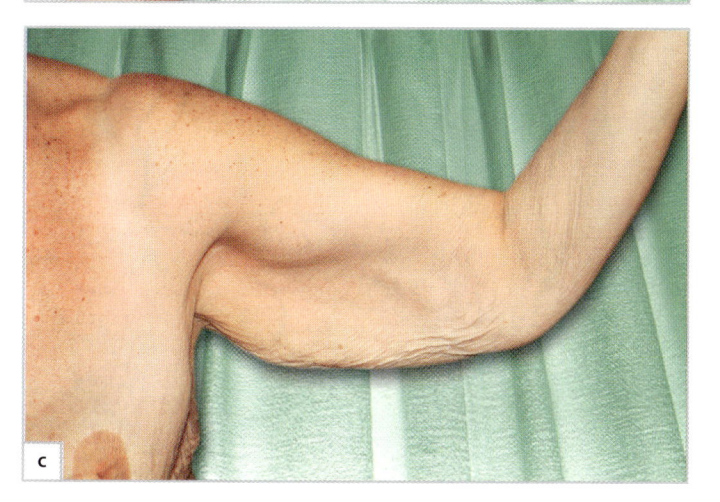

Figure 6.3 (a) This woman lost over 100 lb (45 kg) approximately 5 years before with minimal skin laxity and no lipodystrophy. She is an excellent candidate for minimal proximal brachioplasty. (b) This woman has more significant skin ptosis and minimal lipodystrophy that is focal in the upper arm. She is an excellent candidate for traditional brachioplasty addressing the arm from axilla to elbow. (c) This woman has significant skin excess and ptosis. The skin redundancy continues down the lateral chest wall, and the axillary depression is not distinct. This patient will benefit from a brachioplasty, extending from elbow to axilla and down the lateral chest wall.

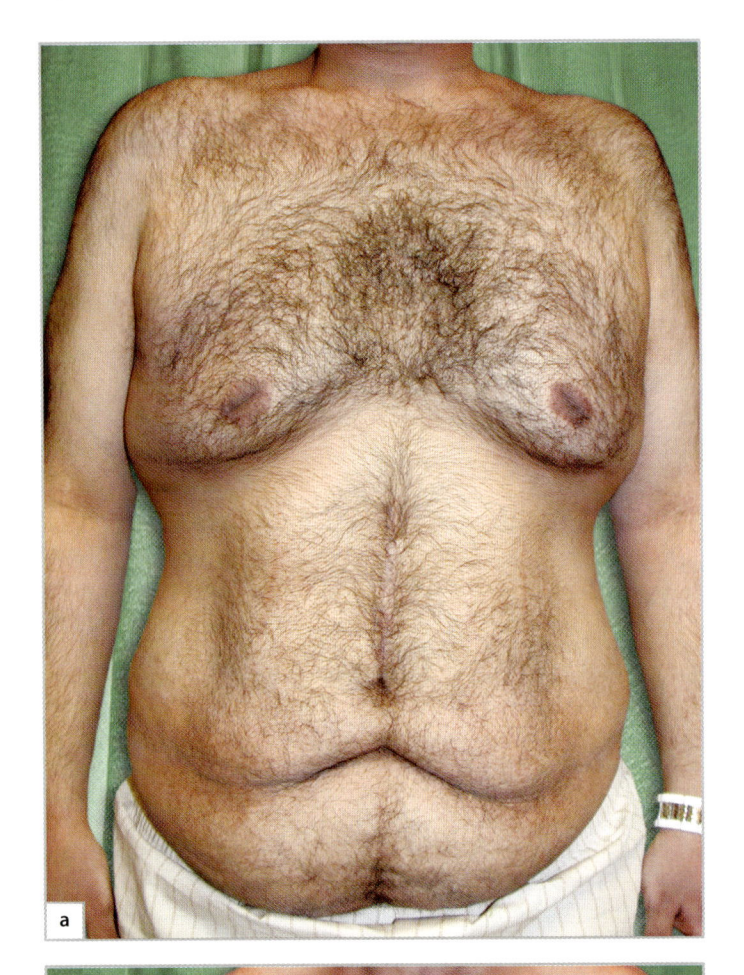

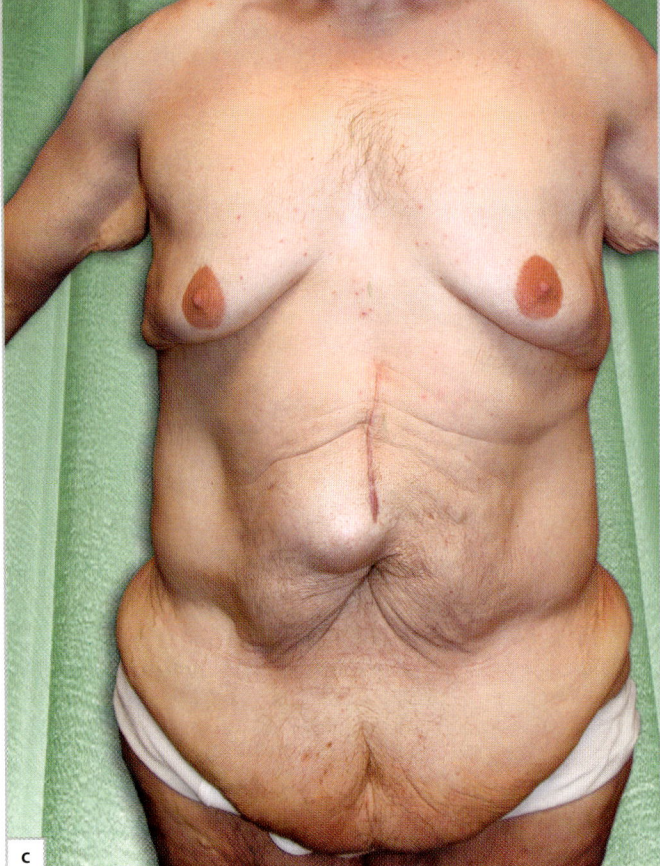

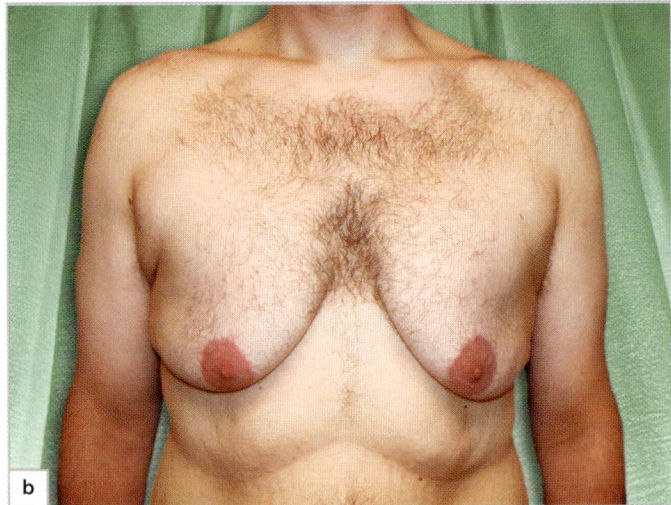

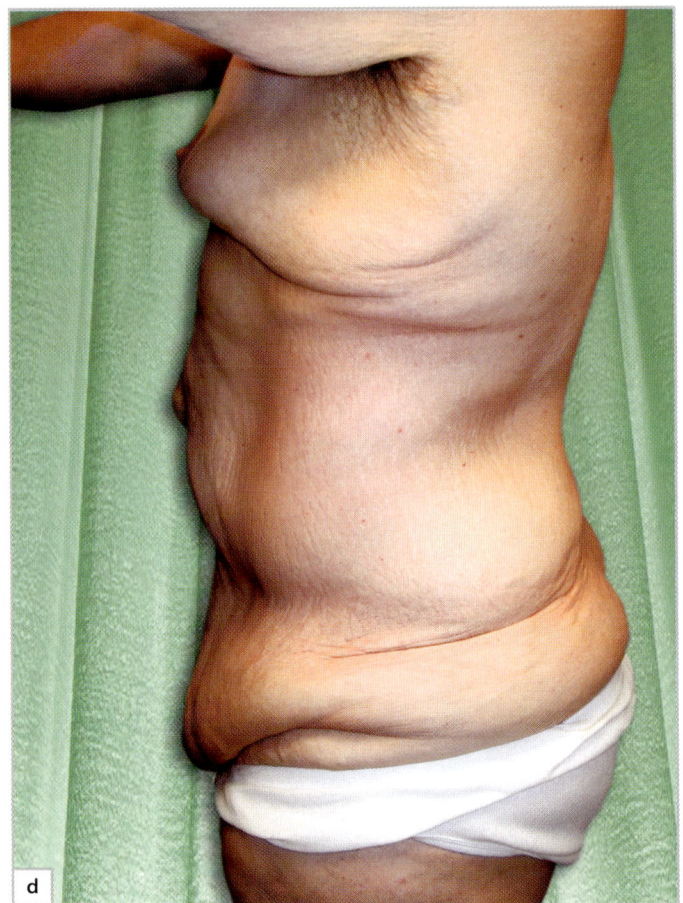

Figure 6.4 (a) This 27-year-old Middle Eastern man had minimal skin redundancy and pseudo-gynecomastia. Liposuction will flatten the chest and provide skin retraction that will provide optimal results with minimal scar. (b) This 30-year-old man lost 200 lb (90 kg) and he has resultant pseudo-gynecomastia with skin excess and fibrous 'breast' tissue. With skin and breast tissue excess and skin redundancy, this man would benefit from resection of skin and subcutaneous tissue with resultant scars on the chest. (c, d) This 35-year-old man has chest fullness with skin redundancy extending to the axilla and upper back, which would benefit most from an upper body lift.

Female breast 29

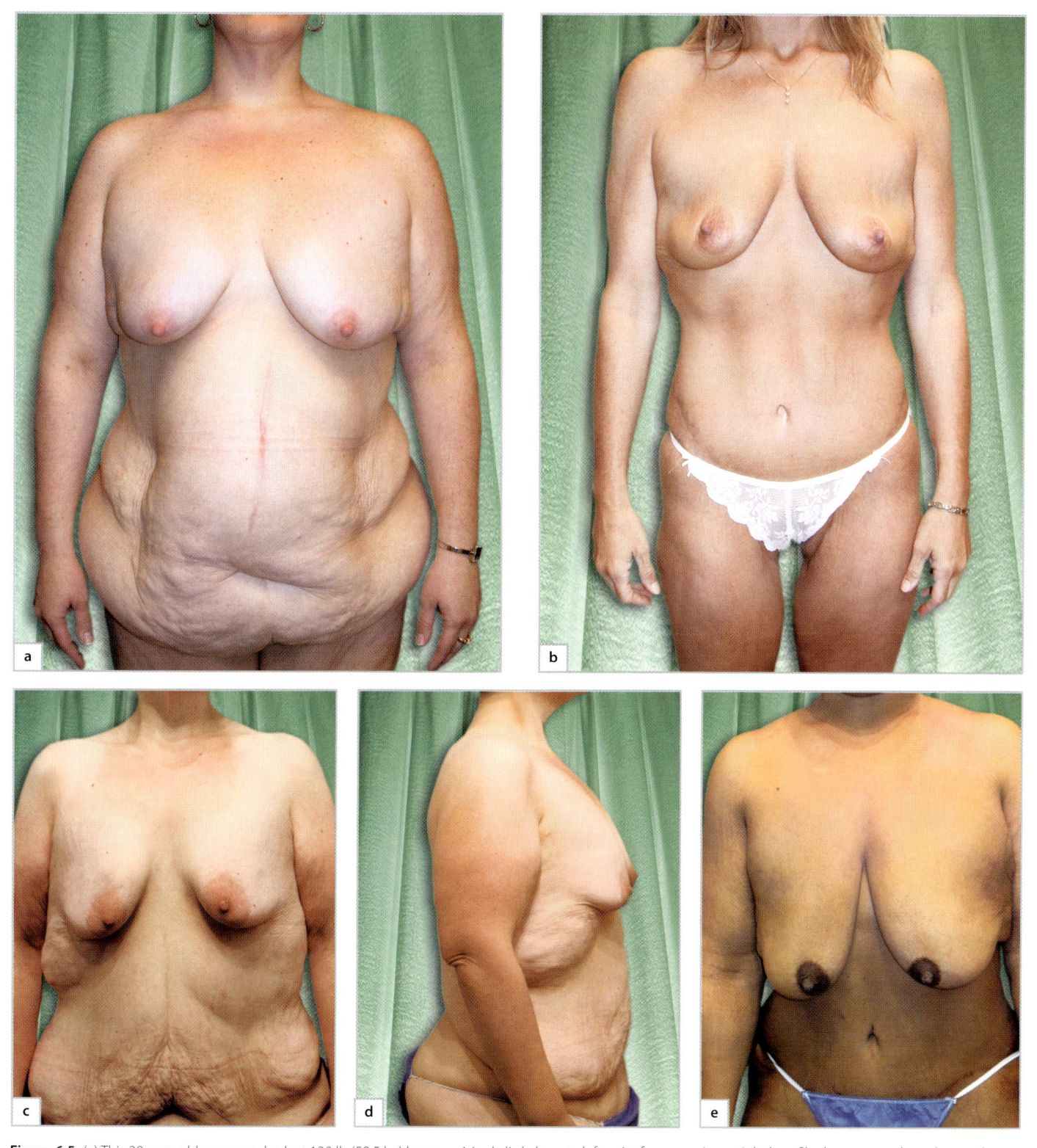

Figure 6.5 (a) This 38-year-old woman who lost 130 lb (58.5 kg) has surprisingly little breast deformity from massive weight loss. She has some volume loss and ptosis, which may respond well with volume augmentation alone. (b) This 30-year-old woman lost 100 lb (45 kg) over 5 years. She demonstrates significant volume loss and ptosis, which would optimally require volume augmentation and lifting techniques. The significant volume loss in the breast reveals underlying skeletal deformity with barrel chest. (c,d) This woman in her mid-20s lost 200 lb (90 kg). She has minimal breast volume paired with minimal skin excess; however, she has a barrel chest, medial nipple–areolar complex (NAC) displacement and significant skin excess of the axilla into the back, making it more complicated. (e) This woman has significant volume loss, ptosis of the NAC with medial displacement, inframammary fold ptosis, and remarkable skin redundancy extending into the axilla and back. This patient would benefit from an upper body lift, comprising augmentation–mastopexy with breast implants, and skin excision of the upper back blending anteriorly into the breast.

approach must be investigated to ensure safety in augmentation–mastopexy to avoid complications.

Approaches to reconstruction depend on presentation and patient goals. Patients may desire improved volume with breast implants and/or fat grafting. MWL patients may also benefit from lifting techniques requiring skin tightening, with scars around the NAC. These may extend vertically down the center of the breast, and possibly across the IMF into the upper back to more adequately address skin excess. Augmentation–mastopexy in MWL patients is a challenging procedure due to chest wall deformities, asymmetries, and unpredictable bottoming out after surgery.

ABDOMEN

The abdomen is the region most frequently addressed surgically after MWL. The abdomen structurally has multiple elements that need to be analyzed in the MWL patient. These consist of skin, subcutaneous fat, muscle, umbilicus, and pubis. Skin quality may range from excellent to poor, with striae, thinning, and overhang. There may be skinfold adhesions, particularly in the epigastric region and at the pubis. The subcutaneous fat layer may range from thin to thick, and there may be focal fat deposits associated with skin folds and adhesions. Muscle tone may be intact or lax, with diastasis or frank herniation from significant weight change and denervation from prior abdominal surgery, including gastric bypass and cholecystectomy. The umbilicus may also have experienced surgical alteration with detachment from prior abdominal procedures, including ventral hernia repair, or may be elongated and stretched from significant weight loss. The pubis is continuous with the abdomen and may have skin excess and focal fat deposits (**Fig. 6.6**). The degree of weight loss may not be the critical factor impacting the degree of abdominal deformity. This is multifactorial, including nutritional issues, age, and genetics.

Many authors have attempted to provide a classification system to guide surgical treatment of abdominal deformities. Generalized systems for classification of abdominal deformities have been developed by Matarasso and Wallach, Bozola and Psillakis, and Nahas.[6-8] Matarasso and Wallach[6] defined aesthetic subunits of the whole torso, seven for women and six for men. These include the upper abdomen, lower abdomen, flank, umbilicus, and mons pubis, as well as the sacrum and dorsal rolls, the latter of which the authors believe do not concern men. This accounts for their smaller number of aesthetic subunits. The dorsal roll is, however, a real issue for men sustaining MWL. This classification system was developed well in advance of the explosion of MWL surgery.

Bozola and Psillakis[7] also developed a generalized abdominal grading system of I–V, with increasing disorder of skin, fat, and muscle. Each grade is paired with a different abdominoplasty technique that the authors advocate to correct it: Type I is lipodystrophy only; type 2 is excess skin but normal muscle; type 3 is skin redundancy and muscle laxity; type 4 has mild skin excess, lipodystrophy, and muscle laxity from xiphoid to pubis; and type 5 has large amounts of excess skin, varying adipose tissue, and muscle weakness.

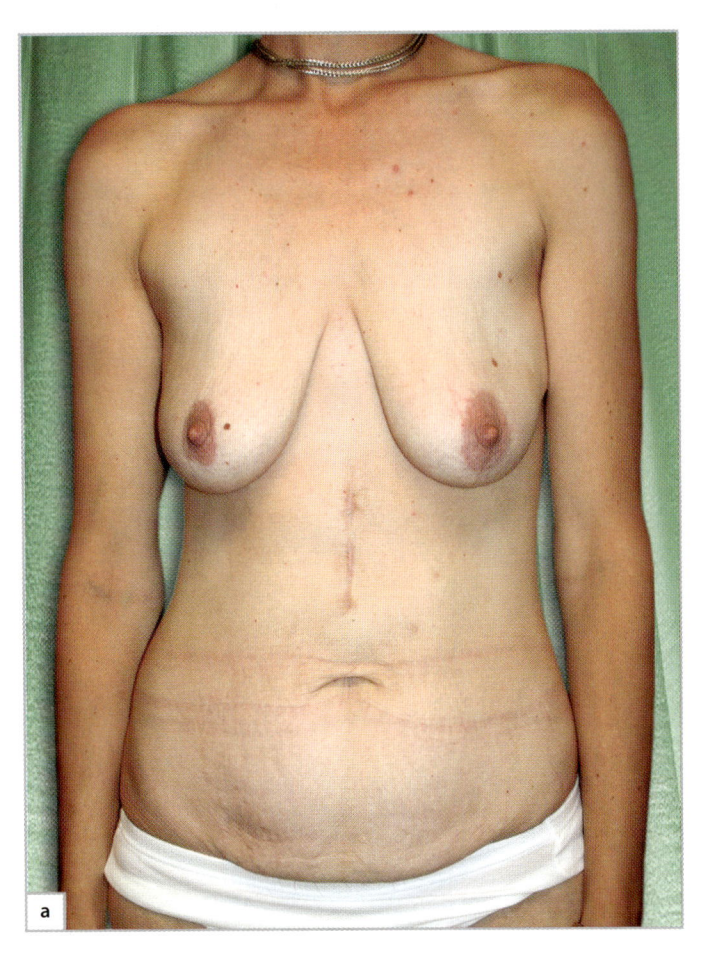

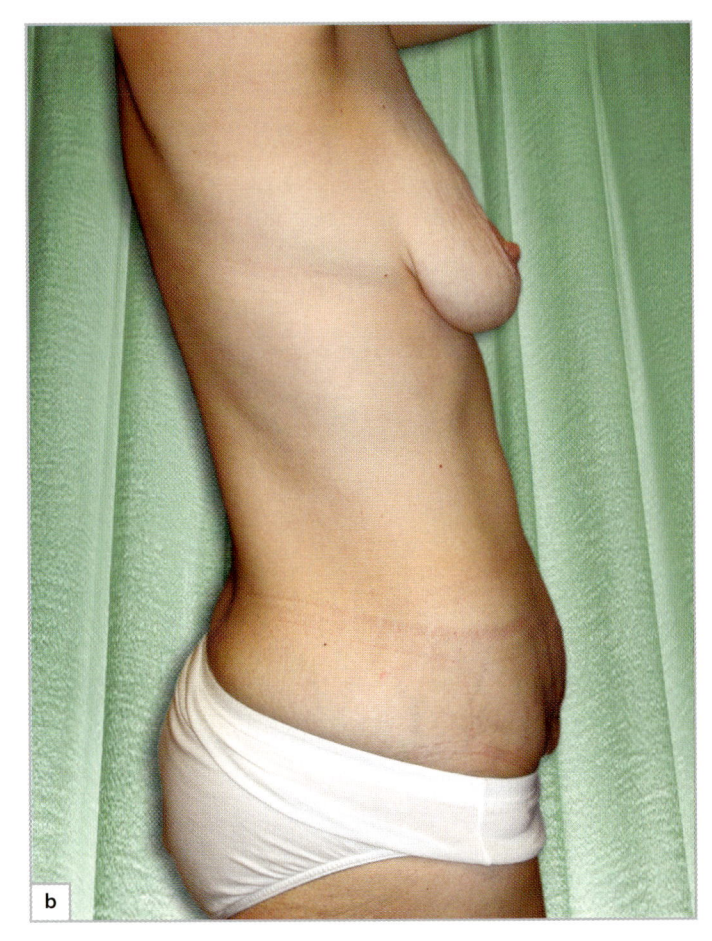

Figure 6.6 The spectrum of abdominal presentation of massive weight loss (MWL) patients. *Continued on pp. 31–33.*

Abdomen

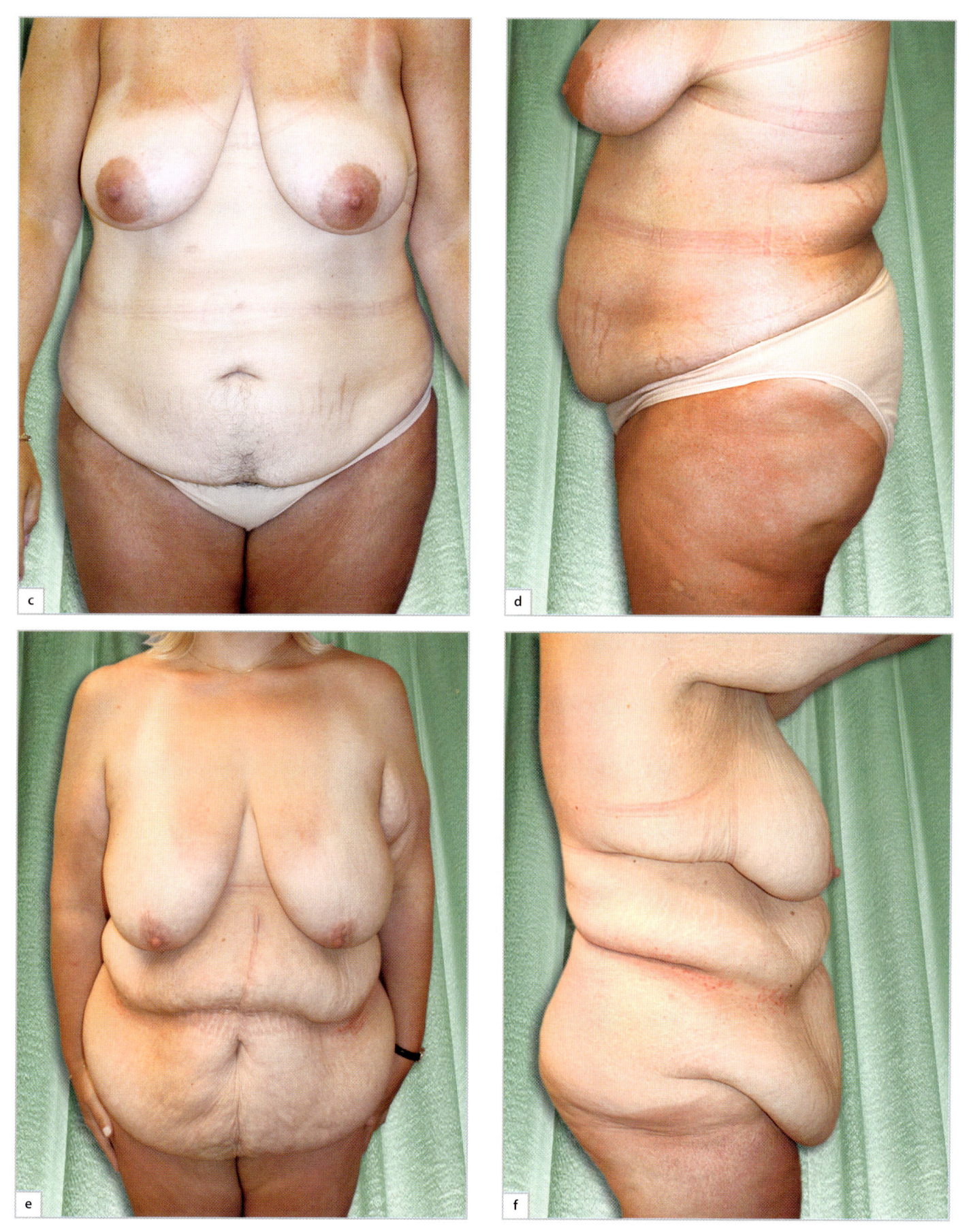

Figure 6.6 The spectrum of abdominal presentation of massive weight loss (MWL) patients. *Continued on pp. 32–33.*

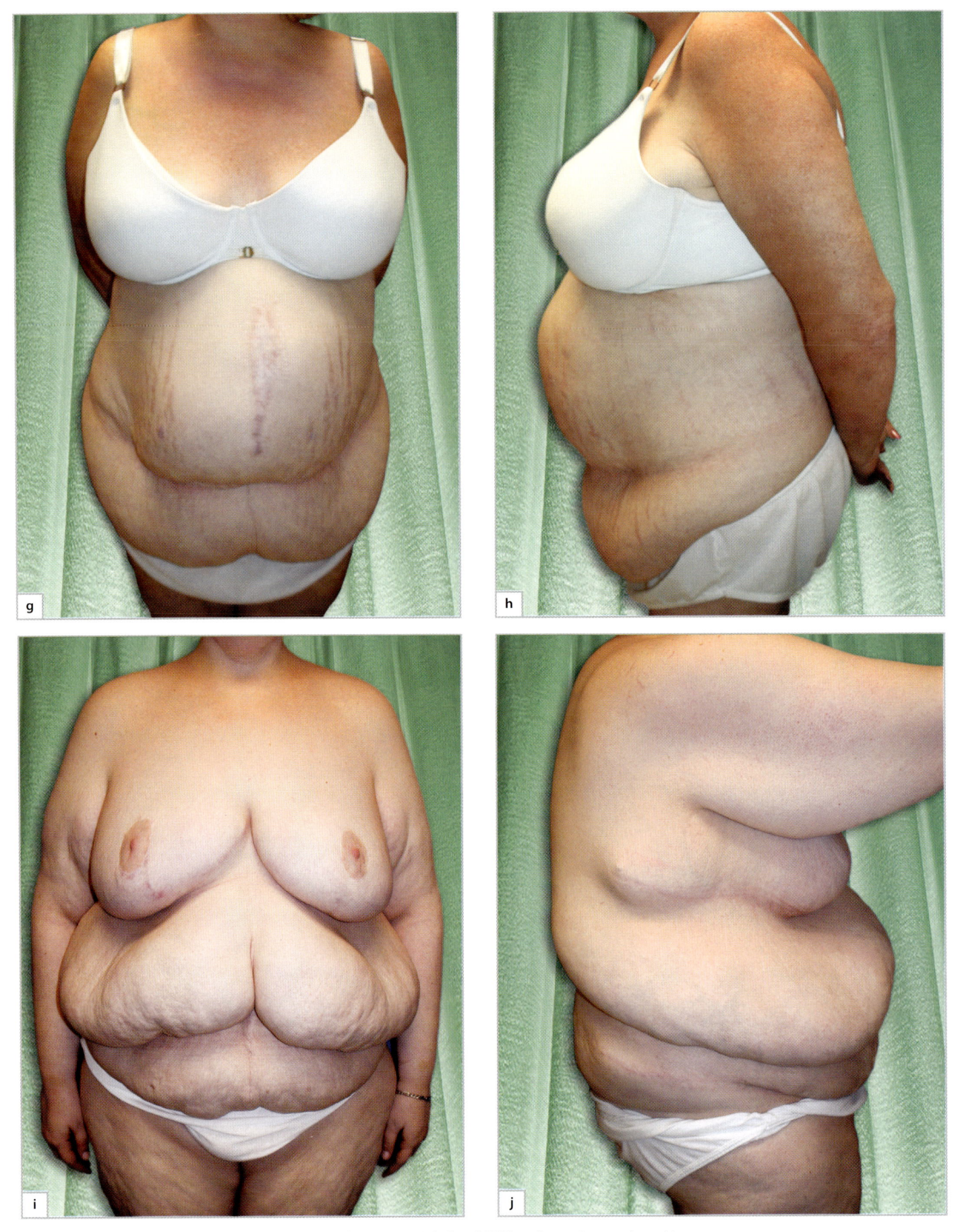

32 ANATOMICAL DEFORMITIES SECONDARY TO MASSIVE WEIGHT LOSS

Figure 6.6 The spectrum of abdominal presentation of massive weight loss (MWL) patients. *Continued on p. 33.*

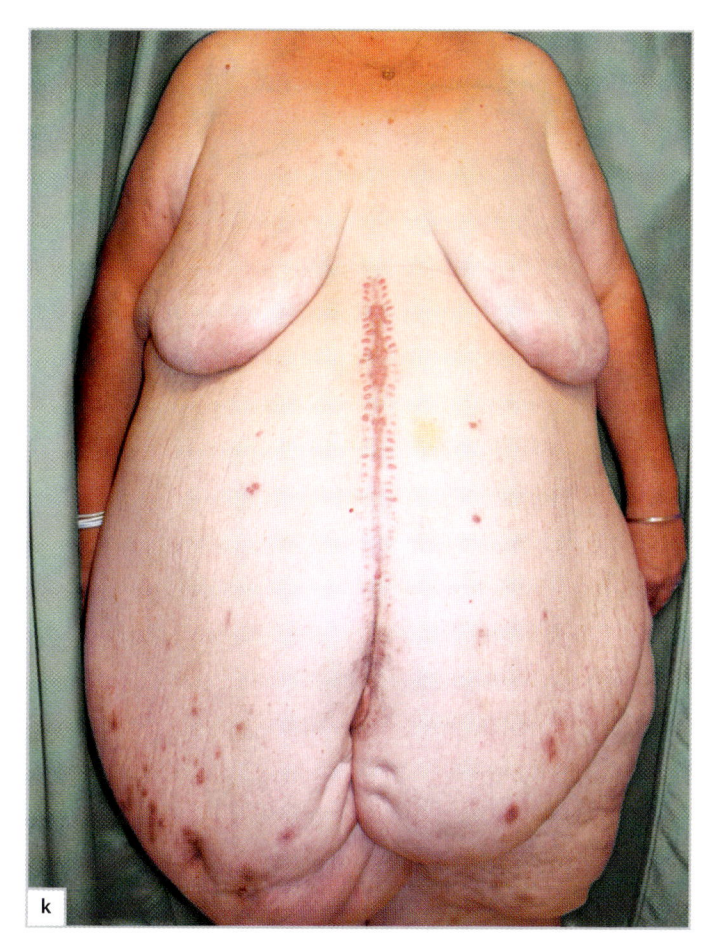

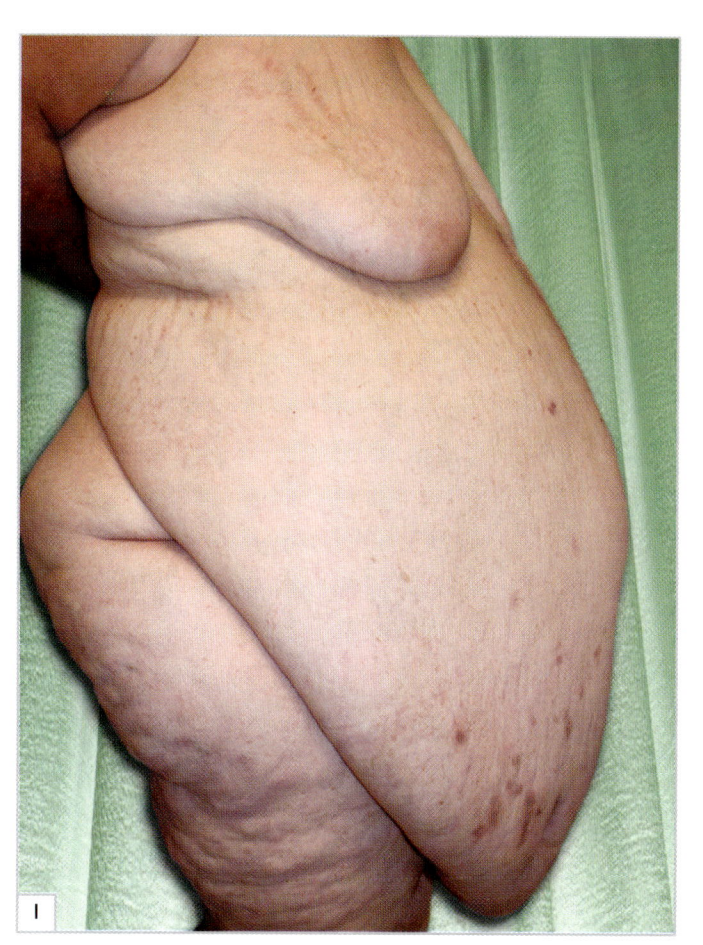

Figure 6.6 The spectrum of abdominal presentation of massive weight loss (MWL) patients. (a,b) Frontal and lateral views of a woman who sustained MWL with skin laxity and minimal subcutaneous lipodystrophy, with minimal abdominal wall laxity. This patient would benefit from standard abdominoplasty. (c,d) Frontal and lateral views of a woman who sustained MWL with minimal skin laxity and good skin quality, with moderate abdominal wall laxity. This patient would benefit from conservative lipoabdominoplasty. (e,f) Frontal and lateral views of a woman who sustained MWL with skin laxity and skinfold adhesions in the epigastric region, with moderate lipodystrophy and muscle laxity. This patient, depending on her medical condition, would ideally benefit from lipoabdominoplasty with release of the abdominal skin flap superiorly to allow release of the skin fold. (g,h) Frontal and lateral views of a woman who sustained MWL with minimal-to-moderate skin overhang and good skin quality, but a large abdominal hernia from her open gastric bypass surgery. This patient will require a fleur-de-lis abdominoplasty with hernia repair. (i,j) Frontal and lateral views of a morbidly obese woman who sustained MWL with skin laxity, significant epigastric skin adhesion, moderate lipodystrophy, and abdominal wall laxity. This is a difficult case in a patient with significant medical comorbidities, meriting a direct panniculectomy mid-abdomen. (k,l) Hypermorbidly obese patient with significant skin overhang, lipodystrophy, and abdominal wall laxity, requiring massive panniculectomy without undermining.

Nahas[8] created a classification based on myoaponeurotic deformities and the surgical therapy necessary to treat them. Within the classification: A describes rectus diastasis secondary to pregnancy (with the need for rectus diastasis repair); B describes laxity of the lateral and inferior abdominal wall with rectus diastasis (with the need for an L-shaped plication of external oblique aponeurosis and rectus diastasis repair); C describes rectus muscles with a lateral insertion on costal margins, leading to increased risk of umbilical and epigastric hernias (needing release and undermining of the rectus muscles and advancement in continuity with the anterior sheath); and D describes poor waistline definition (requiring external oblique rotation and rectus diastasis repair).[8]

Generalized classification systems fall short in their application to the MWL abdomen. Typically the highest grade of these generalized classification systems lumps all MWL abdomens together, although presentation is actually highly variable. Within the Pittsburgh rating scale dedicated to classification of MWL body regions, abdomens are graded as follows: Grade 0 represents a normal abdomen; grade 1 represents redundant skin with rhytides or moderate adiposity without overhang; grade 2 demonstrates an overhanging pannus; and grade 3 demonstrates multiple rolls or epigastric fullness.[1] The Pittsburgh scale is the only system dedicated to the classification of the MWL abdomen, and is therefore the best system currently available to describe the spectrum of deformity of the MWL abdomen; however, as seen in the figures, it is clear that a more comprehensive classification system designed to encompass the full range of encountered deformities would be quite cumbersome.

BACK

The back in the MWL patient must be broken down into upper back and lower back for analysis and treatment. The upper and lower back are two distinct body regions with varying degrees of skin excess and ptosis, rolls with skinfold adhesions, and lipodystrophy. The upper back region is continuous anteriorly with the male chest and the female breast. The lower back is continuous anteriorly with the

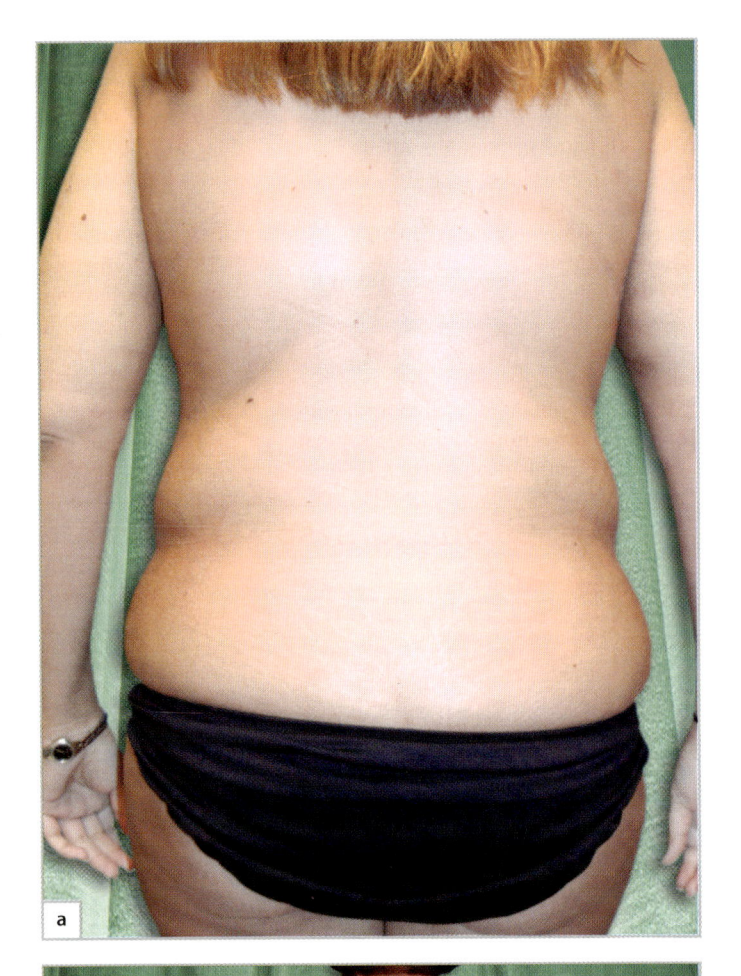

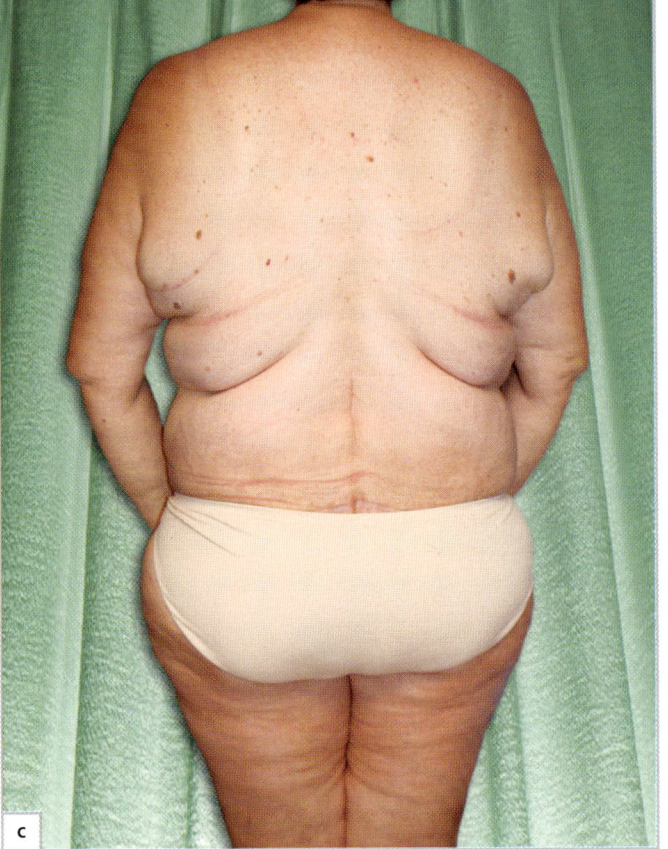

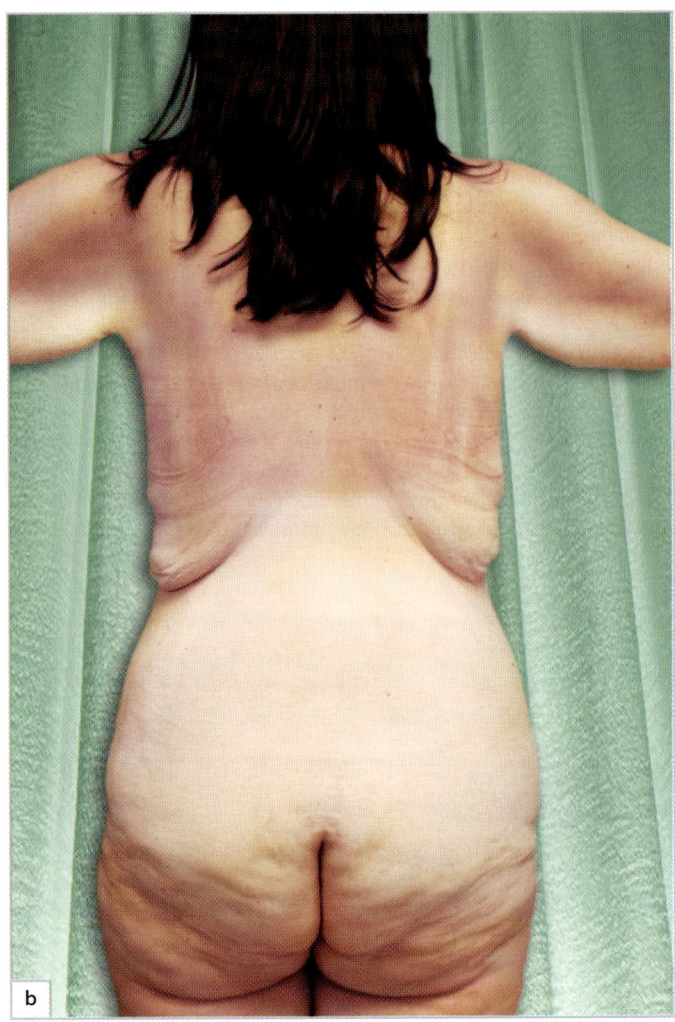

34 ANATOMICAL DEFORMITIES SECONDARY TO MASSIVE WEIGHT LOSS

Figure 6.7 (a) This 27-year-old woman lost 120 lb (54 kg) to reach a BMI of 26. She has fullness of the upper back with minimal skin laxity and no folds. She would benefit from liposuction only of her back to provide better contour with some skin retraction. (b) This 31-year-old woman lost 160 lb. She has minimal lipodystrophy, with skin redundancy and a tight crease. This woman would benefit from direct upper back skin excision without undermining. (c) This 45-year-old woman has more lipodystrophy and a tight adhesion in her upper back with skin overhang. She also would benefit from direct upper back skin excision without undermining.

Back 35

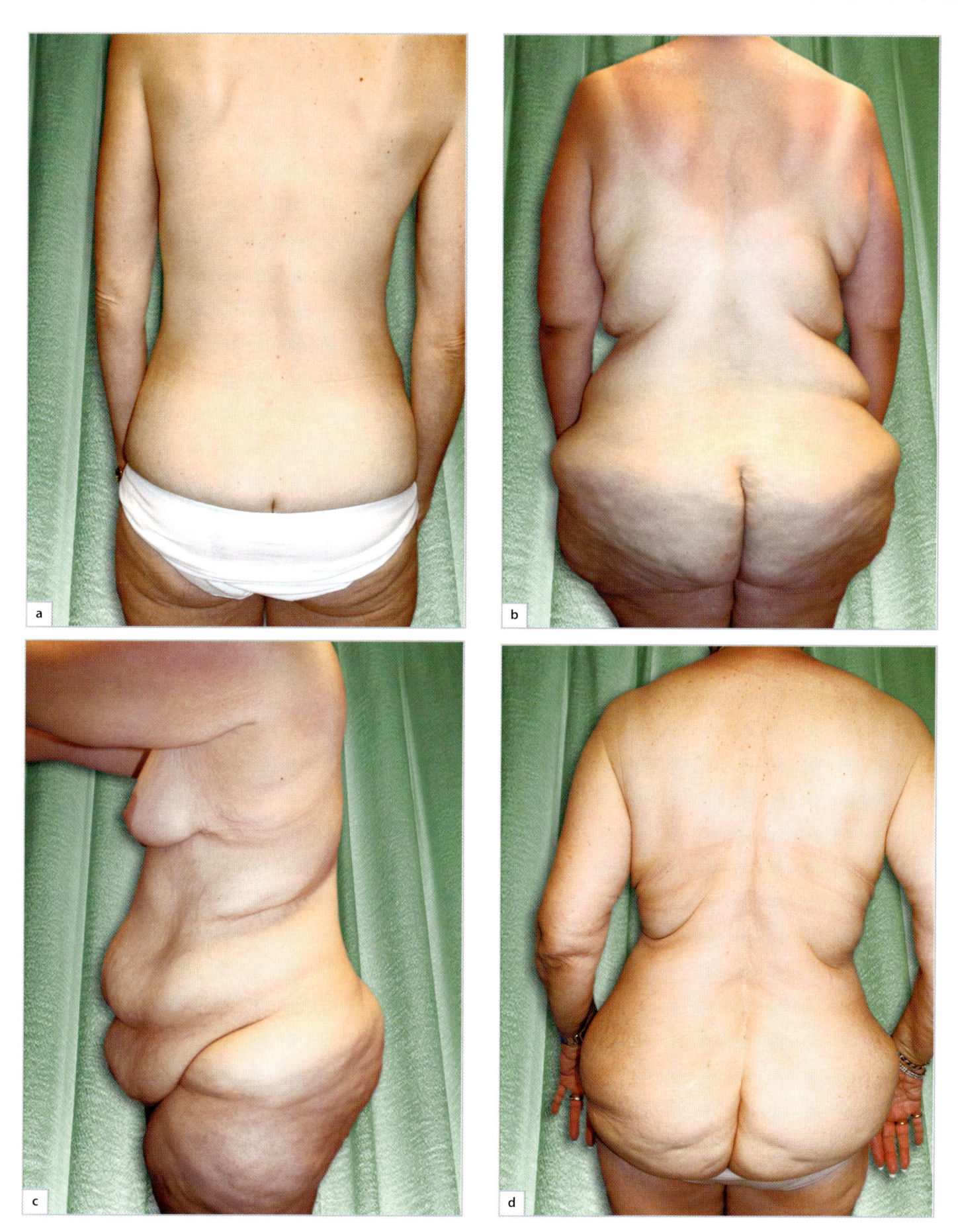

Figure 6.8 *Continued on p. 36.*

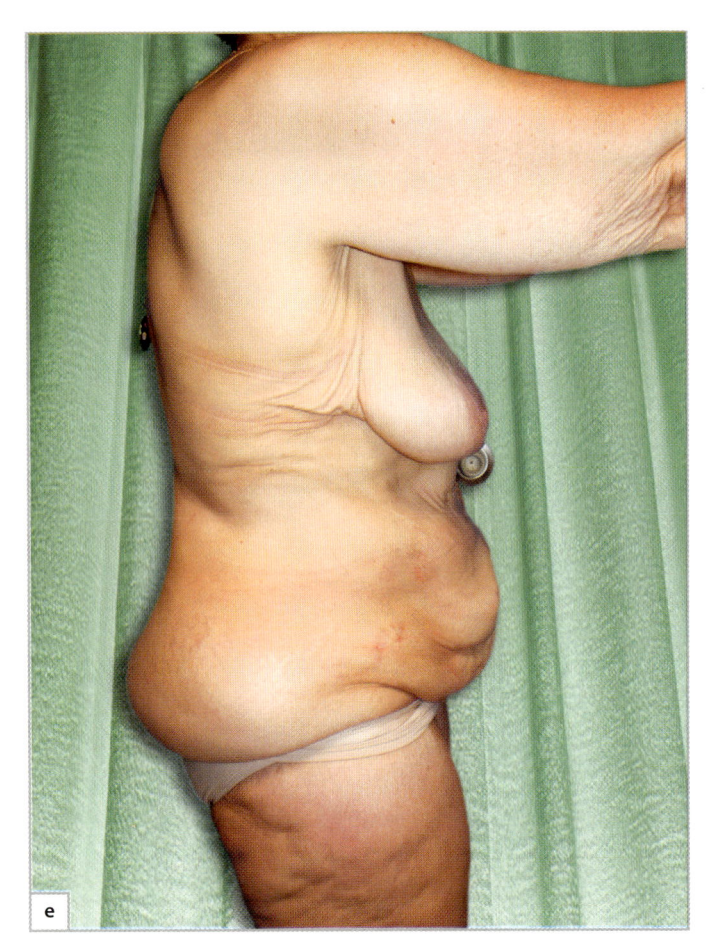

Figure 6.8 (a) This woman lost 130 lb (58.5 kg) to attain a body mass index of 21. Her lower back is lax with minimal lipodystrophy and buttock ptosis. She is an ideal candidate for a circumferential belt lipectomy, including abdominoplasty and lower back lift. (b,c) Frontal and lateral views of a woman who has lengthening of the lower back with significant lipodystrophy but a full buttock. This patient would also benefit from a direct lower back lift. (d,e) This woman has a large thick lower back, which is obscuring her buttock. She has minimal buttock volume under this shelf of skin and fat and would benefit from autologous gluteal augmentation with transposition of perforator flaps from the lower back tissue into the buttock.

abdomen, and also includes the buttocks in its analysis for treatment. The lower back may be particularly elongated in the vertical dimension in MWL patients, requiring direct removal. In some cases, the buttocks are so deflated that the excess tissue in the hip and lower back may be recycled to autoaugment the buttock (**Figs 6.7** and **6.8**).

THIGH

Thigh presentation is broad in the MWL population. They may exhibit variable degrees of skin quality, skin excess, lipodystrophy, adhesive skin folds with focal fat deposits, and panniculi. Knees are often considered in analysis for treatment of the thigh, because there may be lipodystrophy and thickened skin folds over the patella. The calf also needs to be examined for lymphedema or lipoedema, which is fairly common in individuals with a history of morbid obesity. Varicose veins are also common and demand attention before performing excisional surgery on the thigh (**Fig. 6.9**).

Surgical treatments of the thigh can be broken down into proximal excisional techniques with a hidden scar in the groin, possibly extending into the infragluteal crease, and vertical excisional techniques with extended incisions down the inner thigh from the groin to the knee. The latter may result in a powerful outcome but a much higher propensity for postoperative lymphatic derangement. Presentation will mandate which procedure should be performed, weighing the pros and cons of each procedure.

CONCLUSION

Surgery is both an art and a science. Anatomic deformities seen in the MWL population span a wide spectrum of presentations, depending on skin quality, skin excess, lipodystrophy, and skinfolds with focal fat deposits, as well as the patient's medical landscape. Presentation, as demonstrated in this chapter, is highly variable, making it extremely difficult to develop a useful classification system that would assist in exactly determining surgical treatment, allowing appropriate data comparisons in outcome analyses, and improving professional communications. Although the science of body-contouring surgery is evolving, the art of surgical therapy is critical for this patient population, treating each patient specifically and individually to safely achieve their goals.

REFERENCES

1. Song AY, Jean RD, Hurwitz DJ, et al. A Classification of contour deformities after bariatric weight loss: The Pittsburgh Rating Scale. *Plast Reconstr Surg* 2005;**116**:1535–44.
2. Iglesias M, Butron P, Abarca L, et al. An anthropometric classification of body contour deformities after massive weight loss. *Ann Plast Surg* 2010;**65**:129–34.
3. El Khatib HA. Classification of brachial ptosis: Strategy for treatment. *Plast Reconstr Surg* 2007;**119**:1337–42.
4. Simon BE, Hoffman S, Kahn S. Classification and surgical correction of gynecomastia. *Plast Reconstr Surg* 1973;**51**:48–52.
5. Gusenoff JA, Coon D, Rubin JP. Pseudogynecomastia after massive weight loss: detectability of technique, patient satisfaction, and classification. *Plast Reconstr Surg* 2008;**122**:1301–11.
6. Matarasso A, Wallach SG. Abdominal contour surgery: Treating all aesthetic units, including the mons pubis. *Aesthet Surg J* 2001;**21**:111.
7. Nahas FX. An aesthetic classification of the abdomen based on the myoaponeurotic layer. *Plast Reconstr Surg* 2001;**108**:1787–95.
8. Bozola AR, Psillakis JM. Abdominoplasty: A new concept and classification for treatment. *Plast Reconstr Surg* 1988;**82**:983–93.

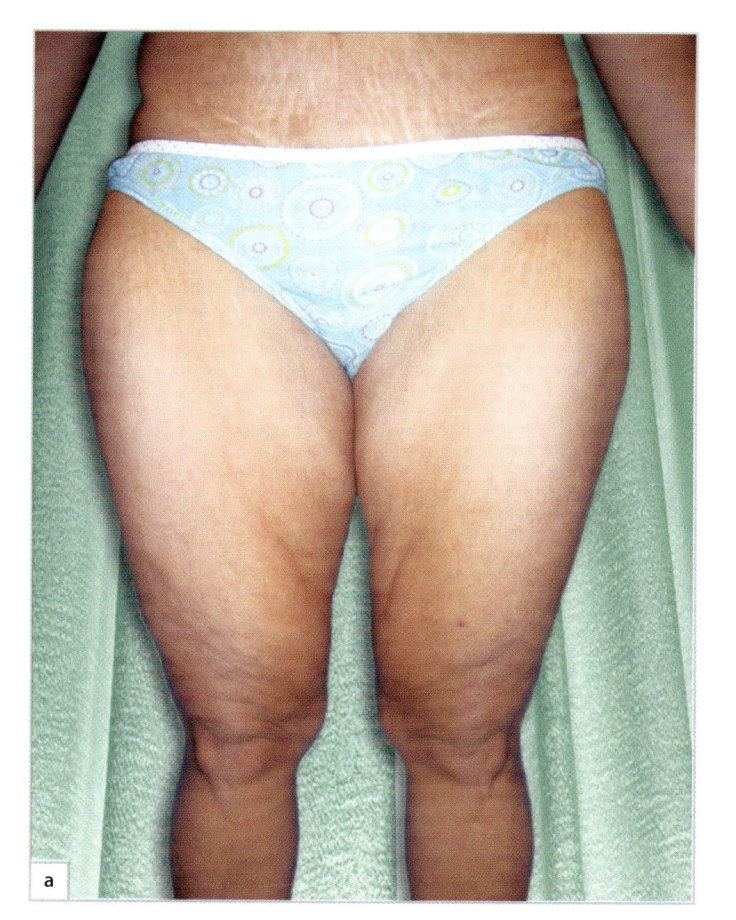

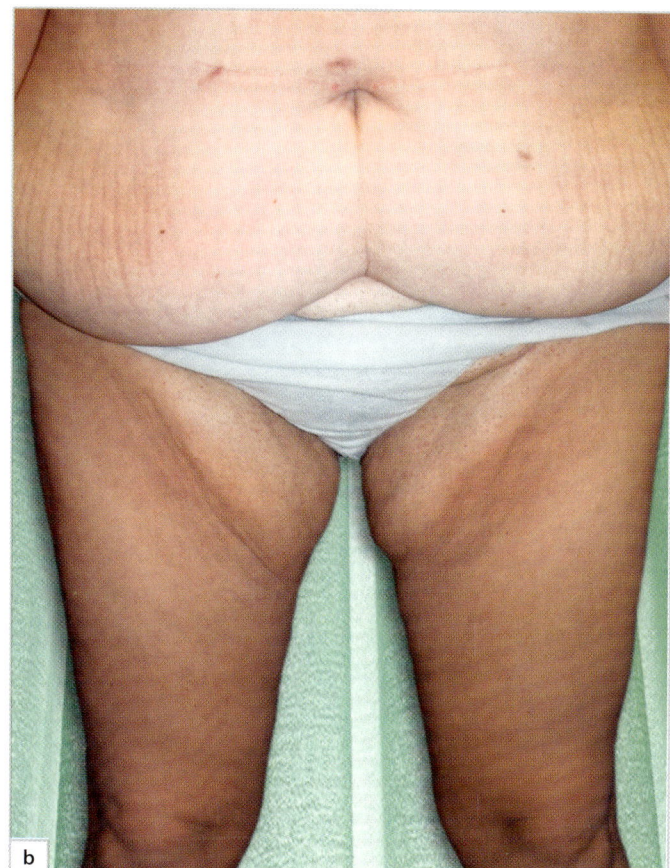

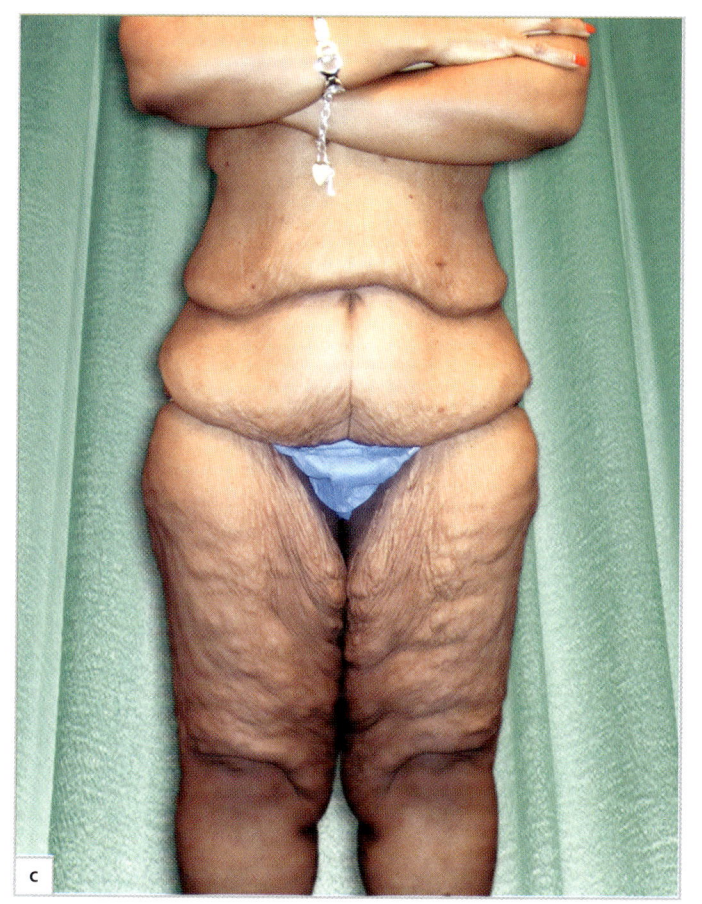

Figure 6.9 (a) This 40-year-old woman lost 100 lb (45 kg) and has some upper inner thigh laxity, without remarkable skin excess, lipodystrophy, or rolls, and good skin quality. She could be a candidate for a proximal incision thigh lift, but also may see enough secondary improvement with abdominoplasty.
(b) This 38-year-old woman has localized pannus of the upper inner thigh after massive weight loss, with good skin quality. She would benefit from a proximal thigh lift, which would allow a hidden scar and excellent result. (c) This 42-year-old woman had a 200-lb (90-kg) weight loss and has marked skin excess, poor skin quality, and diffuse involvement of the whole thigh. She has varicose veins that should be evaluated and treated before thigh-lift surgery. Surgery will require a medial vertical scar extending to the knee.

Chapter 7 Outpatient lower body lift

Richard H. Tholen, Douglas L. Gervais

Obesity has become a national epidemic. Increased prevalence of morbid obesity in our population over the past two decades and recognition of the major health risks accompanying obesity have fueled a concomitant upsurge in bariatric surgery. After massive weight loss (MWL), patients are increasingly seeking body-contouring surgery to deal with their loose skin and still-disappointing body image.

Despite the health advantages of MWL, most postbariatric body-contouring procedures have been classified as elective or 'cosmetic.' This adds supplementary financial burdens to the psychological and physical issues that these patients already confront. Surgery to deal with circumferential truncal cutaneous excess is often the first, largest, and most costly of several operations that MWL patients request. Our plastic surgical solutions need to be safe, effective, and *cost-conscious*.

Outpatient circumferential lower body lift surgery substantially reduces costs and also increases safety, compared with the same operation performed at a hospital with days of inpatient care.

This chapter conveys a comprehensive anesthesia, surgical, and postoperative protocol that has allowed us to successfully perform over 260 circumferential lower body lifts as safe, definitive, and cost-effective outpatient procedures in our accredited Minneapolis office-based surgical facility.

■ OBESITY, BARIATRIC SURGERY, AND BODY CONTOURING

Two-thirds of adult Americans (about 200 million) are overweight or obese (body mass index [BMI] ≤25). Obesity (BMI ≤30) affects over a third of the adult American population (about 72 million Americans).[1] Over 220 000 gastric bypass surgeries were performed in the USA in 2009 (an increase of >600% in past decade).[2]

Over 313 000 body-contouring procedures were performed in 2010 (a 498% increase in the last 13 years; a 19% increase from 2009). Of these, 9,147 lower body lifts were done in 2010 (a 25% increase from 2009). An average surgeon's fee is $7904, the highest for 21 listed surgical procedures.[3] These data shows that >95% of MWL patients have not undergone lower body lifts.

Hospital care can easily add $15 000–30 000 to the surgical fee, totaling ≥$23 000–38 000. These cost estimates vary widely among hospitals and geographic locations. They are substantially higher than the approximate *total* cost of the same exact operation performed in our office surgical facility as an outpatient procedure – around $17 000. These cost savings could increase accessibility to body lifts for more MWL patients.

■ PATIENT SELECTION

Most postbariatric patients lose ≥100 lb (45 kg). They then have new problems from their excess skin. Several of our patients have described themselves as 'bodybuilders with Shar-pei skin.' Without body-contouring surgery, many MWL patients cannot wear stylish clothing or avoid rashes, infections, odor, or chronic irritation from chafing folds of macerated skin. Instead, they must undergo additional costly operations to achieve what they had anticipated their weight loss alone would yield.

Although the distribution and severity of excess skin vary widely in postbariatric patients, the abdomen is often the site of the greatest deformity. Many plastic surgeons are not yet experienced in performing lower body lifts. Instead they offer abdominoplasty. Plastic surgeons who are members of the American Society for Aesthetic Plastic Surgery (ASAPS) performed an average of 0.9 lower body lifts per year. Abdominoplasty, however, is the fourth most commonly performed operation by ASAPS member plastic surgeons – an average of 18.5 procedures per year (2010 data). However, most postbariatric surgery patients are ill-served by abdominoplasty alone. As a result of the severity of the circumferential truncal cutaneous excess in MWL patients, even extended or fleur-de-lis (inverted-T) abdominoplasty (**Fig. 7.1**) often yields unsatisfactory aesthetic results.

Patients still losing weight after their bariatric procedure, or who have residual excess intra-abdominal fat despite weight loss, are not candidates for lower body lift surgery. Prospective patients should maintain a stable, healthy weight for a minimum of 6 months before undergoing circumferential lower body lift. The closer a patient gets to ideal weight, the better the final contour improvements after surgery, and the lower the complication rate.[4–7]

Patients with cardiac or pulmonary disease, diabetes, or psychiatric concerns may not be good candidates for outpatient lower body lift. Patients who smoke are not candidates for this operation unless they can successfully discontinue all tobacco and nicotine products (including exposure to second-hand smoke) for a minimum of 2 weeks before surgery.

Patients who have a history of deep venous thrombosis or pulmonary embolus, or are anticoagulated for these, or who have cardiac concerns are considered unsuitable for outpatient surgery.

Some otherwise healthy appearing, post-MWL patients exhibit asymptomatic bradycardia or anemia, or both. In this subset of MWL patients, left ventricular hypertrophy and cardiac outputs that resulted from decades of morbid obesity could not diminish rapidly enough to compensate for rapid weight loss. The only physiological mechanisms available to counter the substantially reduced perfusion needs are reactive anemia and bradycardia. Structural, functional, and beneficial cardiovascular effects of major weight loss after bariatric surgery are documented in the literature.[8,9] This specific phenomenon merits further study, but no longer disqualifies patients from consideration for outpatient surgery.

Any outpatient lower body lift patient with identified surgical risk factors has their history and physical exam reviewed by our anesthesia provider *before* the day of surgery. Any additional tests or evaluations may be expedited. Failure to do this wastes time, personnel, and patient preparation, which can involve time off work, arrangement of care-giver's schedule, child care, and unreimbursed costs of hundreds to thousands of dollars, aside from the emotional toll of a 'false start.'

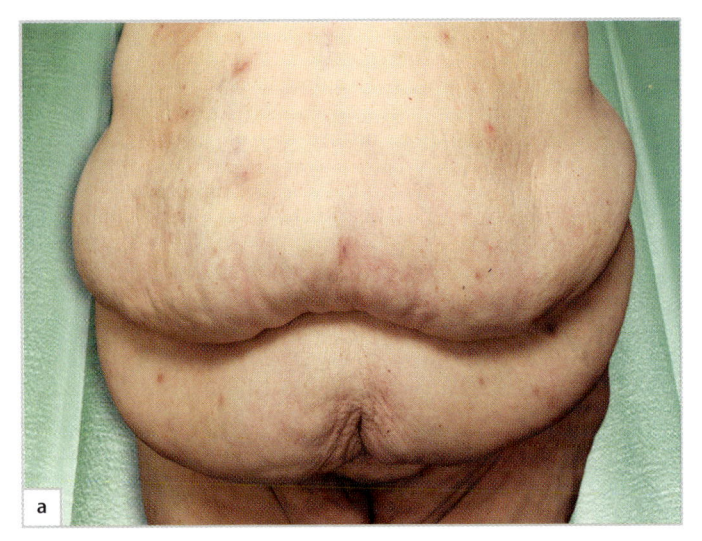

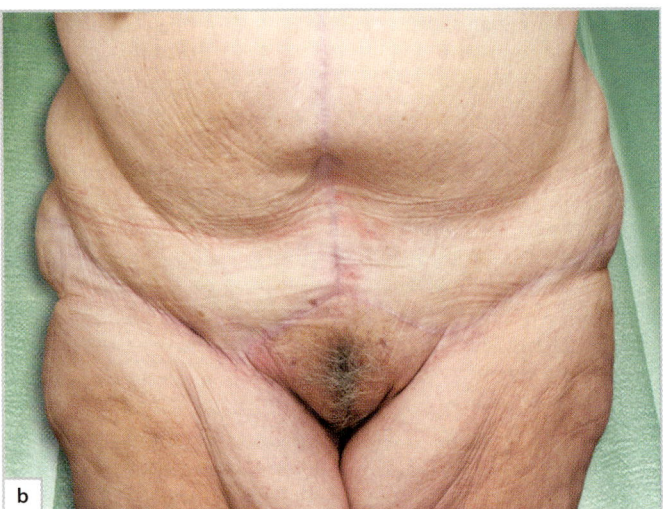

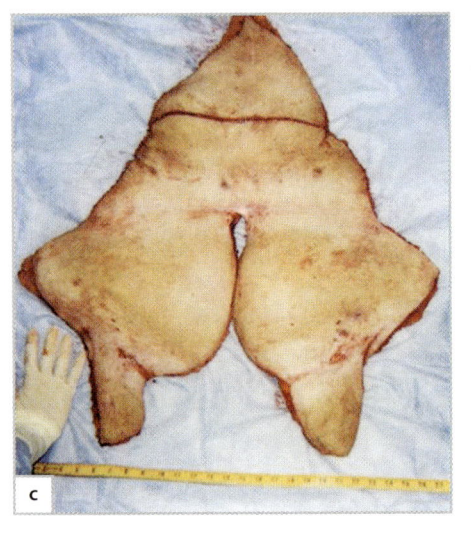

Figure 7.1 Patient 1. (a) A 46-year-old woman after 107 lb (48 kg) weight loss (body mass index [BMI] 42.1); pre-weight loss BMI 58; (b) 16 months after fleur-de-lis abdominoplasty. (c) Surgical specimen (hand and tape measure for reference): 20.1 lb (9 kg).

TERMINOLOGY

Belt lipectomy was originally described half a century ago.[10] Since that time, circumferential surgical resections have been reported by various descriptive names, including type 1 lower body lift[11] and type 2,[12] and belt lipectomy or circumferential belt lipectomy.[13] Belt lift, torsoplasty, and dermolipectomy are other terms that describe circumferential lower body lifts.

We prefer the terms 'circumferential lower body lift' or 'belt lift' to describe single-stage, 360° excisions that combine a 'posterior lift' with either a medial thigh lift (type 1) or abdominoplasty (type 2).

Type 2 circumferential lower body lifts are much more common in MWL patients. In our series of 263 consecutive patients over a 14-year period, 240 underwent a type 2 abdominoplasty plus posterior lift, whereas 23 had a type 1 medial thigh lift plus posterior lift.

PREOPERATIVE MARKINGS

After preoperative photographs and body weight/fat analysis, markings are made in the presurgical area in the upright position. These can vary dramatically with individual patient weight and cutaneous laxity, but several key points will help understanding of **Fig. 7.2**, which shows the markings for type 2 lower body lift:

- Excess tissue resection should be aggressive anteriorly and conservative posteriorly.
- The final scar should be planned to mimic the line formed by a G-string or thong underwear, slanting gently upward laterally, and meeting posteriorly just above (but not within) the gluteal cleft. The degree of rise laterally will be greater for certain (high leg opening) bathing suit styles, and flatter (lower) for women who prefer low-riding 'hip-hugger' jeans or slacks, and men who wish to avoid scar exposure above swim trunks or irritation by clothing waistbands.
- The superior line of abdominal skin resection is not a 'hard' mark, because this may change substantially when the operating table is flexed to take tension off the abdominal closure, and as skin rolls are detached from their abdominal wall attachments.
- Undermining and stretch are superior for the abdomen (fixation to the lower incision superficial fascial system, or SFS, taking into account that the mons pubis is often ptotic and requires elevation and stretch before closure). Undermining and stretch is inferior for the buttocks and lateral thigh (fixation to the lower back and hip SFS). The transition between these anterior and posterior areas is the zone of adherence just above the lateral thigh.
- If the lateral thigh exhibits 'tethered laxity,' release of the musculofascial to SFS and skin fibrous septa via a Lockwood dissector (Byron Medical, Tucson, AZ) (**Fig. 7.3a**) will need to be planned. If the lateral thigh skin is relatively smooth and only loose superiorly, a Lockwood dissection will not be beneficial, and the vertical extent of excision is marked moderately aggressively to yield a smooth lateral thigh/hip line.
- Often what seems to be localized, excess, lateral thigh, fat protrusion in need of liposuction is simply loose skin 'slumping' under gravity to form a 'pseudo-saddlebag.' Firm elevation of the lateral thigh when marking facilitates both an improved smoothness after excision and closure, but will also exhibit the true degree of excess localized fat suitable for liposuction.
- Under-resection can be adjusted for in the operating room, whereas over-resection creates excessive tension, difficulty with closure, wider scars, and a higher potential for dehiscence.
- Vertical cross-hatch or 'registration' marks are made with a tape measure and ruler, not by visual estimation. Once the final superior incision line is marked circumferentially, this length is accurately measured. The planned inferior circumference is also measured. These circumferences will *not* match – the inferior circumference will usually measure 10–15 cm longer than the superior incision circumference, yet accurate closure will need to accommodate these unequal lengths. Once the discrepancy

Preoperative markings 41

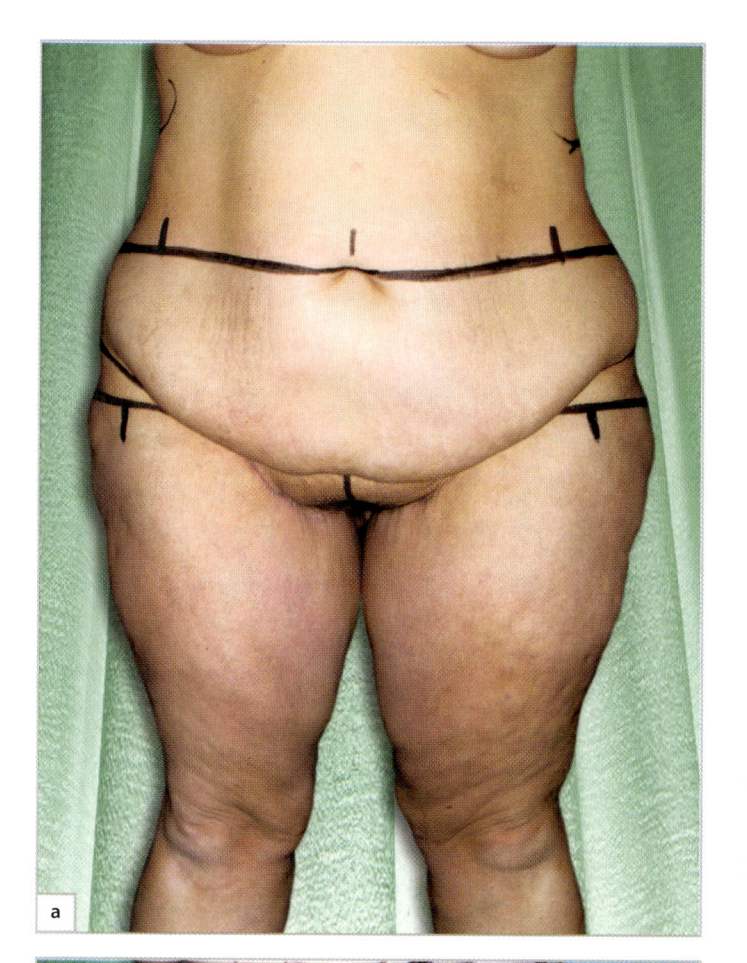

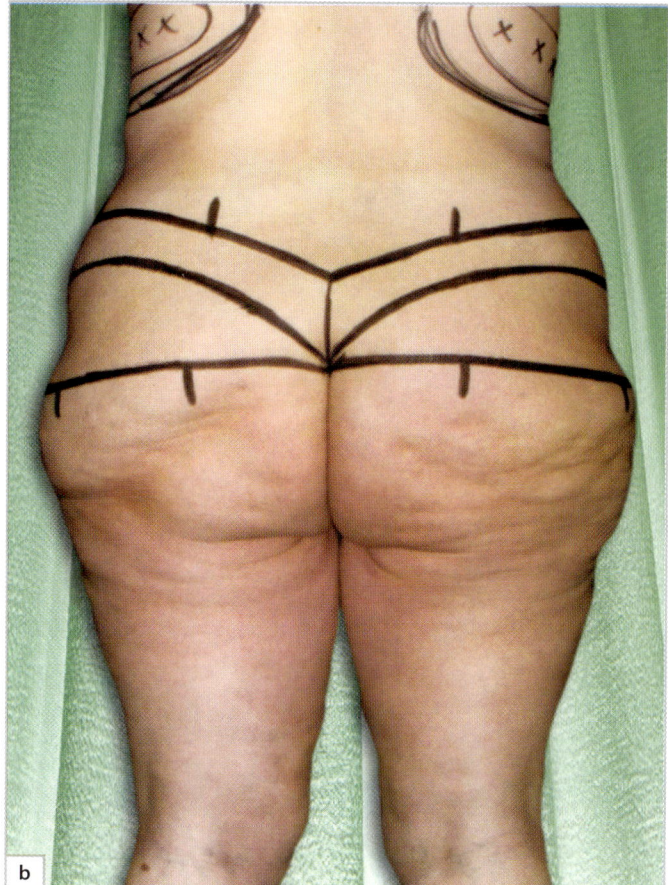

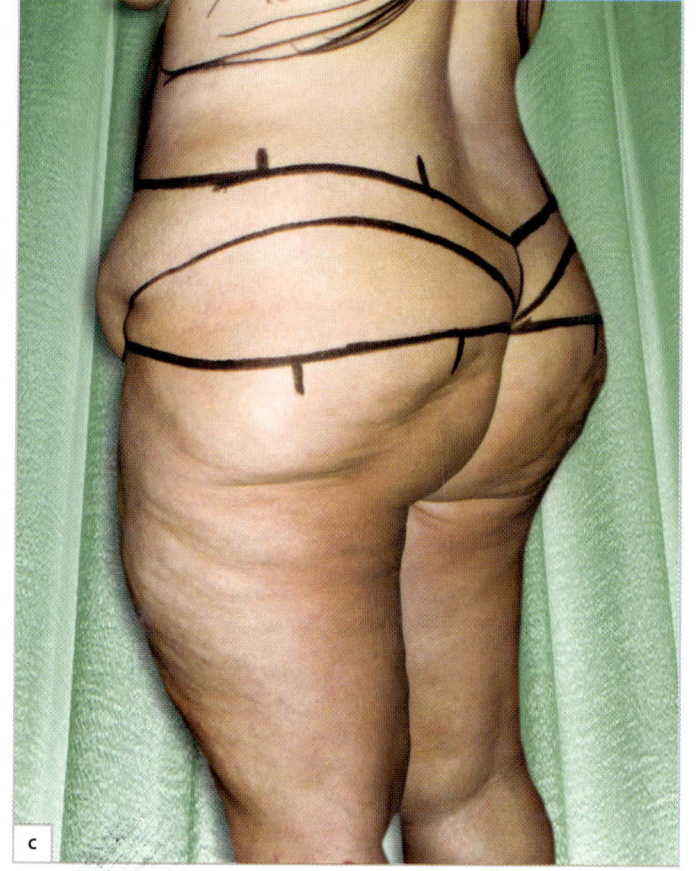

Figure 7.2 Preoperative markings. See text for details.

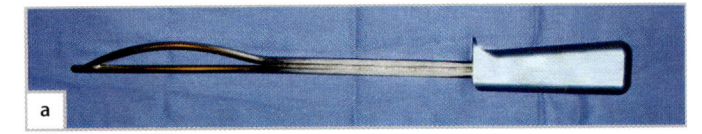

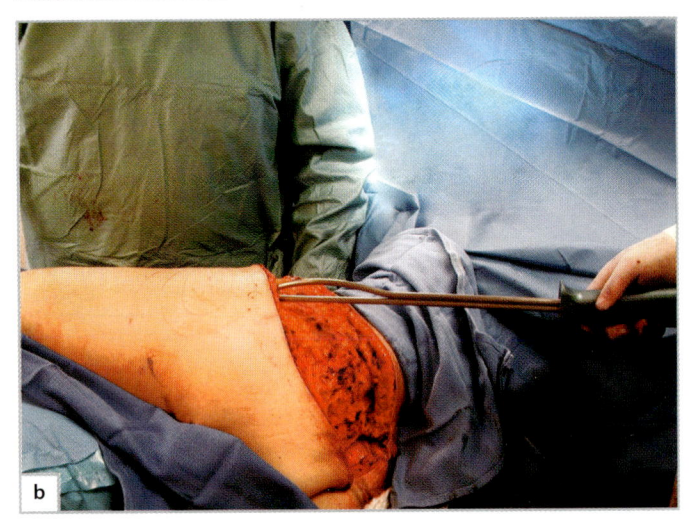

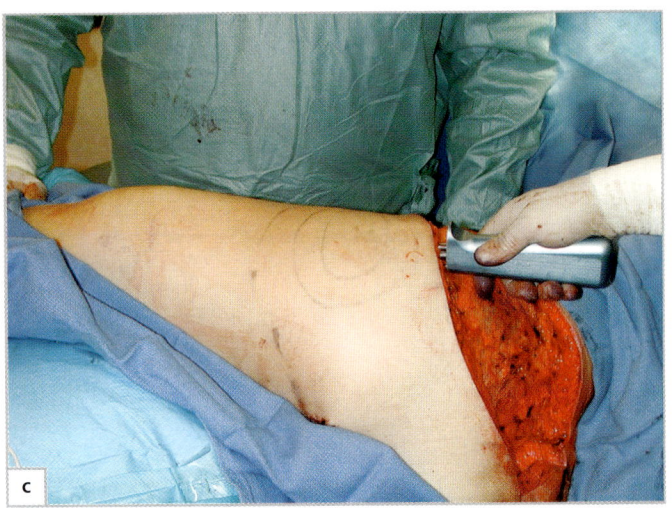

Figure 7.3 Lockwood dissector in use. (a) Lockwood dissector. (b,c) After excision and tumescent infiltration, dissector is inserted above fascia six to eight times along lateral and posterolateral thigh, stretching and releasing musculofascial attachments to allow smoother skin contours.

has been quantified, the vertical alignment marks are made every 10 cm on the inferior incision line mark, starting posteriorly, where accuracy of closure is most critical. As the superior incision line circumference is usually less, the discrepancy is made up by marking the upper vertical cross-hatch mark at 9-cm intervals, e.g. correcting a 10-cm discrepancy over an approximate 100-cm total circumference. Adjustment is made for different patient measurements. Final compensations are made anteriorly, where discrepancies are more easily corrected.

- We recommend that these vertical alignment marks be lightly scratched into the patient's skin with a sterile 30-gauge needle. These scratches will prevent inaccuracies of closure that could occur if marks are lost during the prep scrub and intraoperative position changes.

■ ANESTHESIA: OPTIONS AND STATISTICS

Virtually all reports in the literature to date of lower body lifts describe circumferential lower body lift operations being performed as hospital inpatient procedures, often with a two-surgeon team, and including hospital stays of several days.[12,14,15] Transfusion is not uncommon,[12-14,16] particularly as major tissue removal can include unmeasured blood loss.

Common *hospital* general anesthesia protocols utilize intravenous propofol induction, followed by inhalational anesthetic (isoflurane, sevoflurane, or desflurane plus nitrous oxide) and an opiate (fentanyl or remifentanil) plus an amnesic (diazepam or midazolam). This regimen is safe, effective, and less costly than total intravenous anesthesia (TIVA).

Increasing financial pressures and decreasing reimbursement for non-elective hospital operations may encourage hospital-based anesthesia providers to shift their choices toward inhalational anesthetics, and away from more costly propofol-based TIVA, particularly for long cases.

Although TIVA and balanced inhalational anesthesia are both safe, cost is not the only difference between these two disparate techniques. Multiple studies indicate that postoperative nausea and vomiting (PONV) rates are higher for inhalational anesthetics than for TIVA.[17-20] These studies reported outpatient cases lasting < 3 hours. Nausea and vomiting rates for inhalational anesthetics ranged from 5% to 75% within the first 24 hours after surgery, whereas the TIVA PONV rates ranged from 5% to 17%.

However, the TIVA data included the use of nitrous oxide in 39 of 42 studies in the largest review.[19] Duration of nitrous oxide (N_2O) administration during adult ambulatory surgery has a direct effect on PONV in cases of any duration. In this study,[21] anesthesia times and the percentages of patients exhibiting PONV in the N_2O-free and N_2O-treated groups, respectively, were: < 1 hour, 0% and 6.3%; between 1.0 and 1.9 hours, 35.3% and 36.8%; between 2.0 and 2.9 hours, 24.2% and 66.7%; and between 3.0 and 5.3 hours, 35% and 100%.

This suggests that TIVA without any inhalational anesthetic *or* N_2O administration should exhibit *correspondingly lower* PONV rates for comparable case lengths and types.

■ ANESTHESIA AND PERIOPERATIVE PROTOCOL

We have offered full anesthesia services in our accredited office surgical facility for the past 20 years (since 1991), staffed by a certified registered nurse anesthetist (CRNA) team. Initially, our general anesthetic cases mirrored the anesthesia practices at hospitals and hospital-affiliated outpatient surgical facilities where our CRNAs also worked. Balanced anesthesia with inhalational agents was most commonly used for our elective general anesthetic procedures.

As our CRNAs collect office PONV statistics, we were able to identify and modify those practices that contributed to higher PONV rates. These included use of inhalational anesthetics, N_2O, and opioid analgesics during surgery or recovery, and led us to decrease these accordingly. Addition of one or more antiemetic medications – prochlorperazine, droperidol, scopolamine transdermal, metoclopramide, ondansetron, or dolasetron – in patients with a history of PONV, and eventual elimination of *all* inhalational anesthetics *and* N_2O, led to gradually decreasing PONV rates in our surgical facility.

Between 1991 and 1997, our office facility PONV rates ranged from 5% to 11% (3 or 4 plastic surgeons; average 902 CRNA-staffed cases/year; 25–445 min case duration – average of 137 min/case; average of 9.1% PONV).

Adding preoperative intravenous dexamethasone further reduced PONV. Preoperative oral celecoxib and methocarbamol reduce inflammation, pain, and muscle spasms; these drugs are continued in the early postoperative medication regimen. Bupivacaine with epinephrine is utilized to control muscle spasm and incisional pain.

Between 1998 and 2002, our anesthesia protocols were modified as described, and our case data remained essentially identical, but PONV rates dropped to 3–7% (2–4 plastic surgeons; average 910 CRNA-staffed cases/year; 35–430 min case duration – average of 140 min/case; average of 5.0% PONV).

Since 2002, our statistics (all cases) reflect two plastic surgeons (RHT and DLG) with total fewer cases, longer duration cases, and PONV rates ranging from 2.6% to 3.5%.

This combination of perioperative medications and practices has allowed our lower body lift (and other cosmetic surgical) patients to be routinely discharged from our facility after 1–1½ hours in the recovery room. At discharge our patients have taken oral liquids, been to the restroom and voided, and are dressed and ambulatory (with assistance).

At Minneapolis Plastic Surgery, our present *preoperative* anesthesia regimen (for all outpatient general anesthetic procedures) includes the following:
- 'Pre-emptive' analgesia: Celebrex (celecoxib) 400 mg orally
- 'Pre-emptive' muscle relaxant: Robaxin (methocarbamol) 750 mg orally
- Decadron 10 mg intravenously (i.v.)
- Ancef (cefazolin) 1–2 g i.v. (if not allergic).

If the patient has a history of PONV, add:
- 'Pre-emptive' antiemetic: Zofran (ondansetron) 4 mg i.v.
- Metoclopramide 10–20 mg i.v.

If the patient has a history of motion sickness, add:
- Scopolamine patch (Transderm Scop).

If the patient has reflux or a diagnosis of gastroesophageal reflux disease (GERD):
- Bicitra 30 ml orally.

Our *operative* anesthesia protocol consists of Versed 2 mg i.v. + 1 ml (50 μg) fentanyl pre-induction, no paralytic if laryngeal mask airway (LMA) is used, or Zemuron 0.5 mg/kg if oral endotracheal (OET) intubation is used. Induction is with propofol 1–2 mg/kg, followed by propofol/remifentanil continuous infusion (propofol 100–200 μg/kg per min + remifentanil 0.025–0.200 μg/kg per min). Higher doses of remifentanil are used for 'big/long' cases (0.1–0.2 μg/kg per min); lower doses of remifentanil are used for 'small/short' cases (0.025–0.050 μg/kg per min); most cases will have intermediate doses of remifentanil (0.05–0.10 μg/kg per min) (**Table 7.1**).

Marcaine 0.25% with epinephrine is injected into the rectus sheath, as well as drain exit sites, and lower abdominal skin incision for reduction of postoperative muscle spasm and pain, respectively. We prefer direct injection at the time of surgery over catheter-instilled pain pumps, but use of one of these is imperative, in our opinion, because pain on emergence from anesthesia is not only implicated in delayed discharge, but can precipitate unplanned admission.[22] Ondansetron 4 mg i.v. is administered 30 min before the end of the case, and is re-dosed in recovery if needed. Accurate fluid administration is monitored via a Foley catheter, which is removed in the recovery room so that the patient can successfully void before discharge, and must ambulate for restroom visits after discharge. Low-dose glycopyrrolate can reduce bradycardia-related nausea.

Table 7.1 Propofol/Remifentanil continuous intravenous infusion.

Propofol (μg/kg per min)	100	120	140	160	180	200
0.5 mg remifentanil (1 ml)[a]	0.10	0.12	0.14	0.16	0.18	0.20
0.25 mg remifentanil (0.5 ml)[b]	0.05	0.06	0.07	0.08	0.09	0.10
0.125 mg remifentanil (0.25 ml)[c]	0.025	0.03	0.035	0.04	0.045	0.05

Mix 4 ml intravenous fluid in 2-mg vial of remifentanil = 0.5 mg/ml.
Add 0.25, 0.5, or 1 ml to 50 ml propofol for the following remifentanil concentration (μg/kg per min):
[a] Most cases, use 0.25 mg (0.50 ml) remifentanil.
[b] 'Big/long' cases, use 0.5 mg (1 ml) remifentanil.
[c] 'Small/short' cases, use 0.125 mg (0.25 ml) remifentanil.

Our present TIVA protocol allows rapid emergence from anesthesia due to the short and ultra-short half-lives of propofol and remifentanil, respectively. The antiemetic effect of propofol is not reduced by use of long-acting opioids, and is enhanced by pre-treatment with intravenous dexamethasone and ondansetron. As propofol lacks analgesic properties, pre-treatment with celecoxib, concomitant continuous intravenous infusion with the ultra-short half-life (3–10 min) opioid remifentanil, minimal doses of fentanyl (half-life 3.7 h), and regional local anesthesia (bupivacaine plus epinephrine) provide long-lasting pain relief during and after surgery. Preoperative oral methocarbamol provides long-acting central muscle relaxation and spasm reduction, sometimes a major component of perceived postoperative pain. Judicious intravenous Versed use provides mild-to-moderate sedative and retrograde amnesic effects that are dose dependent and beneficial for restless or agitated patients.

The pharmacokinetics and pharmacodynamics of this protocol are aimed at rapid and comfortable return to consciousness, pain control without the nausea and vomiting induced by long-acting opioids, and avoidance of the odor and rebreathing of volatilized lipid-dissolved inhalational anesthetics that can stimulate PONV, and N_2O-induced dilation of hollow body cavities such as the stomach, gut, sinuses, and middle ear, which can initiate, aggravate, or prolong PONV. As the antiemetics dexamethasone, ondansetron, prochlorperazine, and promethazine all have different metabolic receptors and mechanisms of action, combining one or more of them can provide additive benefits, or improved results when one is less effective.

Postoperative medications include celecoxib 200 mg orally twice daily for 10 days, methocarbamol 750 mg orally every 3 h (while awake) for 10 days, cephalexin 250 orally three or four times daily for 4–5 days, and Vicodin ES (hydrocodone bitartrate and acetaminophen) half to one tablet orally every 2–4 h rather than one to two orally every 4–6 h. A prescription is given (but not filled unless needed) for Zofran 8 mg as an orally disintegrating tablet or prochlorperazine 25 mg as a suppository every 6 h as needed for nausea. One refill authorization is included with each prescription, and drugs/dosages are altered as required for individual patient allergies, sensitivities, or other needs.

■ SURGICAL TECHNIQUE FOR OUTPATIENT LOWER BODY LIFT

After the markings have been completed, the patient is taken to the operating room for a standing, awake Betadine scrub and prep. A more thorough and complete cleansing between ptotic skin folds, around the external genitalia, and in the umbilicus and gluteal folds is possible with the active assistance of an awake patient, compared with an anesthetized MWL patient. 'Prepping as you go' is both disruptive and more likely to suffer contamination than a standing, awake prep.

The patient is carefully assisted onto an already-padded and sterile-draped operating table, sequential foot compression devices are placed, and the patient is covered with sterile drapes. A warming pad is used on the operating table, and a warm forced-air blanket (BairHugger) is used for the head and arms. Anesthesia is induced, a urinary catheter placed, and sterile draping completed. Intravenous and irrigation fluids are warmed, and the ambient room temperature is kept as warm as the surgical team can tolerate.

Initially, for type 2 lower body lifts we preferred prone–supine positioning (**Fig. 7.4**). As we routinely utilize lateral decubitus positioning for liposuction operations, we now prefer lateral-lateral-supine positioning. It has become our preferred lower body lift-positioning regimen for most of the past decade (**Fig. 7.5**).

For type 1 lower body lifts (medial thigh lift with in-continuity posterior lift), we utilize either supine frog-leg positioning (**Fig. 7.6**) or gynecologic stirrups for completion of the medial thigh lifts. After excision with minimal undermining, closure is carried out from posterior to anterior, anchoring the thigh dermis to Colles' fascia with number 1 Ethibond sutures soaked in Betadine, and additional number 0 polydioxanone (PDS) sutures from the deep dermis to Colles' fascia. Bacterial contamination of permanent braided sutures (Ethibond) is always a concern in a warm, moist, bacteria-rich region, and we limit these sutures to three or four per side, using monofilament 0 PDS for the remainder of the tension-holding sutures. Overcorrection is recommended, because the medial thigh/vulva scar always widens and migrates inferiorly, leading to visible scars around swim bottoms, or pubic hair on the medial thighs, both of which cause patient dissatisfaction. Buried interrupted 3/0 PDS and 4/0 Monocryl are used for the dermis and skin closure. An additional skin closure layer utilizes a running 3/0 Prolene for the central thigh–vulva region. Two 10-mm flat Jackson-Pratt drains are usually, but not always, utilized. Each patient is assessed for the possibility of a 'T' or 'V' medial thigh excision – generally needed for patients who lose extreme amounts of weight and exhibit horizontal or circumferential laxity that cannot be satisfactorily addressed via crescentic excision and vertical lift alone. An example of this is seen in **Fig. 7.7**.

As > 90% of our cases (240 of 263) have been type 2 lower body lifts, the remainder of this section describes the specifics for the type 2 lift.

After lateral decubitus positioning, re-measurement and pinch testing are carried out in the lateral thigh/hip and buttocks. Markings are adjusted if necessary to ensure optimum tension after the resection and lift.

Superior and inferior incisions are made from the anterior hip to several centimeters beyond the gluteal cleft and deepened to meet just above the muscular fascia in a 'V' fashion. Preserving the fat layer just above the fascia may help to reduce postoperative seromas. Incisions deepened perpendicular to the skin surface result in a wide-based excision defect (see **Fig. 7.4a**) which remains as a suprafascial dead space when the more superficial layers are sutured together, or else extensive undermining is needed, further contributing to seroma formation. This 'V' modification of the surgical technique decreased seroma rate from 68% in the earliest cases to 39% in later cases.

One additional benefit of the 'V' excision technique is that better buttock contour (less flattening) is achieved. When additional autologous buttock augmentation is desired, the area of planned excision is instead de-epithelialized, mobilized to produce fullness in the desired location, trimmed to the desired size, and appropriate undermining carried out to cover the autologous fat–dermis pedicle with the lifted buttock. Number 0 PDS suture fixation provides immobilization to the gluteal fascia and overlying flap SFS layer.

Once the excess skin and fat have been resected, assessment is made of the degree of lateral thigh laxity and the need for release of the fibrous SFS attachments. About half of lower body lift patients will benefit from stretching of these musculofascial attachments via a Lockwood dissector. This allows improved lifting and smoothing of the posterolateral thigh without significant damage to vessels and nerves. The remaining patients have less preoperative lateral thigh laxity, and will receive little or no benefit from this step.

When the use of the Lockwood dissector is planned, infiltration of the anterior, lateral, and posterior thigh is carried out with superwet (1:1) Hunstad tumescent formula (1 liter lactated Ringer with 50 ml of 1% lidocaine and 1 ml – 1 ampoule – of 1:1000 epinephrine) fluid just above the muscular fascia in the deep subcutaneous fat, along the planned path of Lockwood dissector spreading. If requested, ultrasound-assisted lipoplasty of the lateral thigh, inferolateral buttock, or presacral lower back is carried out after infiltration. Lockwood dissection is then performed, passing the dissector six to eight times along the suprafascial plane until the overlying layers are adequately released (see **Fig. 7.3b,c**).

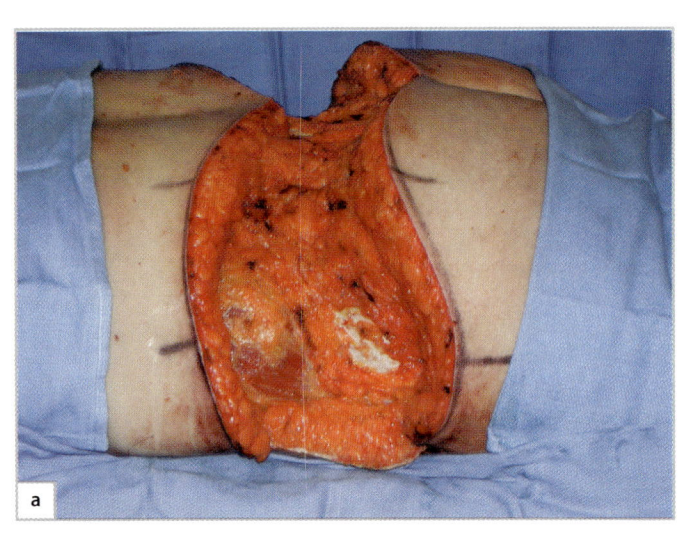

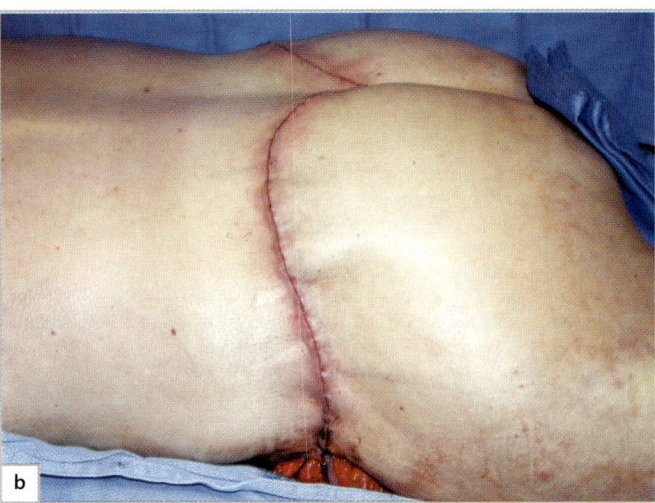

Figure 7.4 Prone–supine position (no longer used). (a) After posterior excision. Note straight-down dissection requires extensive undermining for closure, increasing seroma formation. (b) After everting layered closure; ready for final turn to supine position for abdominoplasty – completion of belt lift type 2.

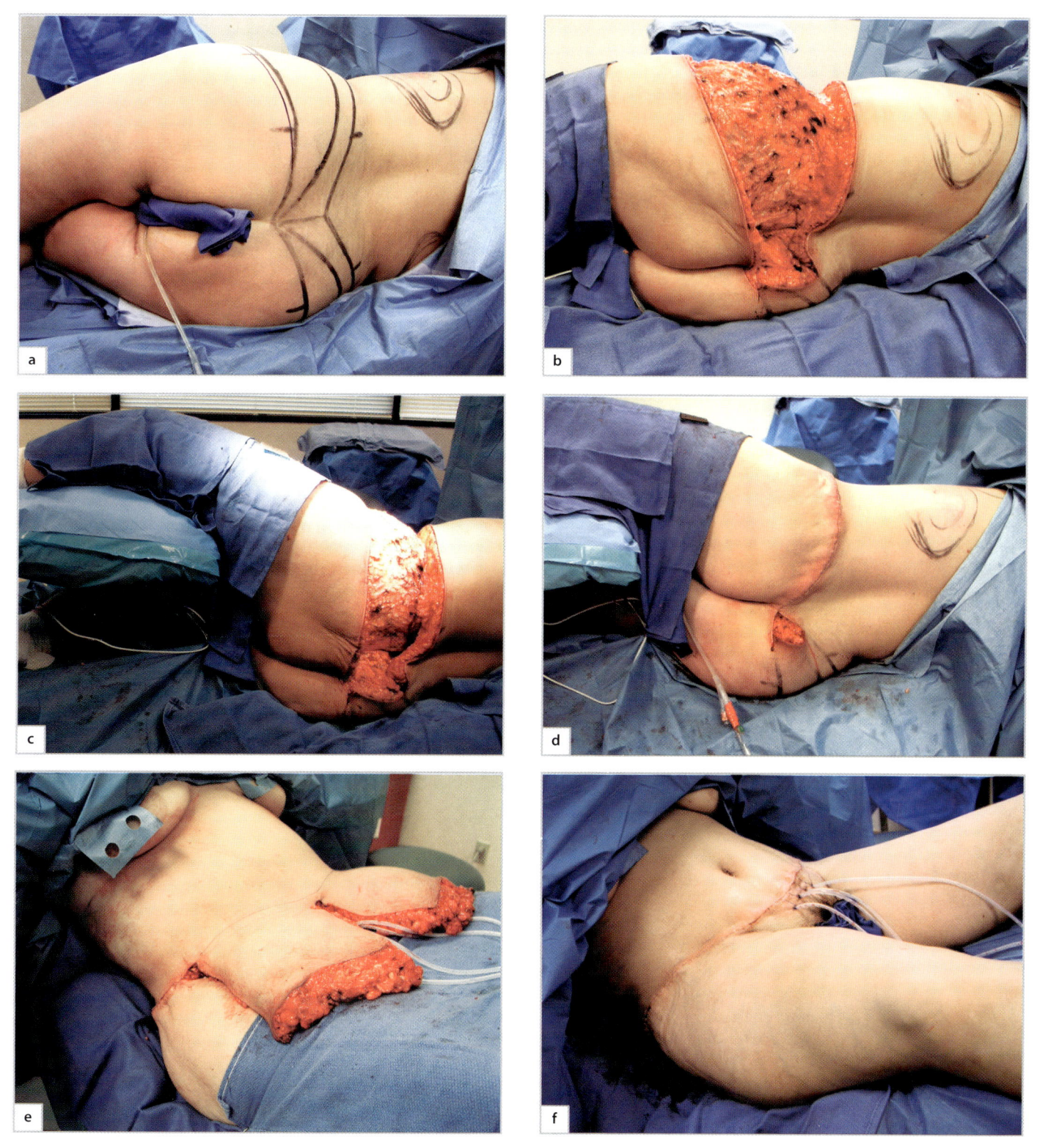

Surgical technique for outpatient lower body lift 45

Figure 7.5 Lateral–lateral–supine position (currently used). (a) Positioned for first half of posterior lift. (b) After completion of first half of posterior excision (leg adducted) and flank liposuction. Note excision extends past gluteal cleft to allow closure to midline. (c) Leg abducted on well-padded, sterile-draped Mayo stand to decrease closure tension. (d) After everting layered closure; ready for turn to opposite lateral decubitus position for second half of posterior lift. (e) Posterior lift completed; supine for completion of abdominoplasty portion of circumferential lower body lift. (f) After completion of type 2 belt lift; liposuction of flanks. Patient is 46 years old, preop body mass index (BMI) 32.1, 19.4 lb (8.7 kg) excised, 5 hours surgical time. Left recovery room in 1 h 45 min; no postoperative nausea and vomiting. Returned for recheck the following morning with makeup on and hair styled.

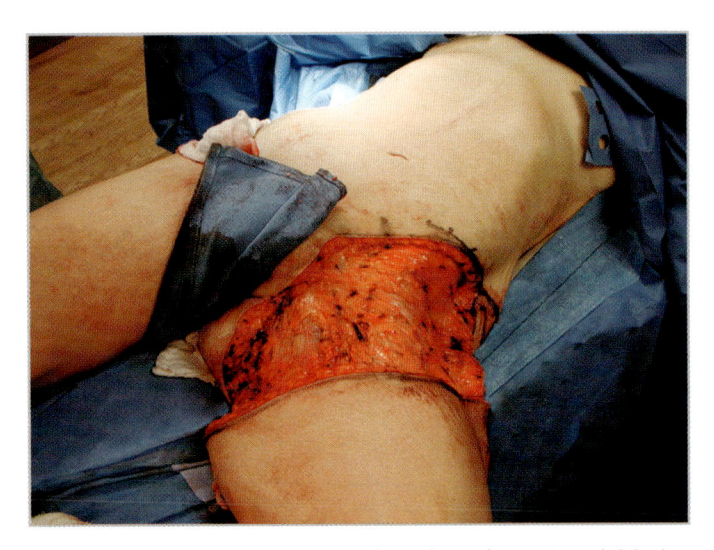

Figure 7.6 Intraoperative lower body lift (Lockwood type 1). Medial thigh lift + posterior lift; first medial thigh lift in frog-leg position.

A 10-mm flat Jackson–Pratt silicone drain is placed in the buttock excision and the drain tubing temporarily secured to the anterior skin.

The leg is then abducted approximately 20° to decrease closure tension, and supported on a well-padded, sterile-draped, adjustable-height Mayo stand (see **Fig. 7.5c**). (A sterile-draped foam wedge is also suitable for leg abduction, but is more difficult to set aside in sterile fashion until needed.) If excessive laxity persists, additional resection is carried out and the additional vertical height measured for contralateral symmetry.

SFS closure is accomplished with Betadine-soaked number 1 Ethibond in double-loop, buried-knot fashion. Starting at the posterior midline, a total of four to five Ethibond sutures are spaced to the anterosuperior iliac spine (ASIS) level, interspersed by additional SFS layer double-loop no. 0 PDS sutures. SFS closure alone should provide good skin–skin approximation without tension.

The deep dermis is closed with buried interrupted 3/0 PDS, and the skin with buried interrupted 4/0 Monocryl. Except for the deepest layer, which utilizes antiseptic-soaked braided permanent sutures, all layers are closed with monofilament sutures. We believe that this reduces the stitch abscesses seen with braided dissolvable skin sutures.

The patient is turned to the opposite lateral decubitus position to complete the remaining half of the posterior lift. We have not seen damage to the already-completed closure with the patient's weight immediately compressing it, at least with the approximate operating time of 60–90 min for each half of the posterior lift, and with a gel pad and warming blanket beneath the patient and sterile drapes. The patient is then returned to the supine position for the anterior portion of the circumferential procedure (see **Fig. 7.5e,f**).

Another BairHugger is placed on the patient's legs, covered with sterile drapes to the pubic level. This helps to keep the patient warmth. The umbilicus is incised in a modified chevron fashion, avoiding a

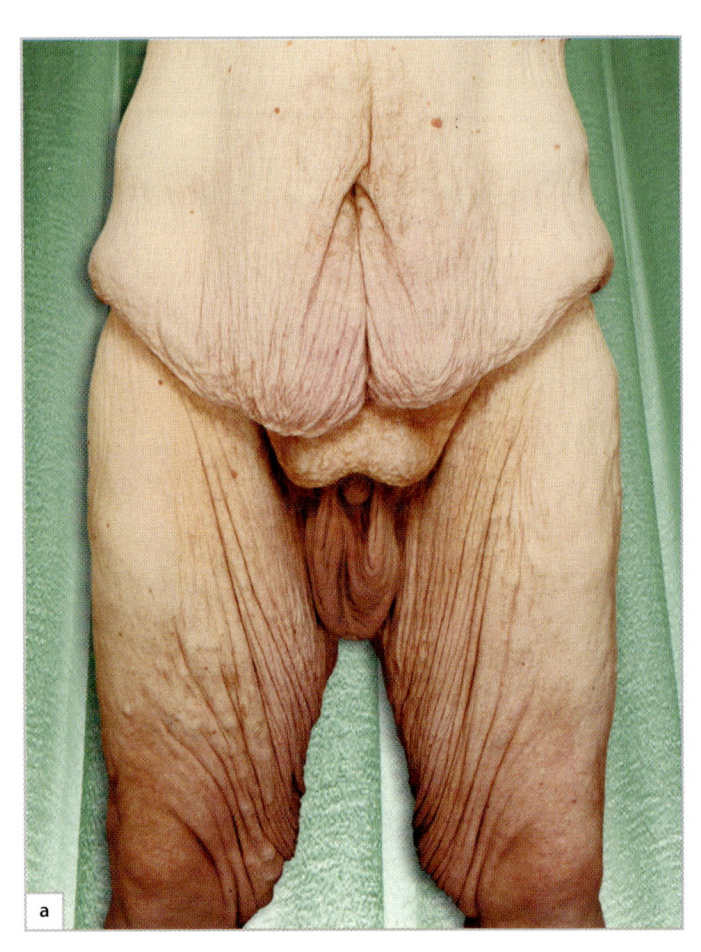

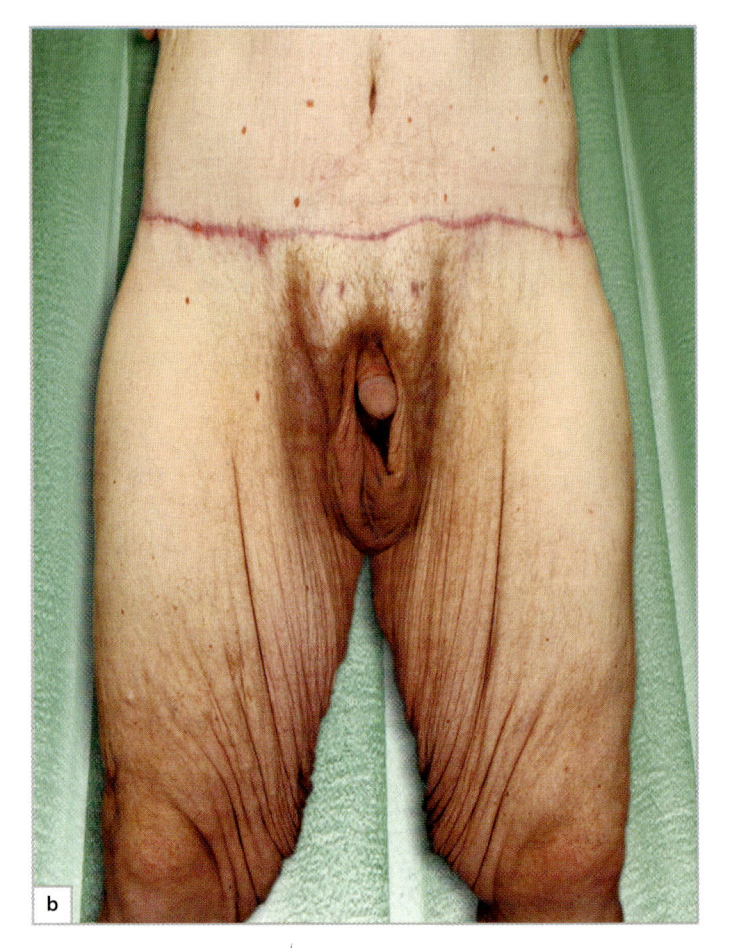

Figure 7.7 Patient 2. *Continued on pp. 47–48.*

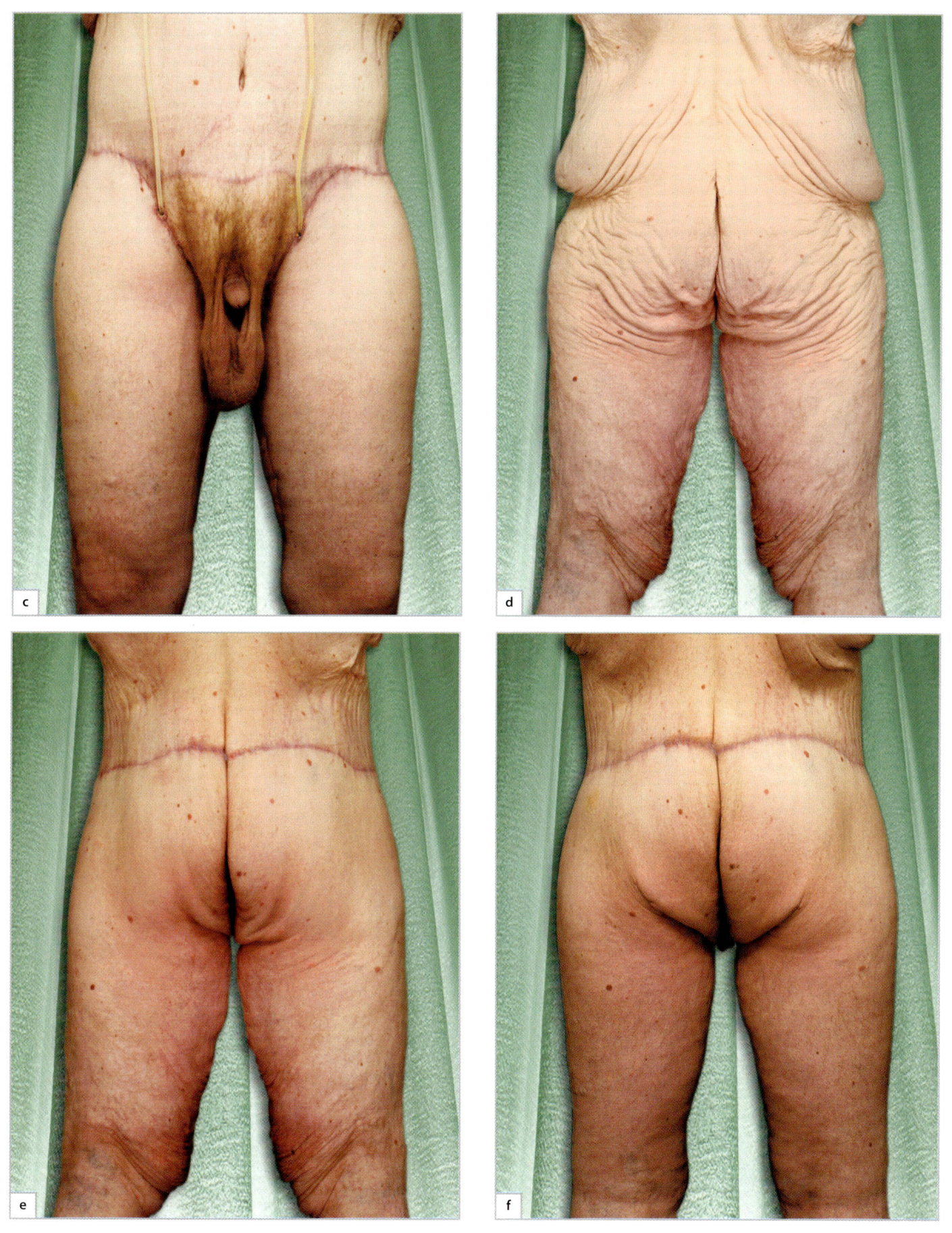

Surgical technique for outpatient lower body lift 47

Figure 7.7 Patient 2. *Continued on p. 48.*

48 OUTPATIENT LOWER BODY LIFT

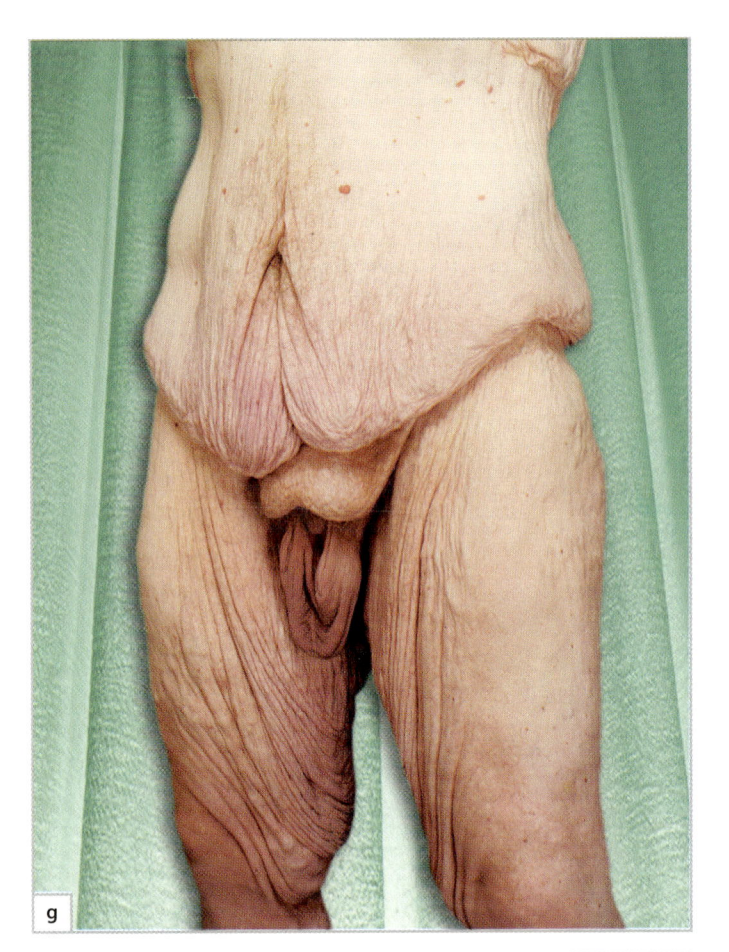

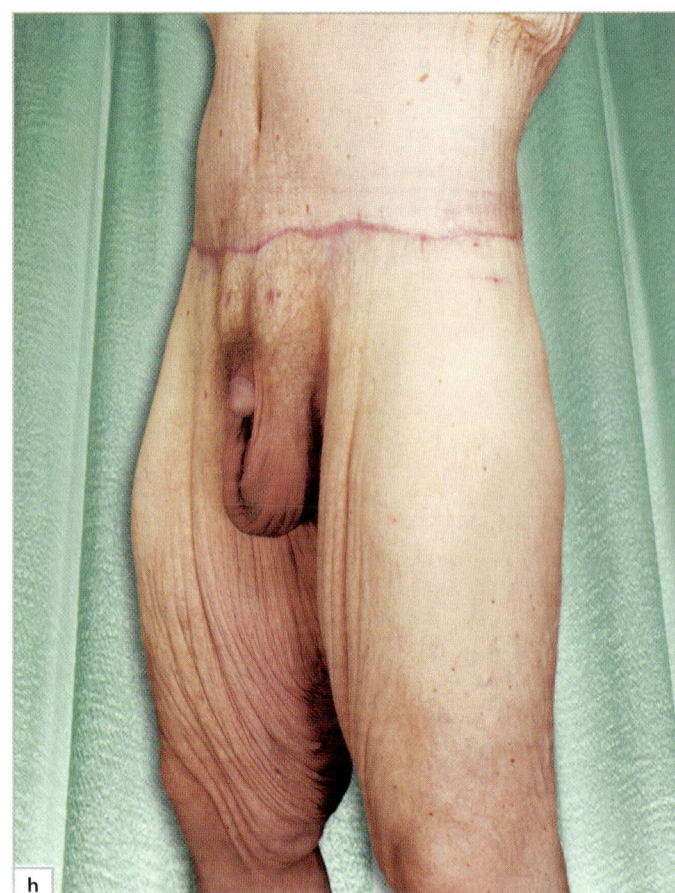

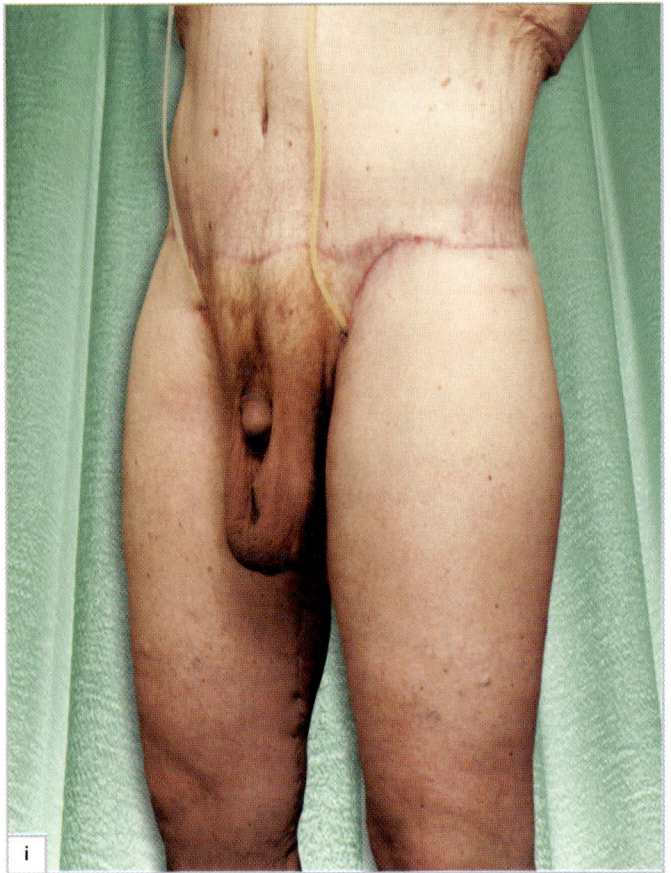

Figure 7.7 Patient 2. (a,d,g) A 39-year-old man after 450 lb (202 kg) weight loss (body mass index [BMI] now 33.4); pre-weight loss BMI 91.2 (6 feet 2 inches tall [1.88 m], 710 lb [319 kg]). (b,e,h) Three months postoperative to circumferential belt lift (type 2): 15.0 lb [6.75 kg] excised, 8 h 30 min surgical time. Outpatient. (c,f,i) Six weeks postop V-to-T medial thigh lift (vertical scar just above knee to groin, posteromedial location to minimize visibility; drains in place): 4385 g (9.7 lb excised), 7 h 35 min surgical time. Outpatient.

circular periumbilical scar. The inferior abdominoplasty incision is made in continuity with the posterior lift incisions on each side. Skin and fat are elevated from inferior to superior, maintaining a thin layer of fat on the abdominal wall fascia for improved lymphatic drainage and decreased seroma formation. From the umbilicus superiorly, elevation is carried out centrally to the xiphoid. This preserves lateral tissue attachments to minimize dead space and maximize circulatory support to the lower abdominal flap. Depending on the degree of truncal redundancy and extent of anterior abdominal rolls, additional lateral dissection may be required. If there are subcostal scars, patients are advised preoperatively of the potential risks, and dissection is limited. We have thus far not experienced healing problems in patients with subcostal scars.

After cefazolin (Ancef) irrigation, aggressive rectus sheath plication is performed according to the surgeon's preference, repairing any ventral or umbilical hernias. The senior author (RHT) prefers a running, locked suture of number 0 PDS, interspersed by triple-loop buried 2/0 Prolene sutures every 2–2.5 cm, from xiphoid to pubis. If the umbilical stalk is excessively long, it is trimmed, and sometimes plicated, to the anterior rectus sheath, depending on the residual anterior layer thickness (after sub-Scarpa fat resection and periumbilical fat contouring). Then 30 ml 0.25% Marcaine with epinephrine is infiltrated into the anterior rectus sheath, drain exit sites, and lower abdominoplasty skin incision.

The operating table flexes the abdomen, and the upper abdominal excess tissue is accurately measured, marked, and resected. The sub-Scarpa fat is excised to equalize flap thickness with pubic flap thickness. The degree of pubic elevation and tension on the abdominal–pubic closure is again determined, adjustments made, temporary suture placed, and the umbilical exit site marked. An inverted-V incision is made approximately 1 cm higher than the anticipated umbilical exit site, because the abdominal flap will descend this additional amount when the layered SFS closure is performed. Tension on the abdominal flap will stretch the inverted-V incision to the modified chevron shape of the incised umbilicus, avoiding a circular scar contracture. The periumbilical fat is excised under direct vision to provide funnel-like invagination which yields a natural umbilical contour.

The two posterior drains exit via lateral pubic escutcheon punctures made several centimeters below the incision line, and the abdominal Jackson-Pratt drains exit via two central punctures (see **Fig. 7.5f**). Prolene (2/0 monofilament) sutures are used for drain fixation. Silk sutures are not used – they are braided. The skin frequently becomes inflamed from bacterial contamination within suture interstices, leading to pain, premature loss of drain fixation, and increased drain site scarring. Posterior drains are frequently required for prolonged periods, so this is not a trivial concern or choice.

Anterior closure is accomplished with buried interrupted no. 0 PDS for the SFS layer, incorporating a deep bite of the abdominal wall fascia to minimize subincisional dead space, isolate the drains from each other, and reduce migration of the scar superiorly. No. 0 PDS quilting sutures can decrease dead space and anterior seroma formation, but prolonged drainage and seroma formation is more common posteriorly.

Subdermal closure is carried out with buried, interrupted 3/0 PDS sutures, and the skin with buried, interrupted 4/0 Monocryl. The umbilicus is exteriorized with buried interrupted 4/0 Monocryl for the subdermal layer, and simple, interrupted 5/0 Prolene sutures for the skin.

Suture lines are cleansed with warmed cefazolin (Ancef) irrigation, and sterile dressings and pads are placed. If Lockwood dissection or liposuction of the lateral thighs is performed, a crotchless compression garment is applied; otherwise, an elastic abdominal Velcro binder is utilized. Thromboembolic deterrent (TED) stockings are left in place until activity levels normalize.

RECOVERY

When appropriate criteria are met, all patients are discharged from our office surgical facility to the care of a responsible caregiver, usually within 60–90 min. Of 263 lower body lift patients, none required admission to a hospital or overnight care facility, and most returned to our office the following day for a recheck. Only sponge bathing is allowed. Ambulation is encouraged, particularly if patients exhibit any lethargy at their first office visit. Conversely, if any patient exhibits inappropriate ebullience, they are warned about complications resulting from overactivity. Liberalization of activity is not allowed if drains remain in place, or if a seroma requires intermittent aspiration. If incision maceration is noted (usually at the gluteal crease suture line in the posterior midline), patients are advised to open their garment daily and dry this area.

Drains are removed when drainage is less than 30 ml/day. Usually dependent on the flap size and amount of tissue removed, and to a lesser extent on patient activity, most patients had their *anterior* drains removed within 1–2 weeks. We stress to our patients that drain removal is volume rather than time related.

Most patients returned to non-strenuous work 3–4 weeks after surgery, usually after the final drains had been removed. In cases of prolonged drainage from posterior drains (or reinsertion after seroma recurrence), patients returned to work with the drains still in place. Exercise was not advised until all drains had been removed with no evidence of recurrent seroma, after which compression was also discontinued.

RESULTS

Between 1997 and 2011, 263 circumferential lower body lifts were performed in Minneapolis Plastic Surgery's AAAASF-accredited class C surgical facility. Of our patients 238 were female, 25 male, with ages ranging from 25 years to 67 years; 240 patients received type 2 lower body lifts and 23 had type 1 lifts, mostly because of previous abdominoplasty.

The weight of resected tissue ranged from 714 g to 14 256 g (1.6–31.4 lb) with a mean of 4062 g (8.9 lb). Liposuction was performed in addition to lower body lift in 32 of 263 patients, with aspirate volumes of 400–3750 ml (mean 910 ml); this was the most common associated procedure. Additional procedures performed are included in **Table 7.2**.

Surgical times ranged from 4.0 h to 8.5 h (mean 5.7 h); anesthesia times averaged an additional 30 min per patient for cleansing, bandaging, and placing compression binder or garment(s), but did not result in longer recovery room times or increased average time to discharge of 60–90 min.

Additional patient results are seen in **Figs 7.8–7.11**.

COMPLICATIONS

Seroma/prolonged drainage was the most common complication, occurring in two-thirds of our first 100 cases. This was usually noted in the posterior drains, and seemed to correlate with increased activity and residual obesity (size of resection). Persistent high drainage amounts were treated by tetracycline sclerodesis (1 g in 50 ml saline), clamping for 15–30 min, and then returning the drain to suction. When daily outputs were <30 ml, the drain was removed.

OUTPATIENT LOWER BODY LIFT

Table 7.2 Associated procedures performed at the same surgical setting and anesthetic as circumferential lower body lift in 263 outpatient cases over a 14-year period (n = 76; 29%).

UAL/SAL thighs, calves, knees, flanks	32
Ventral/umbilical hernia repair	19
Gynecomastia (excision or UAL/SAL)	7
Augmentation mammoplasty	6
Autologous buttock augmentation	4
Brachioplasty	2
Mastopexy/Augmentation	1
Bicoronal forehead lift	1
Submental fat excision/augmentation genioplasty	1
Dermal/fat graft to nasolabial folds	1
Dermal/fat graft lip enlargement	1
Facial dermabrasion	1

SAL, suction-assisted lipectomy; UAL, ultrasound-assisted lipectomy.

Sclerodesis was usually not initiated until about 3 weeks postoperatively, recognizing that the mean length of time for drains to be in place was 29 days (range 4–62 days, except one patient who sought care elsewhere after becoming discouraged). This patient self-referred to a radiologist for alternative care. Although initially lost to our follow-up, she had her surgical drain removed and CT-directed J-tube placed, numerous fluoroscopy-directed contrast studies to assess pseudobursa size, periodic instillations of absolute alcohol or other sclerosants, and treatment of at least two infections. After failure and frustration with this prolonged effort, she returned to our care and underwent near-complete circumferential pseudobursectomy. The resected pseudobursa lining was a thick, nonviable, moist eschar. Her pseudobursectomy course was uneventful.

Sclerodesis was usually well tolerated, but pain or malaise occurred in several patients. Lidocaine added to the sclerosant, oral analgesics, and oral antihistamine (Benadryl) reduced these transient symptoms, allowing these patients to reluctantly accept ongoing sclerodesis, continued weekly until drainage tapered and the drain(s) were removed. Of 263 patients, 103 (39%) underwent sclerodesis for persistent drainage, down from 68% in the first 100 procedures.

The biggest alteration in our practice consisted of changing to a 'V' excision technique described earlier. As Lockwood dissection was performed in about half our patients, we theorized that this might play a role in prolonged seroma/drainage, but no correlation was identified.

Quilting or progressive tension sutures in the anterior skin flaps were rarely utilized, nor were they apparently necessary, because prolonged drainage and recurrent seromas after drain removal were almost exclusively posterior. A third of patients developed recurrent seromas after drain removal; this was treated by serial percutaneous 14-G needle aspirations once or twice weekly. If aspirated amounts tapered, no further treatments were needed. However, if the post-drain seroma persisted despite aspiration, a drain was reinserted under local anesthesia, and sclerodesis initiated. When this failed, a total of

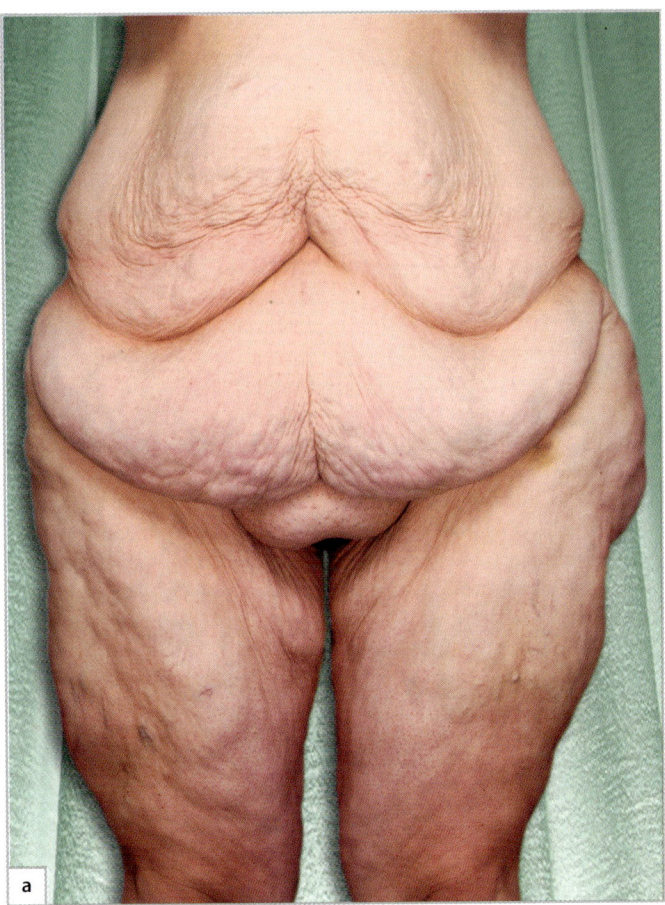

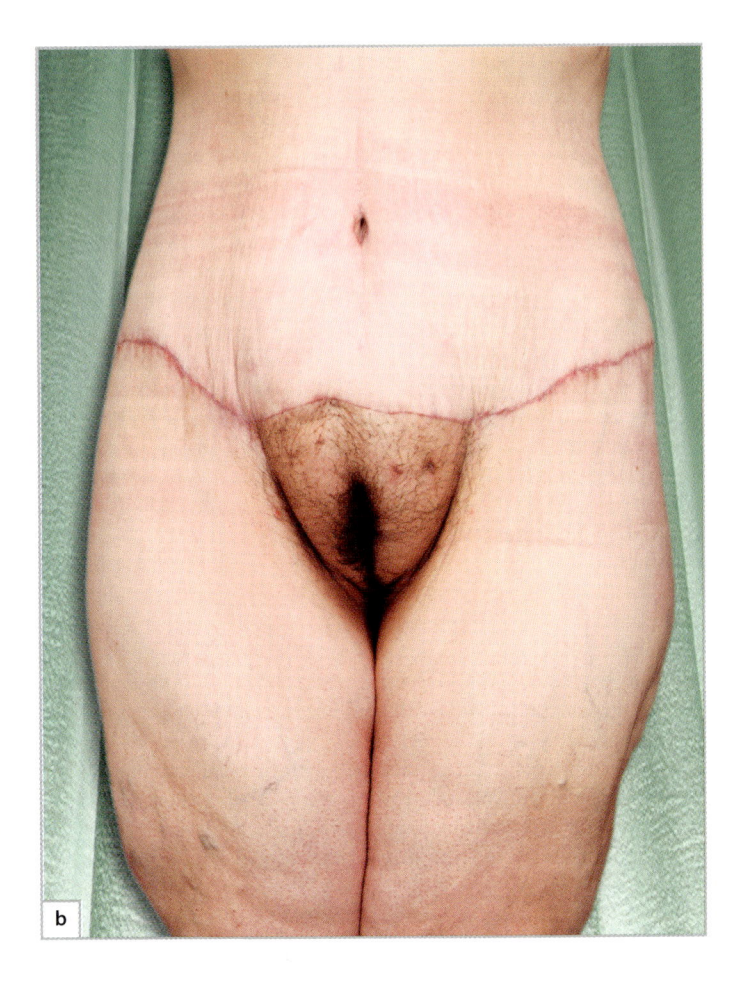

Figure 7.8 Patient 3 *Contd...*

Complications | 51

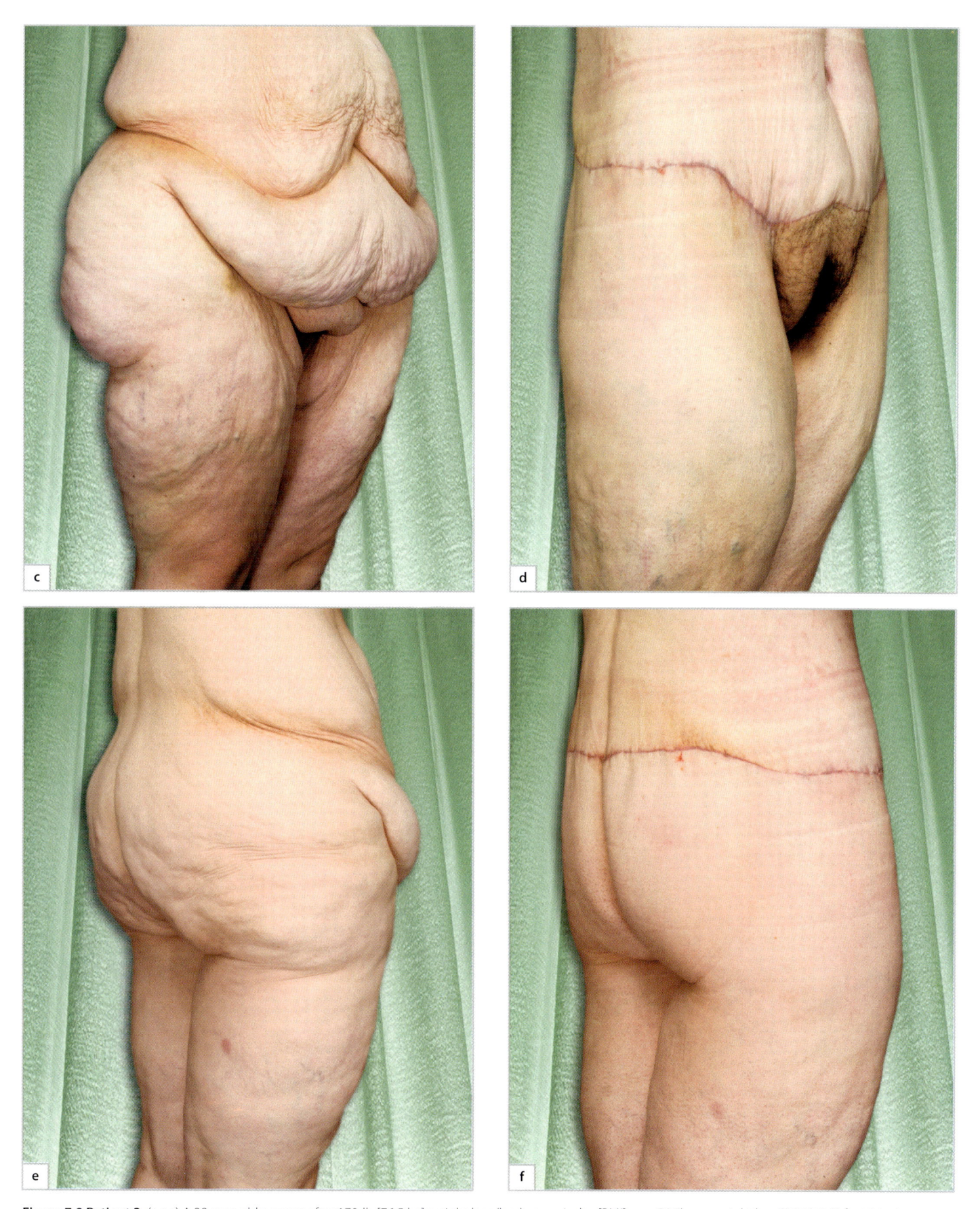

Figure 7.8 Patient 3. (a,c,e) A 38-year-old woman after 170-lb [76.5 kg] weight loss (body mass index [BMI] now 30.7); pre-weight loss BMI 58.1 (5 feet 6 inches tall [1.68 m], 360 lb [162 kg]). (b,d,f) A 6-week postop circumferential belt lift (type 2) plus liposuction of lateral thighs (8110 g excision + 1600 ml suction-assisted lipectomy); 21.4 lb [9.6 kg] removed, 6 h 30 min surgical time. Outpatient.

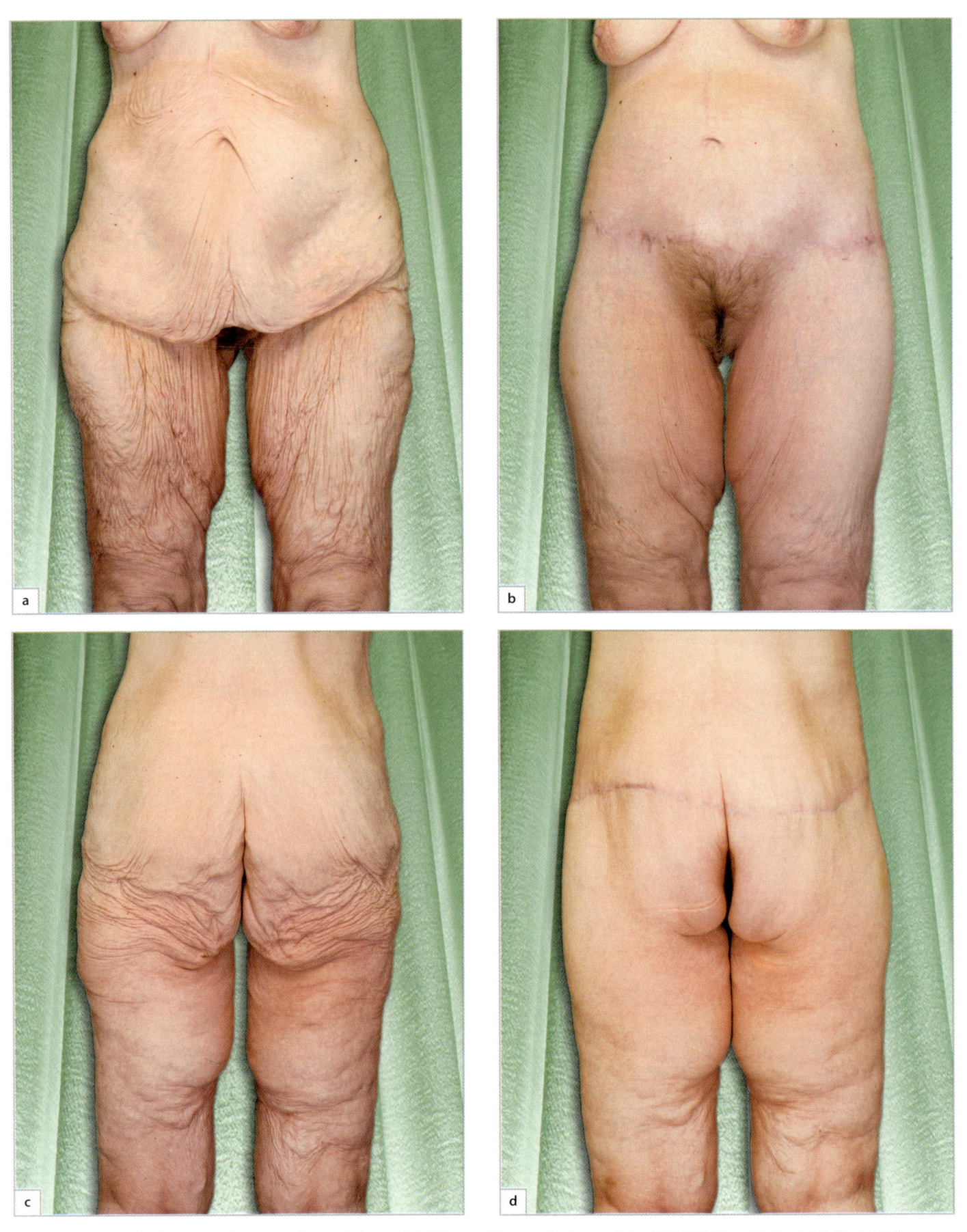

Figure 7.9 Patient 4. (a,c) A 67-year-old woman after gastric bypass in 1979 at age 36; current body mass index (BMI) 25.9 (5 feet 4 inches tall [1.63 m], 153 lb [68.9 kg]). (b,d) Seven months postop circumferential belt lift (type 2): 8.4 lb [3.8 kg] excised, 5 h 15 min surgical time. Outpatient.

Complications 53

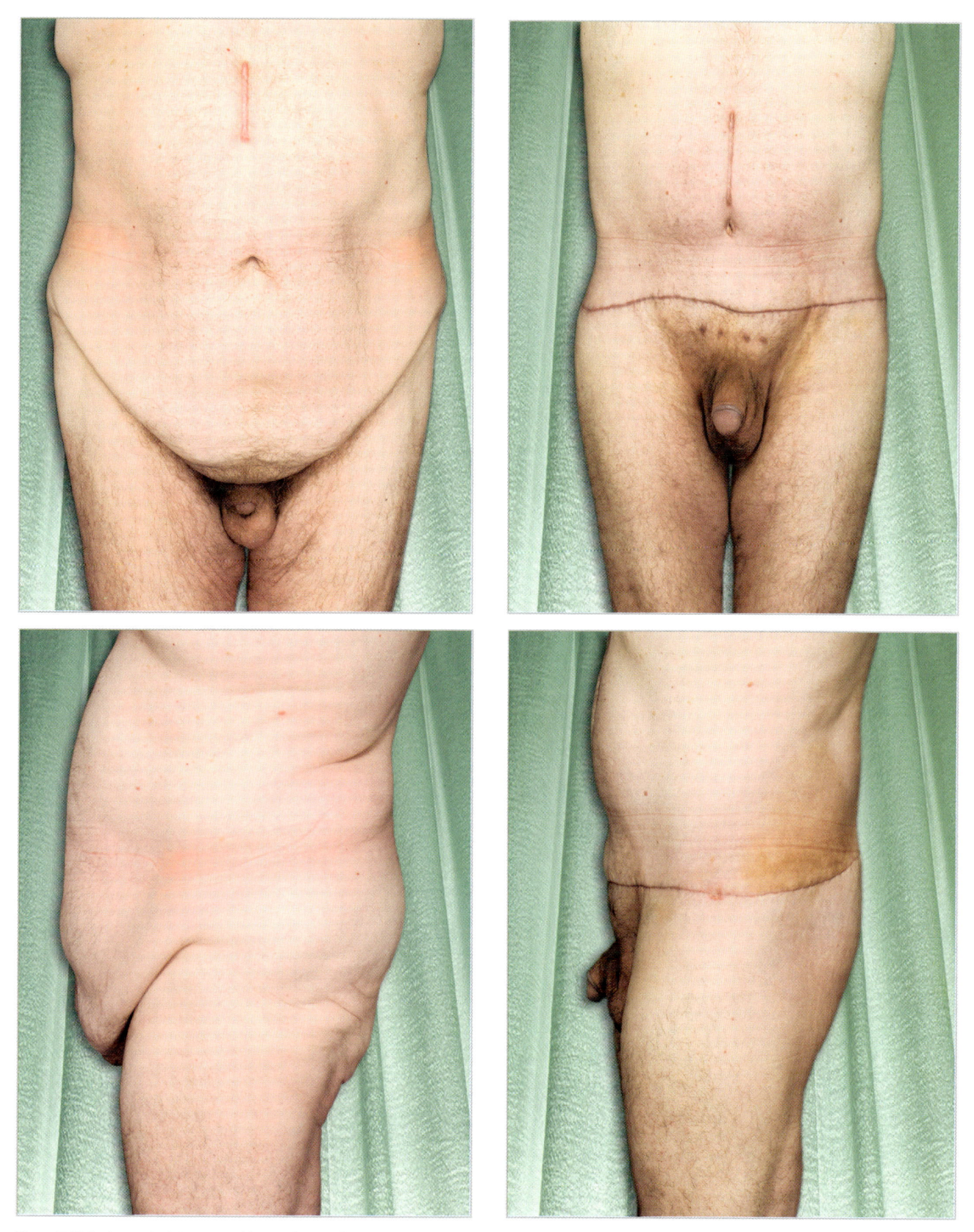

Figure 7.10 Patient 5. (a,c) A 62-year-old man after 110 lb 49.5 kg] weight loss (body mass index [BMI] now 28.1); pre-weight loss BMI 43.9 (5 feet 10 inches tall [1.78 m], 306 lb [162 kg]). (b,d) Ten weeks postop circumferential lower body lift (type 2): 14.0 lb [6.3 kg] excised, 5 h 30 min surgical time. Outpatient.

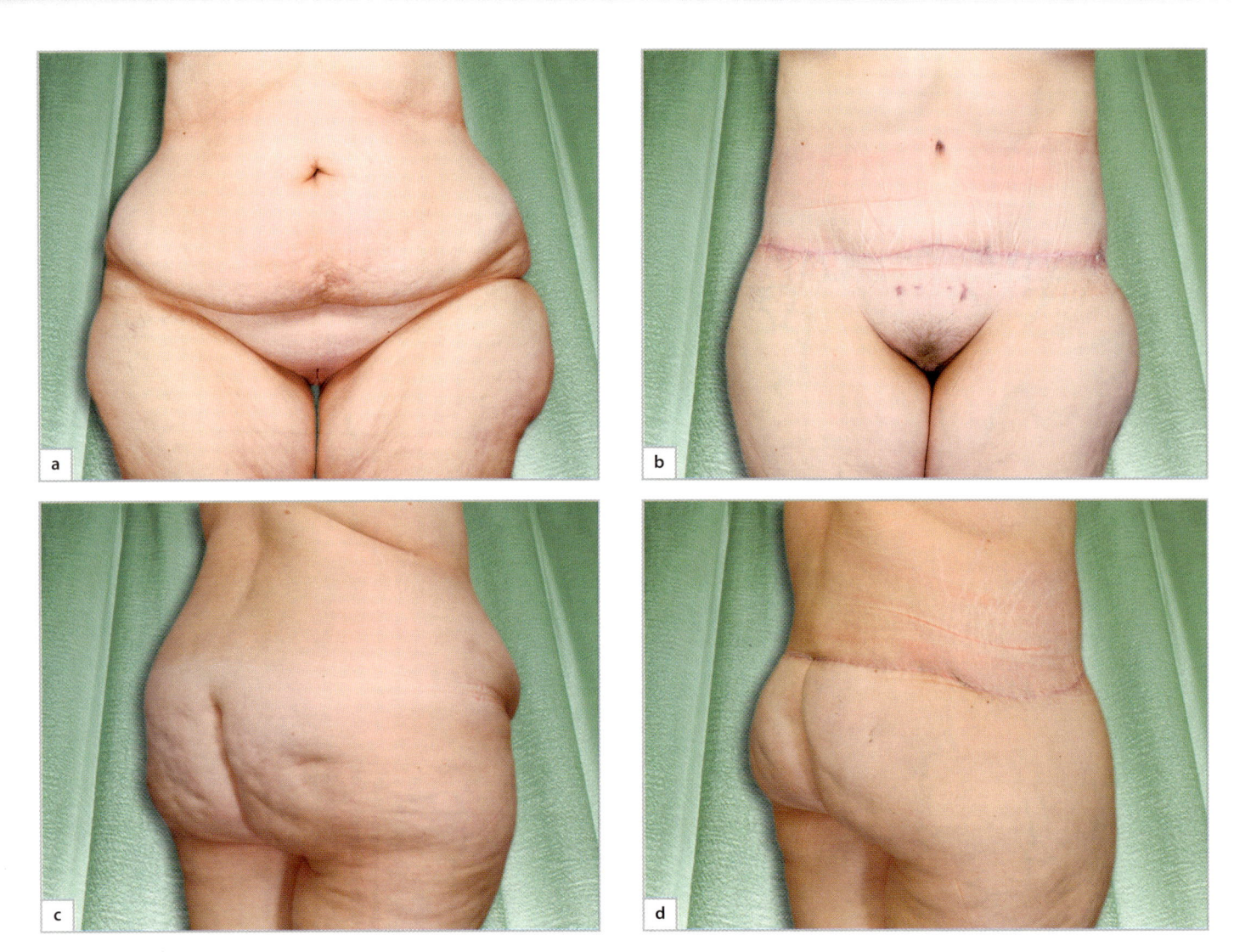

Figure 7.11 Patient 6. (a,c) A 40-year-old woman after 100 lb [45 kg] weight loss (body mass index [BMI] now 28.1); pre-weight loss BMI 42.8 (5 feet 9 inches tall 1.75 m), 290 lb [130.5 kg]). (b,d) Three months postop circumferential lower body lift (type 2) plus liposuction of hips and lateral thighs (9575 g excision + 3750 ml SAL) 29.4 lb [13.2 kg] removed, 7 h 25 min surgical time. Outpatient.

four surgical pseudobursectomies (including the patient managed elsewhere who returned to our care) were required, each healing uneventfully after reoperation.

Other management alterations in later patients who developed persistent drainage/seromas included earlier sclerodesis (after 2 weeks), more concentrated sclerosant (2–4 g tetracycline in 50 ml saline), and earlier drain reinsertion. A compression binder or garment was continued as long as drainage persisted, although this led to another concern – maceration and wound breakdown in the posterior suture line at the gluteal cleft.

Seroma formation and prolonged drainage from the posterior flaps remain a focus of ongoing investigation, because this remains the biggest recovery challenge from the patient's perspective. Additional complications are summarized in **Table 7.3**.

Other than prolonged drainage/seroma, minor wound dehiscence was the most common complication in our series, all but one healing with conservative nonsurgical management. One patient had a posterolateral 18-cm wound dehiscence in the early postoperative period when she kicked her legs vigorously trying to disentangle from her bed sheets. No further healing problems were noted after reclosure.

The most common location for incisional healing problems was just above the gluteal cleft. Excessive tension did not appear to play a role in the wound issues here, but rather skin–skin maceration exacerbated by use of the compression garment. Various methods were utilized to reduce this area of chronic moist irritation, including Benzoin/Tegaderm adherent film placed at the time of surgery (failed frequently due to early loss of adherence), use of dry gauze dressings to prevent/minimize skin–skin contact, and simply opening the compression garment, cleansing the incision line, and using a hair dryer on cool setting to dry this area once or twice daily. Six of seven minor wound breakdowns requiring re-excision and closure under local anesthesia were in this area; one was anterolateral in the thin tissue layer overlying the pelvic rim.

Suture line maceration and early scar widening are also noted for type 1 lower body lifts in the medial thigh–vulva region. This was also the area where yeast/fungal inflammation was noted in several patients. Stopping topical antibiotic ointment and oral antibiotics, topical treatment with clotrimazole and/or oral diflucan, as well as frequent dry gauze dressing changes and cool hair dryer use, prevented any dehiscences requiring reoperation in our 23 type 1 patients. Addition

Table 7.3 Complications associated with 263 outpatient circumferential lower body lift patients over a 14-year period at Minneapolis Plastic Surgery, Ltd.

Seroma:	Drainage 4–62 days[a] (mean 29 days)
Tetracycline sclerodesis with drain(s) in place	68 of first 100 patients (68%)
Tetracycline sclerodesis with drain(s) in place	103/263 (39%)
Recurrent seroma after drain removal	89/263 (34%)
Surgical pseudobursectomy	4/263 (1.5%)
Dehiscence: 14 (minor); 1 (major); 8/15 reclosed	15/263 (5.7%)
Infections: 6 (bacterial); 3 (yeast); 1 debridement (MRSA)	9/263 (3.4%)
Ischemic healing (suprapubic, umbilicus, thigh)	4/263 (1.5%)
Hematoma (1 late, aspirated; 1 transfusion)	2/263 (0.8%)
Phlebitis/DVT/PE[b]	0/263 (0%)
Skin loss	0/263 (0%)
Unplanned hospital admission	0/263 (0%)
PONV	9/263 (3.4%)
Reoperation (other than drain reinsertion):	13/263 (4.9%)
Dehiscence	8 (1 major – general anesthesia; 7 minor – local anesthesia)
Pseudobursectomy	4 (all 4 general anesthesia)
Debridement	1 (for MRSA-infected autologous buttock flap)

[a]One patient treated elsewhere not included.
[b]One pulmonary embolism (PE) 6 weeks postop documented by ventilation–perfusion scan.
DVT, deep vein thrombosis; MRSA, meticillin-resistant Staphylococcus aureus; PONV, postoperative nausea and vomiting.

of a running 3/0 Prolene in this medial thigh–vulva area reinforced the buried interrupted skin closure used in all other areas. This suture is removed at 12–14 days postoperatively.

Infections were infrequent (3.4% overall), with a third being the yeast infections noted above. These all responded to conservative management. Of the six bacterial infections, three were noted to be fecal bacteria, and two of three patients were cat owners. Although this is anecdotal, we now recommend pet-free zones for recovery of our patients. One patient presented with purulent drainage, erythema in the posterior suture line, low-grade fever, and uncharacteristic malaise of several hours' duration. She was taken immediately to the operating room and the wound opened. A portion of one autologous buttock augmentation flap showed signs of ischemic necrosis and, after culture, aggressive debridement was carried out. Irrigation and drainage catheters were placed, and the wound re-closed in layers utilizing only monofilament PDS sutures. The patient showed immediate improvement in the recovery room, and at the time of discharge reported her malaise to be 'gone.' Intraoperative cultures subsequently showed meticillin-resistant *Staphylococcus aureus* (MRSA) for which appropriate therapy was already under way. Other than loss of a portion of the buttock fullness that she wished for, the remainder of her course was uneventful.

When ischemia was noted, topical nitropaste (NitroBID topical) was applied three times daily. All such areas (four, small in size) recovered and healed without reoperation. Although skin flap undermining is often much more extensive in MWL patients, vascularity of the flaps corresponds to the previous bulk of the tissue, and cutaneous circulation seems enhanced, not diminished, after substantial weight loss.

One small hematoma was noted in the same patient who had the dehiscence requiring re-closure, and may have been induced by the same excessive motion causing the wound breakdown. The second hematoma occurred several weeks postoperatively in a patient whose anticoagulants were re-started by his cardiologist while drains were still in place. No healing sequelae or difficulties were seen in this patient until lateral thigh fluctuance was noted after drain removal; several hundred milliliters of liquefied blood were aspirated. This patient's physician ordered transfusion; no further difficulties were encountered in the healing process.

No patient in our series experienced phlebitis, deep venous thrombosis, or pulmonary embolus (PE) within 30 days of surgery. One patient experienced chest pain 6 weeks postoperatively (after returning to work and normal activities), and evaluation identified PE via ventilation–perfusion scan. Treatment was initiated and the patient remains well. Although her PE was more likely related to her daily 1-hour commute (one way) than to surgery, its identification is no less important or cautionary. We utilize sequential compression foot pumps in every general anesthetic case in our office surgical facility, as well as TED hose, early ambulation, and encouraged hydration. We do not routinely use enoxaparin (Lovenox), but employ it where indicated.

CONCLUSION

Although circumferential lower body lift is a lengthy operation (relative to most elective outpatient procedures) with numerous important procedural considerations, at heart it is a skin-fat removal and tightening operation that is not only safe but appropriate for performance as an outpatient. Patients and their doctors who view this as a 'major, potentially-dangerous, risky, and complication-prone' operation tend to reinforce their perception that this is an expensive, extensive, and 'serious' surgery which mandates inpatient care and several days' recovery in the hospital. Hospital anesthesia practices further validate this misconception, and may encourage a patient's perceived need for recovery, immobility, bed rest, and assistance. Hospitals co-validate this perception by providing bed rails, nurse call buttons, bedpans, and activity limitations rather than individualized recovery plans.

We emphasize to our patients that safe and successful outpatient lower body lift is *less* a function of the surgical skill (or speed) of the authors. Anesthesia, in our opinion, is the more critical factor in allowing this operation to be safely carried out as an outpatient, and the attitude, mindset, and preconceptions of the anesthesia provider(s) have profound impact on a patient's acceptance of this paradigm.

Outpatient procedures, besides being significantly more cost-effective, can actually be superior in avoiding exposure to sick patients or resistant nosocomial bacteria, while requiring a baseline of increased ambulation, routine self-care activity, and personal awareness that is often surrendered when hospitalized. Our practice stresses availability of our staff and surgeons to our patients. Patient awareness that they are the focus of our efforts, rather than an 'interruption' of our work, is critical to making outpatient lower body lift surgery not only possible, but safe, effective, and perhaps even better than as an inpatient. Factoring in substantially-reduced costs makes this a pathway to increased availability as well as enhanced outcomes.

REFERENCES

1. Ogden CL, Carroll MD, Curtin LR, et al. Prevalence of overweight and obesity in the United States, 1999-2004. *JAMA* 2006;**295**:1549–55.
2. American Society for Metabolic and Bariatric Surgery. Fact sheet: *Metabolic and Bariatric Surgery*. Available at: http://asmbs.org/asmbs-press-kit (accessed May 2011).
3. American Society for Aesthetic Plastic Surgery. ASAPS Statistics: Complete charts, 2010. Available at: www.surgery.org/media/statistics.
4. Van der Beek ES, van der Molen AM, van Ramshorst B. Complications after body contouring surgery in post-bariatric patients: the importance of a stable weight close to normal. *Obes Facts* 2011;**4**:61–6.
5. Coon D, Gusenoff JA, Kannan N, et al. Body mass and surgical complications in the postbariatric reconstructive patient: analysis of 511 cases. *Ann Surg* 2009;**249**:397–401.
6. Au K, Hazard SW 3rd, Dyer AM, et al. Correlation of complications of body contouring surgery with increasing body mass index. *Aesthet Surg J* 2008;**28**:425–9.
7. Vastine VL, Morgan RF, Williams GS, et al. Wound complications of abdominoplasty in obese patients. *Ann Plas Surg* 1999;**42**:3–39.
8. Garza CA, Pellikka PA, Somers VK, et al. Structural and functional changes in left and right ventricles after major weight loss following bariatric surgery for morbid obesity. *Am J Cardiol* 2010;**105**:550–6.
9. Rider OJ, Francis JM, Ali MK, et al. Beneficial cardiovascular effects of bariatric surgical and dietary weight loss in obesity. *J Am Coll Cardiol* 2009;**54**:718–26.
10. Gonzalez-Ulloa M. Belt lipectomy. *Br J Plast Surg* 1961;**13**:179–86.
11. Lockwood T. Lower body lift with superficial fascial system suspension. *Plast Reconstr Surg* 1993;**92**:1112–22.
13. Aly AS, Cram AE, Chao M, et al. Belt Lipectomy for circumferential truncal excess: the University of Iowa experience. *Plast Reconstr Surg* 2003;**111**:398–413.
14. Hurwitz DJ, Agha-Mohammadi S, Ota K, Unadkat, J. A clinical review of total body lift surgery. *Aesthet Surg J* 2008;**28**:294–303; discussion 304–5.
12. Lockwood T. Lower-body lift. *Aesth Surg J* 2001;**21**:355–69.
15. Spector JA, Levine SM, Karp NS. Surgical solutions to the problem of massive weight loss. *World J Gastroenterol* 2006;**12**:6602–7.
16. Hurwitz DJ. Single-staged total body lift after massive weight loss. *Ann Plast Surg* 2004;**52**:435–41; discussion 441.
17. Shinn HK, Lee MH, Moon SY, et al. Post-operative nausea and vomiting after gynecologic laparoscopic surgery: comparison between propofol and sevoflurane. *Korean J Anesthesiol* 2011;**60**:36–40.
18. Kim GH, Ahn HJ, Kim HS, et al. Postoperative nausea and vomiting after endoscopic thyroidectomy: total intravenous vs. balanced anesthesia. *Korean J Anesthesiol* 2011;**60**:416–21.
19. Gupta A, Stierer T, Zuckerman R, et al. Comparison of recovery profile after ambulatory anesthesia with propofol, isoflurane, sevoflurane, and desflurane: a systematic review. *Anesth Analg* 2004;**98**:632–41.
20. Hachenberg T. Perioperative management with short-acting intravenous anesthetics. *Anaesthesiol Reanim* 2000;**25**:144–50.
21. Smiley BA, Paradise NF. Does the duration of N2O administration affect postoperative nausea and vomiting? *Nurse Anesth* 1991;**2**:13–18.
22. Pavlin DJ, Chen C, Penaloza DA, et al. Pain as a factor complicating recovery and discharge after ambulatory surgery. *Anesth Analg* 2002;**95**:627–34.

Chapter 8

Sequencing and timing of surgery of the postbariatric patient

Dennis J. Hurwitz

▎INTRODUCTION

The strategy for body-contouring surgery after massive weight loss (MWL) matches patient deformity and motivation to an inventory of operations offered by an experienced plastic surgeon. A surgeon should combine clinicial expertese, artistry, technical excellence, and inspiring leadership.[1] At the surgeon's disposal are a set of classic cosmetic body contouring operations such as abdominoplasty, mastopexy, thighplasty and brachioplasty that have been modified to treat extensive after MWL deformities.

After a surgeon becomes proficient in each cosmetic procedure, he or she can proceed to multiple operations in a single session. The goal is not only to skillfully execute but also to efficiently integrate as many operations as deemed safe. Our own prior experience, after receiving self-referred partially treated patients, leads us to believe that frequent surgical sessions are less apt to be well coordinated and achieve anticipated aesthetic goals. Moreover, piecemeal surgery consisting of single or two operations at a time usually fails to complete surgical rehabilitation by virtue of premature physical and/or financial exhaustion of the patient.

Total body lift (TBL) surgery was conceived as a coordinated and artistic reconstruction of the MWL deformity from arms to knees in as few stages as safely possible.[2,3] TBL surgery of MWL patients results in extraordinary physical and psychological transformations.[4] We have extensive experience with all manner of staging TBL surgery, from single to four separate surgical sessions.[5,6] This chapter presents our current approach to staging TBL surgery based on treating over 300 patients since 1999.

▎PRESENTATION

The consultation elucidates the deformity and the patient reaction to it. Although often initiated through the internet, the consultation requires an hour in an office interview and examination. A shorthand form has ben designed to streamline documentation (**Fig. 8.1**). The prospective patient should have been sent a copy of our patient education book, *Total Body Lift*.[7] If read as instructed, the book will help patients rapidly assimilate the repeated information, including the principles behind each procedure, realistic expectations, the postoperative recovery, and risks. Then they simply have to focus on the particulars of their situation. If they have not read the book, they are then given a copy and encouraged to read it carefully later and compare it with the information presented during their consultation.

Anticipating extensive surgery, we explore in detail the candidate's motivations and behavior. Understanding major concerns allows us to design a personalized and coordinated efficient series of procedures that will fit the patient's needs and expectations.

A thorough medical evaluation including assesment of prior common obesity comorbidities such as mental depression, gastric reflux, hypertension, sleep apnea, asthma, diabetes, malnutrition, and anemia is essential.

We analyze the patient deformities in detail. We document and assess them using the Pittsburgh grading scale.[8] We note the location of rolls and folds of the torso, upper arms, and thighs, and ptosis of the breasts, buttocks, and mons pubis. Each specific deformity is placed in the context of neighboring features and the full body. A 360° guided tour through a full-length mirror is revealing to both the surgeon and the patient. Although the patient's awareness of his or her physical disorder may be limited, he or she will readily communicate the emotional and physical impact. We document the pattern and magnitude of skin laxity, fat deposition, and cellulite (skin quality). Discordance between the patient's and surgeon's assessments should be resolved; if that is not possible, consider body dismorphic disorder which requires psychological support. A consensus to the problems leads to a preliminary multistaged treatment plan.

Corrective aesthetic surgery is delayed until after the weight lost has stabilized and there is no further anticipated changes. Predictable stability improves the longer the interval between a stable weight and the scheduled body-contouring surgery. As a general rule, 1 year after bariatric surgery and 6 months after a stable weight loss is an adequate elapse of time. Our clinical observations mirror studies published by bariatric surgeons, in that the rapid weight loss after bariatric surgery reaches a plateau at 18 months and a 20% regain of the excess weight will occur over the next year. On the other hand, the stability of MWL achieved by caloric restriction and exercise is less predictable than after weight loss surgery. As such, we prefer >2 years of stability before initiating body-contouring surgery in the lifestyle weight loss patient. Significant weight gain will mitigate the improved aesthetics of body-contouring surgery.

Patients are assessed for malabsorption and treated. In addition, we seek to identify restrictive eating disorders. Excessive and persistent weight loss is a serious problem that needs investigation. Eating disorders, food intolerances, food eccentricities, supplement excess, vomiting, purging, and diarrhea may result in malnutrition that not only diminishes the aesthetic result, but also causes life-threatening wound healing and infectious complications.[9]

▎OBESITY AND MASSIVE WEIGHT LOSS

Obesity to some extent causes irreversible distension of the tissues as well as local and systemic inflammation. Under this burden, excess subcutaneous adipose permanently stretches the dermis and

Total Body Lift   /   /201
Name   Age
Height   Wgt   BMI
Highest / Lowest Wgt: /
Method/ Date of Wgt loss

Wgt loss Hx
Dress size B/A loss   /
Bra Size B/A loss: /
Belt size B/A loss   /
Clothing
Shoulder/ Neck/ Back pain
Intertigo
Intimacy, Mental, Social
Activity

Hernia
Apnea. Asthma.
Diabetes. HBP.
Arthritis,
Depression.
GERD.
Med/Surg

Supplements
Food Intolerance
Meds
Smoking/ Alc./ Drugs
Breast disease
Bleeding disorders
ROS:

Arms: 0 1 2 3
Skin 0 1 2 3
Fat 0 1 2 3
Axilla 0 1 2 3
Limited Brachio.
 ❏ L Brachio.
 ❏ Liposuction.

Breasts: 0 1 2 3
Chest Symmetry
Breast/ Axillary Mass
Breast Shape
 Symmetry
NAC Symmetry
NAC ptosis I II III
Laxity
Footprint

Surgeon:
Breast Parameters: Right   Left
Sternal Notch to Nipple
Nipple to IMF Fold
Nipple to Midline
Nipple position
Base Width
Areolar Diameter

Breast Reshaping
❏   Peri-areolar
❏   Circumvertical
❏   Wise
❏   Silicone
❏   Dermal Susp.,
❏   Spiral Flap
❏   Lipoaugmentation
❏   Gynecomastia

Mammary Fold
IMF Elevation
Obliteration

Resection/Augmentation
R   cc.   L   cc.

Abdomen: 0 1 2 3
Epigastric Prominence 0 1 2 3
Pannus 0 1 2 3
Mid abdominal adherence 0 1 2 3
Adipose 0 1 2 3
❏   Limited
❏   Standard
❏   Extended
❏   Plication
❏   T
❏   UAL abd flanks hips

Back: 0 1 2 3
Breast
Scapula
lumbar
Lower back roll
❏   Vertical Excision
❏   Upper Transverse Excision
❏   Combination
❏   Liposuction

Flanks: 0 1 2 3
❏   Liposuction
❏   Direct Excision

Obesity and massive weight loss 59

Mons: 0 1 2 3
- ❏ Liposuction
- ❏ Picture Frame

Buttocks: 0 1 2 3
A V Boxy Round
Large, Flat, Ptotic
- ❏ Buttock Lift
- ❏ Adipose flap
- ❏ Lipoaug

Hips/Lat. Thighs: 0 1 2 3
Saddlebag 0 1 2 3
- ❏ Lower Body Lift
- ❏ Liposuction

Medial Thighs: 0 1 2 3
- ❏ Upper Medial
- ❏ Spiral

Lower Thighs, Knees: 0 1 2 3
Medial
Anterior
Posterior
- ❏ Vertical
- ❏ Liposuction

Upper: Arms, Breast, Abdomen, Flank, Back
  1-5 Mild   6-10 Moderate   11-15 Severe

Lower: Mons, buttocks, Hips/Lat thighs, Medial Thighs, Lower Thighs/Knees
  1-5 Mild   6-10 Moderate   11-15 Severe

Total Body:
  1-10 Mild   11-20 Moderate   21-30 Severe

Surgery Plan

Stage 1

Stage 2

Stage 3

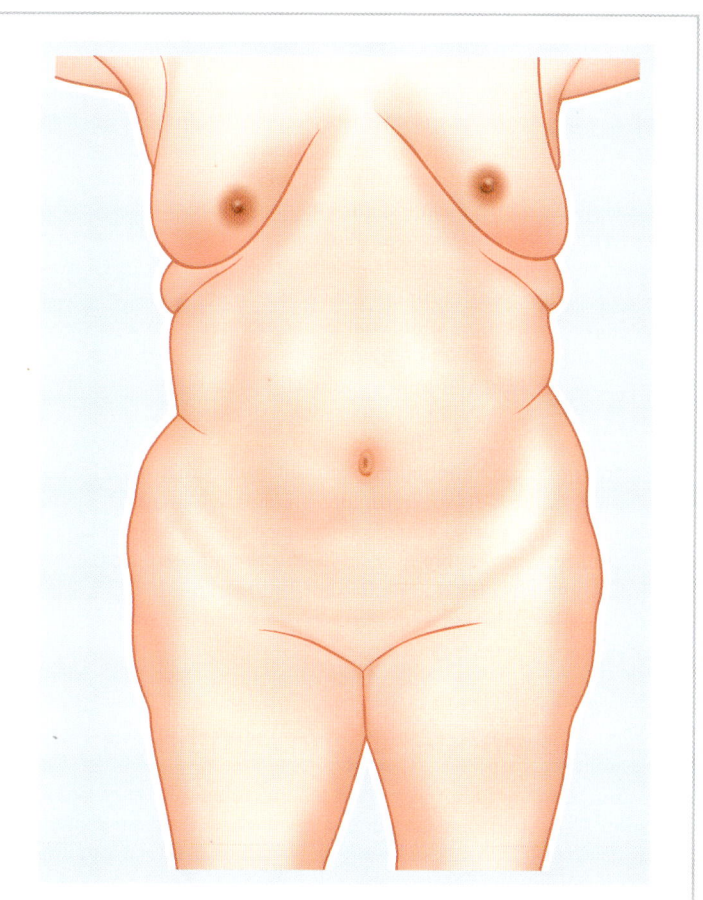

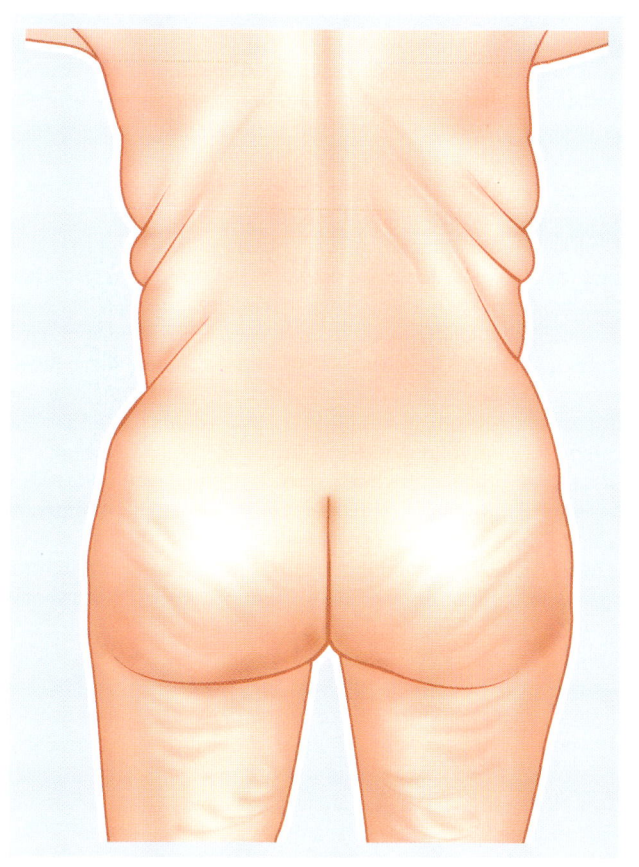

Figure 8.1 Short-hand form for total body lift.

supporting connective tissue. Prolonged food restriction causes a negative caloric balance and then MWL in obese individuals. As the major store of energy, adipose tissue is depleted of triglycerides, causing shrinkage of the individual cells and a reduction in the volume. This deflation is the primary source of skin laxity with undesirable contours. In addition there is some irreversible destruction of collagen and elastin support. These changes occur throughout the subcutaneous tissues of the body, but to a greater degree in previously excessive fat deposits. As women store relatively larger volumes of fat in their subcutaneous tissue, they more dramatically exhibit skin laxity. Nevertheless MWL men do present with profound skin laxity and gynecomastia.

PREPARATION

The patient follows our preoperative preparation protocols before scheduling the initial operations. Looking for psychological, hepatic, hemotological, and nutritional disorders, we obtain a thorough history, exam, and a battery of laboratory studies. Attention is paid to patient activity, illnesses, and skin and mucosal quality.

Correction of anemia and malnutrition

All patients must drink ProCare MD (from Nutressential) twice weekly, which contains a variety of micronutrients including arginine and glutamine.[10] Surgery should be delayed until anemia, nutritional deficiencies, and abnormal lab values are corrected. Oral iron supplements may not be adequately absorbed, necessitating intravenous iron infusions. B-complex vitamins are supplemented. For anemia that inadequately responds to these supplements, we treat with erythropoietin for 2 weeks before surgery.

Close monitoring and treatment of critical laboratory values such as the complete blood count (CBC), electrolytes, total protein, albumin, and prealbumin continue through the early postoperative recovery.

Psychological issues

Residual depression, disabling anxiety, and other psychological disorders are common. If under psychiatric treatment, the patient gives us permission to consult his or her doctor, who will become involved in planning and postoperative support. The medications may need adjustment. As these patients often have dependent and addictive personalities, the surgeon must firmly direct their care. A plan for postoperative pain management is introduced and followed. For opioid medication use beyond 6 weeks, consider management through a pain clinic. Our assistants, during the course of edema and nutriton mangement, seek symptoms of depression and anxiety. They alert us to the possible need for psycholytic medications. Through thoughtful therapeutic interaction, they help elevate the patient's emotions and mood, and perhaps adjust their expectations.

Inquiry is made of disruptive social and domestic issuues. Before initiating elective body-contouring surgery, seek resolution of disturbing discord or loss. Otherwise, the patient may be psychologically unprepared and lack a support system to deal with even minor complications. Also assess for unrealist patient expectations. Appropriate reactions to prior plastic surgery are reasuring; overconfidence in the surgeon's skills is not. A step beyond this is the body dismorphic disorder. Although rare in the MWL patient, BDD frustrates satisfaction and leads to unending requests for revision and inappropriate surgery.

Adjuncts (supplements, dieting and Endermologie)

All our well-nourished patients are instructed to drink two servings a day of ProCare MD for 2 weeks preoperatively and 2 weeks thereafter. Overweight patients are encouraged to lose weight by returning to their bariatric team or on their own. If unable to lose further weight, we offer a variation of the Simeon diet as taught to us by plastic surgeon Hassan Tazi of Morocco.[11] Patients are advised that the US Food and Drug Administration (FDA), through scientific inquiry during the 1980s, found that the hCG/500-calorie restrictive diet ineffective. The independent experiences of Drs Trudy Vogt, Hassan Tazi, and Dennis Hurwitz are otherwise. Through 42 days of human chorionic gonadotropin (hCG) hormone injections and a low-fat and low-carbohydrate 500-calorie a day rigorous diet, we are able to routinely achieve 15–30 lb (6.75–13.50 kg) weight loss, primarily within the abdominal cavity, without complications. Additional significant weight loss can be achieved by a second 42-day session. Further sessions are contraindicated due to pituitary suppression, sexual hormone inbalance, and possible ovarian cysts. Continuous supervision by our caring physician assistant achieves almost uniform patient compliance and satisfaction.

Preoperative preparation also includes a series of Endermologie treatments in our aesthetic center spa. Endermologie softens adipose for the anticipated liposuction, helps reduce postoperative edema, and shapes contours rapidly. We feel that our results are better and a rapport is created with one of the aestheticians, which serves everyone well during the difficult early convalesence.

EXAMINATION

After the patient has discussed their medical history and motivations, the medical assistant escorts him or her to a nearby exam room. From the onset, the surgeon observes her ease in exposing her body and notes excessive discomfort and inhibition. If she has unreasonable disdain, the physician is cautious.

Torso skin adherence and scars related to surgery are noted. Using a Pittsburgh grading scale form, the severity of deformity for each area is noted from 0 to 3 for skin laxity, adiposity, and cellulite, and then the grades are added to obtain a total score of deformity[8] (see Table 7.1). Any additional description is unusual because the photographs document the detail.

The exam is started in the area of most concern to the patient, which is usually the abdomen. As most patients are female we have used that gender. Understandably, males tend to be more relaxed and casual.

Abdomen

The patient stands on the exam table end platform in front of the surgeon in a short toga-like gown clipped at the shoulder. With her permission, the gown is opened as if parting a curtain to expose her abdomen. This presentation is viewed and documented and she is asked to pull up her pannus to reveal the underlying lower abdomen, noting any scars, fat deposits, rashes, post-inflammatory hyperpigmentation, laxity, hanging mons pubis, symmetry, and adherences. All the while the surgeon considers the role of liposuction, retention of adipose tissue, and the incision pattern. Seeing a modicum of new-found comfort, the surgeon asks permission to touch and grasp her skin and, once given permision, proceeds to move her skin to simulate and describe her abdominoplasty in front of a mirror.

Thighs and lower body

After a glance assessment of the thighs, we ask her to turn away, whereupon the surgeon raises her gown over her shoulder to examine the back, buttocks, and posterior thighs. Then he grasps the areas of concern in order to show the patients, with the help of the mirror, the problems that he can see more clearly then she can. By transversely grasping and pinching the hip, lower back, and upper thighs, the effect of a lower body lift and posterior thigh lift is demonstrated. The same is done for the midback. Having achieved rapport and understanding, the surgeon asks her to again stand and face him and pull up her pannus. He sits before her to grasp her inner thighs to simulate an upper and vertical medial thighplasty while looking in the mirror.

Supine abdomen

With the gown closed, she is asked to sit down. She then lies down and raises her straightened legs as the surgeon palpates for abdominal hernias and assesses the contribution of intra-abdominal obesity to her standing contour. This maneuver is explained, and the patient's hands are placed in such a way as to palpate and grasp the abdomen to confirm the exam. In this way, she has a realistic understanding of what her abdominoplasty can achieve.

Breast and upper body

If she desires breast reshaping, the surgeon will observe, comment, and seek accord on the shape, symmetry, and footplate position of her breasts. Linear measurements typically taken for breast reduction, such as sternum to nipple, nipple to inframammary fold, etc. are taken. Then the surgeon palpates for breast lumps and tenderness. After this, she sits up and opens her gown to view her upper torso, breasts, and arms. The rolls and adherences are graded. The need for a reverse abdominoplasty is estimated. The upper body lift procedures of a bra line pinch approximation is compared with the J torsoplasty advancement. Then arm reductions are simulated by pinching skin together to demonstrate the extent of appropriate skin resection and scarring.

In the upper body, there are same considerations for managing loose skin and adipose tissue as in the lower body, except for the added component that the reverse abdominoplasty is suspended to the ribs. The spiral flap augments and suspends the breasts, and this is contrasted with the role of silicone implants. In general, the MWL female (as do we) distains implants and prefers spiral flap reshaping of her breasts.

Gynecomastia

Gynecomastia deformity is fully described to the patient. After MWL, it tends to be extensive with moderate nipple ptosis. We estimate the extent of glandular hypertrophy, which requires direct excision, and the excess fat, which is suctioned from the inferior pedicle to the nipple. We look for pectoralis major development and inquire about the patient's interest in weight training for enhancing pectoral bulk. Usually the masking gynecomastia has discouraged body building. We discuss the various procedures to correct gynecomastia from simple ultrasound-assisted lioplasty, through ultrasound-assisted lipectomy (UAL) with pull-through to perareolar mastopexy. The ultimate skin tightening over pectoralis major gynecomastia correction is UAL with a J-modified bomerang correction. The trade-off is a long chest zig-zag scar with possible hypertrophy.

Brachioplasty

Arm deformity is considered in isolation and as a continuum into the axilla and along the lateral chest. The upper arm excess is folded into itself along the medial aspect, as well as the lateral chest skin excision to simulate the left brachioplasty through the axilla. As we point out the excessive depth of the axilla, patients share the observation and complain of difficulty in shaving. They are elated at the prospect of reducing arm pit concavity at the price of a linear scar. They welcome the elimination of the under-arm chest roll. We expect an incomplete, about 80%, correction of arm excess because of complete reduction hazards over resection and tissue vitality due to early arm swelling. Secondary further skin reduction is a safer option that is explained and easily accomplished.

SHARED ANALYSIS AND PLANNING

Toward the end of the exam, we demonstrate, with the help of a mirror, what we hope to achieve, restating risks of hematoma, seroma, skin and fat necrosis, wound infection, and dehiscence. We also explain how the chosen combination of techniques will maximize contours and minimize risk. We reiterate that the more operations performed together, the more likely the wound healing complications, but the probabilities are additive and not multiplicative during each surgical session.

As the MWL patient is observed in mulitple positions, we consider ourselves as artists observing subject totality along with isolated figure faults. The character and quality of the tissue to be left behind are assessed for probability of recurrent laxity and this estimate is shared with the patient. The role of unalterable underlying musculoskeletal development is assessed and discussed, e.g. large thoracic cages and high riding pelvis due to oversized viscera will thwart creation of a sensual feminine figure. Each operation is considered in relation to its neighboring one in an effort to emphasize the gender-specific outcomes.

Together, the patient and surgeon prioritize treatment options, realizing that certain operations work better together. As the lower central torso tends to be of major concern and is the keystone of the body, abdominoplasty is pre-eminent. When the lower torso is not the main issue, there was a prior abdominoplasty, or the lower body is too large, the upper body, breast, and/or arms are approached first (**Figs 8.2** and **8.3**).

As the MLW deformity affects the entire body, a complete list of operations should be made by the surgeon even though the patient may present only one or two complaints. Most patients are well aware of the myriad of skin laxity issues and are very receptive to a full evaluation of what is wrong and a comprehensive treatment plan. On occasion patients discuss only one or two complaints which are typically about the hanging abdominal pannus, or sagging inner thighs or breasts. Often wary of the potential costs of extensive surgery, they do not reveal concerns about other areas. With their indulgence we perform a complete skin examination. The surgeon must offer an optimal treatment plan with alternatives, even if the patient rejects it.

COMBINING OPERATIONS

When the patient agrees to multiple areas for treatment, operations are combined. Much has been written about combining mulitple body-contouring operations. Which ones and how many are debated.[12-16]

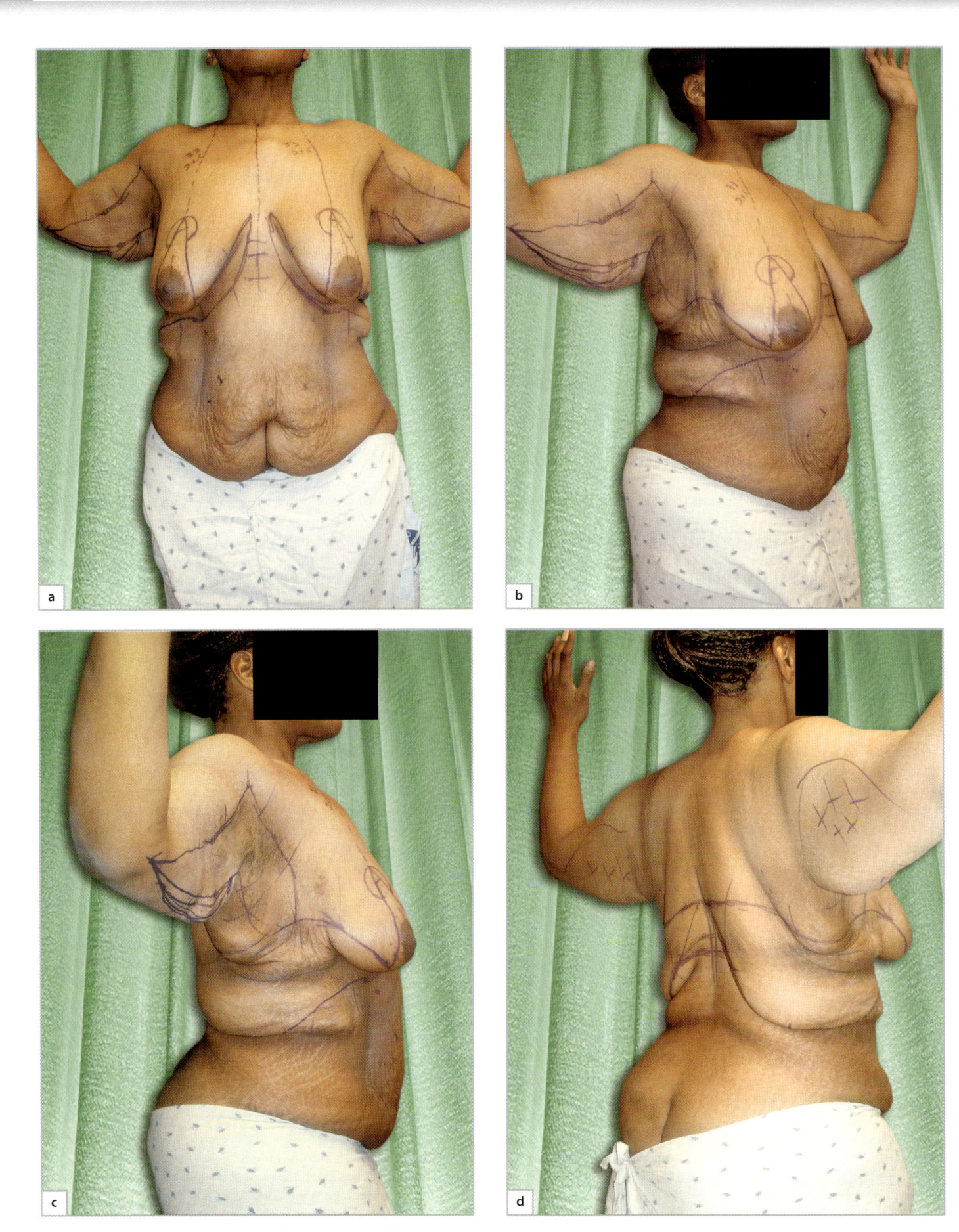

Figure 8.2 Multiple views of a 38-year-old woman. *Continued on p. 63.*

Combining operations

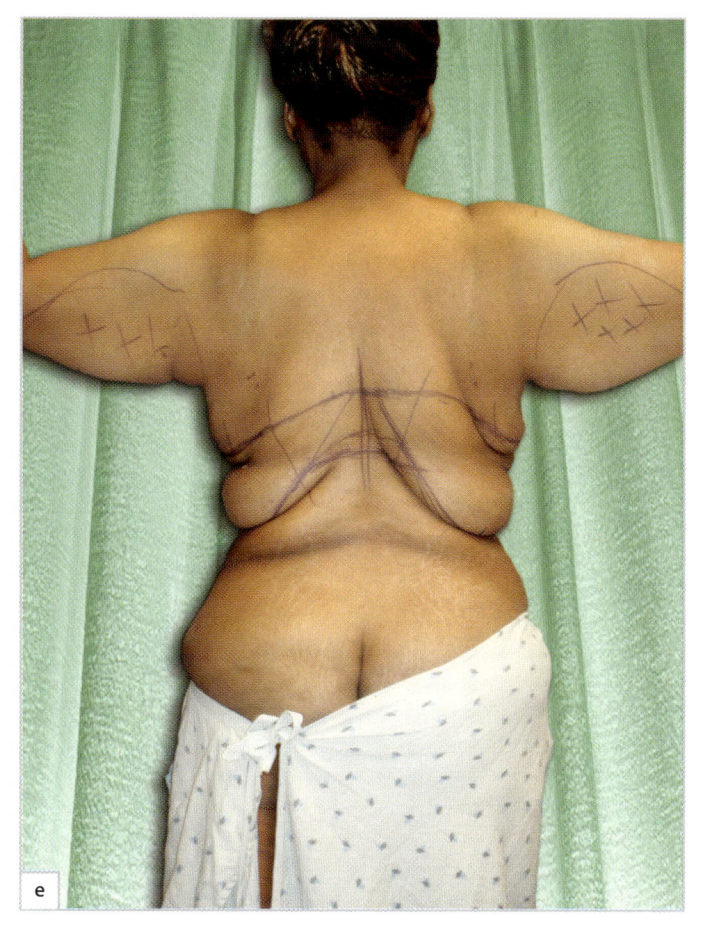

Figure 8.2 Multiple views of a 38-year-old woman, height 5 feet 5 inches (1.65 m), who weighs 225 lb (101 kg; body mass index [BMI] 38.7) after losing 80 lb (36 kg) from gastric bypass surgery. As her lower body is too large for body-contouring surgery, her first stage is marked for an upper body lift, liposuction of the central abdomen, reverse abdominoplasty, spiral flap reshaping of her breasts, and left brachioplasties.

Multiple operatons are reserved for healthy, motivated patients, willing to accept theoretically greater risks of complications. Multiple operations are not for patients with chronic diseases, poorly controlled diseases, such as hypertension, malnutrition, or diabetes, or recurrent acute illnesses. In such cases, in consultation with their primary care physician, we proceed cautiously with a single operation. This tends to be a panniculectomy or abdominoplasty, which would serve as a test to their capacity to recover.

We have no set pattern of operative combinations but we do plan under principles learned through experience.[3,17] For those more organized and regimented in their approach, we have published a series of algorithms, which are a comfortable starting point.[18-23]

There are global and focal considerations. Can the patient physically and emotionally tolerate an extended operation? Will the vectors of closure and reduced blood supply of contiguous operations compromise effectiveness and/or safety? Anticipated interruption of the blood supply during one operation should caution the use of an adjoining operation. An example of this is a fully undermined abdominoplasty combined with an upper body lift which includes a reverse abdominoplasty. This combination would also be of concern because of competing inferior and superior vectors of closure tensions on the epigastric skin, which may lead to wound dehiscence. Those articulated admonitions are ameliorated by the use of discontinuous undermining, with the preservation of cutaneous perforators and

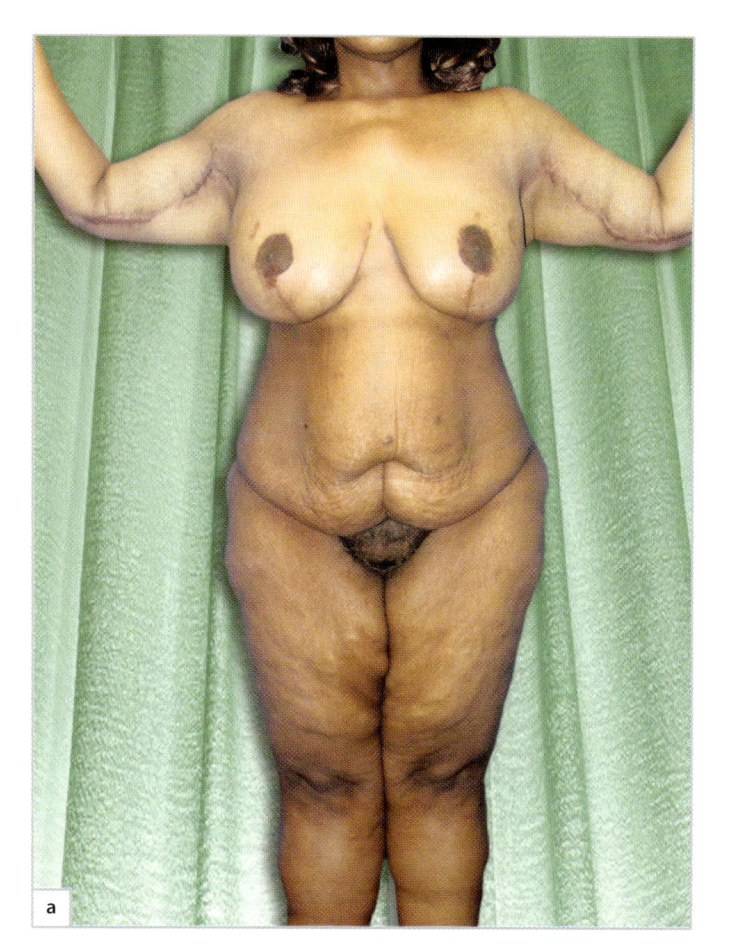

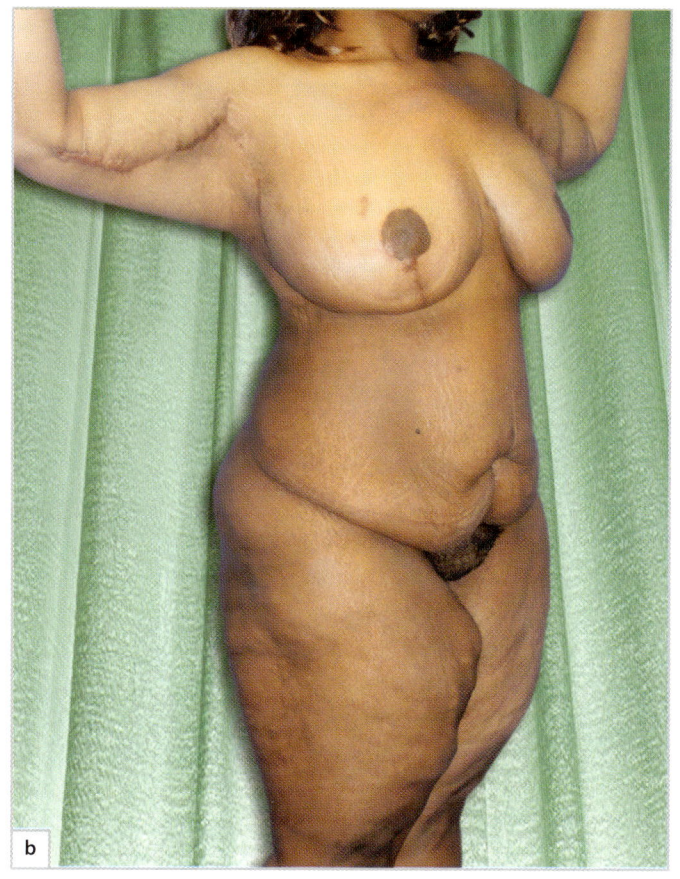

Figure 8.3 Similar views of the same patient 1 year later. *Continued on p. 64.*

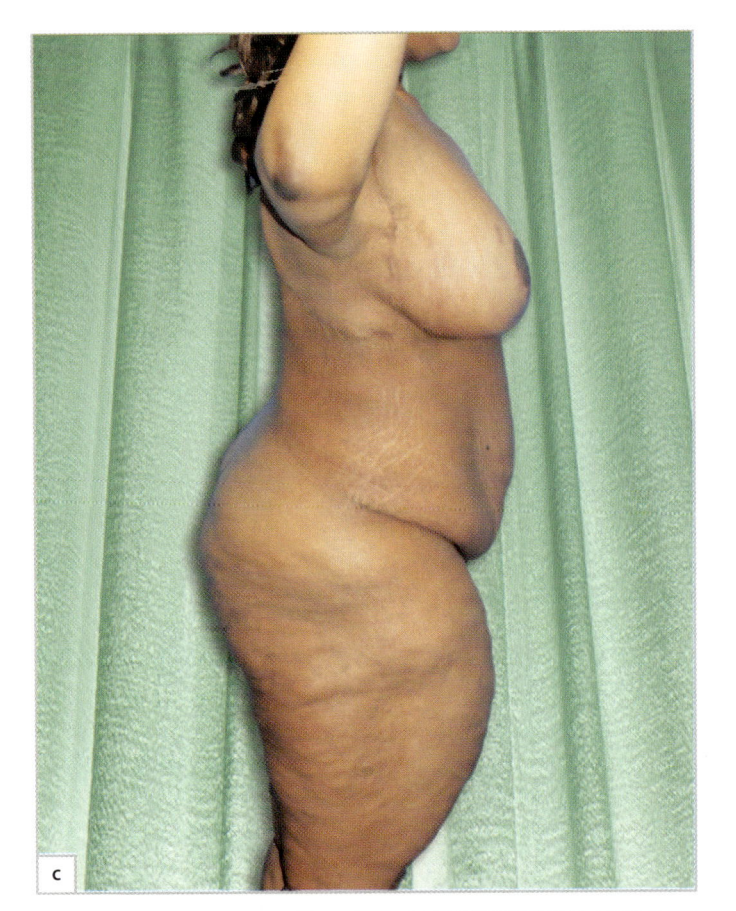

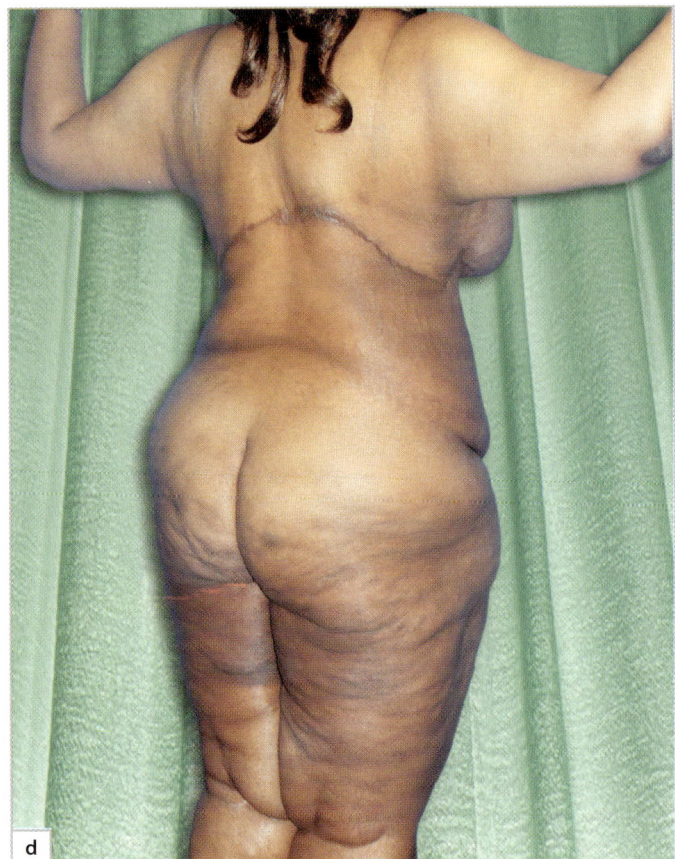

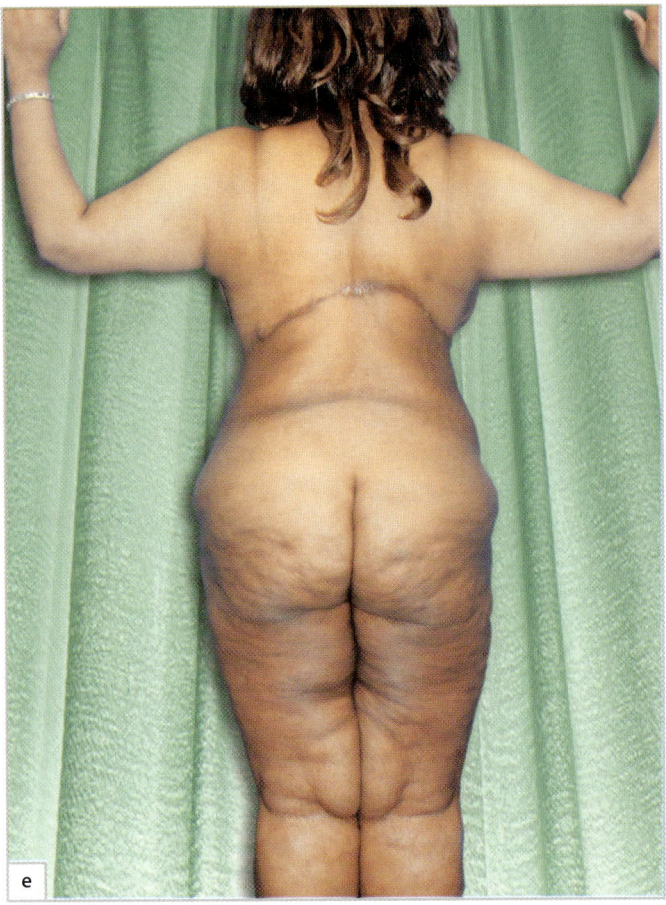

Figure 8.3 The same multiple views of the patient in Figure 8.2 nearly 1 year after upper body-contouring surgery. She had only several limited wound healing issues. She is pleased with the results of each of her operations and her total contouring, and now, 2 years later, unable to lose further weight, she accepts her body shape.

Combining operations

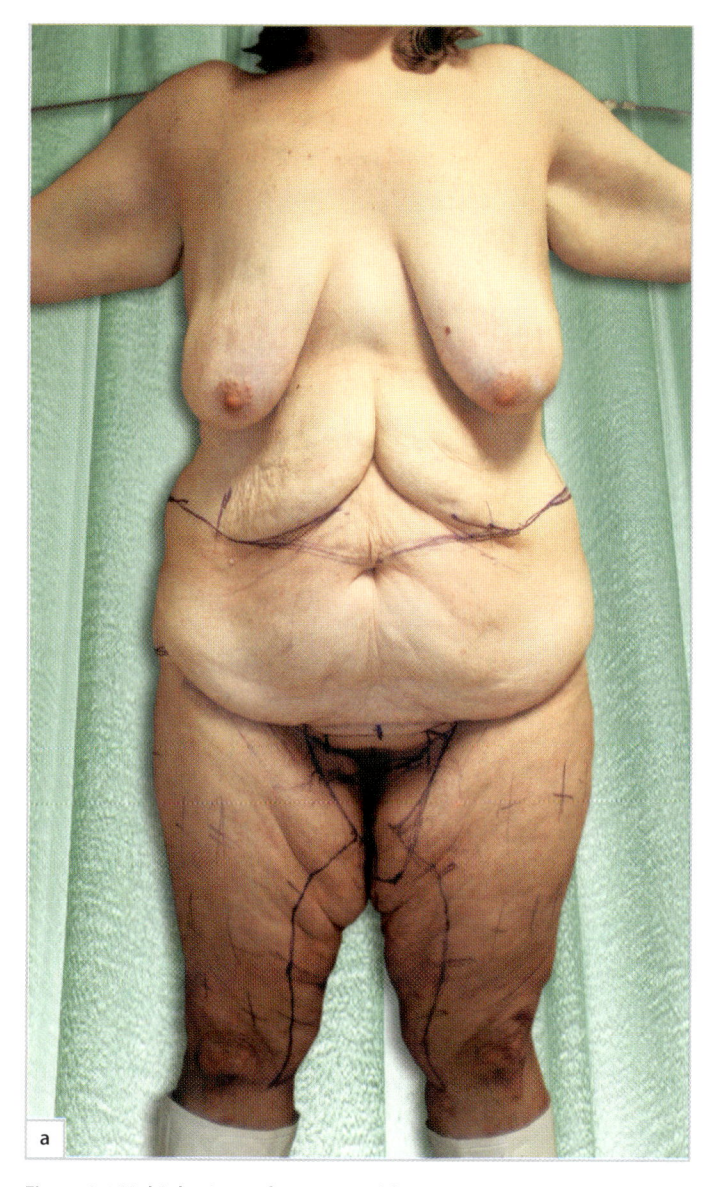

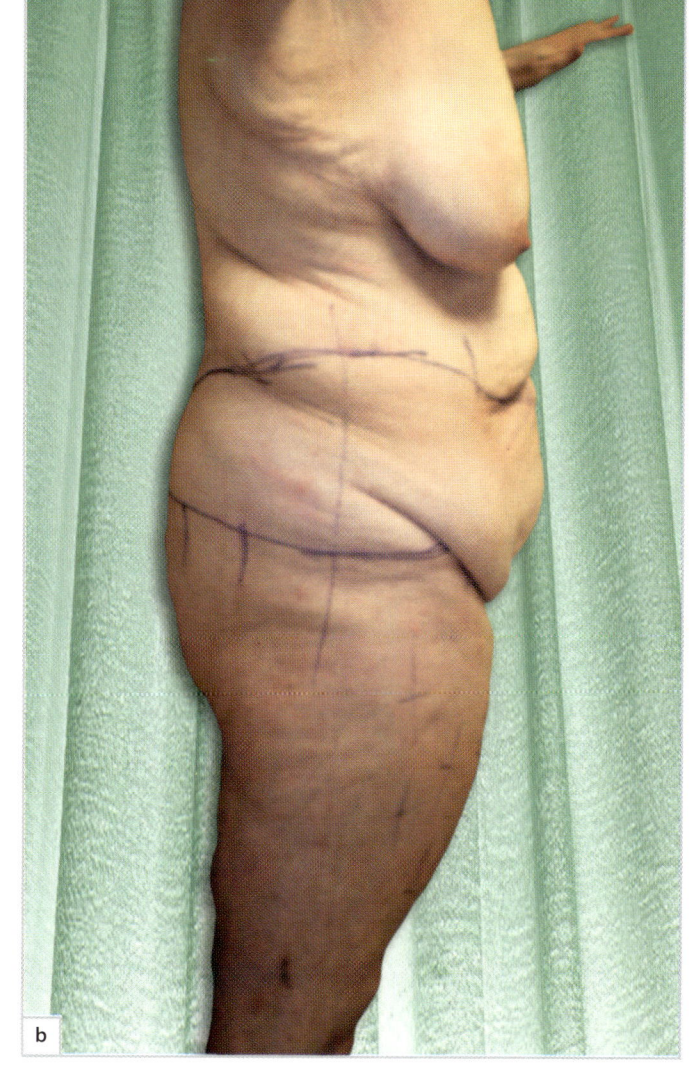

Figure 8.4 Multiple views of a 32-year-old woman. *Continued on pp. 66–67.*

the distancing of excisions beyond the point of competing vectors. As such, in thin patients with long torsos we readily perform lower and upper body lifts during the same surgical session. There must be either no or very limited direct undermining with liberal use of discontinuous dissectors, such as the LaRue distributed by ASSI to preserve perforators to the skin.

Finally, we limit multiple operations in obese patients because these patient are not as healthy and wound-healing complications are higher.[24–27]

Common groupings of operations

Correction of the lower anterior torso is fundamental to total body lifting, and as such abdominoplasty is the centre around which every other operation is built. Abdominoplasty is contiguous with the lower body lift, thighplasty, mons pubisplasty, and upper body lift. These close operations must be anticipated, whether performed at the same time or later. As one of the most impactful procedures that we offer, abdominoplasty in its traditional form, as well as the fleur-de-lys, have reasonable convalescence, low morbidity, acceptable scars, and pleasing results. An exception is the abdomen distended with visceral obesity and further complicated by fascial laxity. Unless the goal is simply a therapuetic panniculectomy, abdominoplasty in these cases should be preceded by further intra-abdominal weight loss, otherwise despite the sizeable resection of skin there will be modest improvement in contour, with epigastric protuberance.

The most common first stage consists of a lower body lift with or without an adipose fascial flap augmentation of the buttocks, a posterior thigh lift along the gluteal thigh crease, an abdominoplasty; and a vertical medial thighplasty (**Fig. 8.4**). The upper horizontal component of the medial thighplasty links the posterior thighplasty through the mons pubis to the abdominoplasty, forming a spiral thighplasty.[28] At this junction between the abdomen and the thighs a three-sided picture frame excision around the mons forms a multidimensional reshaping of a pleasing, slightly convex, appropriately sized, and aesthetic genital area.[29] Despite the admonitions of some expert body-contouring surgeons, we do not feel that the lower body lift and medial thighplasty have

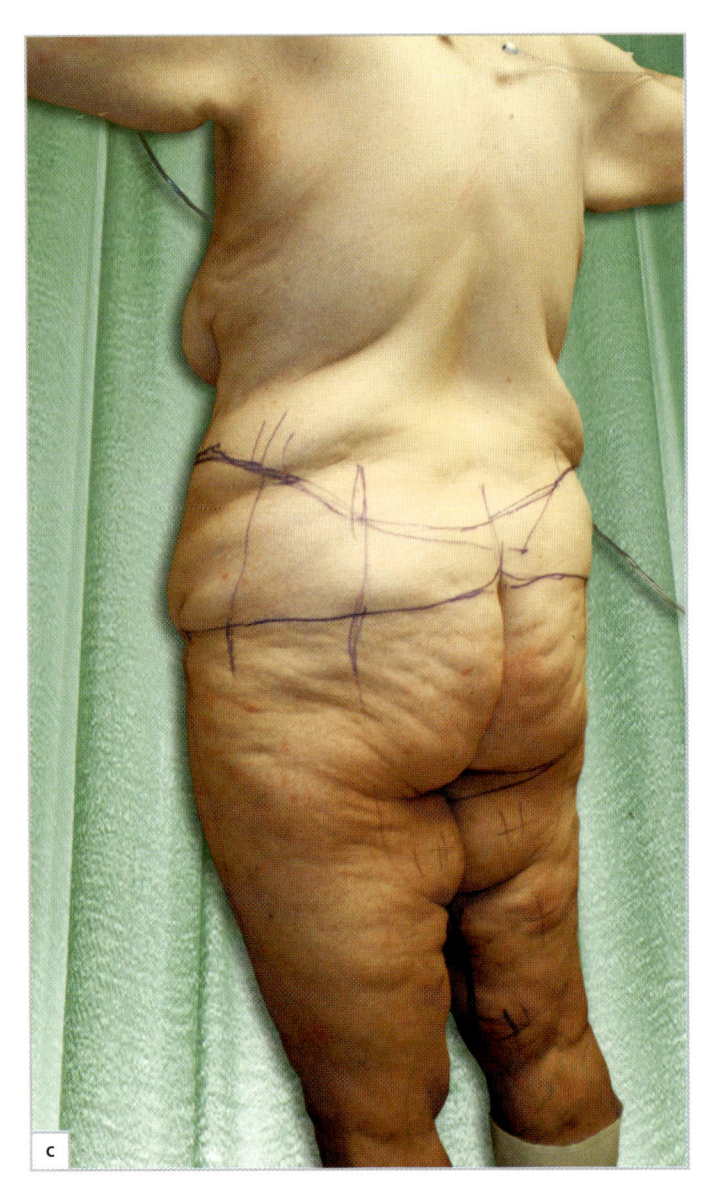

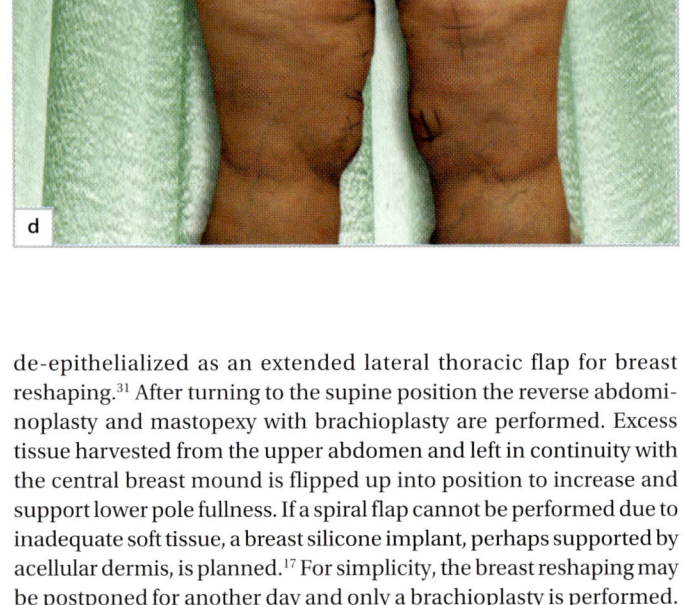

Figure 8.4 Multiple views of a 32-year-old woman. *Continued on p. 67.*

competing vectors.[14] We have described the vectors and diagramed these dynamics (**Fig. 8.5**).[7]

For massive thighs that require liters of liposuction, we do not combine a vertical thighplasty with a lower body lift. The almsot circumferential full-thickness surgical trauma to the upper thighs is of too great a magnitude, leading to unacceptable wound-healing complications such as seroma, wound dehiscence, and prolonged swelling. The lower body lift and thighplasty combination starts prone with the legs abducted on arm boards and the foot of the operating room table dropped. With an assistant at the foot of the table multiple operations can be performed with ease. The patient is turned supine for a team to perform the abdominoplasty and for another team the vertical portion of the medial thighplasty. The operation culminates in the transverse portion of the vertical thighplasty along with the mons pubicplasty.

The second stage or second part of a single stage of a TBL is an upper body lift that sets a higher level for the inframammary fold (IMF) in women and obliterate the IMF in men (**Figs 8.6** and **8.7**).[30] If the upper body lift has a bra line excision then that part had been performed when the patient was prone. The excised tissue can be de-epithelialized as an extended lateral thoracic flap for breast reshaping.[31] After turning to the supine position the reverse abdominoplasty and mastopexy with brachioplasty are performed. Excess tissue harvested from the upper abdomen and left in continuity with the central breast mound is flipped up into position to increase and support lower pole fullness. If a spiral flap cannot be performed due to inadequate soft tissue, a breast silicone implant, perhaps supported by acellular dermis, is planned.[17] For simplicity, the breast reshaping may be postponed for another day and only a brachioplasty is performed.

Intervals between operations

We wait a minimum of three months between lower body and upper body surgery. Over that period of time the wounds have healed and minor issues such as localize superficial dehiscences and minor infections have resolved. Anemia has been adequately treated. The predisposition towards deep vein thrombosis has resolved. Moreover the patient is ready to accept a second major operation. Having said that, after the patient has already gone through an abdominoplasty

Combining operations | 67

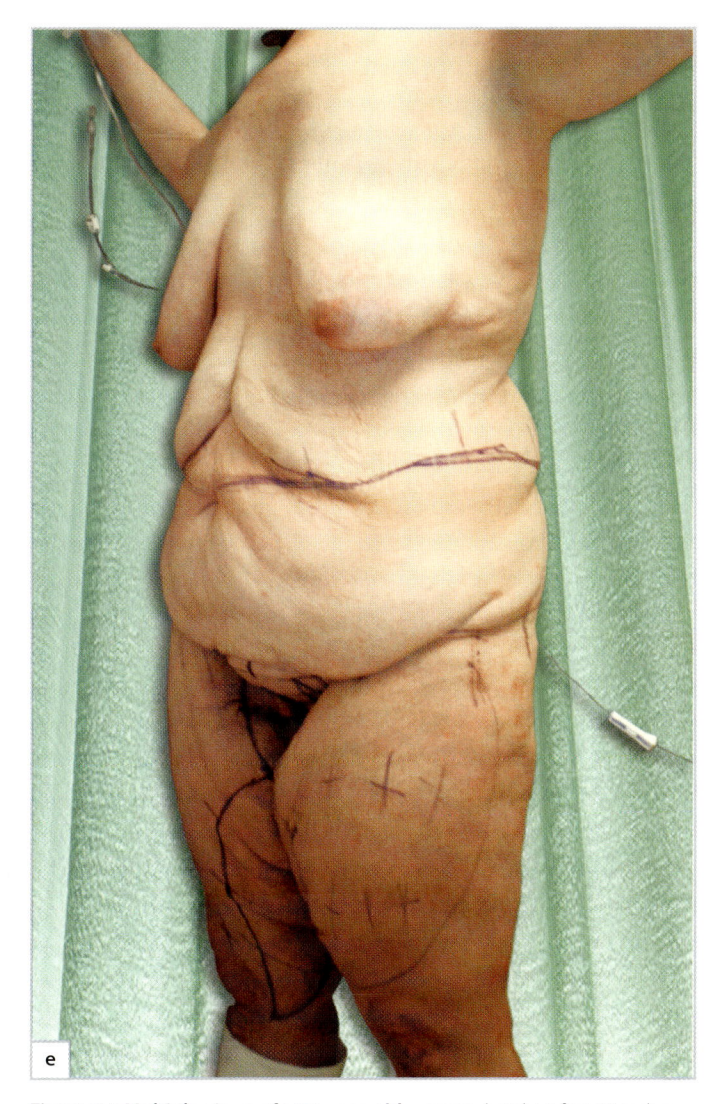

Figure 8.4 **Multiple views of a 32-year-old woman,** height 5 feet 10 inches (1.78 m), who weighs 210 lb (94.5 kg; body mass index [BMI] 32) after losing 150 lb (67.5 kg) from gastric bypass surgery. She is marked for the first stage of total body lift consisting of an abdominoplasty, lower body lift, and vertical medial thighplasty with liposuction.

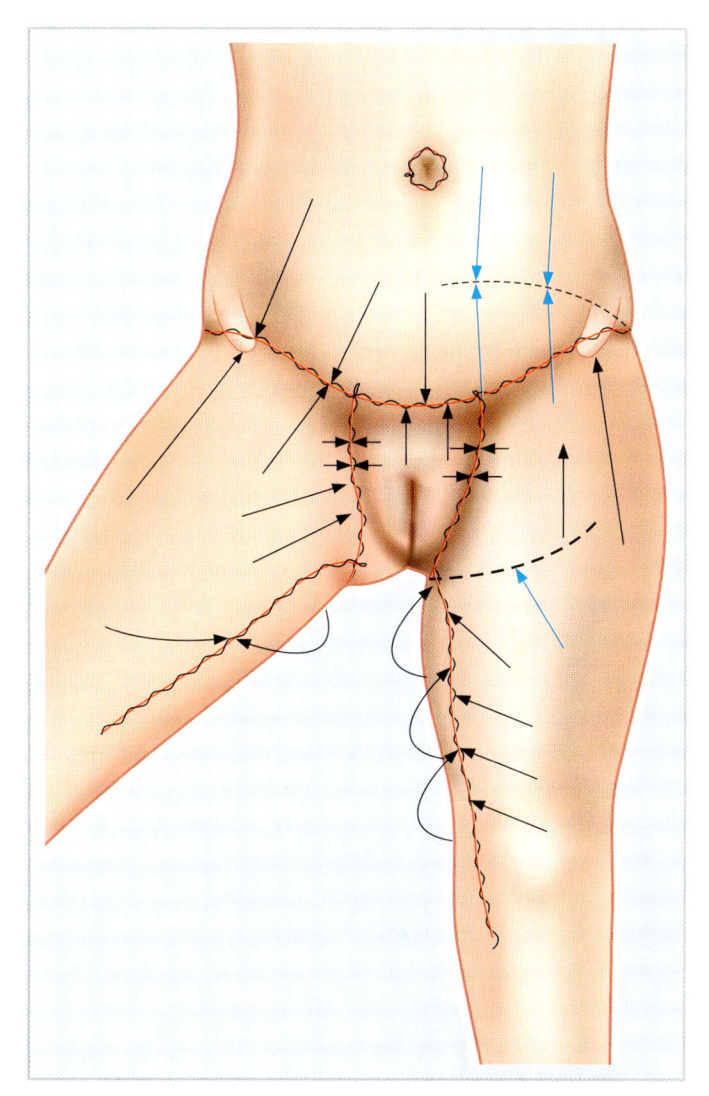

Figure 8.5 **This diagram represents the surgical plan, vectors of force of closures, and resulting scars after combining abdominoplasty, lower body lift with vertical medial thighplasty and mons pubicplasty.** The vectors are do not conflict; hence, one operation does not compromise the healing of another.

lower body lift combination, they should expect a much easier recovery from upper body lift surgery. It appears that the upper body lift combination is of lesser magnitude and is subjected to less hanging weight than the lower body surgery.

Criteria for single-staged total body lift

Early in our body-contouring surgery after MWL experience, we conceived single-stage TBL surgery.[2] Many patients favor this approach because they prefer to avoid several prolonged periods of painful convalescence. Prolonged operations on the skin are well tolerated. Skin surgery, even if extensive, does not induce the extraordinary inflammatory response and overall debilitation as experienced after prolonged operations on viscera or musculoskeletal systems. Furthemore, our cases are elective and well prepared compared with lengthy operations on severely traumatized, chronically ill, and cancer-burdened patients. Although our TBL patients experienced a high (66%) rate of complications, for the most part they were minor and without mortality.[5]

The minor revision rate was fairly high and patients are advised about this. However, these patients are highly motivated to limit convalescence time and expense. Some simply wanted to avoid the unpleasant anticipation of the second major operation. The precedent for such time-consuming complex surgery was experience in craniofacial surgery as well as complex microvascular reconstruction of head and neck, and breast. These patients tolerate the very long operations and we can attest that their adverse response to 8–10 hours of surgery was minimal. Upon entering the recovery room, TBL patients are fully conversant with what has happened, and aside from incisional pain feel very good.

There does not appear to be any aesthetic benefit to a single-stage over a two-stage TBL in women. However, in men performing the boomerang correction of gynecomastia, abdominoplasty at the same time does have a total body-smoothing effect that improves the anterior chest aesthetics.

Due to the shear magnitude of TBL, we most often use the two-stage procedure. As there is a consensus among experts that elective operations lasting longer than 6 hours are to be avoided, single-stage TBLs are now performed only under special circumstances. Our clinical experience has been supportive of the selective use of single-stage TBL. Neverthelss, only patients who meet our strict criteria are considered for single-stage TBL (young [<50], medically, psychologically, and physically fit, normal weight, highly motivated, and thereby willing to accept slightly increased risk of complications).[3]

■ KEYS TO SUCCESS

TBL surgery combines the priorities of the patient with the surgeon's ability to plan and execute the surgical experience. Success comes with proficiency in team work, improving efficiency, avoiding intraoperative hypothermia, and minimizing complications.

■ Team surgery

Team surgery is proficient if the plastic surgeon is secure and ably leads experienced assistants. The surgeon must be confident in the acccuracy of the preoperative markings. The surgical markings of skin excision are conservatively placed with the possibility of tangential excision of more tissue if the closure is loose. With proper attention to detail, surgical markings, which should be adjusted in the exam room until confident, will not need to be significantly altered during the operation. Until the lead surgeon is convinced of the preoperative markings, it is better to limit simultaneous surgery.

As we have found that skilled and experienced assistants can follow the surgical plan and markings to remove the excess fat skin and close while under direct lead surgeon observation, we seek the patient's acceptance. With minimal to no compromise in outcome, extensive surgery can be performed in incredibly short times with experienced teams. The surgeon must be an able leader, planning the entire continuum of the operations and allowing for contingencies. An example of such a problem is a substandard performance of a junior surgical member. Attention to this will distract the surgeon from his or he rassigned duties and delay the operation; however, the assistant's education and/or reasignment is necessary for this and subsequent cases.

At the outset, the surgeon leader advices the assistants of the surgical plan, elucidating the goals and soliciting their optimal particpation. He or she recognizes the assistants skills and limitations and motivates them by encouraging maximum performance, followed by appropriate and timely compliments and criticisms. There should be no hesitation to take over and repeat substandard work. The surgeon sets a hard-working focused example and advances with confidence. Nevertheless, he or she avoids arrogance and overbearance, always being respectful of an assistant's sensitivity and limits. In fact, as a senior surgeon, combining operative intervention with directing junior team members on another section of the body is stimulating and rewarding. You have to be sure of their surgical skills and

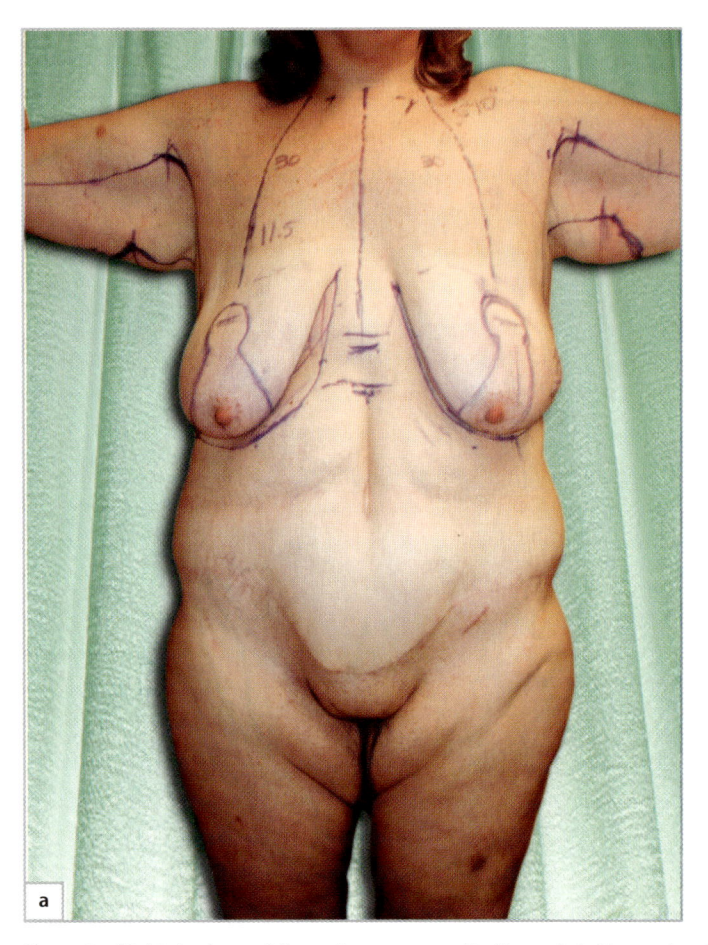

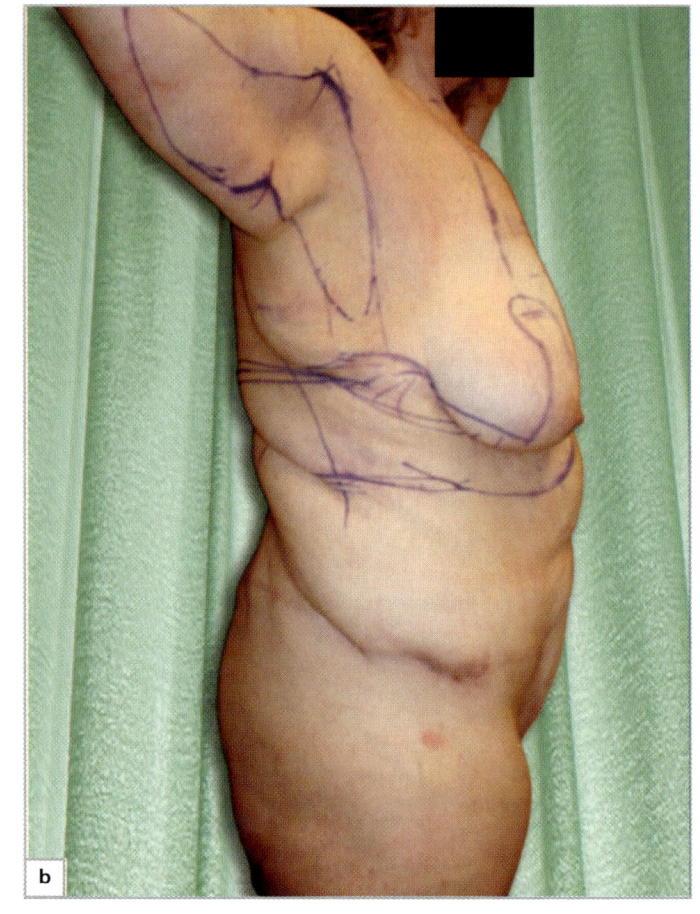

Figure 8.6 Multiple views of the patient presented in Figure 8.4, 10 months after her lower body lift, abdominoplasty, and vertical thighplasty. *Continued opposite.*

Keys to success | 69

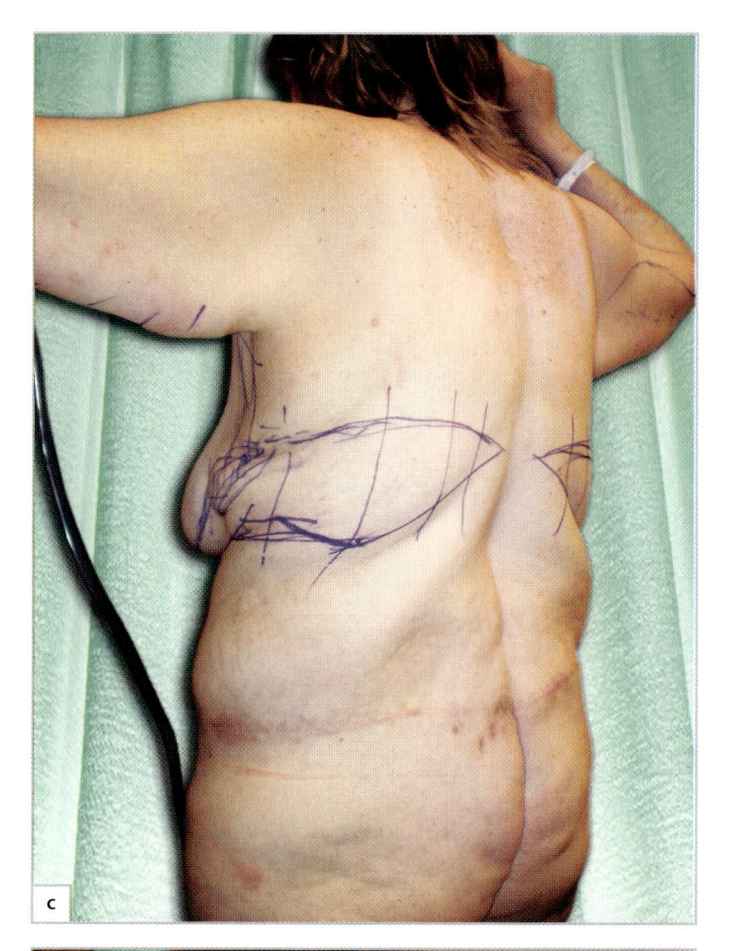

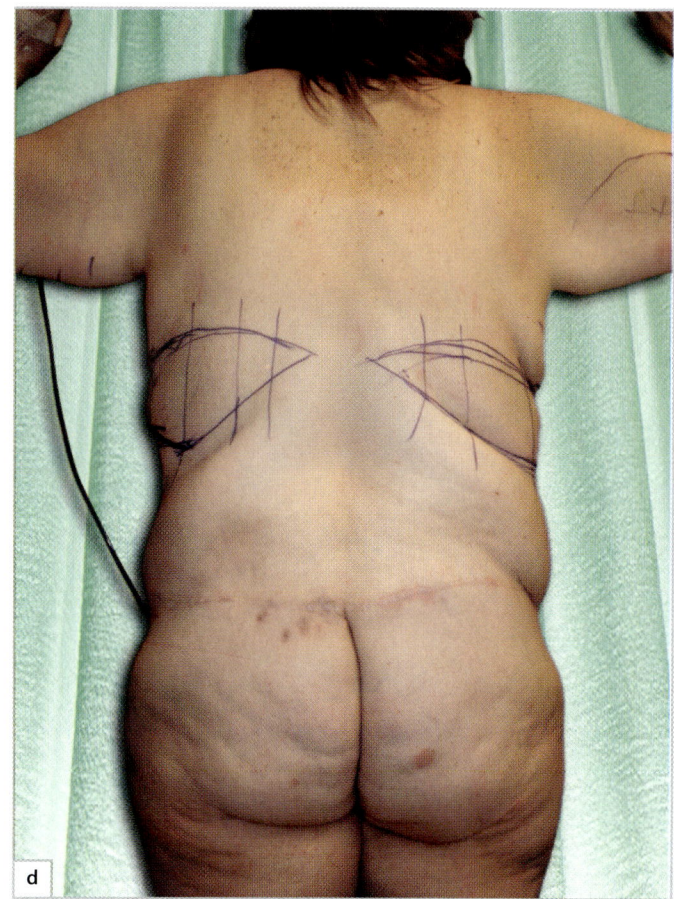

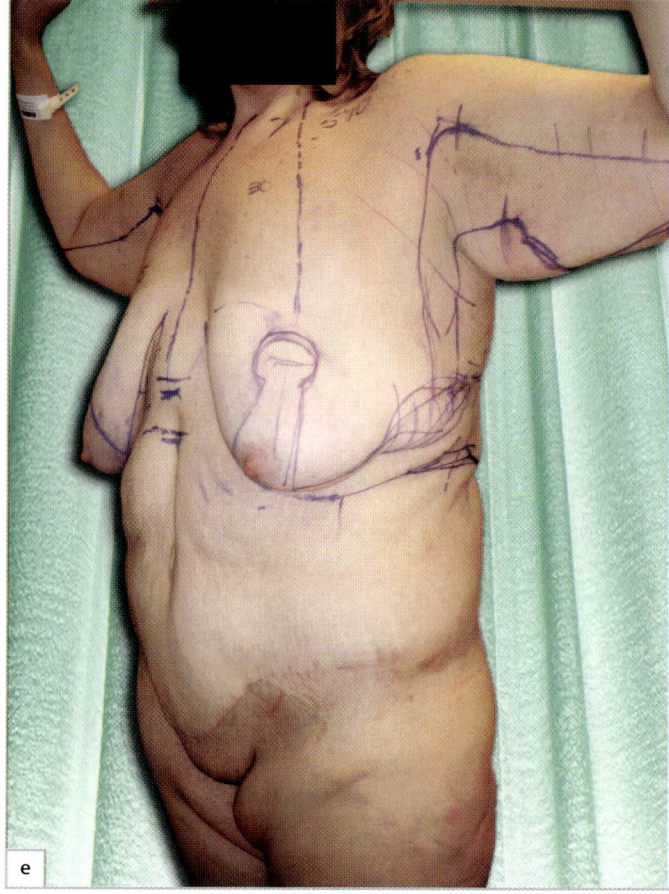

Figure 8.6 Multiple views of the patient presented in Figure 8.4, 10 months after her lower body lift, abdominoplasty, and vertical thighplasty. She is marked for the second stage of her total body lift, upper body lift, reverse abdominoplasty, spiral flap reshaping of her breasts, and left brachioplasties.

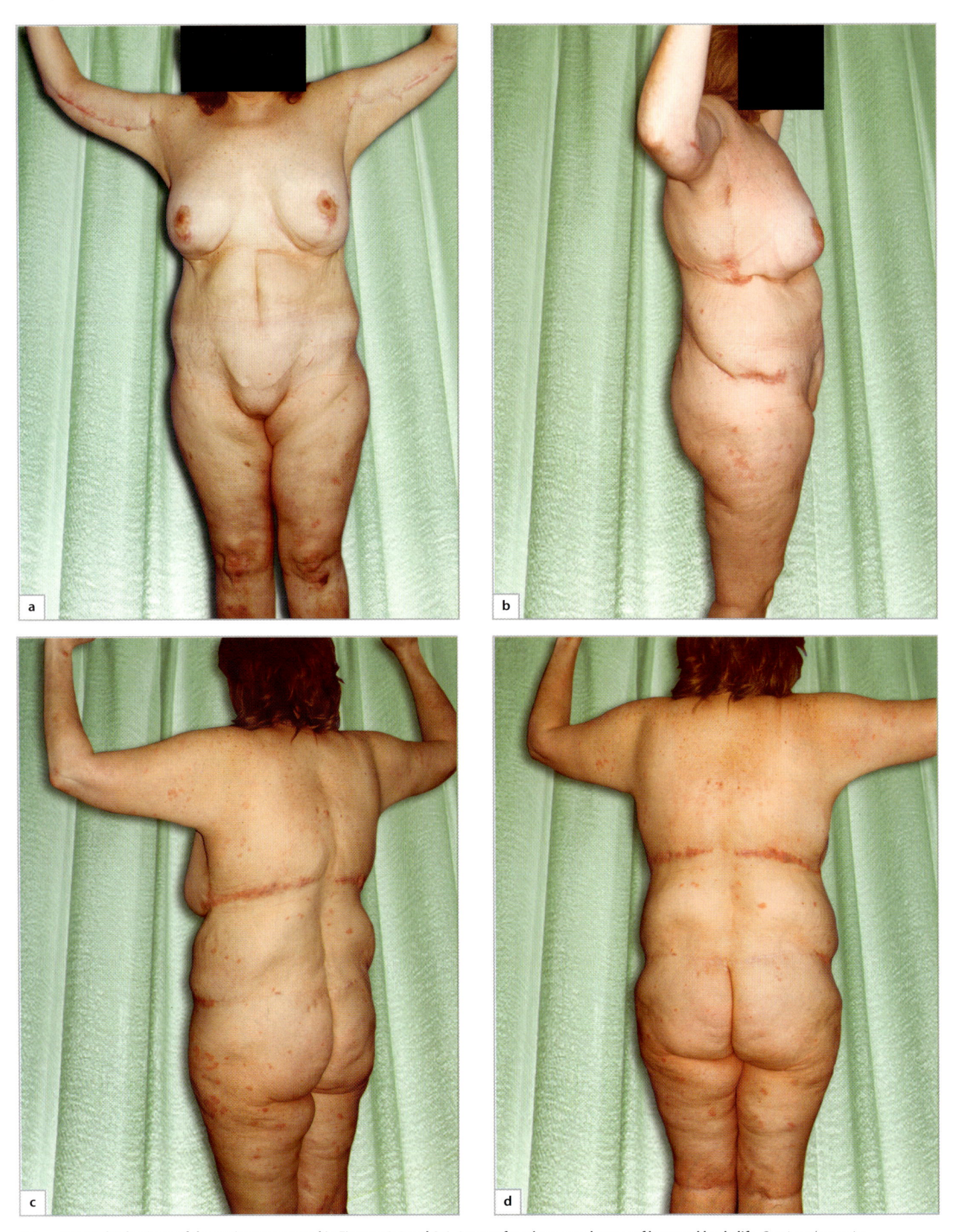

Figure 8.7 Multiple views of the patient presented in Figures 8.4 and 8.6, 1 year after the second stage of her total body lift. *Continued opposite.*

Conclusions

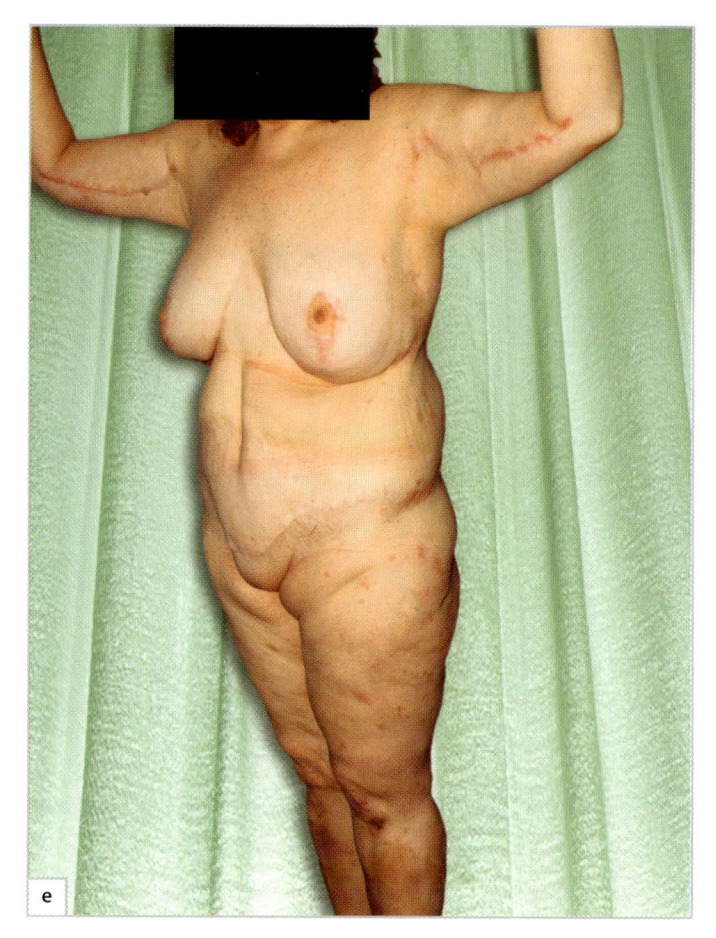

Figure 8.7 Multiple views of the patient presented in Figures 8.4 and 8.6, 1 year after the second stage of her total body lift. First stage was the usual abdominoplasty, lower body lift, and vertical thighplasty, and the second stage was an upper body lift, reverse abdominoplasty, spiral flap reshaping of her breasts, and left brachioplasties.

ongoing attention to detail. In addition you have to keep second and third assistants interested in their task and always learning.

In general the patient is first positioned prone, allowing the circumferential operations such as the lower body lift to be performed bilaterally with every precaution to achieve symmetry. As lead surgeon, this author prefers to proceed slightly ahead of the second surgical team so that they can follow; thereby, the same incisions are made along the wound edge, the same depth is cut, the same degree of undermining performed, and the same quality of closure made. Patients are informed before their operations that, if the surgical team on that day is not deemed to perform at the highest level demanded by the lead surgeon, the totality of the operations scheduled may not be done. Some operations may have to be delayed for another time due to the new excessive length of surgical time. In fact this is a most exceptional situation, demanding a difficult judgment call.

Once the posterior aspect of the operation has been completed, the patient is turned to supine for the abdominoplasty and thighplasty.

■ Improving efficiency

Long multiple operations must be efficient because there are several teams to manage, patient position changes, and adjustments to unforeseen circumstances.

Always looking for improved efficiency in the operating room, a quantum leap forward was taken in 2007 with the introduction of the Quill barb suture device. Large needles at either end of long threads of absorbable bidirectional barbed polydioxanone (PDS) sutures are rapidly run along incisions to securely approximate the subcutaneous fascia under considereable tension. A second intradermal layer is closed with Monoderm.[32] We have cut our surgical times, while at the same time greatly reducing wound-healing complications. Special care and technique are needed to maximize the benefit of the Quill device.

■ Preventing hypothermia

One of the limiting features of simultaneous surgery on different parts of the body is overexposure of the patient. The room should be kept warm, a forced hot air blanket over unoperated areas, warmed intravenous fluids, and cover as much skin as possible, so as to limit hypothermia. Should the patient's temperature go below 36°C, she should be rewarmed and consideration given to stop the session.

■ Reducing complications

In hospitals, postoperative care focuses on patient movement, deep bein thrombosis (DVT) prophylaxis, pain relief, and care of skin closures and early edema. Careful fluid, electrolyte balance, and blood volume restoration is essential. The routine use of of intraoperative blood replacement through normovolemic hemodilution has reduced our need for donor blood transfusion.[6] Most patients are discharged within 3 days. Full nutritional support is resumed.

Outpatient management of swelling is instituted within days, with home use of sequential pneumatic compression tights. Within a week the patient returns to the office for examination and incision care. Through our aesthetic medicine center, aestheticians provide electophysiolymphatic (Hivamat) and manual message throughout the operated areas. Endermologie is resumed as soon as discomfort permits.

We listen and honestly respond to patient concerns. The need for minor surgical revisions is anticipated. Even for major interventions, the patient is reminded that he oer she signed on for a cooperative venture and will accept the surgeon's guidance and work together to correct postoperative disappointments.

■ CONCLUSIONS

Staging of operations to correct the MWL deformity follows a set of principles of patient care and knowledge of the impact of different operations on each other. Most often, the first stage treats the abdomen, lower body, and thighs. After 3 months the upper body, breast, and arms are treated along with minor revisions to the first-stage operations.

REFERENCES

1. Hurwitz DJ, Zewert T. Body contouring surgery in the bariatric surgical patient. *Op Tech Plast Reconst Surg* 2002;**8**:87–95.
2. Hurwitz DJ. Single stage total body lift after massive weight loss. *Ann Plast Surg* 2004;**52**:435–41.
3. Hurwitz DJ. Approach to total body lift surgery. In: Matarasso A, Rubin JP (eds), *Aesthetic Surgery after Massive Weight Lost*. Edinburgh: Elsevier, 2007: 137–57.
4. Hurwitz D. Medial thighplasty. *Aesth Surg J* 2005;**25**:180–91.
5. Hurwitz DJ, Agha-Mohammadi S, Ota K, Unadkat J. A clinical review of total body lift, *Aesth Surg J* 2008;**28**:294–304.
6. Hurwitz DJ. Total body lift surgery. In: Strauch B, Herman CK (eds), The *Encyclopedia of Body Sculpting after Massive Weight Loss*. New York: Thième Medical Publishers, 2011: 63–71.
7. Hurwitz DJ. *Total Body Lift: Reshaping the breasts, chest, arms, thighs, hips, back, waist, abdomen and knees after weight loss, aging, and pregnancies*. New York: MDPublish, 2005.
8. Song AY, Hurwitz DJ, Rubin JP, et al. A classification of contour deformities after massive weight loss: The Pittsburgh rating scale. *Plast Recon Surg* 2005;**116**;1535–44.
9. Agha-Mohammadi S, Hurwitz DJ. Nutritional deficiency of post-bariatric body contouring patients: what every plastic surgeon should know. *Plast Recon Surg* 2008;**122**:604–13.
10. Agha-Mohammadi S, Hurwitz DJ. Potential impacts of nutritional deficiency of post-bariatric patients on body contouring. *Plast Recons Surg* 2008;**122**:1901–14.
11. Hurwitz DJ, Wooten A. Plastic Surgery for the Obese. *Intern J Adipose Tissue* 2007;**1**:5–11.
12. Borud LJ. Combined procedures and staging. In: Matarasso A, Rubin JP (eds), *Aesthetic Surgery after Massive Weight Lost*. Edinburgh: Elsevier, 2007: 159–66.
13. Hallock GG, Altobelle JA. Simultaneous, brachioplasty, thoracoplasty and mammoplasty. *Aesth Plast Surg* 1985;**9**; 233–5.
14. Hurwitz DJ. Approach to the medial thigh after weight loss. In: Matarasso A, Rubin JP (eds), *Aesthetic Surgery after Massive Weight Lost*. Edinburgh: Elsevier, 2007: 113–30.
15. Simon S, Thaller SR, Nathan N. Abdominoplasty combined with additional surgery. *Aesth Surg J* 2006;**26**:413–16.
16. Rubin JP, Gusenoff JA, Cood D. Dermal suspension and parenchymal reshaping mastopexy after massive weight loss: statistical analysis with concomitant procedures from a prospective registry. *Plast Reconstr Surg* 2009;**123**:782–9.
17. Hurwitz DJ. Strategies in breast reduction and mastopexy after massive weight loss. In: Spear SL (ed.), *Surgery of the Breast, Principles and Art*, Vol 2, 3rd edn, Philadelphia, PA: Wolters Kluwer/Lippincott Williams & Wilkins, 2011: 1185–204.
18. Geldwert D, Hurwitz DJ. Upper arm excess. In: Marsh J, Perlyn C (eds), *Decision Making in Plastic Surgery*. St Louis, MO: Quality Medical Publishers, 2010: Chapter 131, pp. 318–9.
19. Geldwert D, Hurwitz DJ. Thigh laxity. In: Marsh J, Perlyn C (eds), *Decision Making in Plastic Surgery*. St Louis, MO: Quality Medical Publishers, 2010: Chapter 132, pp. 320–1.
20. Geldwert D, Hurwitz DJ. Anterior body wall excess after massive weight loss. In: Marsh J, Perlyn C (eds), *Decision Making in Plastic Surgery*. St Louis, MO: Quality Medical Publishers, 2010: Chapter 134, pp. 326–7.
21. Geldwert D, Hurwitz DJ. Posterior body wall excess after massive weight loss. In: Marsh J, Perlyn C (eds), *Decision Making in Plastic Surgery*. St Louis, MO: Quality Medical Publishers, 2010: Chapter 135, pp. 328–9.
22. Geldwert D, Hurwitz DJ. Breast deformities after massive weight loss. In: Marsh J, Perlyn C (eds), *Decision Making in Plastic Surgery*. St Louis, MO: Quality Medical Publishers, 2010: Chapter 136, pp. 330–1.
23. Geldwert D, Hurwitz DJ. Buttock deformities after massive weight loss. In: Marsh J, Perlyn C (eds), *Decision Making in Plastic Surgery*. St Louis, MO: Quality Medical Publishers, 2010: Chapter 137, pp. 332–3.
24. Vastine VL, Morgan RF, Williams GS, et al. Wound complications of abdominoplasty in obese patients. *Ann Plast Surg* 1999;**42**:34–9.
25. Van Uchelen JH, Werker PM, Kon M. Complications of abdominoplasty in 86 patients. *Plast Reconstr Surg* 2001;**107**:1869–75.
26. Shermak MA, Chang D, Magnuson TH, Schweitzer MA. An outcomes analysis of patients undergoing body contouring surgery after massive weight loss. *Plast Reconstr Surg* 2006;**118**:1026–31.
27. Sanger C, David LR. Impact of significant weight loss on outcome of body contouring surgery. *Ann Plast Surg* 2006;**56**:9–13.
28. Agha-Mohammadi, Hurwitz DJ. Spiral thigh lift. In: Strauch B, Herman CK (eds), The *Encyclopedia of Body Sculpting after Massive Weight Loss*. New York: Thième Medical Publishers, 2011: 243–50.
29. Hurwitz DJ, Rubin J P, Risen M, Sejjadian A, Serieka S. Correcting the saddlebag deformity in the massive weight loss patient. *Plast Recon Surg* 2004;**114**:1313–25.
30. Agha-Mohammadi S, Hurwitz DJ. Management of upper abdominal laxity after massive weight loss: reverse abdominoplasty and inframammary fold reconstruction. *Aesth Plast Surg J* 2010; **34**:226–32.
31. Hurwitz DJ, Agha-Mohammadi S. Post bariatric surgery breast reshaping: The spiral flap. *Ann Plast Surg* 2006 **56**:481–6.
32. Hurwitz DJ, Reuben B. Quill™ barbed suture in body contouring surgery: A six year comparison study with running absorbable braided sutures. *Aesth Surg J* 2012 in press.

Chapter 9 Panniculectomy and abdominoplasty

Urmen Desai, Andrew M. Rivera, Bryan R. Wilner, Seth R. Thaller

In the United States, there remains an expanding population who are considered obese (see www.cdc.gov/obesity/data/trends.html). From 1986 to 2000, severe obesity quadrupled from 1 in 200 to 1 in 50 Americans. Similarly, the number of adults who are defined as super-obese in the USA increased by a factor of 5, from 1 in 2000 to 1 in 400.[1] Surgery is often considered as a logical treatment option for the obese patient. Bariatric surgery has increased dramatically over the past 20 years and the number of patients undergoing such surgery continues to rise. Currently, over 200 000 bariatric procedures are performed each year.[2] Factors contributing to this include an increase in the obesity epidemic as well as improvements in the efficacy and safety of bariatric procedures.

After bariatric surgery, many patients display a loss in weight. Although patients experience significant improvements in obesity-associated conditions, they start to present with new problems due to redundant skin and tissue. This large amount of excess skin and fat can lead to many physiological problems such as hygiene, rashes, recurrent infections, and impaired mobility. These compounded problems can severely inhibit patient mental status and affect self-esteem.[3] Body contouring for the massive weight loss (MWL) patient can therefore serve as both an aesthetic and a functional treatment option.

As a result of the rise in MWL patients in the USA, many more patients are presenting to plastic surgeons with large amounts of excess skin on multiple parts of the body. Although patients present with complaints of breast ptosis, upper arm skin redundancy, and facial atrophy, the abdominal apron tends to be the first and greatest disturbance for MWL patients.[4]

The number of MWL patients is expected to grow in the future due to the obesity epidemic. This will result in a greater demand in the number of unique body-contouring procedures offered to these patients. It is important for the body-contouring surgeon to realize that this is a special subset of patients who require treatment needs that differ from those of other patients. After bariatric surgery, many patients expect to be cured of obesity, only to realize that all the redundant skin significantly hinders normal living. Body contouring can significantly improve the daily lives of patients by addressing many of the physiological, aesthetic, and psychosocial conditions associated with massive weight loss.

Historical perspectives

Abdominoplasty has been performed for over 100 years and has undergone a significant amount of technical advancement over time. In 1899, the first attempt to correct excess abdominal skin and fat was made by Kelly.[5] Since then, this technique has evolved with several notable approaches. Thorek (1939) was the first to use a procedure that preserved the umbilicus[6] and in 1967 Pitanguy published a report on the development of abdominal lipectomies.[7] Later that year, Callia[8] described a low incision that extended below the inguinal crease and was the first report of aponeurotic suturing. In 1973, Grazer[9] was one of the first authors to describe the bikini line incision, and 2 years later, Regnault[10] published the W technique. Grazer and Goldwyn[11] first reported complications of this technique in 1977. They reported that, even though aponeurotic suturing in the midline could reduce anterior projection of the abdominal wall, it did not reduce the diameter of the patient's waist. In 1978, Psillakis[12] was able to solve this problem by developing a technique of suture plication of the oblique musculature. This technique allowed for a significant reduction in the diameter of the waist. In 1995, Lockwood[13] described the high lateral tension abdominoplasty. This placed most of the stress of the incision on the anterior thigh region, resulting in a decrease in wound breakdown. Since then, techniques have continued to be refined with improved efficacy and safety.

Unique characteristics in the MWL patient

MWL patients have unique anatomic and physiological challenges. After MWL, patients present with excess skin in almost all areas of the body, including the face, neck, arms, chest, abdomen, thighs, and buttocks. As a result, there is tremendous variation in the presenting deformities. Whereas panniculectomies and abdominoplasties have commonly been performed for purely aesthetic reasons in the past, this is not the case in the MWL patient. Due to the many problems of excess skin in these patients, panniculectomies and abdominoplasties are performed in order to remove the excess skin and improve both physiological function and aesthetic appearance.

Properties of skin in the MWL patient

It is vital for the body-contouring surgeon to understand that MWL patients have both biochemical and mechanical differences in their skin compared with a normal weight patient. MWL patients display stretched skin and the presence of abdominal stria. Postbariatric patients have a decreased collagen network that is more pliable. Skin relaxation can subsequently occur as a result of adipose tissue reabsorption and remodeling, which affect skin strength and elasticity. Ultimately, this affects both immediate and long-term results.[14] However, more studies are needed to fully investigate this relationship.

Quality of life and outcomes

After bariatric surgery, many patients develop a new set of deformities attributed to residual skin redundancy. This loose skin may have a negative impact on both functional status and quality of life of the patient. Functional impairment may be due to persistent rashes, recurrent infection, back and abdominal pain, aesthetic insecurity, and inadequate hygiene which affect overall quality of life.[15] Patients have reported problems with even the most basic day-to-day activities including walking and exercise.[16] It has been reported that excess skin may prevent future weight loss or contribute to additional weight gain.[17]

Many problems associated with obesity and MWL can be improved by body-contouring procedures.[18] Patients have expectations that body-contouring procedures will improve their appearance, quality of life, and ability to be physically active while no longer feeling self-conscious, and reduce feelings of embarrassment.[19] Body contouring has a strong effect on patient self-perception of his or her body.[20] As body-contouring surgery allows patients to return to a more active and functional status, patients display an improved quality of life. Many feel that the positive effects from body-contouring procedures justify the surgical risks associated with these procedures.

We currently live in a society where aesthetic appearance is extremely important. Body contouring can also prove to have psychological benefits in the treatment of disorders often associated with obesity, including depression, alimentary compulsions, preoccupation with one's own appearance, and avoidance of social interactions.[21,22] For a subset of MWL surgery patients who meet criteria for anterior abdominal contouring, patients are able to display improved psychosocial function. By achieving this outcome, patients may be more motivated to maintain weight loss.[23]

Economics of body contouring

Socioeconomic factors play an important role in determining which patients are able to undergo body-contouring surgery after massive weight loss. Postbariatric body-contouring surgery is often not covered by many insurance plans. Many patients are unaware of the actual cost of surgery and do not know the amount of coverage that is provided.[24] Over the last decade, there has been a greater appreciation and awareness of the physiological impairments that MWL patients have. As a result, insurance companies are beginning to change their guidelines for coverage for a suitable insurable surgical procedure.[25] Despite this, it is important to educate patients early about the financial planning of body-contouring procedures after massive weight loss.[24]

Multidisciplinary approach

Obesity is a chronic illness. It affects people in many ways, including both physical and mental deterioration. Despite this, obese patients are often treated by just a single specialist. Therefore it is vital to develop a multidisciplinary team approach for the MWL patient, with the team consisting of various specialists including bariatric surgeons, cardiologists, dermatologists, nutritionists, psychologists, exercise therapists, and plastic surgeons, among others.[26]

Epidemiology

Obesity, which is defined as a BMI >30 kg/m^2, has been increasing in prevalence throughout the USA for many years. Approximately 34% of the American adult population are obese, with an estimated 119 million people categorized as either overweight or obese. This patient population includes not only a third of American adults, but also a sixth of all children and adolescents. More importantly this increased prevalence has been noted among all age, gender, and racial groups throughout the country.[27,28]

Many obese individuals are interested in surgical intervention to correct their deformities, and the number of body-contouring procedures performed has rapidly escalated over the past decade, with such procedures accounting for approximately 30% of operations performed. Bariatric procedures have, however, been recognized as an effective treatment of morbid obesity and the number of bariatric operations performed each year has been increasing steadily from 13 386 in 1998 to 220 000 in 2008.[29]

The exponential growth in bariatric procedures has increased the number of individuals who experience MWL. This, in turn, is associated with a number of severe and diverse body contour deformities that present a significant challenge when attempting a body-contouring surgical intervention.

Pathophysiology

The pathophysiology of obesity and MWL involves a combination of environmental, genetic, behavioral, and molecular factors resulting from an imbalance in food intake and energy expenditure. Although obesity has significant implications in patient health, the pathophysiology of various diseases that develop in each organ system is beyond the scope of this discussion. In postbariatric MWL, changes that affect the physical appearance of patients can be attributed to changes in adipocytes and skin elasticity.[30]

Obesity is associated with changes in skin physiology, collagen structure and function, wound healing, and subcutaneous fat. Although increases in subcutaneous fat storage due to positive energy balance are a well-established and understood result of obesity, the alterations in the skin are not as completely understood. Obese individuals who have experienced MWL have skin with insufficient elasticity and thinned layers of dermal strength. Studies have attributed this to alterations in collage production, function, and deposition. Biochemical studies demonstrate that abdominal obesity in particular results in increased turnover of type III collagen, which is weaker in tensile strength than mature type I collagen.[31] Histological analysis of the redundant skin in patients who have experienced MWL has revealed damage and abnormalities of the extracellular matrix as well. The skin of these patients typically reveals a loose extracellular matrix, with decreased thickness of collagen bundles, and finely dispersed elastin fibers in a disorganized manner. Some have theorized that malnutrition and vitamin deficiencies associated with MWL also contribute to these changes.[32]

Overall, these changes can result in significant aesthetic deformities that can be of concern for patients who have undergone MWL. Abdominal deformities can also lead to medical complications such as intertriginous rashes, dermatitis, and ulcerations. Surgical correction of such deformities is an option and, with regard to the midbody, circumferential abdominoplasty and lipoabdominoplasty are the interventions of choice. A thorough understanding of relevant anatomy is crucial when conducting these body-contouring procedures.

Anatomy and embryology

The abdominal wall is a complex structure defined superiorly by the costal margins, inferiorly by the symphysis pubis and pelvic bones, and posteriorly by the vertebral column. It serves to support and protect abdominal and retroperitoneal structures, and it enables twisting and flexing motions of the trunk. Embryologically it is derived from the mesoderm during fetal development. Sheets of mesodermal tissues in the paravertebral region migrate during weeks 6-7 of fetal development to enclose the future abdominal area. The leading edges of these structures develop into the rectus abdominis muscles, which eventually meet in the midline of the anterior abdominal wall. Before the union of the developing rectus abdominis muscles in the midline, three muscular layers with oblique fiber orientations relative to each other develop to form the internal and external obliques.[33]

Once fully formed, the abdominal wall is divided into layers from superficial to deep. Most superficial is the skin, which can be separated into the epidermis and dermis. Beneath the skin lies the subcutaneous tissue which is a cellular layer consisting of adiposities separated into two layers by the superficial fascia. The areolar layer, which is more superficial, and the lamellar layer, which lies deep to the superficial fascia, are both composed of adipose tissue. The adipose tissue also develops from the mesenchyme and assumes a lobular structure in adults.

The areolar layer varies in thickness with its breadth related to that of the skin. It does not undergo significant changes in obesity but rather has a large number of wide spherical cells with resistance to changes in number and size. The lamellar layer, on the other hand, is composed of small fusiform fat cells with a latent potential to respond when the metabolic situation requires. It is this layer that undergoes significant changes in size in obesity and is the most crucial target in liposuction and lipoabdominoplasty.

Beneath the subcutaneous tissue layer lie the muscle fibers of rectus abdominis anteriorly which are encased within an aponeurotic sheath. The anterior and posterior layers of this sheet are fused in the midline at the linea alba. The lateral borders of the rectus muscles give rise to the surface landmark of the linea semilunaris. There are typically three tendinous junctions:[33]

1. At the level of the xiphoid process
2. At the level of the umbilicus
3. Halfway between the xiphoid process and the umbilicus.

Lateral to the rectus sheath are the obliquely oriented muscle fibers, which make up the external oblique. This muscle originates on latissimus dorsi and serratus anterior muscle laterally and forms a tendinous junction or aponeurosis medially, which is contiguous with the anterior rectus sheath. The inguinal ligament is the inferior-most edge of the external oblique aponeurosis. The internal oblique muscle lies immediately deep to the external oblique muscle and arises from the lateral aspect of the inguinal ligament, iliac crest, and thoracolumbar fascia. The transversus abdominis muscle is the deepest of the three lateral muscles and courses transversely from the lowest ribs, the lumbosacral fascia, and the iliac crest to the lateral border of rectus abdominis.

The blood supply to the anterior abdominal wall is derived mostly from the superior and inferior epigastric arteries. The superior epigastric artery arises from the internal thoracic artery, which descends from the subclavian artery and supplies the thorax. The inferior epigastric artery arises from the external iliac artery and courses upward to anastomose with the terminal branches of the superior epigastric branches. The nerves and arteries that supply the abdominal wall are located in a plane between the internal oblique and transversus abdominis. Direct cutaneous vessels and musculocutaneous perforating branches off the superior and inferior epigastric vessels course medially and laterally, providing the main blood supply to the abdominal wall. In addition, branches of the subcostal and lumbar arteries also contribute to the abdominal wall blood supply. The lymphatic drainage of the abdominal wall is predominantly via the superficial inguinal and axillary areas.[34,35]

Innervation of the anterior abdominal wall is associated with specific spinal levels. The motor nerves to the abdominal wall muscles branch off thoracic spinal nerves at the levels of T6–12. The overlying skin is innervated by afferent branches of the T4–L1 nerve roots, with the nerve roots of T10 providing sensation of the skin around the umbilicus.

PREOPERATIVE EVALUATION

History and physical examination

The preoperative evaluation of a patient for body contouring after MWL should begin with a thorough history and physical examination. In patients who have experienced MWL, it is important to be aware of the specific mechanism of weight loss. Not only should the mechanism be determined, whether by diet and exercise, pharmacotherapy, or bariatric surgery, but also the stability of the weight loss should be determined. This should include weight stability over the previous 3–6 months, particularly in patients who lost weight via diet and exercise, because this group has a greater risk of regaining weight.[36] In patients who have undergone bariatric surgery, weight loss occurs in a predictable pattern, typically reaching a plateau. Although patients may present for body-contouring evaluation before stabilization of their weight, it is best to delay surgery until stability has been achieved for at least 6 months. Maximum and current BMI should be recorded because most body-contouring procedures, other than panniculectomy, are preserved for patients with a BMI ≤35.

The use of pharmacotherapy is important to be aware of as well because various medications have been associated with specific risks in the perioperative period and toward patient health in general. Ginsing tea, for example, is a herbal supplement and component of several health food regimens that has been associated with an increased bleeding risk. Equally important is patient smoking history, because this activity is well established as associated with increased risk of infection, poor wound healing, and thromboembolic events.

Functional disturbances associated with excess skin, such as rashes, sexual dysfunction, and difficulty with exercise, are also important to document, because they can help the patient obtain insurance coverage for at least a portion of their intervention. In addition, comorbidities should be reviewed because obese patients often present for bariatric procedures with several comorbidities serving as indications for their surgical intervention. Once a thorough history has been obtained, a complete physical exam should be conducted to evaluate the degree of deformity.[37]

Nutritional assessment

An assessment of preoperative nutritional status is of particular importance in individuals who have experienced MWL. This patient population has undergone significant changes in their dietary intake in terms of volume and content, and can have major derangements in their levels of vitamins, minerals, and protein. Such derangements can have an impact on perioperative risk and wound healing.

Various nutritional deficiencies that can occur in patients who have experienced MWL can manifest as abnormalities in their clinical presentation as well. The astute clinician should be aware of such abnormalities during the preoperative workup to ensure that all nutritional deficiencies are addressed before proceeding with surgery. Calcium deficiency as well as vitamin D deficiency, for example, can result in osteoporosis, osteomalacia, and increased anesthetic risks. Iron and folate deficiencies result in micro- and macrocytic anemias as well. Zinc deficiency can present with poor wound healing, as well as skin changes and hair loss. Vitamin B_{12} deficiency presents with megaloblastic anemia and peripheral neuropathies, and can also manifest as depression. Vitamin A deficiency can result in night blindness and dry skin in addition. As a result of these important effects, a thorough nutritional assessment is imperative.[38]

Assessment should include an evaluation of both macro- and micronutritive status. Determination of eating behaviors, particularly calorie and protein intake, is important, and the input of a nutritionist can not only aid in these calculations, but also help provide recommendations to promote adequate intake preoperatively. Serum albumin should measure >3.5 g/dl preoperatively, and serial prealbumin levels should be obtained to evaluate any patients with hypoalbuminemia.[39]

Preoperative workup and safety precautions

Standard preoperative workup should also include routine laboratory analysis such as a complete blood count (CBC) with differential, basic metabolic panel to determine levels of electrolytes, prothrombin time (PT), international normalized ratio (INR), and adjusted partial thromboplastin time (PTT). Although these basic labs can reveal underlying nutritional deficiencies, some advocate the assessment of additional vitamin and mineral levels, such as folate, vitamin B_{12}, calcium, iron, zinc, and others that could be deficient as well. A standard 12-lead EKG and chest radiograph should also be obtained to rule out any unknown underlying cardiopulmonary pathology that could increase the patient's risk for perioperative complications.

As with any surgical intervention, routine safety precautions should be taken. These include a review of the patient's medications with particular attention to antiplatelets and any other anticoagulants, which should ideally be stopped before the procedure to reduce the risk of bleeding. All patients should abstain from smoking for 6 months before surgery to reduce the risk of infection, poor wound healing, and venous thromboembolism. Appropriate precautions should be taken to avoid infections, such as perioperative antibiotic prophylaxis, and nutritional status should be optimized as discussed previously.

Photography and photo-documentation

The preoperative evaluation in both reconstructive and aesthetic surgery should also include photographic documentation of all deformities. Pre- and postoperative photographic documentation is an essential part of both reconstructive and aesthetic plastic surgery, not only for assessing the clinical effectiveness of the procedure, but also for use in scientific analysis of interventions. Digital imaging is currently widely used for photo-documentation and offers the advantage of high-quality images that are easily stored and retrieved. In addition, digital imaging provides a significant economic advantage by reducing costs related to film purchasing, development, and printing. Despite the advances in technology and high-quality imaging systems that are currently available, obtaining standardized, consistent, and clinically relevant images requires the use of certain techniques that allow the surgeon to capture the appropriate images.[40]

Photography of the abdomen should include frontal, oblique, and lateral views assessing the area between the inframammary fold and the junction of the upper and medial thirds of the thigh. These areas are the upper and lower limits of the abdomen that can be best visualized if the patient is maintained in an appropriate position. This position includes the arms relaxed, behind the back, with one hand holding the contralateral wrist. The oblique views are obtained with the arms in this same position, turned to a 45° angle, with all references points remaining the same. This should be taken with the patient facing both right and left. The lateral view maintains all positioning and reference points but is taken with the patient rotated 90° to both the right and the left. All postoperative photo-documentation should be obtained with the same patient positioning in all the same views for adequate comparison.[41]

Once adequate imaging has been obtained, photo-editing software is used to photo-augment the original image of the patient and create a new refined image that highlights the areas where changes need to be made until the desired effect can be shown. This allows the surgeon to convey a clear idea of what can be achieved. The use of such software is meant only to simulate a virtual outcome and does not take into account skin changes and scarring associated with surgery. As a result of this, a disclaimer should be signed by patients indicating that they understand that the digitally altered image is not an exact replica of what the postoperative outcome will be.

Preoperative classification system in MWL patients

Once a patient has received all the aforementioned aspects in a routine preoperative evaluation, an assessment of the severity of each patient's deformity should be conducted to help in planning the appropriate surgical intervention. In patients who have experienced MWL, the deformities are not only severe, but can be extremely diverse, disordered, and unpredictable. In addition, as a result of the tremendous amount of variety in the deformities that this patient group can exhibit, the surgical options are numerous as well. Selecting the appropriate surgical interventions can be difficult because many patients require combinations of procedures to address all their deformities. A systematic approach to evaluating each area of the patient's body and quantifying the level of deformity is crucial, and the use of a classification system can allow this. There are several classification systems, Song et al.[42] developed the Pittsburgh Rating Scale, which is a validated measure of contour deformities after bariatric weight loss that can be used to evaluate these patients; it can help not only with preoperative planning, but also in evaluating surgical outcomes. This rating scale targets areas of the body most frequently demonstrating skin laxity and ptosis, with a four-point grading scale to describe common deformities found in each region of the body.[42]

Indications and patient selection

Body contouring by way of circumferential abdominoplasty is indicated in patients who have experienced MWL where the unique deformities related to their condition and involvement of other related anatomic regions cannot be adequately addressed with traditional abdominoplasty techniques. Traditional techniques typically do not address the lateral thigh, hip, and buttock, which are important locations to concentrate on redefining during midbody contouring in this patient population. This technique not only addresses these areas, but also allows for correction of back deformities and abnormalities of the anterior abdominal wall such as hernias or rectus diastasis.

This procedure should be reserved for patients who have had stable weight loss for a period of at least 3–6 months in whom a comprehensive preoperative evaluation that includes all of the aforementioned components reveals that they are adequate candidate for surgery.

Relative contraindications to body contouring in MWL patients includes a history of significant cardiovascular disease, hematological disorders, and thromboembolic disease. Current smokers should stop smoking for a minimum of 3–4 weeks before surgery. Patients considering future pregnancy should have a delay in the procedure because body changes occurring from pregnancy would lead to a recurrence in lax skin and muscular weakness.

Informed consent

As with any surgical intervention it is crucial to obtain informed consent from the patient prior to surgery. In patients who have had MWL, there are a number of key points that need to be included during the preoperative discussion in order to obtain thorough informed consent. Of utmost importance is that the patient fully understands all the associated risks of the surgery. Some of the important associated risks that should be mentioned include bleeding, infection, change in skin sensation, skin contour irregularities, major wound separation, damage to deeper structures such as nerves, blood vessels, muscles, lungs, scarring, allergic reactions, swelling, pain, unsatisfactory results, and deep venous thrombosis associated with cardiac and pulmonary complications.

A detailed discussion of scarring is mandatory and should encompass potential location, color changes, asymmetry, and the possibility of surgical revision or treatment. Skin contour irregularities and depressions can occur and residual deformity at the edge of incisions can be expected because these patients tend to have significant amounts of redundant skin. Furthermore, although good results are expected, a thorough discussion of the possibility of disappointment with the results of the surgery should be conducted. This must highlight the possibility of asymmetry, highly visible scars, persistence of visible deformities, poor healing, wound disruption, and loss of sensation.

Review of these risks with family members and individuals in the support groups of patients undergoing surgery also helps ensure that everyone is fully informed. The use of photographs demonstrating successful results as well as complications can help patients develop a better understanding of what to expect after body contouring.

Also of note in this patient population is a discussion of other important issues related to the surgery. The patient should be made fully aware that insurance may or may not cover all the costs of the procedure. They should be informed of the likely length of the procedure and the likely need for multiple additional procedures to achieve an optimal result. The importance of weight maintenance to prevent further complications or recurrence of deformity is crucial, and the increased risk of complications, infection, wound breakdown, and deep venous thrombosis in smokers should be thoroughly discussed with patients.

Considerations in anesthesia

The use of anesthesia in the morbidly obese patient population is associated with a number of identifiable risks. As the number of bariatric patients increases, so does the number of operations, requiring adequate knowledge of anesthesia in this patient group. Furthermore, as technology has improved, procedures have become less invasive, often being conducted in an ambulatory setting.

The risks associated with morbidly obese patients are many. Of most concern are the following:
- Airway obstruction
- Abnormal respiratory drive
- Cardiac risk factors
- Deep venous thrombosis.

A complete preoperative medical evaluation by a board-certified anesthesiologist is recommended to identify all risk factors before surgery and determine each patient's candidacy for any procedure. This evaluation should include a complete history and physical exam, evaluation of all preoperative laboratory analysis, diagnostic tests, and imaging as previously described, and a separate review of the risks and benefits associated with the use of general anesthesia.[43]

The preoperative anesthesia assessment of patients experiencing MWL should include a careful airway assessment. This is meant to identify individuals who are at risk for obstruction of their airway while under sedation. These individuals may present difficulty in terms of accessing and providing an artificial airway with intubation. Identification of a past medical history of obstructive sleep apnea is a good first indicator of likely airway obstruction during sedation. This problem is significantly more prevalent in the morbidly obese patient population. It is also associated with a number of additional risk factors such as chronic hypoxemia and strain to the right heart. Although formal testing such as polysomnography for obstructive sleep apnea is not necessarily recommended, the risk of airway obstruction in these patients is high and should be evaluated clinically. If a patient is identified as having obstructive sleep apnea the use of continuous positive airway pressure during recovery will assist in oxygenation. Furthermore, delaying extubation until the effect of muscle relaxants and sedatives has completely worn off is crucial.[44]

Morbidly obese individuals and those who have experienced MWL are not only more likely to have problems with airway obstruction during sedation, but also known to have difficulties with ventilation and respiratory drive. These individuals can have chronic hypoxia and retain carbon dioxide, develop pathologically elevated red blood cell counts, and exhibit right heart strain as is seen in the pickwickian syndrome. In addition, they are known to have less lung compliance due to the changes of obesity in the chest wall, with increased work of breathing which can lead to rapid oxygen desaturations. For these reasons, anesthesia in this patient population needs to account not only for changes in airway patency, but also for abnormalities in oxygenation and ventilation that may be present as well.[45]

Most obese patients and those who have experienced MWL also have cardiac risk factors that are important to be aware of during the use of general anesthesia. Hypertension is the most common risk factor seen in these patients and can lead to changes in heart function that can affect cardiac output. For patients with known hypertension, preoperative echocardiography can be useful not only for perioperative monitoring, but also for postoperative evaluation. In addition, coronary artery disease poses a tremendous risk. Some individuals may not be appropriate candidates for surgical interventions such as circumferential abdominoplasty.[46]

Finally, venous thromboembolism is an extremely important consideration in morbidly obese individuals and those who have experienced MWL. Body-contouring procedures increase the risk of venous thromboembolism through changes in vascular resistance and decreased mobilization. Furthermore, studies have shown that BMI at the time of body-contouring surgery can be used as a predictor of thrombotic events. For this reason the use of perioperative deep venous thrombosis prophylaxis is crucial when proceeding with body-contouring surgery in this patient population. This should include the use of sequential compression devices in the perioperative period as well as the use of subcutaneous heparin or low-molecular-weight heparin in patients with known risk factors for thrombosis. This is, however, controversial because some believe that this increases the risk of postoperative bleeding and hematoma formation. Encouraging ambulation on the day of surgery is also important to decrease venous stasis.[47]

SURGICAL TECHNIQUES

Introduction: Surgical approach to the MWL patient

Traditional surgical procedures such as panniculectomy and abdominoplasty only partially address the aesthetic and functional changes associated with postbariatric MWL. The conventional surgical indications are associated with only redundancy of anterior abdominal wall skin, stria, and a rectus diastasis. However, MWL patients often have excess skin along the anterior abdominal wall, flank, hip regions, continuing posteriorly along the thighs, and upper and lower buttocks. To achieve an optimal aesthetic result and resolution of symptoms, a comprehensive circumferential approach is often required which includes lateral thighs, lower back, and upper buttock region. However, despite this, many patients are not surgical candidates for such comprehensive procedures. Some postbariatric patients are not medically stable to undergo a lengthy procedure under general anesthesia which may be considered too extensive or aggressive. Others may not be interested in a lengthy procedure because it is often associated with a lengthy postoperative recovery period. Still others may not have sufficient financial resources for such procedures. Thus, a large subgroup of the MWL population choose to address only the anterior abdomen. Nonetheless, it is important for the plastic surgeon to have sufficient experience and knowledge of a wide range of surgical options in their surgical armamentarium, ranging from the standard panniculectomy to total body lifting.

Abdominoplasty and lipoabdominoplasty

Most cases of abdominal deformity after MWL result in circumferential skin and fat changes, which are often best managed with a circumferential procedure. However, some patients are better served with an anterior-only procedure because their skin redundancy is isolated to the anterior abdomen, or they have a personal or medical reason to undergo a procedure that addresses only the anterior abdomen.[48]

In 1980 came the introduction of suction lipectomy with blunt cannulas, which represented one of the most important innovations in the field of body contouring. This allowed for major redefinitions through minimally noticeable incisions. Lipoabdominoplasty, a term initially described by Saldanha,[49] was developed as an alternative approach to the MWL patient as a safe and functional surgical technique that combines both traditional abdominoplasty and liposuction in the same surgical procedure, in order to take advantage of both approaches. This combined approach goes further than simply performing liposuction as an additive to traditional liposuction. Rather, it gives the surgeon a complete appreciation and requires an understanding of the entire abdominal anatomy.[50] Traditional undermining performed with elevation of flaps is replaced with selective undermining using a cannula, which helps preserve blood supply from the abdominal perforating vessels. It has been determined that 80% of the perfusion to the abdominal wall comes from the abdominal perforating branches of the superior and inferior epigastric arteries.[51] The additional 20% arises from the intercostal arteries, and upper external iliac arteries.[52]

In the MWL patient, traditional abdominoplasty has been prolonged with high rate of complications, due to the necessity to elevate large flaps, transection of the abdominal perforating vessels, and preventing trauma to additional neurovascular structures.[53] Resection of adipose tissue by way of liposuction, selective undermining, and maintenance of Scarpa fascia with deep fat permit improved preservation of vascular, lymphatic, and nervous tissue. This, as a result, has been what has led to the decrease in complications postoperatively.[52] Historically, the combination of abdominoplasty and liposuction has been slow to be accepted, because this combined approach was initially perceived as having greater complications than abdominoplasty alone.[54] Despite this, over the last two decades, the number of procedures with significant undermining has decreased, whereas the literature reporting the number of postoperative complications associated with undermining such as sarcoma, hematoma, and flap necrosis has also decreased.[53] Selective undermining of only approximately 30% of traditional undermining, strictly along the internal borders of the rectus muscle to adequately preserve the abdominal perforating vessels, has dramatically helped decrease the incidence of complications. This combined approach to the anterior abdomen is believed to have a steep learning curve, particularly in surgeons who have become facile in both procedures performed separately.

Surgical technique

Patients are marked 1 day before surgery and confirmed in the immediate preoperative period in order to ensure proper surgical planning. Additional adjustments are also often made intraoperatively. With the patient in the standing position, the midline of the anterior abdomen is marked. Marking for the planned lower incision is made initially with a transverse line across the mons at the level of the suprapubic crease. If, in fact, the mons needs to be lifted, the marking should be made 2–3 cm inferior to the hairline. The transverse line should be extended laterally toward the anterosuperior iliac spine. The lateral extent of the incision is patient dependent and variable, depending on the degree of lateral skin and fat redundancy. Areas of liposuctioning are then marked in the upper and lower abdomen, as well as the flank region and mons if needed.

After surgical markings are made, the patient is placed over a beanbag in a supine position on the operating table. Sequential compression device, thromboembolic deterrent (TED) stockings, perioperative antibiotics, and bladder catheter are then placed. After the patient has been intubated and general anesthesia initiated, the patient is prepped and draped in a sterile fashion. A tumescent technique is used with infiltration of the abdomen, initiated using 1 liter lactated Ringer solution infused with 25 ml 1% lidocaine with 1:100 000 epinephrine, plus an additional ampoule of epinephrine 1:1000. The tumescent is allowed to set for a total of 10 min in order to allow for adequate vasoconstriction and to ensure a bloodless lipoaspirate. Liposuctioning is initiated using 3-mm and 4-mm Mercedes tip cannulas, and fat is subsequently suctioned in the intermediate and deep planes to ensure the prevention of contour deformities superficially. Liposuctioning is performed in the upper and lower abdomen, as well as the flank region and mons if needed. The end-limit is determined by improved contour as well as onset of bloody aspirate (**Fig. 9.1**).

After adequate liposuctioning is been performed, the lower abdominal incision is made over previous surgical markings. Complementary open liposuction is performed to remove additional fat deep to Scarpa fascia. Selective undermining of a tunnel in the midline of the upper abdomen is performed between the internal borders of the rectus muscle, thus preserving the abdominal perforating vessels. The lateral extent of supraumbilical liposuctioning should not traverse lateral to the edges of the rectus fascia. Undermining of the tunnel continues until the level of the xiphoid process is reached (**Fig. 9.2**). Vertical midline rectus sheath plication is then performed 2 cm laterally from midline, using 0 Ethibond suture in interrupted fashion from the xiphoid process to the umbilicus, then from the umbilicus to the pubic symphysis. Next, a running 1-0 Prolene suture is placed, again from the xiphoid process to the umbilicus, and then from the umbilicus to the pubic symphysis (**Fig. 9.3**). After rectus plication, an incision is made after re-draping the upper abdominal flap for new placement of the umbilicus. The placement of this midline entry site for the umbilical stalk is at the level of the iliac crests. Umbilicoplasty is then performed as an inverted V-shaped skin incision, and the umbilical stalk is advanced thorough and secured with 3-0 Monocryl deep dermal and 4-0 Monocryl subcuticular sutures. After re-draping of the abdominal flap, any anterior excess of skin can be redistributed anteriorly over the lower skin incision. Two Jackson–Pratt drains are placed, exiting on either side of the midline pubic symphysis. The lower abdominal incision is then closed in layered fashion using 0 Ethibond to approximate the Scarpa fascia, 3-0 Vicryl, 3-0 Monocryl sutures are placed in a deep dermal plane, whereas 4-0 Monocryl sutures

Surgical techniques

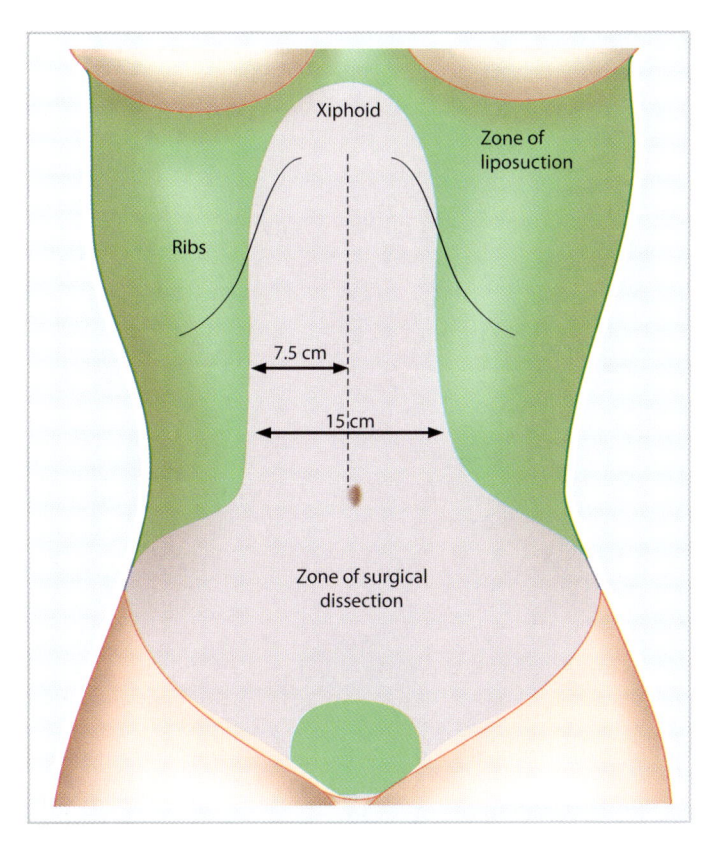

Figure 9.1 Areas of liposuction versus surgical dissection highlighting selective undermining of a tunnel in the midline of the upper abdomen between the internal borders of the rectus muscles, thus preserving the abdominal perforating vessels. Undermining of the tunnel continues until the level of the xiphoid process is reached.

Figure 9.2 Selective undermining of a tunnel in the midline of the upper abdomen is performed between the internal borders of the rectus muscle, thus preserving the abdominal perforating vessels. The lateral extent of supraumbilical liposuctioning should not traverse lateral to the edges of the rectus fascia. Undermining of the tunnel continues until the level of the xiphoid process is reached.

are placed in a subcuticular plane. Dermabond is then placed over the anterior skin incision, followed by an abdominal binder placed around the patient. The patient is then transferred to the recovery bed in supine position with the bed flexed at the hips and knees.

Complications

Saldanha et al.[53] presented 445 patients who underwent lipoabdominoplasty over an 8-year period. They report an incidence of epitheliolysis in four (0.1%), skin necrosis in four (0.9%), deep vein thrombosis or pulmonary embolism in four (0.9%), hematoma in four (0.9%), sarcoma in two (0.4%), and wound dehiscence in two (0.4%) patients. Similarly, Matos et al.[52] performed 209 lipoabdominoplasty procedures. Poor outcomes consisted of epidermolysis in three (1.5%), sarcoma in two (1%), hematoma in two (1%), and necrosis in two (1%) patients. Weiler et al.[54] reported higher complication rates in their experience of 173 consecutive patients undergoing lipoabdominoplasty. Complications included infection requiring antibiotic therapy in 13 (7.5%), partial skin dehiscence and necrosis in 12 (7%), sarcoma in 6 (3.4%), deep vein thrombosis in 5 (3%), and pulmonary emboli in 2 (1%), skin flap necrosis requiring re-advancement of the abdominal flap in 2 (1%), suture granuloma in 1 (0.5%), and major fat necrosis requiring local debridement in 1 (0.5%) patient. Finally, Espinosa-de-los-Monteros et al.[48] report their experience with 60 patients over a 5-year period who underwent lipoabdominoplasty. They report six (10%) patients with partial wound dehiscence, three (5%) patients with epidermal necrolysis, two (3%) patients who developed seromas, one (2%) patient with postoperative abscess, and one (2%) patient with a postoperative wound infection.

Reverse abdominoplasty

The upper abdomen is well known to be a challenging area for the surgeon. In this region, residual fat can be addressed with liposuction, but in the MWL patient, redundancy of skin in this region can be addressed *only* surgically. The first description of the reverse abdominoplasty was described in 1977 in a systemized approach through the inframammary sulcus but it has not gained significant popularity until recently.[55] This technique differs from traditional approaches to abdominoplasty because it involves the direct excision of skin and fat from the upper abdomen along the inframammary fold. The reverse abdominoplasty can be performed by a single W-shaped incision or as two separate inframammary crescentic excisions.

The reverse abdominoplasty should be considered a therapeutic option in the MWL patient who has excess soft-tissue redundancy isolated to the upper abdomen and epigastric region relative to the lower infraumbilical abdomen. The ideal candidate is the MWL patient who has previously undergone conventional abdominoplasty or liposuction, and has residual skin laxity in the upper abdomen. In addition, the redundant upper abdominal tissue can be used to autoaugment the breast tissue if the patient requests a mastopexy–augmentation together with the abdominoplasty. With MWL and breast ptosis, the inframammary fold often becomes loose and

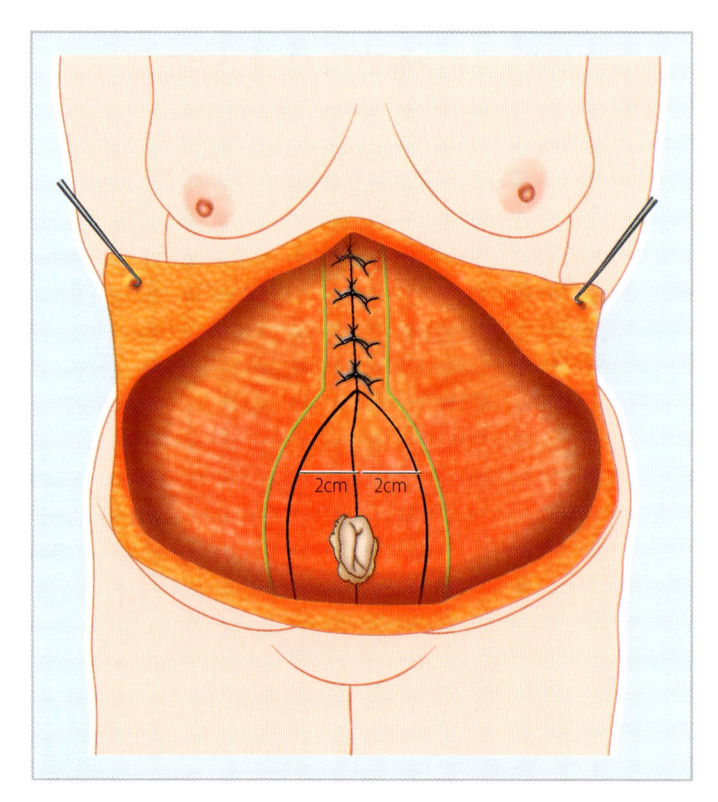

Figure 9.3 Vertical midline rectus sheath plication is then performed 2 cm laterally from midline using 0 Ethibond suture in interrupted fashion from the xiphoid process to the umbilicus, then from the umbilicus to the pubic symphysis. Next, a running 1–0 Prolene suture is placed, again from the xiphoid process to the umbilicus, then from the umbilicus to the pubic symphysis.

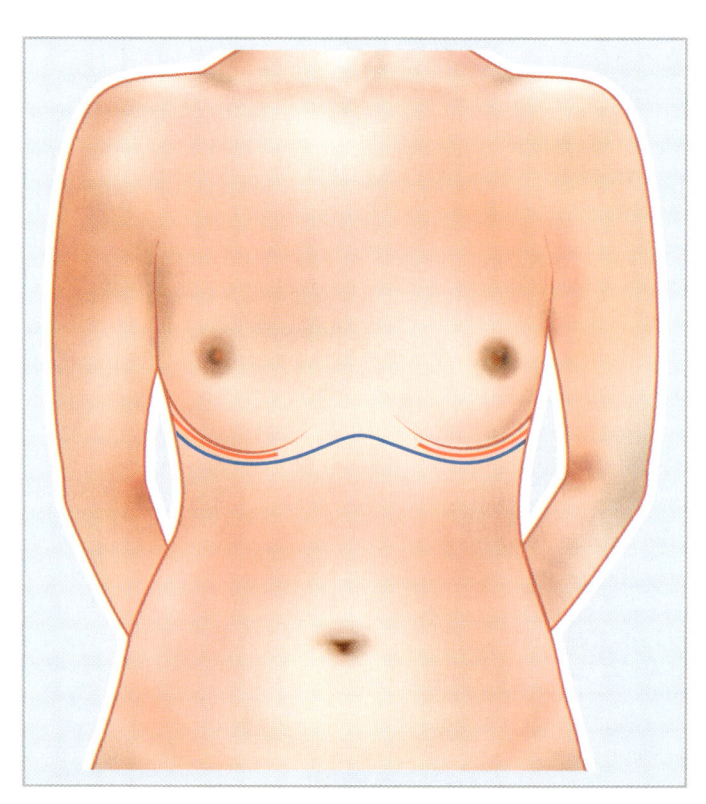

Figure 9.4 Excision of soft tissue is then excised as two crescent inframammary incisions (red) or a single W-shaped incision (blue).

descends infralaterally. The reverse abdominoplasty has a limited surgical indication in a highly select group of patients who previously have undergone MWL. This approach is ideal for the patient with pre-existing scars in the inframammary region and with redundancy of the upper abdominal wall tissue after previous abdominal wall contouring procedures. This technique should be considered in circumstances where traditional abdominoplasty would not adequately result in an improved aesthetic effect. It should be retained in the surgeon's armamentarium as an option to address upper abdominal fat and skin excess.

Surgical technique

Patients are marked 1 day before surgery and confirmed in the immediate preoperative period to ensure proper surgical planning. Additional adjustments are also often made intraoperatively as well. With the patient in the standing position, the inframammary folds and edges of the upper torso are marked. A pinch test is performed by pulling the redundant skin in the cephalad direction from the upper abdomen to the epigastric region, after which the lower border is marked. Excision of soft tissue then occurs as two crescent inframammary incisions or a single W-shaped incision (**Figure 9.4**).

After surgical markings have been made, the patient is placed in supine position on the operating table. Sequential compression device, TED stockings, perioperative antibiotics, and bladder catheter are then placed. After the patient has been intubated and general anesthesia initiated, the patient is prepped and draped in sterile fashion. First, the superior incision is made with a no. 15 blade, with dissection down to the level of the rectus sheath, taking care to preserve the inframammary fold.[56] Dissection continues down to the umbilicus at the level of the rectus fascia. The excess skin is then pulled superiorly and excised so that the planned final closure will have minimal tension. Vertical midline rectus sheath plication is performed 2 cm laterally from midline using 0 Ethibond suture in an interrupted fashion from the xiphoid process to the umbilicus. Next, a running 1-0 Prolene suture is placed, again from the xiphoid process to the umbilicus. After meticulous hemostasis, two Jackson–Pratt drains are placed, exiting along the lateral aspect of the inframammary incision. Next, tacking sutures are placed between the abdominoplasty flap and the rectus sheath to limit the degree of tension placed on the inframammary incisions. The inframammary incisions are closed while ensuring that the inframammary fold is recreated to avoid loss of definition and prevent future lowering due to gravity. Deep superficial fascial suspension sutures are placed from the Scarpa fascia of the abdominoplasty flap down to the perichondrium of the ribs over the inframammary sulcus. The inframammary incision is closed in layered fashion using 0 Ethibond to approximate the Scarpa fascia, 3-0 Vicryl, 3-0 Monocryl sutures are placed in a deep dermal plane, whereas 4-0 Monocryl sutures are placed in a subcuticular plane. Dermabond is then placed over the inframammary fold incision, followed by an abdominal binder placed around the patient. The patient is then transferred to the recovery bed in a supine position with the bed flexed at the hips and knees.

Complications

Agha-Mohammadi and Hurwitz[57] found in their series of 88 patients undergoing reverse abdominoplasty within the context of combined or staged circumferential abdominoplasty. They present five (6%) patients with major wound dehiscence, two (2%) with wound infections, and two (2%) requiring revisions for persistent laxity. Deos et al.[58] presented their work after 18 consecutive reverse abdominoplasties were performed. A single (5%) patient who underwent reverse abdominoplasty, requiring an incision unification at the midline, ended up with a postoperative skin redundancy resulting in synmastia due to insufficient resection at the midline. An additional patient (5%) in the dual unilateral mammary sulcus group had asymmetric resection of dermal fat excess resulting in unilateral skin redundancy. Finally, two (11%) patients had persistent upper abdominal laxity as the final result. In a review by Pacifico et al.,[56] who presented a case series of 14 consecutive patients who underwent body contouring with a reverse abdominoplasty over a 5-year period, found minimal complications. Only a single (7%) patient who underwent a simultaneous breast augmentation developed a breast sarcoma that required removal of the prosthesis, whereas two (14%) additional patients developed areas of hypertrophic scarring, and one (7%) final patient experienced minor delayed wound healing. Halbesma and van der Lei[59] presented their series of seven patients who underwent a reverse abdominoplasty. They report three (42%) patients who presented with complications, one (14%) patient who had a postoperative sarcoma, and another (14%) who had slight wound dehiscence. One (14%) final patient had a poor aesthetic result due to necrosis of the abdominal flap secondary to aggressive undermining.

Monsplasty

A youthful mons pubis is narrow, with elasticity and strong skin tone, and a moderate degree of fat in the subcutaneous plane to provide padding against the bony symphysis.[60] Often with massive weight gain, the mons pubis tends to enlarge, protrude, and descend. After subsequent weight loss, this particular region tends to remain descended and continue to contain a significant degree of excess skin and fat. This area can cause residual functional problems such as difficulty with intercourse, maintenance of hygiene, and discomfort when wearing clothing.[61] As a result, this can lead to significant psychosocial stress and impairment of quality of life.[62] From an anatomic standpoint, the superficial fascia inserts onto the pubic bone, which supports the skin and fat component of the mons pubis. In patients who were previously obese, the supportive architecture of the superficial fascia is lost due to previous distension and loss of elasticity.[62]

Patients who have undergone MWL are often classified into one of three classifications as determined by the Pittsburgh Rating Scale.[42] Patients in group 1 have deformities with only moderate mons ptosis without fat excess; group 2 comprises patients with fat excess and a more pronounced degree of mons ptosis, with occlusion of a portion of the external genitalia; group 3 is characterized by significant fat excess, and mons ptosis of the entire pubic and genital area.[42] For many years, surgical correction of the mons pubis has been poorly understood, and is thus often a neglected aspect of body contouring after MWL. Historically, the mons has been surgically addressed with excision of fat by either liposuction or open excision, together with a pubic skin lift. However, this often results in an unsuccessful lift with residual mons ptosis. Other surgeons prefer to excise redundant fat and skin from the midline, which often results in an aesthetically displeasing vertical T-shaped midline scar. To achieve a long-lasting lift of the mons pubis, the excess suprapubic skin and fat removed from the mons must be performed together with tacking of the fibrofatty tissue of the pubis to the rectus fascia.[61] This surgical technique results in lifting of the vulvar commissure and positions the clitoris in its natural topography without displacing the urethral meatus, which thus effectively harmonizes the pubogenital area.[62]

Monsplasty can be performed together with simultaneous abdominoplasty, or as a separate procedure after abdominoplasty. Others advocate performing monsplasty simultaneously with a vertical medial thigh lift.[63] Traditional abdominoplasty techniques do not adequately address the mons region. Failure to recognize this will result in residual fullness of the pubic area, ptosis, and an appreciable step-off between the mons and the upper abdominal flap.[64] When the mons pubis is overlooked in abdominal contour surgery, this can result in a fatty, loose, or wide mons pubis which is stretched and disproportionate.[60] This will often result in relative lengthening of the mons pubis, creating an imbalanced transition from the newly contoured abdomen. To achieve ideal harmony during body contouring, the lower abdomen should be viewed as being composed of several aesthetic units, in a similar fashion to how subunits of the face and nose are defined.[60] Only recently have normal dimensions and angles of the mons been defined in the literature, and only limited data have described the mons as a separate subunit.[65] However, despite this, treating the mons region as a distinct aesthetic unit will lead to an improved aesthetic result and a high patient satisfaction.[64]

Surgical technique

Patients are marked 1 day before surgery and confirmed in the immediate preoperative period to ensure proper surgical planning. Additional adjustments are also often made intraoperatively. With the patient in the standing position, the abdominal pannus is elevated for better examination of the mons. If the monsplasty is being performed together with the abdominoplasty, excess tissue excision can be removed only after the resection planned during the abdominoplasty. A pinch test is performed on the redundant pubic skin and fat to lift the pubogenital region in order to align the anterior vulvar commissure to the lower edge of the pubic bone. This soft tissue is elevated over the pubic hairline to determine how much excess soft tissue will need to be excised in the vertical axis. A crescent-shaped pattern is marked with a surgical marker and placed just inferior to a fold of the pannus or blended within a previous abdominoplasty scar (**Fig. 9.5**). Alternative markings in the shape of a trapezoid have been used as well.[62] The lateral aspect of the crescent should be marked to span the lateral edge of redundant soft tissue, with the lateral limit of the incision being the anterosuperior iliac spine.

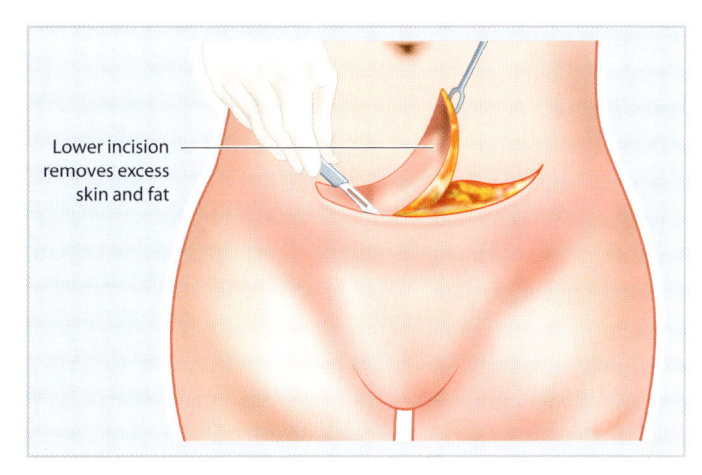

Figure 9.5 A crescent-shaped pattern is placed just inferior to a fold of the pannus or blended within a previous abdominoplasty scar.

After surgical markings have been done, the patient is placed in supine position on the operating table. Sequential compression device, TED stockings, perioperative antibiotics, and bladder catheter are then placed. After the patient has been intubated and general anesthesia initiated, the patient is prepped and draped in sterile fashion. First, a no. 15 blade scalpel is used to make a skin incision along the upper aspect of the skin crescent. Double-prong skin hooks are used to assist with dissection down through the skin and subcutaneous tissue, down to the fascia of rectus abdominis. Next, the dissection continues in a superior to inferior direction while elevating fat off the rectus fascia. Once the level of the inferior border of the crescent markings is met, the underlying skin and fat are excised while tapering the incision toward the pubic symphysis. If liposuctioning of the mons is to be performed together with monsplasty, then infiltration of the mons is initiated using 1 liter lactated Ringer solution infused with 25 ml 1% lidocaine and 1:100 000 epinephrine, plus an additional ampoule of epinephrine 1:1000. The tumescent is allowed to set for a total of 10 min to allow for adequate vasoconstriction and ensure a bloodless lipoaspirate. Liposuctioning is initiated using 3-mm and 4-mm Mercedes tip cannulas, and fat is then suctioned in the intermediate and deep planes to ensure the prevention of contour deformities superficially. The end-limit is determined by improved contour as well as onset of bloody aspirate. Additional open fat excision is performed if liposuction techniques alone do not achieve a smooth contour. Approximately 2 cm of fibrous subcutaneous tissue must be preserved for adequate resuspension. An aesthetically displeasing pubic concavity can be avoided by lateral feathering with liposuction. In addition, caution must be taken during liposuction in the inguinal region to prevent formation of genital lymphedema. A single Jackson–Pratt drain is placed exiting the lateral aspect of the pubis. Next, tacking sutures using 0 Ethibond are placed in transverse interrupted fashion, with a row from the pubic superficial fascia to the fascia of the abdominal flap, and anchored to the aponeurosis of the anterior rectus abdominis muscle. Caution must be held to prevent tethering of the labia majora, dimpling of pubic skin, distortion of clitoral hood, and exposure of the urethral meatus.[61,62] Additional 3-0 Vicryl, 3-0 Monocryl deep dermal sutures are placed, followed by 4-0 Monocryl sutures in subcuticular fashion. Dermabond is then placed over the pubic incision, followed by an abdominal binder placed around the patient. The patient is transferred to the recovery bed in a supine position with the bed flexed at the hips and knees.

Complications

It is believed that, as long as excision of fat from the mons is excised superior to the pubic symphysis, no change in sexual sensation will occur, because there will be no trauma to the clitoris. Drastic elevation of the mons could potentially create an abnormal escutcheon, with resulting secondary deformities of the labia majora and clitoral hood.[61] A pubic concavity could also result with overly aggressive excision of liposuction of the mons fat. El-Khatib[66] presented one of the largest series of monsplasty to date, containing 132 patients monitored over a 6-year period. He noted that two patients (1.5%) presented with postoperative skin laxity due to further weight loss and poor skin tone; an additional two patients (1.5%) experienced postoperative edema of the mons requiring abdominal pressure garments applied to the entire abdomen. One final patient (1%) experienced a 2-cm area of wound dehiscence secondary to a superficial infection, which was managed with local wound care.[62] Marques et al.[66] looked at a series of 23 women who underwent previous MWL and presented with pubogenital ptosis and underwent monsplasty. Prolonged edema was noted to be the most common postoperative complication, seen in 16 (70%) patients. They attribute high incidence of postoperative edema to the fact that the pubogenital region is the lowest and most dependent portion of the trunk, and gravity results in a delay in resolution of this local edema. Additional postoperative complications included hypertrophic scarring in five (22%) patients, distortion of the position of the clitoris in a single patient (4%), enlargement of the labia majora in an additional patient (4%), and surgical wound infection in a final patient (4%).[62] Rezak and Borud[63] present seven patients who underwent simultaneous monsplasty with vertical medial thigh lift. They found only one (14%) patient with a small wound dehiscence in the groin region, which required intravenous antibiotics, and another (14%) who displayed prolonged lower extremity edema for 8 weeks. No sarcomas, hematomas, or lymphedema resulted. Michaels et al.[64] report performing over 400 mons rejuvenation procedures in the MWL patient over a 7-year period. Complications included self-limiting edema and mons fullness secondary to conservative defatting, and a single case of suture granuloma from permanent suture requiring excision.

Fleur-de-lis abdominoplasty

MWL patients are known to have redundant skin and residual fat in both the horizontal and the vertical planes. As a result of this phenomenon, traditional abdominoplasty techniques may not adequately correct the horizontal laxity in this patient population. The presence of abdominal scars or hernia from open bariatric surgery further adds an element of complexity in surgical planning.[67] In order to adequately surgically address this, a fleur-de-lis vertical excisional component has been included with the traditional abdominoplasty approach. The best candidates for this surgical approach are MWL patients who have a significant degree of epigastric skin laxity and present with a double-roll deformity. As the fleur-de-lis abdominoplasty results in an increased scar, the procedure is most often approved for patients with a pre-existing upper abdominal scar from original bariatric procedure. Many patients who have minimally invasive gastric bypass performed with four or five stab incisions often prefer this approach because of the contour improvements that it offers.[68] Similarly, patients who have had traditional approaches to gastric bypass already have an upper abdominal scar that may hinder re-draping of the soft tissues in traditional abdominoplasty, by tethering the superior flap as it is pulled inferiorly during final tailoring. Older patients who have greater laxity will not need significant lateral tissue undermining, which maintains better vascular perfusion of the flap. In patients who have previous subcostal scars, the vertical skin excision encompasses the scar to decrease the risk of devascularization of the flap. Patients must have an understanding that they will receive improved contour in the epigastric region, flank, and waist at the expense of an anterior vertical scar. In addition, patients should be warned that the umbilicus, as a result, will lie within the vertical scar and can widen postoperatively.

Surgical technique

In the fleur-de-lis abdominoplasty, resection in both the vertical and the horizontal planes is required. Patients are marked 1 day before surgery and confirmed in the immediate preoperative period to ensure proper surgical planning. Additional adjustments are also often made intraoperatively. With the patient in the standing position, the midline of the abdomen is marked. A full abdominoplasty pattern is initially marked from 5 cm to 7 cm, from the vulvar commissure to the top of the mons pubis, traversing laterally to the anterosuperior iliac spine. The vertical component of the abdominoplasty is then marked as an inverted 'V' to address planned excision of abdominal skin and fat, with the widest portion being at the base of the triangle as determined by a confirmatory pinch test (**Figure 9.6**).

After surgical markings are performed, the patient is placed supine position on the operating table. Sequential compression device, TED stockings, perioperative antibiotics, and bladder catheter are then placed. After the patient has been intubated and general anesthesia initiated, the patient is prepped and draped in sterile fashion. First, a circumumbilical incision is made with the assistance of a no. 15 blade scalpel and single-prong skin hooks. Metzenbaum scissors are used to dissect the umbilical stalk. This dissection is continued down to the fascia with caution so as not to exit from the umbilical tract skin. The lower abdominal incision is then made to the abdominal wall fascia. Subsequent elevation is performed from the medial to the lateral direction, and subsequently in the superior direction to the level of the umbilicus. At this point, caution must be made so as not to transect the umbilical stalk. Next, the lower abdominal flap is divided along the midline to assist with further dissection cephalad to the umbilicus. Dissection then continues to the level of the costal margins and xiphoid process in the midline.

After traditional abdominoplasty approaches and fascial plication, a pinch test is performed in both planes. Once the redundant tissue has been excised off the anterior skin flap in the vertical plane, the vertical incision is made from the supraumbilical region caudally to the xiphoid process. Preservation of lateral perforators is made with minimal undermining in the superolateral directions along the abdominal fascia, but with enough dissection to resolve the epigastric and lateral flank redundancy. To best define the horizontal line of resection, three sharp towel clamps are placed along the vertical incision on either side of the midline. The skin flaps are pulled inferomedially, and the points where the clamps can be palpated are marked with a marking pen on the anterior abdominal skin. An en bloc resection is subsequently performed.[69] Epigastric fullness and the presence of a standing-cone deformity are addressed with subcutaneous debulking at the apex of the incision. The umbilicus is inset within the vertical incision. Reapproximation of the superficial fascial system of the vertical incision, and circumferentially around the new position of the umbilicus, is made with skin incisions closed in layered fashion using 0 Ethibond to approximate the Scarpa fascia, 3-0 Vicryl, 3-0 Monocryl deep dermal sutures are placed followed by 4-0 Monocryl sutures in subcuticular fashion. Dermabond is then placed over the pubic incision, followed by an abdominal binder placed around the patient. The patient is transferred to the recovery bed in supine position with the bed flexed at the hips and knees.

Complications

Although there has been much success with the fleur-de-lis approach to the anterior abdomen, many surgeons continue to be hesitant to perform the vertical excision due to previous high complication rates. Several authors have reported that the fleur-de-lis approach to the anterior abdomen results in a superior aesthetic result in select MWL patients; however, these results may be at the expense of wound-healing problems in the postoperative period. This was most often seen at the trifurcation point where the horizontal incisions meet the vertical incision. Friedman et al.[70] compared the overall complication rates in 154 patients who underwent fleur-de-lis abdominoplasty with those of 345 patients who underwent traditional abdominoplasty. They concluded that overall complications in the former patients were higher than with traditional abdominoplasty (30.5% versus 24.6%); however, this difference was not statistically significant ($p = 0.16$). Thus, complication rates for fleur-de-lis abdominoplasty and traditional abdominoplasty were found to be similar.[70] The fleur-de-lis approach to the anterior abdomen can be performed safely with complication rates similar to those of traditional abdominoplasty in the MWL patient.

■ Circumferential abdominoplasty

Circumferential abdominoplasty is an approach that is tailored to the MWL patient. Often when patients with circumferential truncal redundancy undergo traditional abdominoplasty procedures, the upper and lower trunks are not adequately addressed. Circumferential abdominoplasty is a more ideal procedure for these patients because it integrates an abdominoplasty with circumferential excision of skin and fat. Traditional abdominoplasty techniques are quickly recognized as being inadequate to address the functional as well as the aesthetic concerns, which are different in this patient population. The circumferential abdominoplasty directly addresses an improved midbody contour with abdominal wall tightening and a circumferential incision, abdominal plication, undermining of the back, and suspension of the superficial fascial system. The midbody and abdominal areas are often the region of the body that is of greatest concern in the MWL patient. The redundant skin in this region presents as both a functional and an aesthetic concern, because patients often complain of skin breakdown and intertrigo, which are often chronic and persistent despite continuous hygiene attention and medical treatments. It has become quite clear that traditional abdominoplasty approaches do not address the areas of excess skin and fat from the lateral thigh, upper buttock, and back. These must be surgically addressed at the same time as dealing with mid-abdominal redundancy. The circumferential abdominoplasty is efficient in providing a lateral thigh and buttock lift. The plastic surgeon can resuspend the superficial fascial system to achieve a more ideal anatomic correction of the abdomen, lateral thighs, and back.[71] Bariatric patients also display areas of redundancy in the back, which can be surgically corrected. The lower back roll

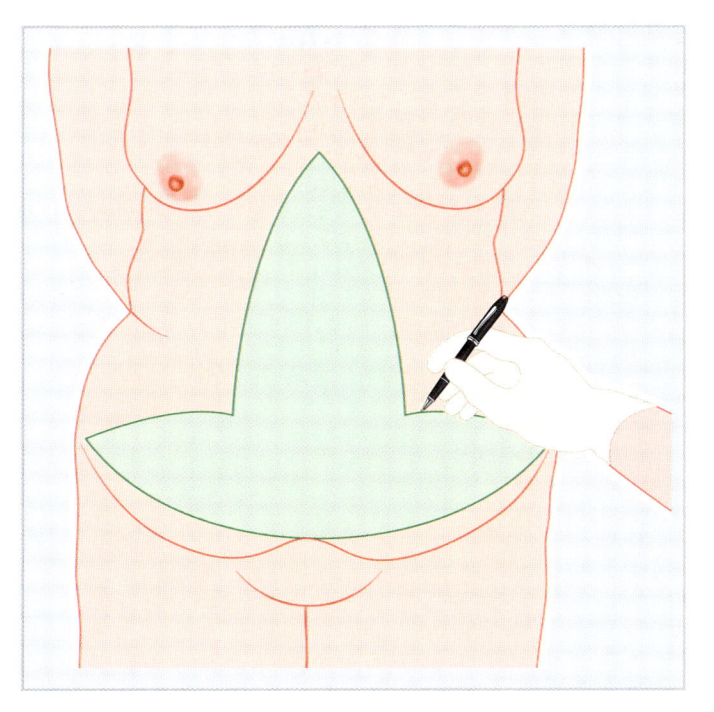

Figure 9.6 The vertical component of the abdominoplasty is then marked as an inverted 'V' (in blue) to address planned excision of abdominal skin and fat with the widest portion being at the base of the triangle as determined by a confirmatory pinch test.

can be addressed together with circumferential abdominoplasty. In addition to including surgery of redundant back tissue in circumferential abdominoplasty, surgery of the buttocks and lateral thighs can be blended into surgery of the abdomen. Despite the inclusion of associated surgical procedures, circumferential abdominoplasty should directly address the anterior abdomen, rectus muscles, and transposition of the umbilicus, as well as any concomitant deformities including ventral, incisional, and umbilical hernias.

Surgical technique

Patients are marked one 1 before surgery and confirmed in the immediate preoperative period to ensure proper surgical planning. Additional adjustments are also often made intraoperatively. With the patient in the standing position, the midlines of the abdomen and back are marked. Marking for the planned lower incision is made first. A transverse line is made across the mons at the suprapubic crease. If, in fact, the mons needs to be lifted, the marking should be made 2–3 cm inferior to the hairline. The transverse line should be extended laterally toward the anterosuperior iliac spine. Markings should continue posterolaterally to the midline of the back. The height of this marking is determined by the degree of lower back and upper gluteal resection needed (**Fig. 9.7**). Next, the planned upper incision is marked out. The pinch technique is used to accurately gauge the volume of skin and fat to be resected and still have a tension-free closure. Anteriorly, the superior extent of the abdominal incision is marked 2–3 cm superior to the umbilicus. It is expected that, after abdominal flap re-draping, this superior marking may be adjusted so a more accurate indication of the degree of tension can be assessed. Posteriorly and laterally, the areas of resection are marked with the patient bent forward at the waist to better determine the degree of laxity to prevent dehiscence and achieve tension-free closure. Surgical markings are then measured and confirmed for symmetry. Vertical marks are then made circumferentially to ensure a more accurate closure.

After surgical markings are performed, the patient is placed over a beanbag in supine position on the operating table. Sequential compression device, TED stockings, perioperative antibiotics, and bladder catheter are then placed. After the patient has been intubated and general anesthesia initiated, the patient is prepped and draped in sterile fashion. First, a circumumbilical incision is made with the assistance of a no. 15 blade scalpel and single-prong skin hooks. Metzenbaum scissors are used to dissect the umbilical stalk. This dissection is continued down to the fascia with care not to exit the umbilical tract skin. The lower abdominal incision is then made to the abdominal wall fascia. Subsequent elevation is performed from the medial to the lateral direction, then in the superior direction to the level of the umbilicus. At this point, care must be taken not to transect the umbilical stalk. Next, the lower abdominal flap is divided along the midline to assist with further dissection cephalad to the umbilicus. Dissection then continues to the level of the costal margins and xiphoid process in the midline. Next, the abdominal flap is lowered and the superior incision is completed, after reassessment of the degree of tension has been made when lowering the flap at the level of the superior incision. The skin flaps are then dissected laterally on both sides to the posterior axillary line. Pre-existing abdominal wall hernias are next addressed through placement of mesh or biologic material. Vertical midline rectus sheath placation is performed 2 cm laterally from midline using 0 Ethibond suture in an interrupted fashion, from the xiphoid process to the umbilicus, then from the umbilicus to the pubic symphysis. Next, a running 1-0 Prolene suture is placed, again from the xiphoid process to the umbilicus, and then from the umbilicus to the pubic symphysis. After rectus plication, an incision is made after re-draping the upper abdominal flap for new placement of the umbilicus. The placement of this midline entry site for the umbilical stalk is at the level of the iliac crests.

Umbilicoplasty is then performed as an inverted V-shaped skin incision is excised, and the umbilical stalk is advanced thorough and secured with 3/0 Monocryl deep dermal and 4/0 Monocryl subcuticular sutures. After re-draping of skin, any anterior excess of skin can

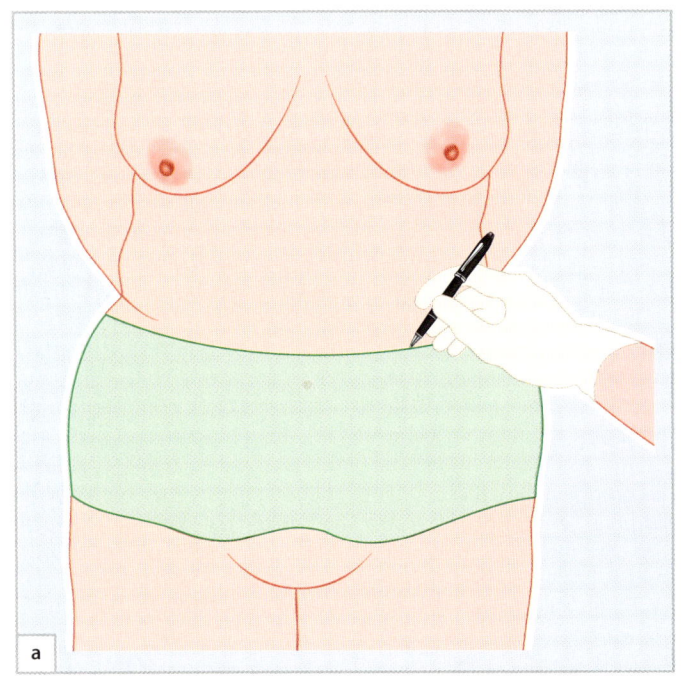

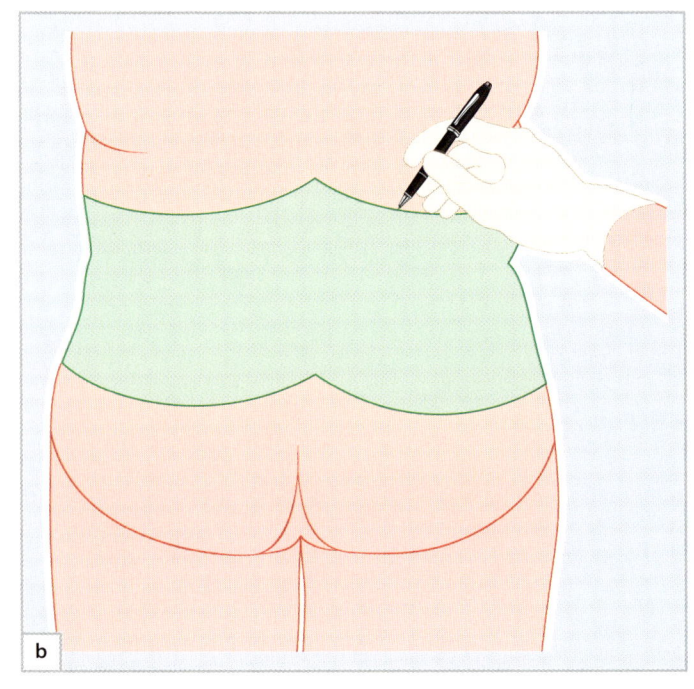

Figure 9.7 A transverse line is made across the mons at the suprapubic crease. If the mons needs to be lifted, the marking should be made 2–3 cm inferior to the hairline. The transverse line should be extended laterally toward the anterosuperior iliac spine. Markings should continue posterolaterally to the midline of the back. The height of this marking is determined by the degree of lower back and upper gluteal resection is needed.

be redistributed circumferentially over the lower skin incision. Two Jackson–Pratt drains are placed exiting on either side of the midline pubic symphysis. The lower abdominal incision is then closed in layered fashion using 0 Ethibond to approximate the Scarpa fascia, 3-0 Vicryl, 3-0 Monocryl sutures are placed in a deep dermal plane, and a 4-0 Monocryl suture is placed in a subcuticular fashion. Dermabond is then placed over the anterior skin. Patients are rotated into the prone position while maintaining a sterile field. Incisions are carried out from previously made lateral incisions, extending medially down to the level of the fascial plane of the deep back musculature. Minimal undermining of the lower back or upper gluteal regions should be made to avoid sarcoma formation. After complete medial dissection, the skin flap is excised. Two Jackson–Pratt drains are placed exiting the lateral incisions. The upper and lower abdominal incision is then closed in layered fashion using 0 Ethibond to approximate the Scarpa fascia, 3-0 Vicryl, 3-0 Monocryl sutures are placed in a deep dermal plane, while 4-0 Monocryl sutures are placed in a subcuticular plane. Dermabond is then placed over the anterior skin incision, followed by an abdominal binder placed around the patient. The patient is transferred to the recovery bed in a supine position with the bed flexed at the hips and knees.

Complications

The complications seen with this surgical technique are similar to those of traditional abdominal procedures. Strauch et al.[72] reported their complications after 75 consecutive circumferential abdominoplasties over a 5-year period. They report no operative perioperative mortalities, or incidence of deep venous thrombosis or pulmonary emboli. Aly et al.[73] reported an incidence of 3 patients (9%) in 32 operations. Seroma formation is often seen as the most frequent complication with circumferential abdominoplasty. Only 1 patient (1.4%) in Strauch's series resulted in a postoperative seroma formation and rates as high as in 12 patients (37%) by Aly et al. The incidence of partial- and full-thickness wound-edge necrosis was seen in five patients (7%) who healed by secondary intention by Strauch et al., compared with four patients (12.5%) by Aly et al.

■ Total body lifting

Many patients who have undergone MWL are candidates for the surgical procedures discussed previously in this chapter. However, there remains a small subset of patients who are in need of body contouring that a circumferential abdominoplasty does not completely address. Total body lifting has emerged as a series of surgical procedures to provide comprehensive surgery under as few general anesthetics as safely as possible. Total body lifting in the MWL patient combines multiple surgical approaches to both the upper and the lower regions of the body. Candidates for total body lifting are in a lower age demographic, generally healthy, and dedicated to improving their self-image.[74] The ideal patient has lost a significant amount of weight and is left with only a residual degree of excess redundant skin (**Fig. 9.8**). Ideally, this can occur after at least 18 months after the original bariatric surgical procedure and at least 3 months of stability in weight. Most often, total body lifting procedures occur in multiple stages of two or three. At least 3–4 months should be separated between surgical procedures in order for the patient's weight to stabilize.[75] When staging procedures, it should be decided between the surgeon and patient which procedures to combine. The areas of most concern should be addressed first, because this will give the patient the greatest amount of satisfaction and motivation to proceed

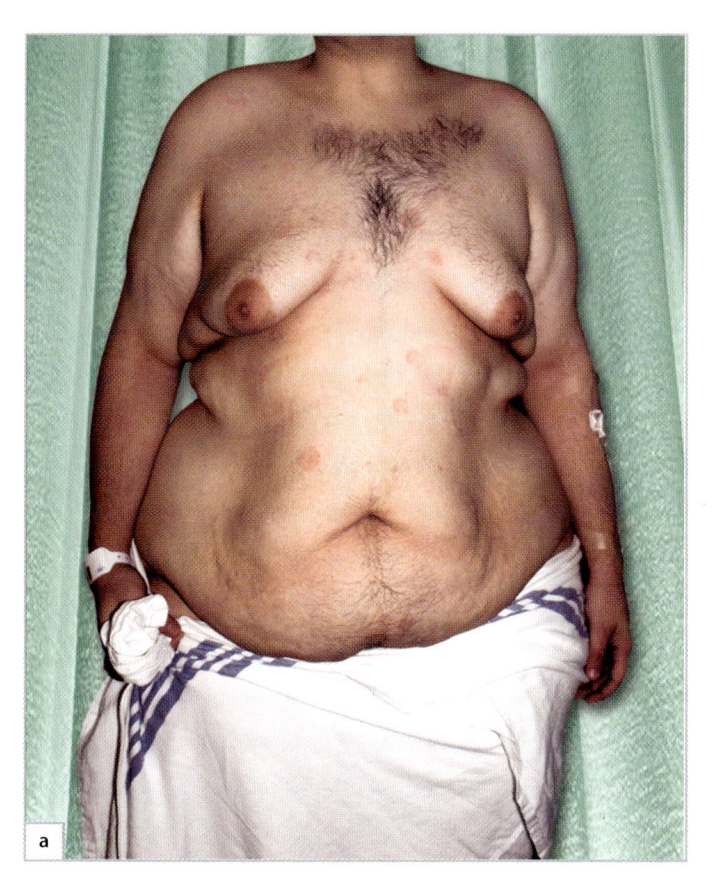

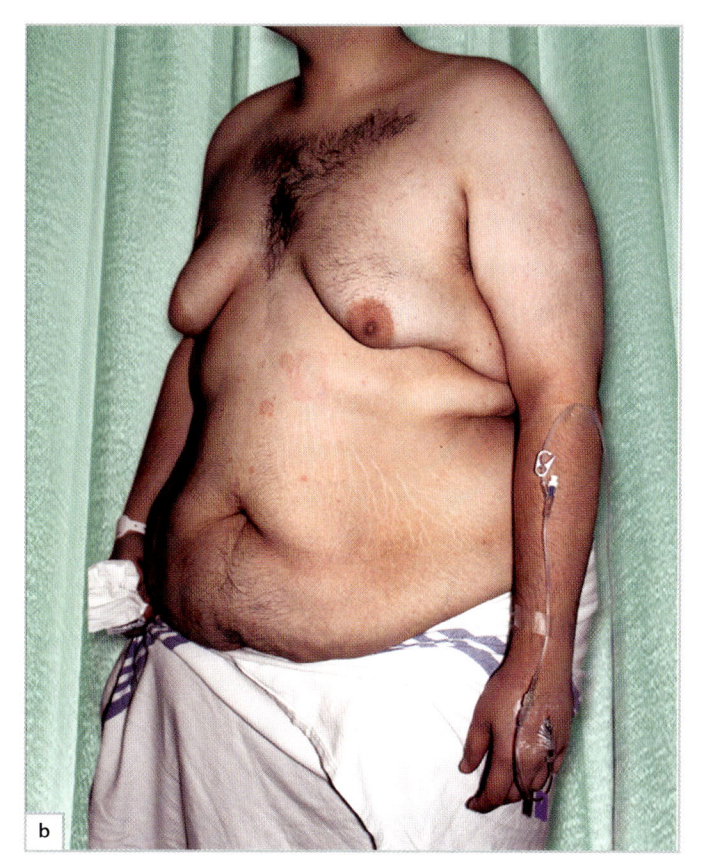

Figure 9.8 The ideal patient has lost a significant amount of weight and is left with only a residual degree of excess redundant skin. *Continued overleaf.*

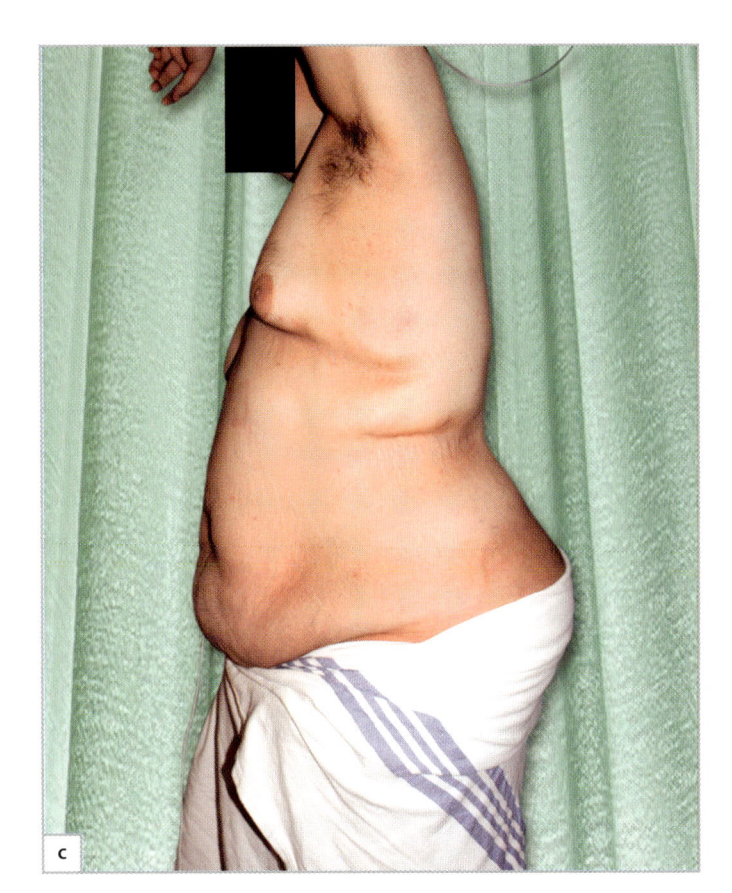

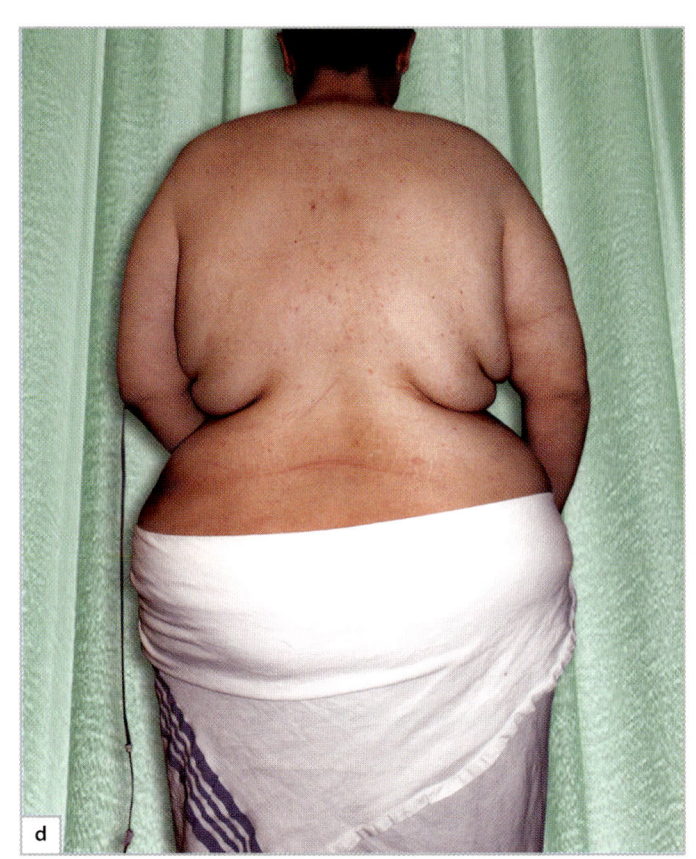

Figure 9.8 The ideal patient has lost a significant amount of weight and is left with only a residual degree of excess redundant skin.

with the subsequent procedures. In addition, if these areas of focus need further revisions, performing the original surgery in the first stage allows for this in the second and third stages. The initial surgical procedure most often includes an abdominoplasty with lower body lift. The second stage usually includes a medial thighplasty, with back roll excision, brachioplasties and mastopexies, as well as any revisions needed from the initial stage.[76] Total body lifting is discussed in detail in Chapters 8 and 10.

CONCLUSIONS

With an increasing number of bariatric procedures occurring each year, as a result there is an ever-expanding population of MWL patients who are in search of the ideal body-contouring procedure that is tailored to the specific needs of the patient. Body contouring after MWL is an expanding field that has seen an exponential rise over the last 10 years.[24] Over this time period, it has become clear that traditional anterior abdominal procedures are not adequately designed for this patient population. Such surgery should not be indicated for these patients; they are deemed inadequate solutions because this population presents unique anatomic and physiological challenges. Over the last decade or so, a number of surgical procedures have emerged to adequately address the concerns of the MWL patient. Although MWL patients have facial aging changes with MWL which, unlike abdominal redundancy, cannot be easily concealed with clothes. Preoperative assessment of patients will determine the ideal surgical approach and the extent of body-contouring procedures. Midbody contouring has become vital in the surgical care of the MWL patient, and an important area of further study and technical advancements in the field of plastic surgery. Body contouring can significantly improve the daily lives of patients by curing many of the physiological, aesthetic, and psychosocial conditions associated with MWL. If performed with strict patient selection criteria, adequate surgical planning and intricate surgical technique, surgery of the midbody can be performed in a safe manner without surgical complications and ideal patient satisfaction.

REFERENCES

1. Sturm R. Increases in clinically severe obesity in the United States, 1986–2000. *Arch Intern Med* 2003;**163**:2146–8.
2. Lee SM, Pryor AD. Future directions in bariatric surgery [Review]. *Surg Clin North Am* 2011;**91**:1373–95, x.
3. Pecori L, Serra Cervetti GG, Marinari GM, et al. Attitudes of morbidly obese patients to weight loss and body image following bariatric surgery and body contouring. *Obes Surg* 2007;**17**:68–73.
4. Fraccalvieri M, Datta G, Bogetti P, et al. Abdominoplasty after weight loss in morbidly obese patients: a 4-year clinical experience. *Obes Surg* 2007;**17**:1319–24.
5. Kelly HA. Excision of fat of the abdominal wall lipectomy. *Surg Gynecol Obstet* 1910;**229**.
6. Thorek M. Plastic reconstruction of the female breast and abdomen. *Am J Surg* 1939;**43**:268.
7. Pitanguy I. Abdominal lipectomy: An approach to it through an analysis of 300 consecutive cases. *Plast Reconstry Surg* 1967;**40**:384.
8. Callia WE. Uma plastic para cirurgiao genal. *Med Hosp* 1967;**11**:40.
9. Grazer FM: Abdominoplasty. *Plast Reconstr Surg* 1973;**51**:617.
10. Regnault P. Abdominoplasty by the W technique. *Plast Reconstr Surg* 1975;**55**:265–74.
11. Grazer FM, Goldwyn RM. Abdominoplasty assessed by survery, with emphasis on complications. *Plast Reconstr Surg* 1977;**59**:513–17.
12. Psillakis JM. Abdominoplasty: Some ideas to improve results. *Aesth Plast Surg* 1978;**2**:205.
13. Lockwood T: High-lateral tension abdominoplasty with superficial fascial system suspension. *Plast Reconstr Surg* 1995;**96**:603.
14. Orpheu SC, Coltro PS, Scopel GP, et al. Collagen and elastic content of abdominal skin after surgical weight loss. *Obes Surg* 2010;**20**:480–6.
15. Erdmann D. Resection of panniculus morbidus: a salvage procedure with a steep learning curve. *Plast Reconstr Surg* 2008;**122**:1290; author reply 1290–2.
16. Manahan MA, Shermak MA. Massive panniculectomy after massive weight loss. *Plast Reconstr Surg* 2006;**117**:2191–7; discussion 2198–9.
17. Zuelzer HB, Baugh NG. Bariatric and body-contouring surgery: a continuum of care for excess and lax skin. *Plast Surg Nurs* 2007;**27**:3–13; quiz 14–5.
18. Fotopoulos L, Khagias I, Kalfarentzos F, et al. Dermatolipectomy following weight loss after surgery for morbid obesity. *Obes Surg* 2000;**10**:451–9.
19. Kitzinger HB, Abayev S, Pittermann A, et al. After massive weight loss: patients' expectations of body contouring surgery. *Obes Surg* 2012;**22**:544–8.
20. Song AY, Rubin JP, Thomas V, et al. Body image and quality of life in post massive weight loss body contouring patients. *Obesity (Silver Spring)* 2006;**14**:1626–36.
21. Friedman KE, Reichmann SK, Costanzo PR, et al. Body image partially mediates the relationship between obesity and psychological distress. *Obes Res* 2002;**10**:33–41.
22. Sarwer DB, Cohn NI, Gibbons LM, et al. Psychiatric diagnoses and psychiatric treatment among bariatric surgery candidates. *Obes Surg* 2004;**14**:1148–56.
23. Bolton MA, Pruzinsky T, Cash TF, et al. Measuring outcomes in plastic surgery: body image and quality of life in abdominoplasty patients. *Plast Reconstr Surg* 2003;**112**:619–25.
24. Gusenoff JA, Pennino RP, Messing S, et al. Post-bariatric surgery reconstruction: patient myths, perceptions, cost, and attainability strategies. *Plast Reconstr Surg* 2008;**122**:1e–9e.
25. Sati S, Pandya S. Should a panniculectomy/abdominoplasty after massive weight loss be covered by insurance? *Ann Plast Surg* 2008;**60**:502–4.
26. Datta G, Cravero L, Margara A, et al. The plastic surgeon in the treatment of obesity. *Obes Surg* 2006;**16**:5–11. Review.
27. Baskin ML, Franklin AF, Allison DB. Prevalence of obesity in the United States. *Obes Rev* 2005;**6**:5–7.
28. Longo DL, Fauci AS, Kasper DL, et al., eds. *Harrison's Principles of Internal Medicine*, 18th edn. New York: McGraw-Hill, 2012.
29. Dumon KR, Murayama KM. Bariatric surgery outcomes. *Surg Clin North Am* 2011;**91**:1313–38.
30. Yosipovitch G, DeVore A, Dawn A. Obesity and the skin: skin physiology and skin manifestations of obesity. *J Am Acad Dermatol* 2007;**56**:901–16. quiz 917–20.
31. Light D, Arvanitis GM, Abramson D, et al. Effect of weight loss after bariatric surgery on skin and the extracellular matrix. *Obes Surg* 2010;**20**:1422–8.
32. Rasmussen MH, Jensen LT, Andersen T, et al. Collagen. Metabolism in obesity: the effect of weight loss. *Int J Obes Relat Metab Disord* 1995;**19**:659–63.
33. Seymour NE, Bell RL. Abdominal Wall, omentum, mesentery, and retroperitoneum. In: Brunicardi FC, Andersen DK, Billiar TR, et al. (eds), *Schwartz's Principles of Surgery*, 9th edn. New York: McGraw-Hill, 2010: Chapter 35.
34. Nahai F, Brown RG, Vasconez LO. Blood supply to the abdominal wall as related to planning abdominal incisions. *Am Surg* 1976;**42**:691–5.
35. Taylor GI. The angiosomes of the body and their supply to perforator flaps. *Clin Plast Surg* 2003;**30**:331–42.
36. Anderson JW, Konz EC, Frederich RC, et al. Long-term weight loss maintenance: a meta-analysis of US studies. *Am J Clin Nutr* 2001;**74**:579–584.
37. Colwell AS, Borud LJ. Optimization of patient safety in postbariatric body contouring: a current review. *Aesthetic Surg J* 2008;**28**:437–442.
38. Davison SP, Clemens MV. Safety first: precautions for the massive weight loss patient. *Clin Plast Surg* 2008;**35**:173–183.
39. Beck FK, Rosenthal TC. Prealbumin: a marker for nutritional evaluation. *Am Fam Physician* 2002;**65**:1575–8.
40. DiSaia JP, Ptak JJ, Achauer BM: Digital photography for the plastic surgeon. *Plast Reconstr Surg* 1998;**102**:569–73.
41. DiBernardo BE, Adams RL, Krause J, Fiorillo MA, et al. Photographic standards in plastic surgery. *Plast Reconstr Surg* 1998;**102**:559–68.
42. Song AY, Jean RD, Hurwitz DJ, Fernstrom MH, Scott JA, Rubin JP. A classification of contour deformities after bariatric weight loss: the Pittsburgh Rating Scale. *Plast Reconstr Surg* 2005;**116**:1535–44.
43. Adams JP, Murphy PG. Obesity in anaesthesia and intensive. *Br J Anaesth* 2000;**85**:91–108.
44. Young T, Palta M, Dempsey J, et al. The occurrence of sleep-disordered breathing among middle-aged adults. *N Engl J Med* 1993;**328**:1230–5.
45. Gross JB, Bachenberg KL, Benumof JL, et al., American Society of Anesthesiologists Task Force on Perioperative Management. Perioperative management of patients with obstructive sleep apnea: a report by the American Society of Anesthesiologists Task Force on Perioperative Management of patients with obstructive sleep apnea. *Anesthesiology* 2006;**104**:1081–93, quiz 1117–18.
46. Hubert HB, Feinleib M, McNamara PM, et al. Obesity as an independent risk factor for cardiovascular disease: a 26-year follow-up of participants in the Framingham Heart Study. *Circulation* 1983;**67**:968–77.
47. Hatef DA, Kenkel JM, Nguyen MQ. Thromboembolic risk assessment and the efficacy of enoxaparin prophylaxis in excisional body contouring surgery. *Plast Reconstr Surg* 2008;**122**:269–79.
48. Espinosa-de-los-Monteros A, de la Torre JI, Rosenberg LZ, et al. Abdominoplasty with total abdominal liposuction for patients with massive weight loss. *Aesthetic Plast Surg* 2006;**30**:42–6.
49. Saldanha OR, De Souza Pinto EB, Mattos WN Jr, et al. Lipoabdominoplasty with selective and safe undermining. *Aesthetic Plast Surg* 2003;**2**:322–7.
50. Saldanha OR, Azevedo SF, Delboni PS, et al. Lipoabdominoplasty: the Saldanha technique. *Clin Plast Surg* 2010;**37**:469–81.
51. Moon HK, Taylor GI. The vascular anatomy of rectus abdominis musculocutaneous flaps based on the deep superior epigastric system. *Plast Reconstr Surg* 1988;**82**:815–29.
52. Matos WN Jr, Ribeiro RC, Marujo RA, da Rocha RP, da Silva Ribeiro SM, Carrillo Jiminez FV. Classification for indications of lipoabdominoplasty and its variations. *Aesthet Surg J* 2006;**26**:417–31.
53. Saldanha OR, Federico R, Daher PF, et al. Lipoabdominoplasty. *Plast Reconstr Surg* 2009;**124**:934–42.
54. Weiler J, Taggart P, Khoobehi K. A case for the safety and efficacy of lipoabdominoplasty: a single surgeon retrospective review of 173 consecutive cases. *Aesthet Surg J* 2010;**30**:702–13.
55. Rebello C, Franco T. Abdominoplasty through a submammary incision. *Int Surg* 1977;**62**:462–3.
56. Pacifico MD, Mahendru S, Teixeira RP, Southwick G, Ritz M. Refining trunk contouring with reverse abdominoplasty. *Aesthet Surg J* 2010;**30**:225–34.
57. Agha-Mohammadi S, Hurwitz DJ. Management of upper abdominal laxity after massive weight loss: reverse abdominoplasty and inframammary fold reconstruction. *Aesthet Plast Surg* 2010;**34**:226–31.

58. Deos MF, Arnt RA, Gus EI. Tensioned reverse abdominoplasty. *Plast Reconstr Surg* 2009;**124**:2134–41.
59. Halbesma GJ, van der Lei B. The reverse abdominoplasty: a report of seven cases and a review of English-language literature [Review]. *Ann Plast Surg* 2008;**61**:133–7.
60. Matarasso A, Wallach SG. Abdominal contour surgery: treating all aesthetic units, including the mons pubis. *Aesthet Surg J* 2001;**21**:111–19.
61. Alter GJ. Management of the mons pubis and labia majora in the massive weight loss patient. *Aesthet Surg J* 2009;**29**:432–42.
62. Marques M, Modolin M, Cintra W, Gemperli R, Ferreira MC. Monsplasty for women after massive weight loss. *Aesthetic Plast Surg* 2012;in press.
63. Rezak KM, Borud LJ. Integration of the vertical medial thigh lift and monsplasty: the double-triangle technique. *Plast Reconstr Surg* 2010;**126**:153e–4e.
64. Michaels J 5th, Friedman T, Coon D, Rubin JP. Mons rejuvenation in the massive weight loss patient using superficial fascial system suspension. *Plast Reconstr Surg* 2010;**126**:45e–6e.
65. Seitz IA, Wu C, Retzlaff K, Zachary L. Measurements and aesthetics of the mons pubis in normal weight females. *Plast Reconstr Surg* 2010;**126**:46e–8e.
66. El-Khatib HA. Mons pubis ptosis: classification and strategy for treatment. *Aesthet Plast Surg* 2011;**35**:24–30.
67. Borud LJ, Warren AG. Modified vertical abdominoplasty in the massive weight loss patient. *Plast Reconstr Surg* 2007;**119**:1911–21.
68. Wallach SG Technical refinements of the vertical mammaplasty: a modified lejour approach. *Aesthet Surg J* 2006;**26**:179–87.
69. Eisenhardt SU, Goerke SM, Bannasch H, Stark GB, Torio-Padron N. Technical facilitation of the fleur-de-lis abdominoplasty for symmetrical resection patterns in massive weight loss patients. *Plast Reconstr Surg* 2012;**129**:590e–3e.
70. Friedman T, O'Brien Coon D, Michaels J, et al. Fleur-de-lis abdominoplasty: a safe alternative to traditional abdominoplasty for the massive weight loss patient. *Plast Reconstr Surg* 2010;**125**:1525–35.
71. Lockwood T. Lower body lift with superficial fascial system suspension. *Plast Reconstr Surg* 1993;**92**:1112–22; discussion 1123–5.
72. Strauch B, Rohde C, Patel MK, et al. Back contouring in weight loss patients. *Plast Reconstr Surg* 2007;**120**:1692–6.
73. Aly A, Cram M, Chao M, et al. Belt lipectomy for circumferential truncal excess: the university of Iowa experience. *Plast Reconstr Surg* 2003;**111**:398–413.
74. Rohrich RJ, Gosman AA, Conrad MH, Coleman J. Simplifying circumferential body contouring: the central body lift evolution. *Plast Reconstr Surg* 2006;**118**:525–35.
75. Hurwitz DJ. Single-staged total body lift after massive weight loss. *Ann Plast Surg* 2004;**52**:435–41; discussion 441.
76. Nemerofsky RB, Oliak DA, Capella JF. Body lift: an account of 200 consecutive cases in the massive weight loss patient. *Plast Reconstr Surg* 2006;**117**:414–30.

Chapter 10

Belt lipectomy and total body lift

Megan C. Jack, Martin I. Newman

INTRODUCTION

As morbid obesity progresses to epidemic proportions, so do bariatric surgical procedures as a means to cure the problem. The result is a growing population of patients interested in or needing body-contouring procedures. In the postbariatric/massive weight loss patient, simply removing residual fat is inadequate because these patients are often left with excess, draping skin. It has been shown that the skin of bariatric patients has altered histological characteristics, including a loose extracellular matrix, poorly organized collagen, fewer dermal fibroblasts, and a decrease in the integrity and number of elastin fibers.[1] As a result of this abnormal architecture, the skin does not shrink as the individuals lose fat. They typically exhibit a 'deflated' appearance: aesthetically, pleasing contours are left obscured by these residual, hanging skinfolds (**Fig. 10.1**). Despite their successful efforts to lose the excessive weight, these patients often do not feel comfortable wearing clothing suited to highlight their new, smaller bodies. In addition, many patients have a variety of medical maladies associated with an excessive and inelastic skin envelope, including intertrigo, breakdowns, and related disorders of bone and muscle. Finally, as they are often left with striae attributable to their prior morbidly obese habitus, they require removal.

In the torso, abdomen, and groin/pelvic regions, a hanging pannus is particularly problematic because these areas set up a chronically moist environment and are prone to fungal and bacterial infections, difficulties with proper hygiene, and rashes. To address these issues, plastic surgeons are increasingly asked to use their creative and artistic skills by recreating the natural, slim body contours through surgical resection of the residual excess skin and fat after massive weight loss. This chapter focuses on the means to do so using belt lipectomy and total body lift procedures.

HISTORY OF THE PROCEDURE

Belt lipectomy

Patients afflicted with the resulting deflated appearance after massive weight loss do not typically have excess skin and soft tissue isolated to the anterior trunk. These rolls are often circumferential, extending to the posterior trunk. Thus, a simple abdominoplasty or panniculectomy alone is insufficient to provide satisfactory improvements in the aesthetic contour for many patients. It may, in fact, exaggerate the flank and back panni. To better address this circumferential issue the 'belt lipectomy' has evolved. This is interchangeable with the terms 'circumferential abdominoplasty' and 'circumferential dermatolipectomy.'[2] The term 'belt lipectomy' was first used by Gonzalez-Ulloa in the early 1960s as a surgical modality to treat obese patients by excising serial wedges of truncal excess. The technique became more sophisticated in the 1980s and 1990s by more efficient use of surgeon *teams*, concomitant liposuction, abdominal wall plication, and position changes.[2-7] Perhaps one of the most significant contributions to the concept of body-contouring surgery and lift was Lockwood's description of the superficial fascial system and the need to anchor this layer during closure to allow for improved scarring and longer-term results.[8] The goal of this procedure is to treat the circumferential aesthetic unit of the abdomen by removal of panni, restoration of contours, and treatment of abdominal wall laxity.

Total body lift

Lockwood emphasized the concept of the trunk as a circumferential aesthetic unit extending from the breasts to the knees, with the abdomen as the 'cornerstone.' It should be treated as such in attempts at restoration of contours.[9] He stressed that treatment of massive weight loss (MWL) patients with global skin excess via belt lipectomy alone will often produce unsatisfactory results because it does not adequately address ptosis of the buttocks and thighs. The total body lift procedure was described initially by Dennis Hurwitz.[10] To address the residual excess skin left over from smaller individual body-contouring procedures, and to avoid 'piecemeal' operations to achieve a desired result, he championed combining individual procedures into one larger comprehensive total body lift. This can be performed in one or two stages, depending on patient needs and desires, together with surgeon preference, or in the minimal number of stages that are safely possible for any given patient. Patients often favor this approach rather than face the laundry list of surgeries needed to achieve their goal. The total body lift addresses the global skin/soft tissue excess problem of the torso and thighs. It may include circumferential abdominoplasty, lower body lift (buttocks and thighs), upper body lift (back and upper abdominal

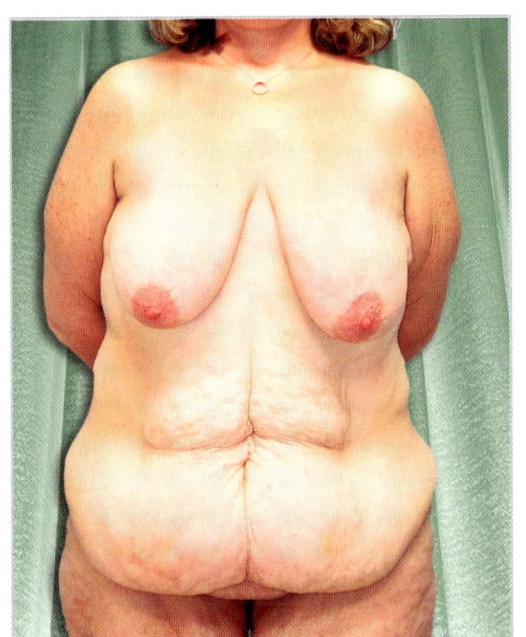

Figure 10.1 Image of a patient after successful massive weight loss surgery. This patient exhibits the classic 'deflated' appearance with hanging panni and obscured aesthetic contours.

region), and breast reshaping. It 'sculpts' the body by excision of excess and reconstruction of what remains into pleasing contours.[10]

RELEVANT ANATOMY

The abdominal wall is composed of skin, subcutaneous fat, the Scarpa (superficial) fascia, deep fat, and the rectus sheath overlying the rectus muscles. The posterior trunk has similar layers with a similar fascia overlying the lower back musculature. A pannus results from a zone of adherence, or a fascial attachment between the dermis and the underlying fascia. These points of adherence act to prevent skin migration away from the fascia, in contrast to those areas without adherence points that are allowed to bulge or sag.

Abdominal blood supply

The blood supply to the anterior abdominal wall originates from the perforators from the superior and inferior epigastric system which penetrate through the rectus muscle.[11-14] The superior epigastric artery originates from the internal mammary (thoracic) artery and its perforators supply the upper abdominal wall skin and soft tissue. The vessel enters the posterior aspect of the rectus abdominis muscle superiorly before branching further into muscle and skin vessels. The inferior epigastric artery originates from the external iliac artery and provides perfusion to the lower abdominal skin and soft tissue. The inferior epigastric artery tends to be the dominant blood supply to the lower rectus abdominis muscle and overlying skin and subcutaneous tissue; however, if either the superior or inferior epigastric artery is transected, the remaining vessel can typically accommodate to supply the entire abdominal wall via the choke system and anastomoses between the two systems. A secondary blood supply originates from subcostal, intercostal, and lumbar vessels, with interconnections to both superior and inferior epigastric arterial systems.

Posterior trunk blood supply

The back has multiple sources of interconnected arterial supply.[11,14] Perforators from the transverse cervical artery off the subclavian artery pierce the trapezius muscle and supply its overlying skin of the upper back. Perforators from the thoracodorsal artery branch from the subscapular artery off the axillary artery and supply the upper, middle, and lower back. These areas are additionally supplied by perforators from the posterior intercostal vessels coursing parallel to the ribs along their inferior border, as well as the lumbar vessels.

Chest/Breast blood supply

The skin overlying the breast is largely supplied by perforators from the internal mammary artery (dominant) and the anterior intercostal arteries.[11,14] Laterally, the chest wall is supplied by the thoracoacromial and lateral thoracic arteries, branches typically from the axillary artery which supplies the lateral chest wall skin, pectoralis major and minor, and the lateral breast.

PREOPERATIVE CONSIDERATIONS

Examination

As in any patient consultation, a thorough history and physical exam are routine. Elements of the history that we find helpful in this context include, but are not limited to, the items listed in **Table 10.1** When performing the physical exam the surgeon should assess areas of skin excess and the estimated amount of soft tissue feasible for resection and closure without undue tension. The exam should look for signs of lymphedema and abdominal hernias, and intertriginous areas should be evaluated for signs of rashes, fungal/bacterial infections, and/or skin breakdown. If abdominal hernias are identified, the approximate size, number, and location are noted. It is critical for the surgeon to rule out hernias. If present, they can be repaired concomitantly. However, concomitant repair of hernia and body contouring is a complex issue, and it brings into play a number of factors and is beyond the scope of this chapter (see Chapter 11). Abdominal wall laxity (rectus diastasis or separation of the rectus muscles from the midline) can be assessed by palpating the rectus and the umbilicus with the patient coughing while in the standing position, by performing a Valsalva maneuver, or by asking the patient perform a partial sit-up while in the supine position. Hernias and rectus diastasis may be difficult to assess in MWL patients but attempts to do so should be made and noted. In addition, it is important to note the quality of the skin, the quantity of subcutaneous tissue present, and any remote or hypertrophic scars or keloids. In addition, the location of scars should be noted because they may affect abdominal wall perfusion.

Finally, preoperative patient photographs are taken, including frontal, bilateral side, posterior, and oblique torso views. The surgeon photographs any intertriginous areas with evidence of rash, infection, or breakdown by asking the patient to elevate the affected pannus to reveal the site. The surgeon may also wish to take more focused images of specific regions to be surgically addressed. Photographic standards recommendations can be found on the American Society of Plastic Surgeons website through the Plastic Surgery Education Network for reference.[15] In addition, a review of photography in body contouring specifically is available.[16] Photographs are added to the medical record.

Table 10.1 Components of history during initial truncal body-contouring consultation.

• Problem area(s) for which patient desires treatment
• Prioritization of areas for which patient desires treatment
• Method of weight loss (e.g. diet, exercise, gastric bypass)
• Maximum weight before weight loss
• Minimum weight after weight loss
• Current weight
• Time patient has been at current weight
• Symptoms specifically related to panni (rashes, wounds, hygiene, clothing fit, self-esteem, pain, arthritis, etc.)
• Current exercise regimen and exercise tolerance
• Current nutrition regimen, including whether patient has a nutrition counselor
• Current medications
• Past medical and surgical history (specifically looking for comorbidities)
• Personal or family history of bleeding disorders, blood clots, keloids, hypertrophic scarring, or wound-healing difficulty
• Tobacco/Alcohol use
• Review of systems – headache, fever, vision changes, chest pain (exertional or at rest), shortness of breath, dyspnea on exertion, night time apnea, productive cough, abdominal pain, nausea/vomiting, dumping syndrome, gastroesophageal reflux, constipation/diarrhea, etc.

Workup and preoperative testing

Before proceeding to the operating room, preoperative testing is ordered based on the history and physical examination findings. These may include chest radiographs in patients with a history of tobacco use or pulmonary disease, electrocardiogram (especially for patients aged > 50 or with a history of cardiovascular disease and/or diabetes). If a hernia has been detected or is suspected, an oral contrast computed tomography (CT) scan of the abdomen may prove helpful. Preoperative laboratory studies in our practice may include a complete blood count (CBC), a comprehensive metabolic panel, nutritional studies (iron, albumin, prealbumin, vitamin B_6 and B_{12} levels, calcium, folate, thiamine), a coagulation profile, and type and screen/cross. Women in their child-bearing years should have a pregnancy test preoperatively and, in many operating rooms, this is mandated by hospital policy. Patients are referred to the primary physician and any indicated specialists (cardiology, pulmonology, etc.) for medical clearance preoperatively and an anesthesia consult if indicated.

Patient selection and timing

For both patient *and* surgeon, it is crucial to properly select patients who are candidates for body contouring. MWL patients should ideally be at a weight loss plateau for at least 3–6 months before considering a belt lipectomy or total body lift. Most often this is anywhere from 18 months to 24 months after a bypass type of bariatric surgical intervention,[17] and may be longer for other types of procedures. This 'waiting period' serves two purposes: First, to ensure that the weight loss is not temporary and, second, that patients will likely not lose additional weight and so will have adequate amounts of excess skin and soft tissue resected. This will optimize their outcomes with respect to the postoperative contours. Some plastic surgeons require that patients achieve and maintain their weight such that they meet a certain body mass index (BMI) cutoff. In our practice a BMI of ≤ 30 is a common goal, with the understanding that there are exceptions to every rule. Some dispute the necessity of such requirements; however, several authors have published the utility of having these patients closer to their ideal weight preoperatively.[3,18-22] A lower BMI has also been shown by these authors to lower the risk of postoperative complications, including wound dehiscence and infections. In one study, the authors found a direct correlation between BMI and complication rates, finding an increase in major and minor complications to 68.7% for super-obese individuals (BMI > 40), 38.1% for morbidly obese indivdiuals (BMI 36–40), 41.7% for obese individuals (BMI 31–40), 27.3% for overweight (BMI 25–30), and 10% for ideal individuals (BMI < 250).[21] For patients who have met a plateau of BMI >30 and remain inhibited from exercise due to large breasts/panni or chronic panniculitis, some favor temporizing procedures such as breast reduction and panniculectomy to allow the patient better success at exercise to promote further weight loss.[22] After a BMI ≤ 30 is reached, further plans may proceed .

As discussed in Chapter 2, a psychosocial assessment proves to be an important componenet when determining whether the patient can cope with the psychological effects of extensive body contouring after massive weight loss. It is helpful for the surgeon to determine patients' level of motivation for achieving theie goals as well as the surrounding support system to help them through this process. This can in part be gauged by the surgeon from their weight loss history, weight loss maintenance, current diet/exercise regimen, and family/friends who attend visits with the patient.

Women in the child-bearing years are questioned about history of and future plans for pregnancy. Pregnancy has significant hormonal and physical effects on the body and often results in wide fluctuations in body habitus. Consideration may be given to the option of waiting until after the patient completes her child bearing before proceeding with her procedure(s) in some cases. If she is not interested in waiting until completion of child bearing, the patient is reminded that future pregnancies may compromise her long-term results.

It is well appreciated that postbariatric patients are at risk for wound-healing issues including dehiscance, seroma, and infection. This may be due to the metabolic effects from their prior morbid obesity and/or the weight loss itself.[17] Despite a history of obesity, these patients may in fact be malnourished; malabsorptive procedures may also play a role. Patients can be optimized from a nutrition standpoint and ideally continue to see a dietician with monitoring of their nutrition laboratory studies under the direction of their bariatric surgeon. Medications that could potentially negatively impact wound healing (e.g. steroids, immunosuppressants) are minimized or discontinued by their primary physician if possible.

Finally, comorbid conditions certainly must be considered – cardiac disease, pulmonary disease, thromboembolic disease, diabetes, and others are common in bariatric patients. They are often improved after massive weight loss; however, the risks of surgery in the setting of any comorbid condition(s) must be weighed against the benefit of this non-urgent procedure. If the plastic surgeon feels that the risk is too great, the patient should be referred back to the appropriate medical specialists for treatment of their other disease processes and optimization for surgery.

Procedure choice

Often, patients present to their plastic surgeon with a focused area to be addressed. For patients who present with complaints of circumferential excess skin and hanging panni without other areas of concern or resources that allow them only a single operation, circumferential abdominoplasty is an appropriate choice. However, when many patients are questioned they often reveal dissatisfaction with the appearance of multiple areas. This is often the case for MWL patients, because many of them are plagued with more global skin excess. Although some patients require/desire a focused, limited intervention, others are very motivated to achieve their goal of an 'extreme makeover' through one solitary operating room visit. Patients with an interest in addressing, for example, improvement in contour of the abdomen, back, breasts, thighs, and buttocks all at once may be good candidates for a total body lift procedure. However, many patients may not be good candidates for such an extensive procedure. Therefore, it is important to understand patient desires and to prioritize areas of dissatisfaction to fashion a coordinated and organized surgical plan. This is particularly important in patients who are not good candidates for extensive intervention and are willing to undergo staging of their procedures. In our practice it is preferable to stage numerous procedures for a number of reasons. Opposing tension lines may be associated with combining some procedures (e.g. augmentation–mastopexy) and this *may* negatively impact scarring. Another reason to stage multiple procedures is the length of surgery. Limiting surgical time may help to limit risks. Finally, a planned return to the operating room for subsequent stages offers the opportunity for minor revisions which can be helpful when trying to manage skin that has lost its elasticity. Notwithstanding the aforementioned cautions, we acknowledge that it is possible for selected, healthy, physically fit patients to undergo a single-stage total body lift with careful attention to lines of tension, patient safety, and potential revisions.

Counseling

Counseling for bariatric patients begins when they start the process for weight-loss surgery. In addition to the surgical counseling patients receive before their weight loss procedure, it is often helpful for patients to be counseled by their weight-loss medical team as to the impact of bariatric surgery on their body habitus, including the expected residual skin and soft tissue excess that will remain despite fat loss. Ideally, the bariatric surgeon would discuss with patients preoperatively that plastic surgeons are an available resource to treat the excess skin and soft tissue after their bariatric procedure, and possibly even make the plastic surgeon a part of the weight-loss team to allow a preoperative meeting.

At their first and subsequent visits in the plastic surgeon's office during preoperative planning, the patient may be counseled on several factors to optimize the results and provide realistic expectations for results. First and foremost, patients need to understand that the tradeoff for removal of this problematic excess tissue and improved body contours is scarring – and this can be unpredictable. In many bariatric patients, to restore or at least provide significant improvement in the aesthetic contours, the scarring may be significant. Surprisingly, many patients in this population willingly accept scars that non-bariatric patients would consider unacceptable. In addition, patients who have a history of poor wound healing or hypertrophic scarring and keloids should be counseled accordingly.

As discussed above, it is helpful to reinforce the importance of good nutrition such that weight can be maintained and wound healing will be optimal – both of which will optimize chances of good results after their body-contouring procedure. Patients are reminded to continue their nutritionist/dietician visits on a regular basis throughout and after this process. In addition, as with any other elective procedure, the benefits of smoking cessation should be emphasized. Part of the preoperative discussion may also include the implications of taking certain medications (e.g. steroids, hormones), non-compliance with diet and exercise, future pregnancy, and weight regain, which may all negatively impact the long-term results of their body-contouring procedure.

As with any operation, risks, benefits, and alternatives are discussed. Risks may include, but are not limited to, wound-healing problems, infection, hematoma, pain, seroma, scars (normal, hypertrophic, keloids, scar migration), numbness, injury to adjacent structures, need for reoperation, and bleeding requiring transfusion. Patients should be counseled to avoid medications that may contribute to bleeding (**Table 10.2**) for 2 weeks before and 2 weeks after surgery. By no means is this list comprehensive – the surgeon should take a thorough medication history and research the effects of medications if unknown. Dietary supplements with unknown effects on coagulation should be discontinued. It may also be helpful to provide patients with a handout listing the more common medications that should be held or stopped before surgery.

Finally, expectations are addressed and must be realistic. If they are unrealistic, the surgeon should be cautious about proceeding without further counseling, if at all. Patients are reminded that perfect results are unlikely and secondary procedures may be required to fine-tune certain areas and scars. It may be helpful for the surgeon to have a group of patients who previously underwent a belt lipectomy or total body lift who can serve as a resource for the preoperative body-contouring patient to fully obtain a comprehensive grasp of the surgical expectations and recovery. Allowing the preoperative patients to contact postoperative patients and giving them time to consider these patient-to-patient discussions can be a helpful adjunct to both patient and surgeon.

Table 10.2 Medications and herbal supplements that may increase perioperative bleeding risk.[10,23]

Medications	Herbal supplements
Aspirin and aspirin-containing medications	Bilberry
Carisoprodol	Dong quai
Clopidogrel	Echinacea
Enoxaparin	Ephedra
First-generation antipsychotic agents (e.g. haloperidol)	Feverfew
	Fish oil
Goody/BC powders	Garlic
Heparin	Ginger
Ibuprofen and ibuprofen-containing medications	Ginko
	Ginseng
Indometacin	Glucosamine
Monoamine oxidase inhibitors	Goldenseal
Nabumetone	Kava
Naproxen	Licorice
Other nonsteroidal anti-inflammatory medications	Omega-3 fatty acids
	St John's wort
Piroxicam/Meloxicam	Valerian
Propoxyphene	Vitamin E
Selective serotonin release inhibitors	
Sulindac/Diclofenac	
Sumatriptan/Avitriptan	
Toradol	
Warfarin	

These medications or those including these medications should be stopped or held for 10–14 days pre- and postoperatively. This list is meant as a guide and should not be considered comprehensive.

TECHNIQUE

Belt lipectomy
Marking (Figure 10.2)

Before surgery, a final assessment of the patient is made by the operating surgeon and markings are made. Patients are typically best assessed starting in the upright standing position with the legs spread to shoulder width. The surgeon ensures that the patient is not slouching, shifting to the side, or dropping a shoulder unilaterally because this will potentially cause the markings to be asymmetric and/or fall off the horizontal plane. After the initial markings are made (as described below), the surgeon may wish to reassess the markings in the supine and prone positions to ensure adequacy of resection and observe the changing effect of gravity. The anterior vertical midline is marked from the level of the sternal notch to the anterior labial commissure inferiorly. The position of the anterosuperior iliac spine (ASIS) is noted bilaterally. The superior aspect of the mons pubis hair is noted and a horizontal line marked at this point or, if is to be lifted, slightly inferior to this line.

Sometimes, the surgeon will have to use the non-marking hand to lift the mons tissue cephalad to determine the amount of lift needed. Different patients will require different marking based on their habitus. One common pattern that may be applicable to many candidates is a 'lazy W'. From the bilateral edge of the vertical midline mark at the pubis, an S-shaped line is made obliquely toward and connecting to the ASIS. The surgeon then pinches the abdominal skin or pannus

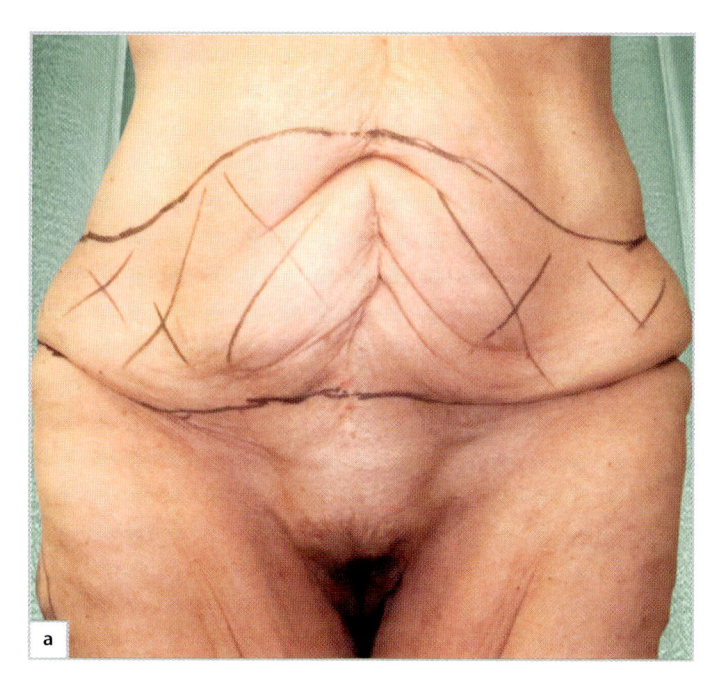

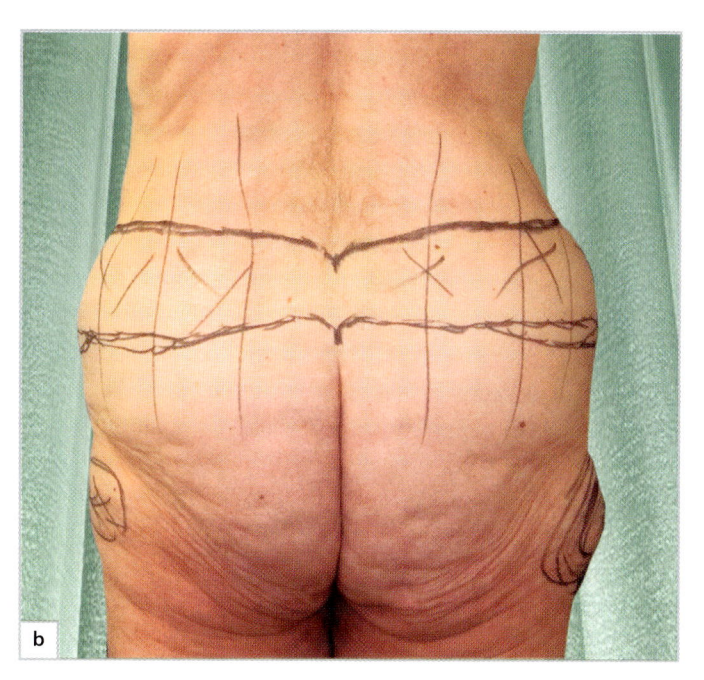

Figure 10.2 Preoperative markings for circumferential abdominoplasty. (a) Anterior and (b) posterior views of the preoperative markings in preparation for circumferential abdominoplasty. Note the 'lazy W' course of the line anteriorly, transition to the flank laterally, and the 'V' posteriorly. This patient will also receive additional suction-assisted liposuction of the posterolateral thighs as indicated by the circle and hashed markings on posterior view (b).

to determine the appropriate amount of tissue to be resected, both centrally and in the lateral trunk. Aly advocates an aggressive lateral resection to truly improve the curving contours in this region.[3] The upper line of the abdominal excision can then be drawn, as typical in abdominoplasty, from just cephalad to the umbilicus centrally to the midaxillary line laterally. Unlike abdominoplasty, however, the upper line will not connect to a point in elliptical fashion; rather as the surgeon pinches the midaxillary line tissue, a point of maximal resection is determined in this area and the line is connected to this point.

The patient is then turned placing the back to the surgeon and the process is repeated on the back. The vertical midline is noted and marked. The lateral extents of both the upper and lower lines are continued posteriorly to meet in the midline; all the while the surgeon checks the amount of skin that can reasonably be resected by pinching. Having the patient bend forward at the hips during the posterior trunk marking can be very helpful at this point. The upper lines will course obliquely and inferiorly slightly until the point that they meet in the midline, forming a wide 'V'. The lower line will be drawn obliquely and superiorly at a slightly steeper course and, when nearing the midline, should be curved back downward to make a more acute 'V'. It is often helpful to make vertically oriented hash marks, with alternating colors connecting the upper and lower lines circumferentially, to help keep the surgeon oriented at the time of closure. It is feasible to offer the patient supplemental suction-assisted lipectomy at the time of their belt lipectomy for focused problem areas (e.g. saddle bags). If this is to be done, these sites are marked per the surgeon's preference at this time. Intravenous antibiotics are administered, patient warming can be initiated, and sequential compression devices are placed on the bilateral lower extremities.

Positioning

Through the years, there has been much discussion regarding proper patient positioning for this circumferential procedure. 'Side–side–supine', 'lower extremity abduction' and 'prone–supine' have all been proposed. In our practice, we are comfortable with the 'prone–supine' approach. The patient is taken to the operating room and general anesthesia is administered and a urinary catheter sterilely inserted. The patient is then placed in the prone position on the operating table. The surgical and anesthetic teams should work together to ensure that the patient is positioned properly to avoid possible nerve injury. All pressure points are carefully padded. The back, buttocks, and thighs are then prepped down to the level of the operating table bilaterally and sterilely draped.

Operation

The inferior line of resection is incised from as far toward anterior as possible bilaterally and then taken down almost to the muscular fascia with electrocautery. A thin layer of fat and areolar tissue on the muscular fascia is preserved. Similarly, the upper line is incised and the tissue between the two is undermined in that areolar plane in its entirety, and is transected at the anterior-most aspect of the incisions bilaterally. Some surgeons may prefer to test the tension before making the superior incision. In this situation, before making the superior incision towel clips can be used to bring the superior line in approximation to the inferior incision. It may be necessary to perform some minor undermining before performing this test, but in our practice we try to avoid undermining the posterior trunk skin when possible. If desired, liposuction of indicated posterior and posterolateral areas can be performed using the existing incision for access at this point. Hemostasis is critically appraised, the site is irrigated with warm saline, and, if the surgeon desires, a topical thrombin spray applied. Two closed suction drains are then placed and brought out through the incisions laterally and the wound is closed in layers to avoid undue tension. This includes closure of the Scarpa layer, deep dermis, and subcuticular levels with absorbable monofilament sutures. Dressings are applied by surgeon preference and in our practice include sterile liquid adhesive skin glue. In preparation for turning, we close the bilateral transition points with staples and cover these areas with large, clear, sterile, occlusive dressings.

Then, the patient is carefully repositioned to supine with attention to the positioning factors mentioned above.

Pressure points are padded, monitors are checked, and then the entire abdomen, mons, and thighs are prepped to the level of the operating table bilaterally. Preparation is inclusive of the occlusive clear dressings placed before repositioning. The patient is sterilely draped, and the occlusive dressings are removed. Similar to descriptions above, the inferior line of excision is incised first, continuing from the transition points laterally, and electrocautery is used to carry this incision down to the areolar plane just above the muscular fascia. Superficial epigastric vessels (as well as other perforating vessels to the skin) tend to be prominent in obese or formerly obese patients to supply the increased body area. It is important to identify these if they prove to be prominent and to ligate them with hemoclips or suture. Similarly the superior marking is incised and dissected to the muscular fascia, preserving a thin layer of adipose. A circular incision is made surrounding the umbilicus leaving a 2- to 4-mm cuff of skin circumferentially. A marking stitch is placed at the 12 o'clock position on this cuff and a long tail left to aid in umbilicoplasty at the end of the procedure. Blunt scissors are then used to spread and dissect a small cuff of tissue circumferentially around the umbilical stalk, down to its base. In our practice a small cuff of fat surrounding the stalk is preserved. Suspicion for a previously undiagnosed umbilical hernia should be high, and this dissection should proceed with appropriate caution with respect to this possibility. Once the base has been reached the skin between the upper and lower incisions is then elevated off the muscular fascia in the areolar plane.

The superior skin flap is then elevated using skin retractors and electrocautery is used to undermine approximately to the xiphoid in the midline and the subcostal margins bilaterally. This flap is then re-draped over the abdomen and if the need arises mobilized further to allow for taut closure while avoiding excessive tension. The rectus muscles are then evaluated and, if found to have laxity, are plicated in a fashion similar to typical abdominoplasty. Some authors advocate 'defatting' of the superior skin flaps in select patients with persistent excess fat deep to the Scarpa layer using sharp dissection.[4] Any additional liposuction necessary (e.g. lateral thighs, flank) can be performed at this time through the existing wound, with attention to the blood supply of the abdominal flap. Although we acknowledge that literature exists to the contrary, these additional maneuvers may impart additional risk to flap perfusion and should be carried out with attention to this notion.

The abdominal flap is then re-draped, held on tension at the position for closure, and the new position of the umbilicus marked. In our practice, the flap is held in position with penetrating towel clips. The umbilical position is marked by using the surgeon's non-dominant hand beneath the flap to indicate the umbilical position on the abdominal wall. The marking hand palpates the skin of the abdominal flap overlying the non-dominant hand to find the appropriate location. A horizontal marking is made indicating this level. The midline, as marked preoperatively, should pass through this horizontal line. However, if this marking were lost during the procedure, or, should alteration of the midline occur, it should be re-approximated between the sternal notch and anterior labial commissure with a marker. Two closed suction drains are then placed and can be brought out through the wounds laterally or through stab incisions and secured with drain stitches. Hemostasis is confirmed and the site is irrigated with warm saline. At this time, the operating room table should be placed in the semi-flexed position to aid in closure and the abdominal skin flap can be tailor tacked to test the tension. If it is too taut, the bed may need to be flexed more sharply, but undue tension on the closure should be avoided during the preoperative marking process. If the tension is inadequate, additional skin may be resected from the abdominal skin flap where necessary. The wound is then closed in layers as described above.

During the closure, efforts should be directed at reducing the possibility of 'dog ears' laterally. If noted, the lateral skin of the abdominal skin flap can be 'walked' medially to redistribute the excess tissue more medially. If this is not sufficient to avoid a dog ear, additional skin resections may be necessary during closure. Having said this, we understand that some redundancy manifesting as a 'dog ear' is sometimes unavoidable. Finally, the mons pubis can also be lifted during the medial incision closure. One suture is placed in the midline from the abdominal wall flap to the mons. The corners of the mons (indicated by the end of the hairline typically) are noted and a stitch is placed in each, pulling them laterally and securing them to the abdominal skin flap. If further mons lift is desired, additional skin may be resected from this area. It is inadvisable to mobilize the deep tissue of the mons to facilitate lift however, as this tends to be painful to the patients and may increase the risk of seroma formation in this dependent area. A lift of the corresponding tissue in male MWL patients may help minimize the 'buried penis' phenomenon of such patients.

Umbilicoplasty is then performed at the site marked on the abdominal skin flap. Our preferred technique is to make a semicircular incision from approximately the 10 o'clock to the 2 o'clock position, arcing upward and then downward like a 'frown'; this may need to be extended if the umbilicus is sizeable. Extremely long umbilical stalks may require truncation at a portion of the distal margin. The fat is dissected bluntly and the Scarpa fascia dilated with thin, deep retractors such as an Army–Navy retractor, to reduce the possibility of constricting the stalk. The umbilicus is delivered through the incision. The marking stitch is then used to orient the 12 o'clock position on the umbilicus to the midline of the new position on the abdominal wall flap. The cuff of skin surrounding the umbilicus is trimmed as needed to allow for inversion at closure and it is inset using buried 3/0 monofilament, absorbable, interrupted suture and the skin closed with 5/0 fast-absorbing suture (**Fig. 10.3**).

Variations of the above, including shape and location of incisions, as well as sequence of positioning, are available in the literature. Aly and colleagues[2] published their experience with a variation of the above technique using supine–lateral–lateral positioning, and provide a nice description of their technique. Their average operating time was 5.75 hours and they achieved good results in 32 patients with 94% improvement in body contour, 97% in abdominal wall laxity, and 78% in mons pubis ptosis. In addition they describe an added benefit to the patient with buttock ptosis, in that a greater lateral flank excision will result in a moderate lift of the buttock, especially reorienting the lower buttock crease to a more oblique rather than a horizontal position.[2,3] Occasionally, pre-existing scars may require a variation in the technique. For patients with a midline supraumbilical scar, this scar can be resected and reclosed to surround the newly positioned umbilicus. A subcostal scar may be repositioned more inferiorly with this technique and it is important to discuss this with the patient preoperatively, plus any possible options to treat this depending on its orientation. More vertically oriented subcostal scars may be incorporated into a vertical excision component with closure around the newly positioned umbilicus. Alternatively, if this is of great concern to patients and they are candidates, reverse abdominoplasty/upper body lift in addition to or instead of lower body lift may be an option.

Figure 10.3a Circumferential abdominoplasty. Anterior, oblique, lateral, and posterior photographs of a patient preoperatively. *Continued on p. 96.*

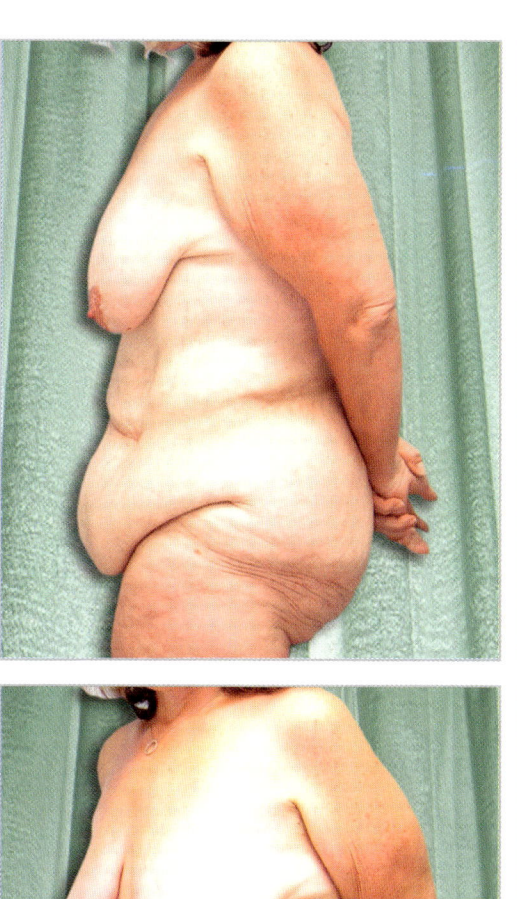

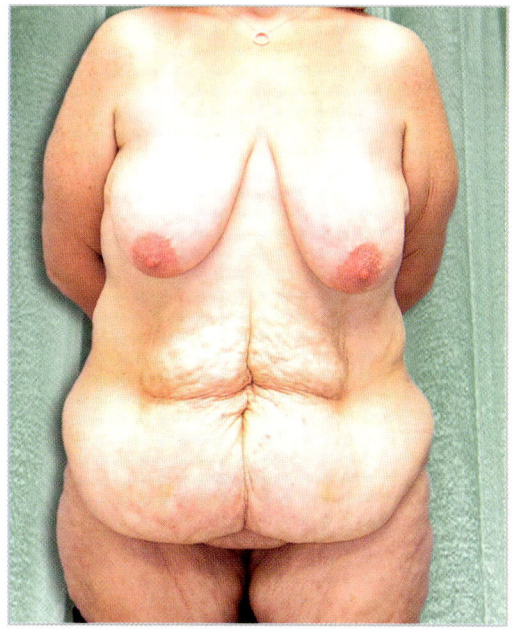

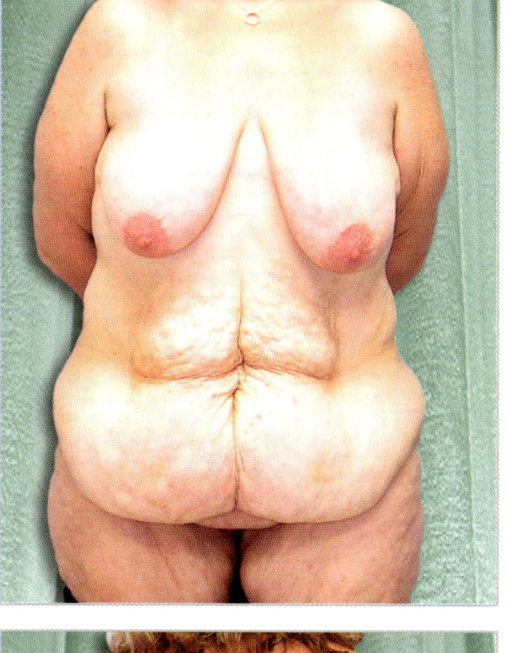

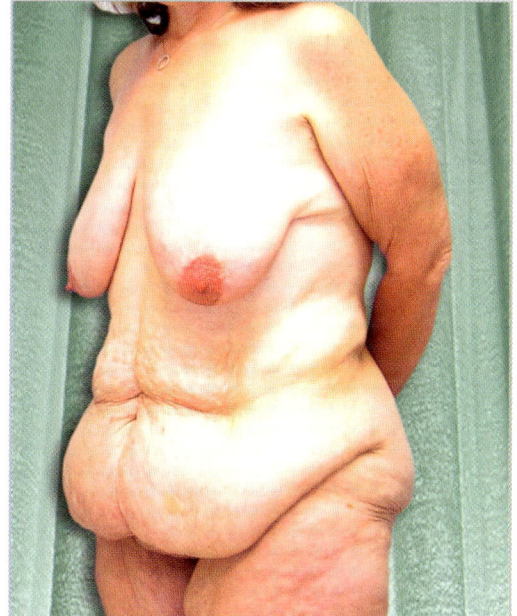

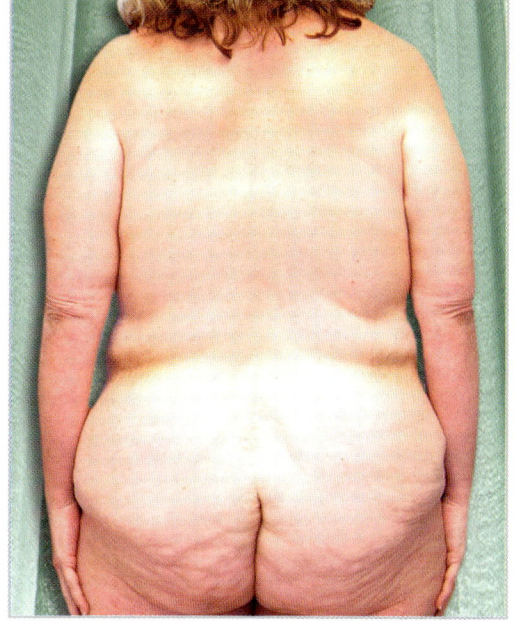

Total body lift

Marking

The total body lift encompasses breast reshaping, upper and lower body lift, and circumferential abdominoplasty performed in a single or several prioritized stages. In selected patients (younger, healthy, motivated), a single stage is feasible. The patient is assessed by the surgeon for final marking 1 day before surgery or in the preoperative holding suite on the same day. Patients are best evaluated with them in the standing position and the surgeon at eye level to the area being marked. The skin of the sites being addressed are pinched and critically appraised by the surgeon to determine the amount of skin to be resected, while allowing for taut re-draping of skin without undue tension on the closure. Others are proponents of marking patients while in the supine position. Incisions are generally marked in an elliptical or crescenteric shape to allow for closure that minimizes dog ears, and ideally lines of closure are situated such that they are hidden by undergarments or in areas less exposed to the public eye. However, this is not always possible and we appreciate the fact that scars may migrate. It is often helpful to have the patient or an assistant elevate the pannus to allow the surgeon complete, hands-free visualization of the site for marking.

In addition to the circumferential abdominoplasty marking as described above, if a medial thigh lift is to be performed this is marked. These may follow a 'crescent' pattern or a 'medial thigh' pattern. For the 'crescent' pattern, marking can be performed in the standing or lying position. In the standing position, the patient will need to stand with feet spread widely; if in the lying position having the patient lie laterally and elevating the top leg will allow for adequate exposure on each side. First the groin crease is marked bilaterally

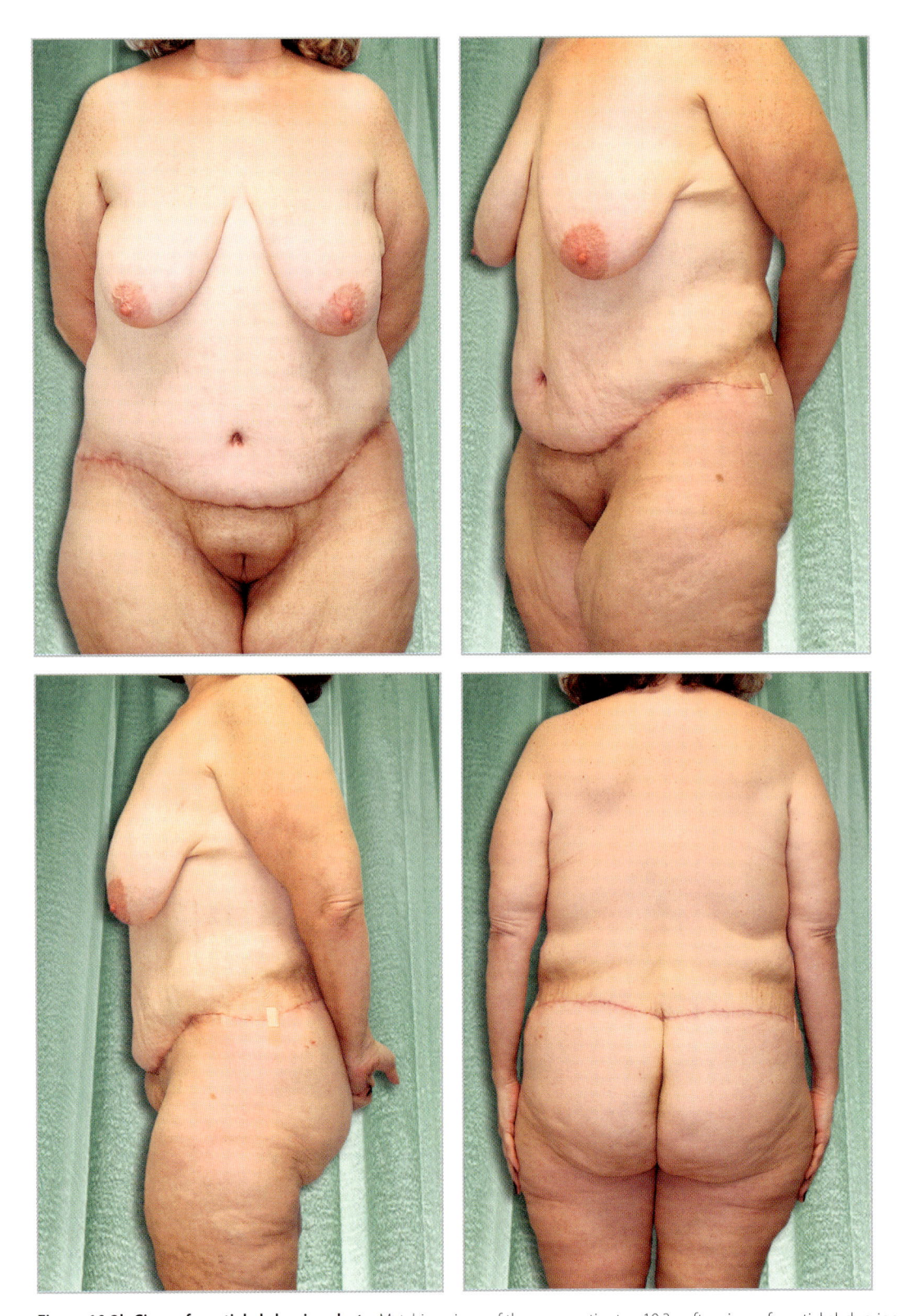

Figure 10.3b Circumferential abdominoplasty. Matching views of the same patient as 10.3a, after circumferential abdominoplasty, showing removal of the pannus and improvement in the aesthetic contour of the lower abdomen and back.

from the ASIS to the posterior aspect of the medial thigh and continued posteriorly to the gluteal crease. The skin is then pinched and the lower line of excision is marked using the same endpoints to form a crescent shape of skin to be excised. If there is excess skin in the vertical plane, the lower skin incision can be modified to a V-shaped lower line while orienting the vertical line of closure more posteriorly on the thigh. This vertical extension of the medial thigh lift can sometimes be extended from the level of the knee to the transition zone between the labia and perineum posteriorly on the thigh. This latter, more extended pattern is sometime referred to as the 'medial thigh' pattern. In practice, we hold that 'tightening' is more durable when achieved by capturing and resecting skin in the horizontal plane (as is achieved with the medial thigh pattern). As well, contouring of the lower extremity is best applied to redundant skin only, and not to excess adipose or soft tissue that may contain (and disrupt) lymphatics and/or venous return.

For upper body lift markings, first the inframammary fold is marked by elevating each breast cephalad and marking the fold in the skin from the point where it meets the sternum medially to the mid to posterior axillary line laterally, depending on where the breast tissue ends. For patients with subaxillary fat/skin rolls this line will likely extend more posteriorly. The excess skin below this line is pinched and the inferior aspect marked in a horizontal line to each posterior axillary line bilaterally. Patients who have upper back rolls may very well be candidates for a circumferential excision. Similar to the markings for circumferential abdominoplasty, the back rolls are pinched to determine the maximum amount of skin/fat to feasibly be excised and two horizontal lines of excision are drawn, meeting the points of the reverse abdominoplasty and breast reshaping markings laterally. If possible the lower line on the back is drawn within the bra line (female patients) to better conceal scarring, with the understanding that this is not always feasible and scars can migrate.

Positioning

In the operating room and after general anesthesia has been initiated, the patient is then placed in the prone position on the operating table. As with all surgery, the surgical and anesthesia teams should work together to ensure that the patient is positioned to avoid possible injury. All pressure points are carefully padded and sequential compression devices, activated before induction, should be continued if at all possible. Intravenous antibiotics should be administered within 30–45 min of incision and a urinary catheter sterilely inserted. As with belt lipectomy, when possible warm air blankets should be applied to non-surgical areas. The back, buttocks, and upper thighs are then prepped down to the operating table bilaterally and draped sterilely to allow for wide exposure.

Operation

The posterior aspects of all areas being treated (upper and lower body lift, circumferential abdominoplasty) are addressed in this position in a fashion similar to that described above. The incisions are closed to the extent possible in the prone position into the transition zone to the anterior torso. The transition zone is the covered with an adherent dressing (e.g. Tegaderm, OpSite) and the patient is then repositioned to the supine position, adhering to caveats as above. The anterior torso and thighs are then prepped to the operating table bilaterally and sterilely draped. All remaining areas to be treated on the anterior torso/thighs are then addressed in this position. If performing a medial thigh lift, the legs may be abducted. Depending on the anticipated surgical time and what other procedures are being performed with the thigh surgery, options for leg placement in the supine position include frog-leg, padded hand tables, and stirrups.

To optimize scar healing and postoperative aesthetics, wounds should be closed in layers – Scarpa, deep dermal, and subcuticular. Subcuticular suturing with absorbable monofilament suture is preferred by many but is admittedly not the only option. Finally, during closure of all sites attention should be paid to 'dog ears' at incisional apices. Preoperative marking may help minimize these, by making the apices of the elliptical incisions more acute if possible. Redistribution of tissue may be achieved by starting closure at the apex (rather than centrally) and walking the tissue from lateral to medial, thereby minimizing dog ears. If dog ears remain despite these attempts, further local skin resection from the apex may be needed to eliminate these unsightly areas. Specific details for each area potentially addressed are discussed below.

Circumferential abdominoplasty is performed as described as above and together with a lower body lift in patients who desire minimization of surgical stages.

Lower body lift

The areas treated by lower body lift portion of the procedure include the thighs, buttocks, abdomen, back, and mons pubis and is often concomitantly performed with circumferential abdominoplasty. At completion of the belt lipectomy and to eliminate the saddlebag deformity of the thighs, the skin of the thighs can be extensively undermined via liposuction or long dissecting instruments (e.g. liposuction cannulas, Lockwood undermining cannulas). Lockwood emphasizes in his technique the importance of undermining to release the lateral thigh zones of adherence especially in the trochanteric region.[9] Release of the sites of dermal attachment to the underlying skeletal structure will aid the surgeon in adequately lifting the thighs at closure. Once undermining is complete, the thigh skin is stretched and re-draped cephalad and excess skin/soft tissue resected. The amount of skin can be determined with specialized instruments (e.g. Lockwood marking clamp) or estimating using penetrating towel clamps. Closed suction drains can then placed and brought out through stab incisions laterally or within the superior mons and secured with drain stitches. The wounds are then closed in layers including a deep Scarpa layer, deep dermal stitches, and subcuticular running suture all with absorbable monofilament suture. Depending on the patient's body habitus, the surgeon may offer a medial thigh lift to address medial thigh skin laxity as it will not necessarily be adequately addressed with a lower body lift.

Upper body lift

This aspect of the procedure can include reverse abdominoplasty, inframammary fold resuspension, breast reshaping, and removal of excess mid-torso skin. While the patient is prone, the posterior markings are incised and the skin between the two horizontal lines is excised, leaving a thin layer of adipose tissue on the fascia. The upper and lower back subcutaneous fat remaining is then undermined in the suprafascial plane, with the extent of undermining determined on an individual basis with the knowledge that this region can be prone to the development of problematic seroma formation (e.g. latissimus dorsi flaps). The upper and lower flaps are then brought together, ideally in the bra line and closed in layers with absorbable monofilament sutures. When all posterior steps have been completed, the patient can be flipped into the supine position with proper attention to detail and precautions as above. The anterior upper body lift markings are then incised and the skin and fat between the lines excised. The superior abdominal skin is undermined to the subcostal margin to allow for adequate mobilization for the lift, and 2/0 absorbable monofilament sutures are serially placed bilaterally, securing the Scarpa fascia to the abdominal wall at the level of the sixth rib – to help obliterate the dead space and add durability to the lift. The inframammary fold is then raised to an appropriate level if needed (approximately the sixth rib). Similarly, the Scarpa fascia can be secured to the periosteum of the sixth rib. This later step should be performed only by the surgeon who is experienced in these maneuvers, with knowledge of the risks and implications for postoperative pain. The inframammary fold incision can then approximated to the upper body lift abdominal incision and closed in layers with absorbable monofilament suture over at least one closed suction drain on the right and left sides beneath the skin flap. It is often helpful to use penetrating towel clamps or staples for tacking to properly line up these two skin edges.

Breast reshaping

Breast reshaping in the MWL patient can be especially problematic and prone to significant dissatisfaction on the part of the patient and surgeon. After massive weight loss, many patients are left with flat, deflated breasts with excess skin and a paucity of breast tissue or fat. Women often have a subaxillary skinfold in the transition zone between the breast and the back which can be pointed out and discussed preoperatively. The choice of procedure, however, as with any patient, depends on the residual shape of the breast after stabilization of her weight. For patients without ptosis who desire a restoration of volume, implant-based augmentation can sometimes be adequate. However, in our practice we have found this presentation to be the exception. Most patients whom we encounter present with significantly ptotic breasts as well as the aforementioned deflation. In these individuals, a staged augmentation with mastopexy can rejuvenate with the mastopexy performed first, and the augmentation preformed at an appropriate later date. A single-staged augmentation--mastopexy in this population is likely to carry a greater revision rate than this difficult operation carries in the non-MWL population. Patients desiring no increase in volume may benefit from traditional mastopexy techniques. Finally, in women with persistently large and ptotic breasts who desire reshaping and reduction, a traditional reduction mammoplasty can be performed. The choice of skin resection for such patients (vertical versus Wise pattern) continues to be debated among plastic surgeons as to the best approach to achieve improved shape. However, the traditional Wise pattern is preferred in our practice for its ability to contour the subaxillary region and its durability in our hands.

In select patients, excess skin and fat from adjacent areas (e.g. subaxillary, upper abdomen) can be utilized for autologous breast reshaping and augmentation. The tissue in these cases is not excised and discarded, but rather de-epithelialized and raised as flaps that can be rotated or advanced into the breast to achieve the desired shape. Upper abdominal tissue can be used to fill and reshape the inferior pole whereas subaxillary tissue can be rotated to provide a full curved lateral breast or the upper pole. As the flaps are rotated into position they can be secured to the pre-pectoral fascia or costal periosteum, adhering to the caveats above for this maneuver. Depending on the deformity and preoperative discussions, implant augmentation can be done at the same time or, as outlined above, more ideally in a staged fashion after recovery from the total body lift procedure. A point of contention is the position of the implant in the subpectoral versus suprapectoral position and should be based on patient body habitus and surgeon preference. Closure can be performed in layers to minimize epidermal tension and is usually done over closed suction drains in each area treated. A surgical bra is placed at the conclusion of the procedure and - after trading for a cotton sports bra - worn for the first 4–6 weeks in our practice. Patients are reminded that underwire bras may cause pressure and wound-healing complications on any inframammary incisions. Figure 10.4 shows an example of a total body lift transformation.

For male patients, breast reshaping is addressed somewhat differently from female patients. The surgeon should beware of pathological causes of gynecomastia and address them (either alone or in consult) before surgical intervention. For men with small amounts of excess skin, a 'donut'-shaped skin excision in the periareolar region can be adequate and leave a more inconspicuous scar. The skin can be pinched here and marked to determine the width of the donut excision needed, and the parenchyma and skin closed in layers with absorbable monofilament suture. For patients with skin excess that cannot be adequately treated with a simple periareolar resection, an ellipse of skin can be taken from the inframammary fold and again closed in layers; however, this leaves a long scar that is more difficult to hide in the male breast. Men with breast tissue or excess fat can concomitantly be treated with excision (direct or with traditional or ultrasound-assisted liposuction) before the skin resection.

POSTOPERATIVE CARE

Immediate inpatient postoperative care

Postoperative admission to a floor bed, a step-down facility, or an intensive care unit is at the discretion of the operating surgeon with input from anesthesia where appropriate. For patients with medical issues, it may be helpful to obtain a hospital or medical consult for management of their medical issues while hospitalized and to adjust any medications as appropriate. Patients can be kept with the bed in a semi-flexed position to take tension off the skin closure while in bed. In most (but not all) cases they should be encouraged to ambulate the evening of surgery or the next morning. When they initiate ambulation, many will likely wish to walk in the semi-upright position until they feel more comfortable about standing and walking erect. In our experience, this usually takes between 1 and 2 weeks. Patients can be safely started on a liquid diet and advanced to a regular diet as appropriate. Until they can tolerate adequate oral intake, they are maintained on intravenous fluids.

Postoperative analgesia is administered according to protocol. In some cases, subcutaneous catheters are placed at surgery to deliver local anesthetic. We have found these helpful but do not consider them a complete replacement for opioid analgesics which can be administered by patient-controlled analgesia pumps, intraveneously, or orally on an as-needed basis.

Vital signs and urine output are closely monitored to assess perfusion because this is vital for skin flap viability; vasopressive agents should be avoided if at all possible. Laboratory values (e.g. CBC, basic metabolic panel) can be checked daily until stabilized and as appropriate, and any abnormal values replaced as needed. The daily output and content of all drains are monitored. Sequential compression boots should be continued for deep venous thrombosis (DVT) prophylaxis and similar chemophalaxis is begun according to protocol, with the understanding that this differs from institution to institution. Hourly use of an incentive spirometer is helpful for expanding the lungs, perhaps decreasing the risk of postoperative pneumonia after a prolonged intubation.

For discharge, patients should be instructed to continue frequent ambulation and incentive spirometry. Again, postoperative DVT chemoprophaxis varies from institution to institution and from practice to practice. Patients will likely feel fatigued and should be reassured that this is the normal process after a major operation. In our practice, patients may shower with drains; however, the wounds should not be submerged under water until completely healed to avoid healing or infectious complications. The patients and family/caregivers should be alerted to signs of infection, DVT, and other potential outcomes, and can be given care instructions for managing the closed suction drains.

Postoperative care 99

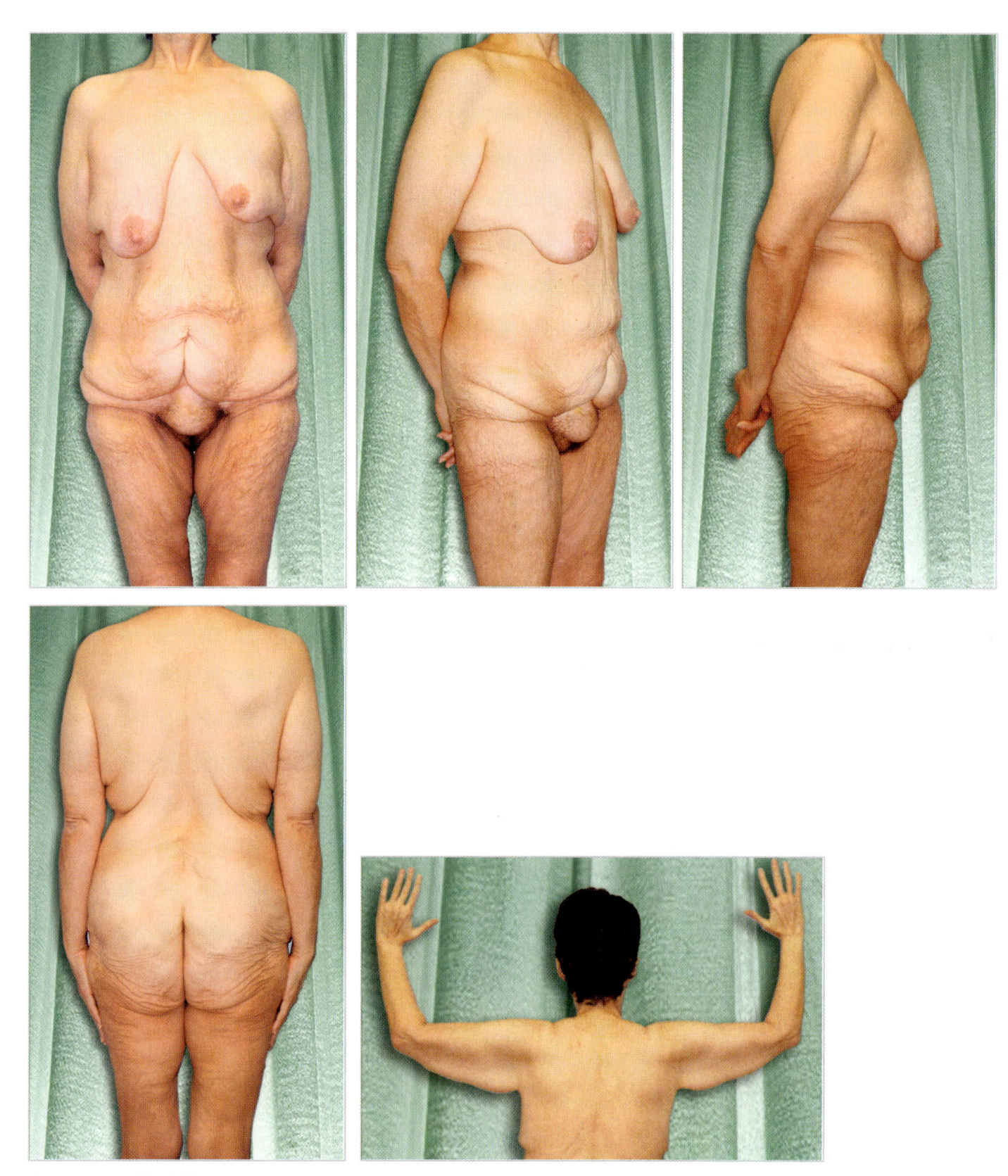

Figure 10.4a Total body lift. Massive weight loss patient: preoperative views. *Continued on p. 100.*

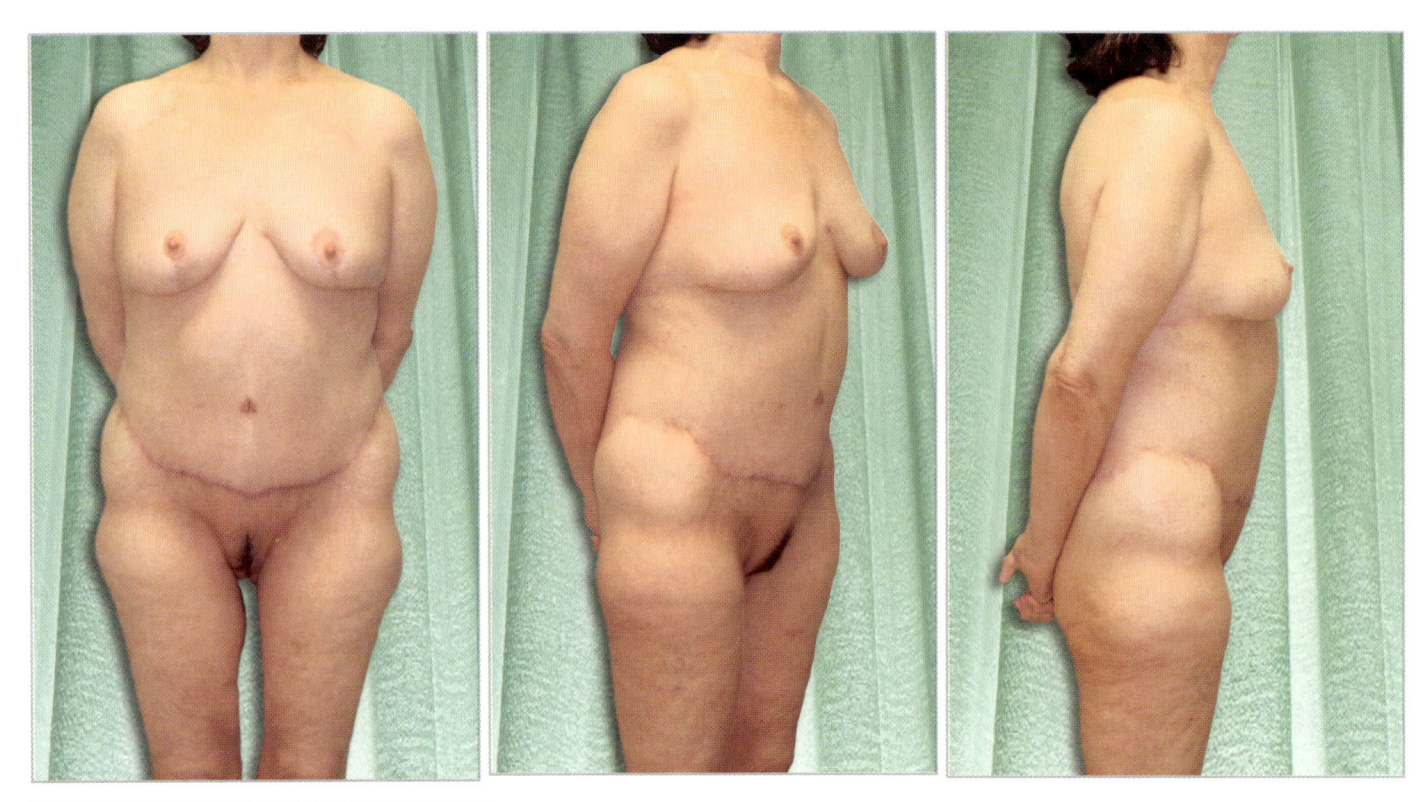

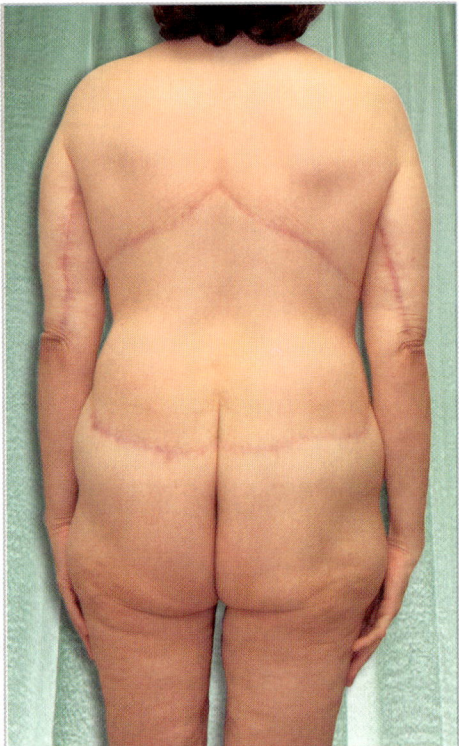

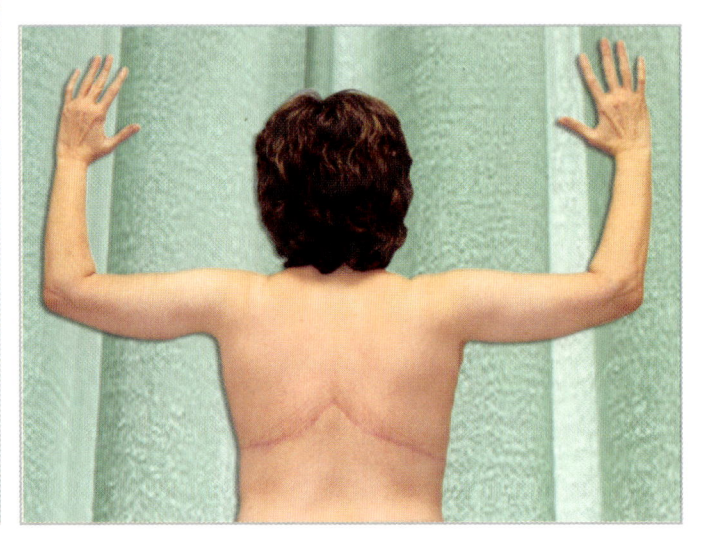

Figure 10.4b Total body lift. The same patient as in part (a): postoperative views after total body lift including circumferential abdominoplasty, upper body lift, breast reshaping, and brachioplasty.

■ Long-term postoperative care

Closed suction drains are typically left in place at our institution until output is minimal (< 20–30 ml/24 h). Once wounds have healed, a scar care regimen can be provided including massage, avoidance of sun exposure, and the surgeon's preference for any scar-minimizing ointments or sheeting if desired. Patients are limited to rest and light activity for the first 2 weeks after surgery and no lifting more than 5–10 lb (2.25–4.5 kg) or strenuous activity for the first month postoperatively to optimize healing. A light walking program after the first few days is advisable to maintain cardiac exercise.

At each postoperative visit the surgeon ensures that the patient is following these recommendations, as well as following appropriate nutritional and exercise regimens to maintain their newly achieved contour. Once the drains have been removed, compression garments can be applied to assist in resolution of postoperative edema. We avoid immediate placement of such garments to circumvent any potential skin flap perfusion issues.

COMPLICATIONS

Many undesirable outcomes can be avoided by careful patient selection, preoperative counseling, and patient optimization, as well as intraoperative measures as described in the earlier section 'Technique' (e.g. pressure point padding, positioning to avoid nerve injury, warm air blankets, antibiotics, and DVT prophylaxis). Despite these maneuvers, however, undesirable outcomes may arise – even in the best of hands – and surgeons should be prepared to address them. The more commonly observed complications are discussed below.

Seroma is a common event after any surgery with a large surface area or dead space, and is one of the most common complications of the above procedures. Rates range from 2% to 37.5% in the literature.[2,3,18,19,21,24–26] Strategies to decrease their incidence include undermining to the minimal extent possible, leaving a thin layer of fat and areolar tissue on the muscular fascia, tissue glues (controversial), and placement of closed suction drains in areas of dead space (especially in sites of dependency), etc. Some have found that the use of quilting or progressive tension sutures from the skin flap to the muscular fascia is helpful in decreasing seroma formation, but the literature is somewhat controversial.[4,24,27] This is generally performed by securing the Scarpa layer to the muscle fascia with absorbable sutures placed at intervals, starting superiorly and moving inferiorly. Closed suction drains are left in place until the output is minimal (<20–30 ml/day) and patients/caregivers should be given instructions for drain care (frequent tube stripping and emptying). Compression garments may be provided after drain removal, as above. If seromas occur despite the above preventive efforts, some surgeons may wish to sterilely aspirate these collections. If collections are recurrent, or if needle aspirtion can not be safely performed in an office setting (e.g. surrounding a breast implant), the surgeon may wish to consider ultrasound-guided drainage and catheter placement.

Thromboembolism is a devastating and often preventable complication of major surgery and body-contouring surgery is no exception. The literature reports rates of 0–5% for DVT and 0–9% for pulmonary embolism (PE) for body-contouring patients depending on the procedure.[2,18,19,24,26,28] Patients with a known history of DVT or PE may be candidates for placement of temporary inferior vena caval filters. Hatef et al. published a report comparing enoxaparin to no enoxaparin for patients undergoing excisional body-contouring procedures with patients ranging from the low to the highest risk for thromboembolism.[28] They found enoxaparin prophylaxis to be useful for patients undergoing circumferential procedures and patients with a BMI >30, because these patients have a higher risk than other body-contouring procedure patients. Similar findings for increased DVT risk in BMI >35 were identified by Shermak et al.[26] They advocate weighing DVT risk against bleeding risk and using risk-stratification methods such as the revised Davison–Caprini model. Most recently, the Venous Thromboembolism Prevention Study was funded by the Plastic Surgery Foundation and conducted at four tertiary institutions.[29] Using the Caprini risk-assessment model as a guide, they performed a retrospective review of patients deemed high risk for DVT ($n = 3334$). Elevated Caprini score and length of hospitalization ≥4 days were found to be independently associated with venous thromboembolism, and postoperative enoxaparin dosing in high-risk patients was protective at 60 days. Patients who are diagnosed with DVT postoperatively should have a hematology consult for management of anticoagulation.

Bleeding complications can often be avoided by preoperative investigation of risk factors as described earlier. If there is any question of a bleeding risk, consultation with a hematologist is warranted and any medications or supplements that increase bleeding should be stopped 10–14 days preoperatively and held for 10–14 days postoperatively if possible. Intraoperatively, judicious use of local anesthetics with epinephrine, hemostasis with electrocautery and hemoclips, use of thrombotic sprays, as well as meticulous confirmation of hemostasis before closure, may help to decrease the risk. At our institution, we favor placing a moistened, open lap sponge over the area being assessed, and watch for areas of bleeding on the white sponge. We then locate the source beneath the sponge and use cautery for hemostasis. We also utilize topical thombotic spray agents as an adjunct at the time of closure. However, extensive body-contouring procedures require extensive dissection and some blood loss is inevitable. If necessary, and the patient becomes symptomatic as a result of blood loss, intra- or postoperative blood transfusion should be utilized. It may be helpful to have cross-matched blood available for these patients in case transfusion becomes necessary. Reported rates of hematoma range from <1% to 5% in the literature.[2,18,19,21,24,25,26] Hematoma may result from confined bleeding and impair wound- and skin-flap healing. A hematoma can be diagnosed clinically or with ultrasonography or CT of the area.

Wound healing is known to be impaired by a host of factors – tobacco use, steroid use, diabetes mellitus, obesity, poor nutrition. Preoperative counseling on relevant patient characteristics or habits that increase wound-healing complications are made clear to the patient. Efforts for risk reduction are made preoperatively and such interventions are given time to take effect – often several weeks – before proceeding with surgery. In addition, hematoma, seroma, wound infections, and undue tension on skin closure may also contribute, and the above measures to reduce these complications will decrease the risk of wound complications.[22] It is inevitable that some degree of skin necrosis, wound dehiscence, and infection will occur, especially in the obese population. Reports in the literature range from 0% to 22% for wound dehiscence, 2% to 10% for skin necrosis, and 1% to 14.7% for wound infections.[2,19,19,21,24,26] Simple cellulitis may be treated with a course of oral antibiotics. If this fails, admission for intravenous antibiotics and workup for possible underlying seroma, hematoma, or abscess is warranted. If wound separation occurs early in the postoperative period it may be possible, in some cases, to reapproximate the wound after washout and sterile reclosure, with close follow-up to watch for signs of infection. More often, however, we offer a course of wound care and offer scar revision after complete healing by secondary intention. Traditional wound care may be the surgeon's preference, and this may include debridement, gauze packing, and/or vacuum-assisted therapy.

Inadequate reshaping, assymmetry, and unsatisfactory scars may occur and often secondary procedures are needed. For residual excess fat or asymmetry, further suction-assisted lipectomy or composite resection may be required. Fat-grafting techniques can be employed to fill in contour irregularities and depressions and scar revisions will treat unsightly or widened scars for select patients. Other less common complications may include paraesthesias and lymphedema. These complications should be discussed preoperatively and intra- and perioperative measures to reduce the risk instituted – including patient positioning, careful dissection in appropriate planes, and properly fitting compression garments.

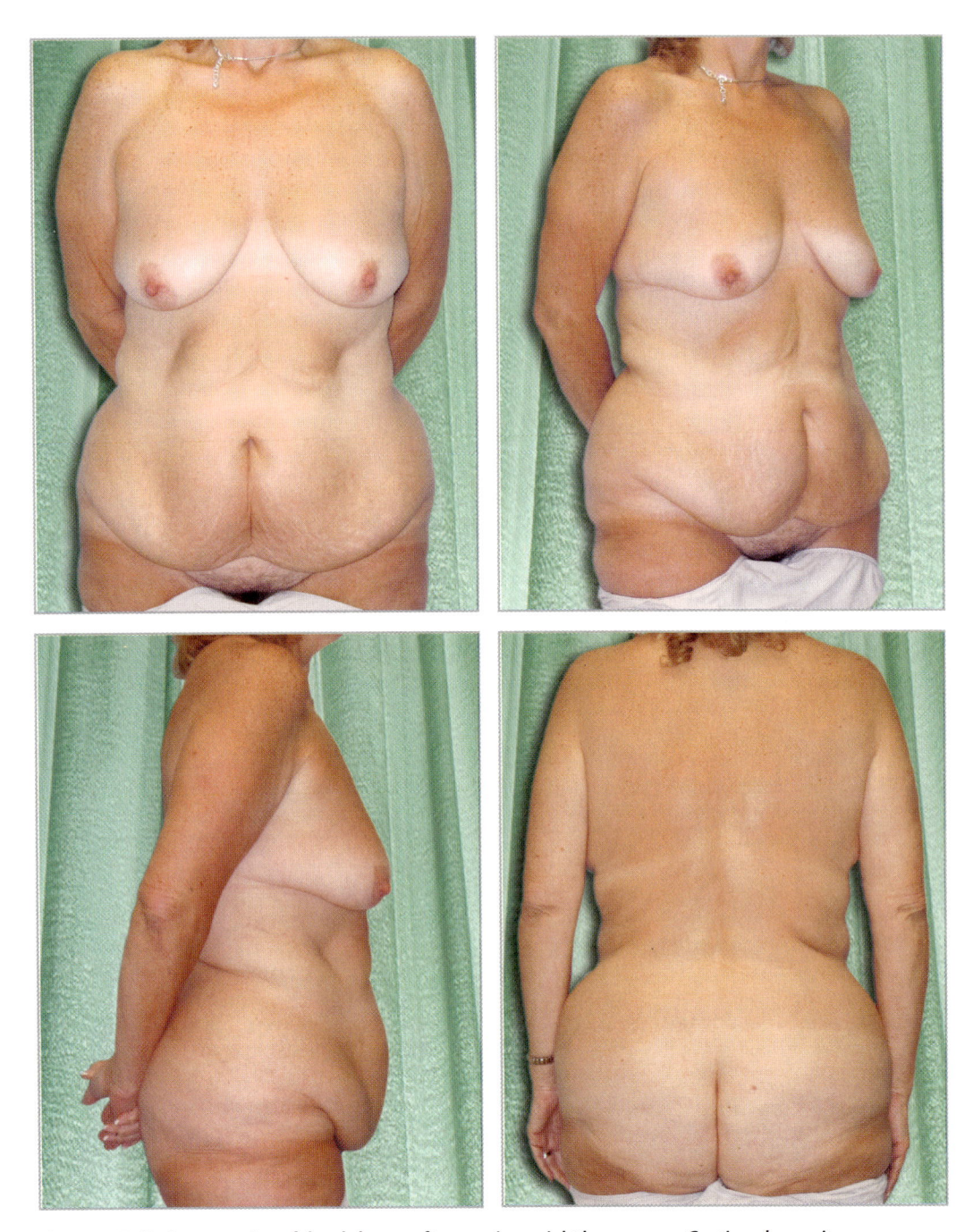

Figure 10.5a Body contouring of the abdomen after massive weight loss surgery. *Continued opposite.*

■ CONCLUSION

Belt lipectomy and total body lift are safe but not risk-free treatment modalities for MWL patients. Thorough preoperative assessment, patient counseling, and outcome optimization, together with the surgeon's meticulous attention to marking and body-contouring principles can allow for spectacular transformations and satisfied patients (**Fig. 10.5**). However, continued evolution of MWL patients, medical and surgical treatments, and body-contouring principles are inevitable and ideally will continue to improve our results.

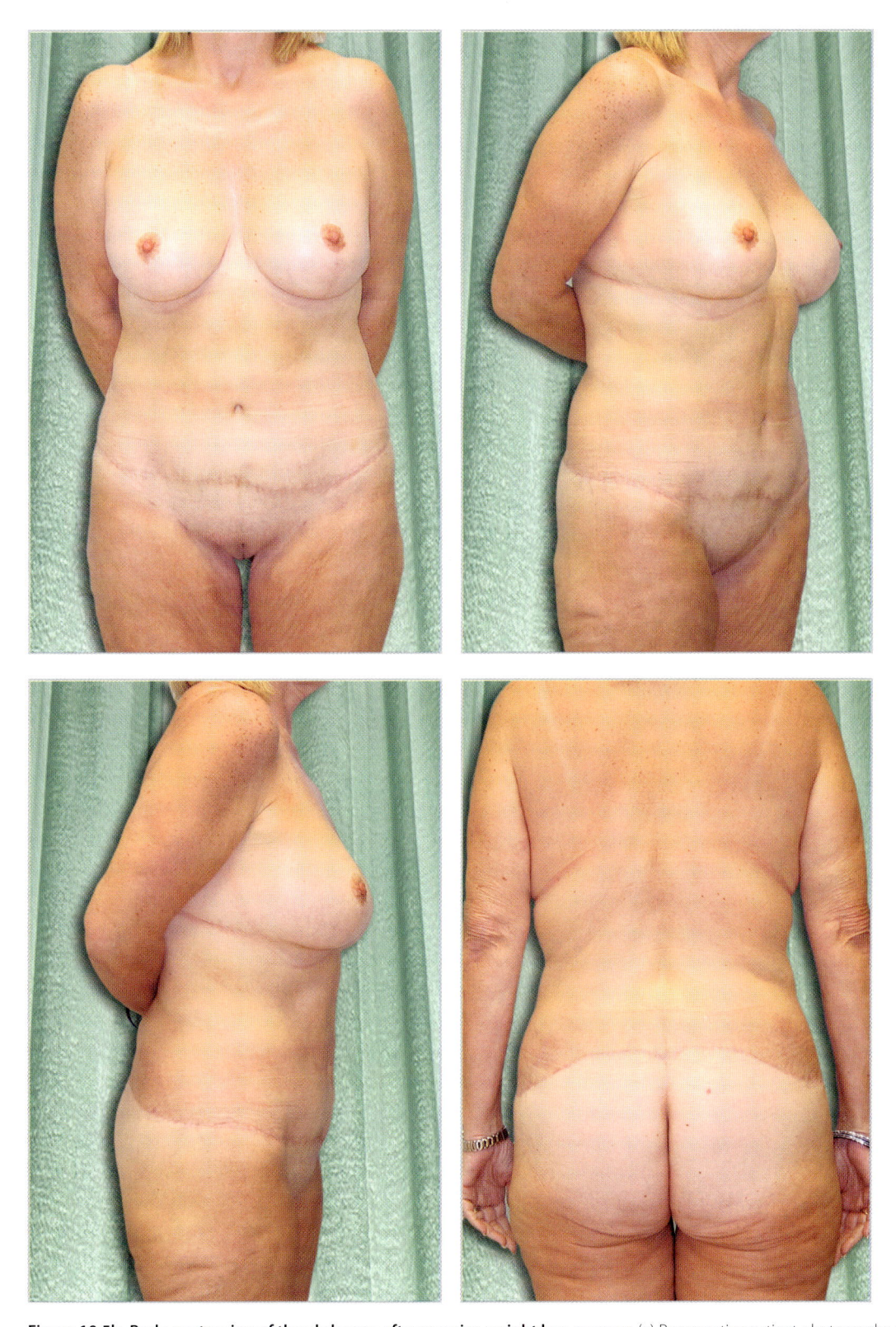

Figure 10.5b Body contouring of the abdomen after massive weight loss surgery. (a) Preoperative patient photographs showing an unsatisfactory appearance. (b) After body contouring, this patient has improved contours and a more aesthetically pleasing appearance in exchange for scars.

REFERENCES

1. Light D, Arvanitis GM, Abramson D, Glasburg SB. Effect of weight loss after bariatric surgery on skin and extracellular matrix. *Plast Reconstr Surg* 2010;**125**:343–51.
2. Aly AS, Cram AE, Chao M, et al. Belt lipectomy for circumferential truncal excess: The University of Iowa experience. *Plast Reconstr Surg* 2003;**111**:398–413.
3. Aly AS, Cram AE, Heddens C. Truncal body contouring surgery in the massive weight loss patient. *Clin Plast Surg* 2004;**31**:611–24.
4. Hamra ST. Circumferential body lift. *Aesth Surg J* 1999;**19**:244–51.
5. Hunstad JP. Body contouring in the obese patient. *Clin Plast Surg* 1996;**23**:647–70.
6. Baroudi R. Body contouring surgery in the 90s. *Advances in Plastic and Reconstructive Surgery*. (Vol. 9; pp. 1–37). St Louis, MO: Mosby-Year Book, 2003.
7. Dardour JC, Vilain R. Alternatives to the classic abdominoplasty. *Ann Plast Surg* 1986;**17**:247–58.
8. Lockwood TE. Superficial fascial system (SFS) of the trunk and extremities: A new concept. *Plast Reconst Surg* 1991;**87**:1009–18.
9. Lockwood TE. Maximizing aesthetics in lateral-tension abdominoplasty and body lifts. *Clin Plast Surg* 2004;**31**:523–37.
10. Hurwitz DJ. *total body lift*. New York: MDPublish.com, 2005.
11. Taylor GI. The angiosomes of the body and their supply to perforator flaps. *Clin Plast Surg* 2003;**30**:331–42.
12. Matarasso, A. Abdominoplasty: a system of classification and treatment for combined abdominoplasty and suction-assisted lipectomy. *Aesthetic Plast Surg* 1991;**15**:111–21.
13. Matarasso, A. Abdominoplasty. *Clin Plast Surg* 1989;**16**:289–303.
14. Mathes SJ, Nahai F. *Clinical Atlas of Muscle and Musculocutaneous Flaps*. St Louis, MO: CV Mosby Co., 1979.
15. DiBernardo BE, Adams RL, Krause J, et al. Photographic standards in plastic surgery. *Plast Reconstr Surg* 1998;**102**:559–68.
16. Gherardini G, Matarasso A, Serure AS, et al. Standardization in photography for body contouring surgery and suction-assisted lipectomy. *Plast Reconstr Surg* 1997;**100**:227–37.
17. Agha-Mohammadi S, Hurwitz DJ. Potential impacts of nutritional deficiency of postbariatric patients on body contouring surgery. *Plast Reconst Surg* 2010;**122**:1901–14.
18. Michaels JV, Coon D, Rubin JP. Complications in postbariatric body contouring surgery: Strategies for assessment and prevention. *Plast Reconstr Surg* 2011;**127**:1352–7.
19. Michaels JV, Coon D, Rubin JP. Complications in postbariatric body contouring: Postoperative management and treatment. *Plast Reconst Surg* 2011;**127**:1693–700.
20. van der Beek ES, van der Molen AM, van Ramhorst B. Complications after body contouring surgery in post-bariatric patients: the importance of stable weight control. *Obes Facts* 2011;**4**:61–6.
21. Au K, Hazard SW 3rd, Dyer AM, et al. Correlation of complications of body contouring surgery with increasing body mass index. *Aesthet Surg J* 2008;**28**:425–9.
22. Rubin JP, Nguyen V, Schwentker A. Perioperative management of the post-gastric-bypass patient presenting for body contouring surgery. *Clin Plast Surg* 2004;**31**:601–10.
23. Chin SH, Cristofaro J, Aston SJ. Perioperative management of antidepressants and herbal medications in elective plastic surgery. *Plast Reconst Surg* 2009;**123**:377–86.
24. Antonetti JW, Antonetti AR. Reducing seroma formation in outpatient abdominoplasty: Analysis of 516 consecutive cases. *Aesthet Surg J* 2010;**30**:418–25.
25. Coon D, Gusenoff JA, Kannan N, et al. Body mass and surgical complications in the postbariatric reconstructive patient: analysis of 511 cases. *Ann Surg* 2009;**249**:397–401.
26. Shermak MA, Chang DC, Heller J. Factors impacting thromboembolism after bariatric body contouring surgery. *Plast Reconst Surg* 2007;**119**:1590–6.
27. Andrades P, Prado A, Danilla S, et al. Progressive tension sutures in the prevention of postabdominoplasty seroma: A prospective, randomized, double-blind clinical trial. *Plast Reconst Surg* 2007;**120**:935–46.
28. Hatef DA, Kenkel JM, Nguyen MQ, et al. Thromboembolic risk assessment and the efficacy of enoxaparin prophylaxis in excisional body contouring surgery. *Plast Reconstr Surg* 2008;**122**:269–279.
29. Pannucci CJ, Dreszer G, Wachtman CF, et al. Postoperative enoxaparin prevents symptomatic venous thromboembolism in high-risk plastic surgery patients. *Plast Reconst Surg* 2011;**128**:1093–103.

Chapter 11

Hernia repair in the massive weight loss patient

Jason W. Edens, Ergun Kocak, Carmen S. Ceron, Liliana Camison, Christopher J. Salgado

INTRODUCTION

Obesity is an increasingly important epidemic in the USA. It affects both adults and children. An alarming increase in the prevalence of obesity has been observed in the USA in the last decade, and it is one of the leading public health concerns worldwide. According to the Centers for Disease Control (CDC), it is has been estimated that around a third of the adult population in the USA is obese, and approximately 17% of children are obese. Further demonstrating this public health concern is that approximately 5% of people are morbidly obese. This is defined as having a body mass index (BMI) ≥ 40 kg/m^2, or ≥ 35 kg/m^2 with a significant secondary disease such as hypertension, diabetes, hyperlipidemia, severe atherosclerosis, or pulmonary dysfunction.[1] As morbid obesity causes or aggravates a multitude of health problems, multiple options have become available for patients seeking assistance with weight loss. These include diet control, exercise, pharmacotherapy, and bariatric surgery.

As non-surgical therapies have consistently failed to achieve significant weight loss, attention has turned to bariatric surgical procedures in treatment of this disease. Surgery offers the best chance to lose a significant amount of weight, to maintain weight loss, and to improve the quality of life in these patients. Results of surgery have been impressive, and many studies have demonstrated improvements and resolution of many of the major comorbid conditions as previously described. As such, the number of bariatric surgical procedures has increased dramatically over the past decade, and many clinicians will be caring for these patients after their bariatric surgical procedure. The options and types of surgical procedures have been discussed in earlier chapters.

Surgical management of the morbidly obese patient has ushered in new hope for treatment of this illness. As more and more patients are being treated with surgery, the potential complications from the surgery will need to be addressed. Although the performance of laparoscopic gastric bypass has been increasing dramatically over the past decade, there are still many instances of open gastric bypass surgeries. The open approach to bariatric surgery is still the preferred method for extreme BMI and for revision of gastric bypass patients. Although not the most common complication associated with gastric bypass surgery, incisional hernias do occur. They will be the most common long-term sequelae that the plastic surgeon will encounter in this patient population. As patients lose a significant amount of weight after gastric bypass surgery, they will likely inquire about body-contouring procedures. Generally, these will include an abdominal component such as abdominoplasty or panniculectomy. When examining these patients, abdominal wall hernias may frequently be encountered. When found, they will require surgical repair with or without the body-contouring procedure. With this in mind, it is important for plastic surgeons to understand the indications and techniques for the repair of incisional hernias after gastric bypass surgery.

ANATOMY OF THE ABDOMINAL WALL

To fully understand incisional hernias, an appreciation of the anatomy of the abdominal wall is required. All hernias arise from some form of defect or weakening of the abdominal wall.

The anterior abdominal wall is a hexagonal area defined superiorly by the costal margin and xiphoid process, laterally by the midaxillary line, and inferiorly by the symphysis pubis, pubic tubercle, inguinal ligament, anterosuperior iliac spine (ASIS), and iliac crest. It is made up of multiple layers, including, from superficial to deep, skin, subcutaneous tissue, superficial fascia, deep fascia, muscle, extraperitoneal fascia, and peritoneum. The superficial fascia of the abdominal wall consists of the Camper and Scarpa fascias. These two entities are fused into a single layer above the umbilicus, but below the umbilicus they are separate and distinct. The Camper fascia is the more superficial fatty outer layer that is continuous with the superficial thigh fascia caudally and extends into the scrotum in males and the labia majora in females. The Scarpa fascia is the membranous inner layer that fuses inferiorly with the fascia lata of the thigh and continues posteriorly to the perineum becoming Colles fascia. The Scarpa fascia is usually visible, and it can be closed separately during various abdominal wall surgical procedures to achieve a more optimal scar result.[2]

The deep fascial layers of the abdominal wall include the linea alba, rectus sheath, external and internal oblique fascias, and transversalis fascia. The linea alba is the midline of the abdominal wall. It forms from the fusion of the anterior and posterior rectus sheaths extending cranially from the xiphoid process to the pubic symphysis caudally. The most important concept in repair of midline incisional hernias is restoration of the linea alba, where all the lateral abdominal wall musculature inserts through the rectus sheath. The arcuate line, which is located midway between the umbilicus and pubic symphysis, is an area of transition that becomes important for abdominal wall repair. Superior to the arcuate line, the anterior rectus sheath consists of the external oblique fascia and the anterior portion of the internal oblique fascia, whereas the posterior rectus sheath consists of the posterior leaf of the internal oblique fascia and the transversalis fascia. Inferior to the arcuate line, the external and internal oblique fascias merge to form the anterior rectus sheath, whereas the posterior rectus sheath consists only of the transversus abdominis fascia. This posterior layer is extremely thin and has only minimal strength. This is important to understand in lower abdominal wall hernias. Laterally, the rectus sheath merges with the aponeurosis of the external oblique muscles to form the linea semilunaris (**Fig. 11.1**).

The musculature of the anterior abdominal wall consists of rectus abdominis, external oblique, internal oblique, transversus abdominis, and pyramidalis (**Fig. 11.2**). Rectus abdominis is a paired muscle and is the principal flexor of the anterior abdominal wall. It functions to

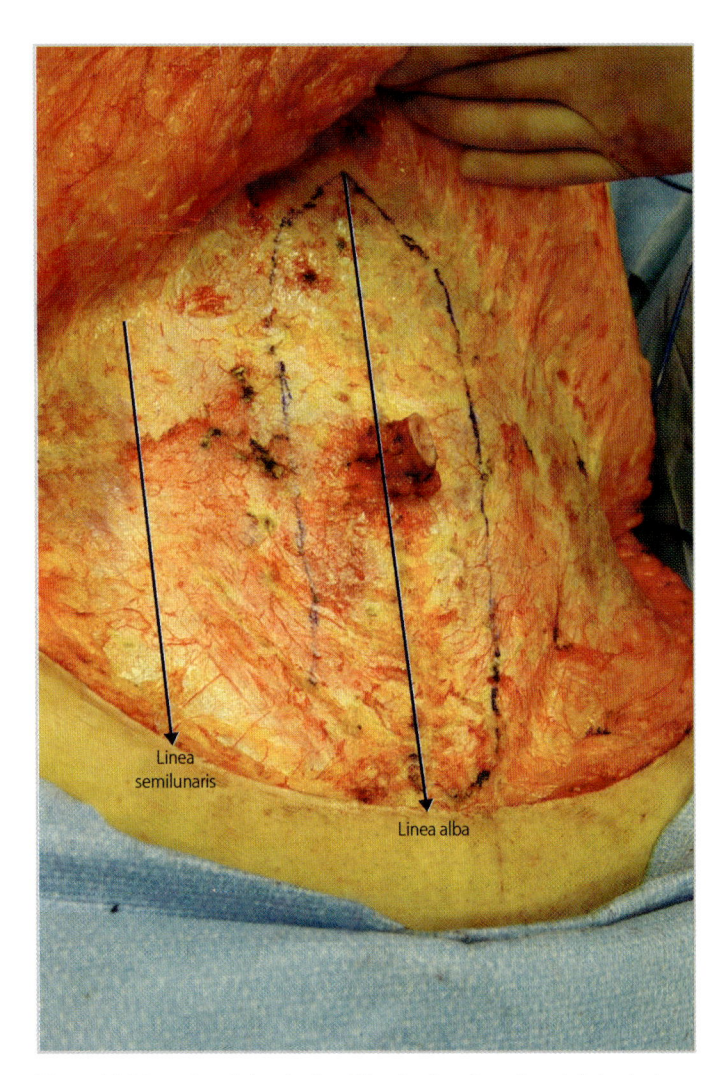

Figure 11.1 Anterior abdominal wall fascia after dissection of abdominal wall skin and subcutaneous tissue using an abdominoplasty incision, showing the linea alba and linea semilunaris.

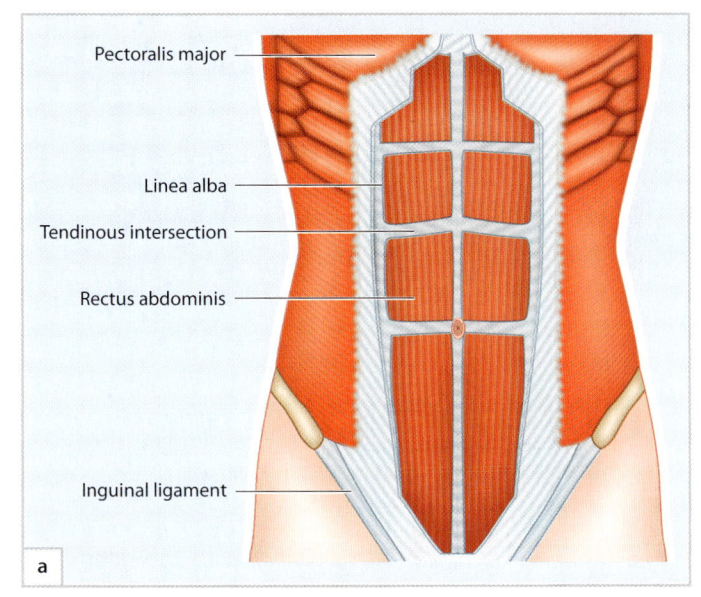

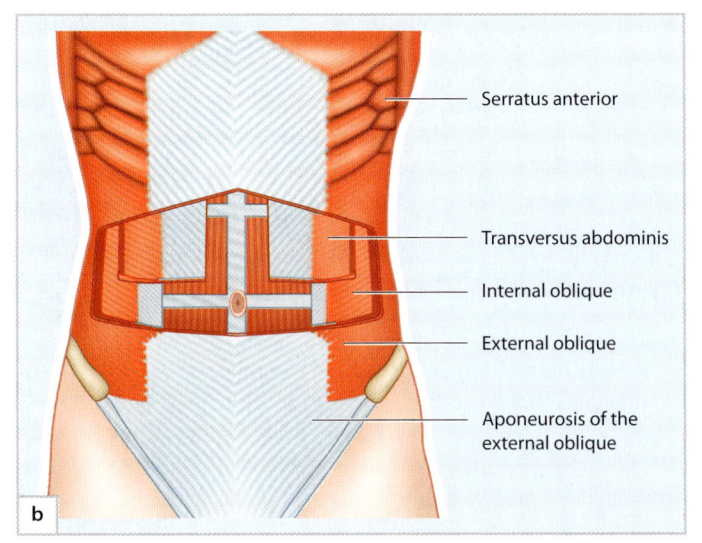

Figure 11.2 Coronal section of the anterior abdominal wall musculature.

stabilize the pelvis while walking, protects the abdominal organs, and aids in forced expiration. Its origin is from the pubic symphysis and pubic crest, and the muscles then insert on to the anterior surfaces of the fifth, sixth, and seventh costal cartilages and xiphoid process. There are three to four tendinous inscriptions that interrupt rectus abdominis along its length and adhere to the anterior rectus sheath. The external oblique muscles are the most superficial and thickest of the three lateral abdominal wall muscles. They originate from the lower eight ribs and course in an inferomedial direction to insert medially on the pubic crest. Inferiorly, they fold on themselves to form the inguinal ligament which extends between the ASIS and pubic tubercle. The internal oblique muscles are deep to the external oblique muscles. Their fibers course in a superomedial direction, perpendicular to the external oblique muscles, and originate from the thoracolumbar fascia, anterior two-thirds of the iliac crest, and lateral half of the inguinal ligament to insert on the inferior and posterior borders of the tenth to twelfth ribs superiorly. Transversus abdominis is the deepest of the lateral abdominal wall muscles and courses in a horizontal direction. It originates from the anterior three-quarters of the iliac crest, lateral third of the inguinal ligament, and inner surface of the lower six costal cartilages, interdigitating with fibers of the diaphragm. Its insertion is medially in a broad, flat aponeurosis, merging above the arcuate line with the posterior lamella of the internal oblique aponeurosis and linea alba, and below the arcuate line into the pubic crest and pectineal line. Pyramidalis is a small, triangular muscle found anterior to the inferior aspect of rectus abdominis and is absent in approximately 20% of the population. It originates from the body of the pubis and inserts into the linea alba inferior to the umbilicus.

The vascular supply of the anterior abdominal wall has been divided into three zones.[3] Zone I consists of the upper and mid-central abdominal wall and is supplied by the vertically oriented superior and deep inferior epigastric arteries. These arteries travel along the posterior aspect of rectus abdominis, supplying the muscles and overlying skin and subcutaneous tissue through musculocutaneous perforators. Zone II consists of the lower abdominal wall and is supplied by the epigastric arcade, superficial inferior epigastric arteries, superficial external pudendal arteries, and superficial circumflex iliac arteries. Zone III consists of the lateral abdominal wall and is supplied by the musculophrenic arteries, lower intercostals arteries, and the lumbar arteries. Veins draining the anterior abdominal wall run as venae comitantes and accompany the main arteries, draining into the azygous venous system and external iliac veins.

Sensory innervations of the anterior abdominal wall are derived from the anterior braches of the intercostals and subcostal nerves from T7 to L1, with T7–9 supplying the skin superior to the umbilicus. T10 supplies the skin around the umbilicus, whereas T11–L1 innervates the skin inferior to the umbilicus. Lateral cutaneous branches of the intercostals supply the lateral areas of the abdominal wall. Motor innervation to the abdominal wall is supplied by the seventh to twelfth intercostal nerves, iliohypogastric nerve, and ilioinguinal nerve. Rectus abdominis is innervated by the ventral rami of the lower six intercostal nerves, the external obliques are innervated by the lower six thoracic and upper two lumbar anterior rami, the internal obliques by the lower thoracic intercostal nerves, iliohypogastric nerves, and ilioinguinal nerves, and transversus abdominis by the lower intercostal nerves, iliohypogastric nerves, and ilioinguinal nerves.

INCISIONAL HERNIAS

Incisional hernias continue to be a challenge in the surgical management of morbid obesity, with the incidence ranging from 0–2% in the minimally invasive patients, to up to as high as 26% in the open approach.[4] In addition, incisional hernias develop in approximately 10% of all midline laparotomies, and they can be extremely difficult to manage, with recurrences after repair ranging from 8% to 55%. Although incisional hernias can occur in any patient, morbidly obese patients and massive weight loss (MWL) patients have been shown to be at a higher risk for the development of incisional hernias than patients of normal weight. Obesity, in and of itself, is a known risk factor for wound complications and the development of an incisional hernia, and the incidence of incisional hernias has been shown to be directly proportional to BMI.[5] Morbidly obese patients are at higher risk for fascial dehiscence at the time of their initial gastric surgery. Other factors associated with morbid obesity that may lead to the development of an incisional hernia include increased intra-abdominal pressure from increased abdominal girth, poor tissue quality due to comorbid conditions, and both nutritional deficiencies and malnutrition following the physiological changes associated with weight loss surgery. Intra-abdominal pressure has been shown to be two to three times higher in morbidly obese patients than in non-obese patients.[6]

Surgical site infection at the time of the gastric bypass procedure is also a known high risk factor for the development of incisional hernias. Incisional hernias may develop after either open or laparoscopic gastric bypass surgery, but the extent of the hernia may be completely different. Incisional hernias will develop within the limitations of the initial incision, so the open approach will oftentimes result in a much larger hernia. This will also factor into the surgical strategy for repair of the hernia, because smaller hernias may be satisfactorily repaired primarily, whereas larger hernias may require mesh repair with or without component separation for complete coverage of the defect. The approach to surgical repair of hernias is discussed later in the chapter.

Incisional hernias may result in functional impairment as well as cosmetic concerns. The abdominal wall functions to protect, compress, and retain the contents of the abdomen. In addition, it aids in forced expiration and is used for flexion and rotation of the trunk. There is a significant functional disability associated with incisional hernias because patients may develop significant life-limiting symptoms. These include prolonged hernias that cause abdominal discomfort and nausea due to the stretching of the mesentery through the defect, respiratory derangements, gait and postural difficulties due to the constant pressure on the abdomen from the hernia, and difficulties with expulsive functions that include coughing, micturition, and defecation.[7] These can become sufficiently severe for patients to be restricted from adequately performing normal daily activities, and some hernias may even prevent patients from going to work. As herniation leads to a failure of critical functions and disabling pain, patients can also have cosmetic concerns. The appearance of a large bulge in the abdomen can be unsightly for patients, and patients may have to find larger, looser-fitting clothing. In addition, as the size of the hernia increases and contains the contents of the abdomen, visible peristalsis may be evident. These factors may lead to psychiatric disturbances including decreased self-esteem and depressive symptoms. Another indicator for surgical intervention for incisional hernia is pain. This should be recorded preoperatively using a visual analog scale.[8]

The natural history of an incisional hernia is for it to increase in size because intra-abdominal pressures will continue to apply pressure to the weakness of the abdominal wall at the site of the hernia. As it enlarges, the chances of complications arising are enhanced. These include incarceration and strangulation of intra-abdominal contents, loss of abdominal domains, thinning of the subcutaneous tissues and overlying skin, and ulceration of the skin with breakdown, leading to fistula formation. As the hernia continues to expand, the lateral abdominal musculature and tissue will further retract and become fibrotic, which adds further to the overall size of the hernia. The most feared complication is that the intra-abdominal contents within the hernia sac become acutely incarcerated or strangulated. This could result in bowel ischemia, necrosis, and possibly frank perforation. Although the optimal timing for hernia repair is not always apparent, in instances of acute incarceration or strangulation of intra-abdominal contents, emergency hernia repair is necessary. In instances where the hernia is uncomplicated, the repair of the hernia becomes elective, with preoperative optimization of the patient a priority. Weight loss after gastric bypass surgery will greatly improve the outcome of hernia repair. Surgery will become easier because there is less soft tissue, allowing for easier closure as well as decreased intra-abdominal pressure. This scenario leads to decreased recurrence rates. If the patient remains symptomatic from the hernia, elective repair needs to be performed in a timely fashion because delays in the repair of hernias can lead to increased morbidity as well as increased difficulty in hernia correction.

PREOPERATIVE EVALUATION

Patients considered medically appropriate for elective hernia repairs should undergo a complete history and physical examination. Clinicians should focus on the size of the hernia defect, associated abdominal symptoms, duration of the hernia, and consideration of patient expectations. In cases where preoperative optimization is required, the use of an abdominal binder may be the most rational treatment option until surgery can be safely performed. In cases of large hernias where additional techniques, such as component separation, are used, it is important to assess skin laxity and integrity overlying the hernia, as well as the amount of subcutaneous fat present. Patients should be greatly encouraged to quit the use of all tobacco products. In instances where a cosmetic procedure is added to the hernia repair, such as abdominoplasty, the patient's weight needs to have reached a plateau, and to have been stable for some time. Occasionally, radiographic adjuncts such as computed tomography can be utilized to assess the fascial defect, or defects. These may aid subsequent repair.

In cases where the procedure may be conducted more efficiently and with fewer complications after pannus resection, the patient's insurance company is then typically approached for coverage for a panniculectomy procedure.[9]

OPTIONS FOR INCISIONAL HERNIA REPAIR

Many options exist for the repair of these hernias, including open primary (or suture) repair, open repair with the use of mesh (biologic or synthetic), laparoscopic repair, or autogenous tissue transfer.

Multiple approaches and techniques are available for the repair of incisional hernias. This likely stems from historically high recurrence rates, which have led to the development of new procedures directed toward improving overall results. Recurrence rates have been reported as high as 50%, mostly with primary suture repairs. Primary suture repair can lead to excessive tension on the surrounding tissues and edges of the defect. This can result in local tissue ischemia, leading to increased rates of subsequent wound dehiscence and recurrent herniation. In a prospective, randomized, multicenter study, Luijendijk et al. compared mesh repairs with suture repairs in first-time incisional hernia repairs. For hernias repaired with mesh, the mesh was placed in a retrofascial, preperitoneal fashion, with approximately 2–5 cm of overlap between the mesh and fascia.[10] The study by Luijendijk demonstrated a 43% recurrence with suture repair, and a 24% recurrence rate with mesh repair.[11] The use of mesh was superior with regard to the recurrence of hernia, regardless of the size of the defect. This study led to a new paradigm suggesting that a tension-free mesh repair is the standard of care for incisional hernia repair. Mesh has been found to be superior in larger defects, and some authors have advocated that primary closure for incisional hernias should be considered only in patients whose abdominal defects are <2–5 cm and lack risk factors that would preclude appropriate healing.[12] This finding also applies to the postbariatric patient in whom there is usually an excess of fascia and subcutaneous tissue. In small hernias, this excess fascia can be plicated. This allows a stable, tension-free, primary herniorrhaphy.[13] Large hernias will ultimately require mesh closure for the reasons described above.

Initial open incisional hernia repairs utilized mesh applied in an inlay fashion, with the mesh placed underneath the hernia defect but above the posterior rectus sheath, keeping it off of the abdominal viscera. This was due to the concerns about adhesions and ingrowth between earlier meshes and intra-abdominal organs. As the properties of the meshes used have advanced, they can now be safely placed in contact with abdominal viscera, allowing for the intraperitoneal placement of mesh. This has been done both laparoscopically and in an open manner. Numerous studies have focused on the placement of mesh, whether it be in an onlay, inlay, or underlay fashion. The underlay method has been demonstrated to be superior to these other methods,[14] and has led to its adoption by most surgeons with regard to hernia repair. The use of mesh in the underlay position allows for a tension-free hernia repair, which may explain its low recurrence rate.

Open repairs may theoretically have an advantage over laparoscopic repairs in that, in open repairs, the rectus muscles can be reapproximated at the midline, leading to improved coverage of the mesh as well as improved cosmesis and abdominal wall function. Laparoscopic repairs tend to leave the hernia sac in place, with coverage only of the defect and without muscle coverage of the mesh. However, the open repair does require extensive soft-tissue dissection around the hernia, with risks to underlying bowel from the development of adhesions to the hernia sac as well as the abdominal wall. In addition, this dissection can cause the devascularization of the surrounding tissues, which can lead to higher rates of infection and hematoma formation. The laparoscopic approach limits the amount of soft-tissue dissection, because the mesh is placed into the peritoneum and along the underside of the anterior abdominal wall. In this fashion, the mesh is held in place by the outward force of the intra-abdominal pressure. In a large review of the current literature, Rudmik et al. demonstrated that the laparoscopic repair appears to decrease recurrence rates and lower complication rates associated with incisional hernia repair.[15] The technical detail of the laparoscopic approach to incisional hernia repair is beyond the scope of this text; however, plastic surgeons must be knowledgeable about the technical approach and familiar with the details of the open approach to incisional hernias.

In instances where there are extremely large incisional hernias, methods of repair with mesh alone may not suffice. In addition, prosthetic mesh cannot be utilized for hernia repair in infected of contaminated fields. As an alternative to the use of mesh, manipulating the anatomy of the abdominal wall with mobilization of its structures can be performed for the repair of incisional hernias. In 1990, Ramirez first described a tension-reducing hernia repair utilizing a patient's own tissues with his development of the component separation technique.[16] This followed a study by Ger and Duboys who showed that innervated and vacularized musculofascial flaps were superior to the use of prosthetic materials in the repair of large hernia defects.[17] This method is based on the enlargement of the abdominal wall by movement of its muscular layers to the midline. The advancement of this autologous muscle tissue provides fascial continuity and closure in a tension-free manner as well as dynamic support of the abdomen. This technique utilizes release of the external oblique aponeurosis for mobilization of the rectus muscles into the midline. It restores the normal intra-abdominal pressure by reattaching the abdominal wall musculature at the linea alba, which may prevent later diaphragmatic dysfunction (**Fig. 11.3**). Loss of external oblique function is not important. Weakness in the abdominal wall may develop in this area, and some surgeons have reinforced these areas of release with mesh. The initial description of the procedure by Ramirez was based on cadaveric specimens, and it did not utilize the incorporation of mesh, which has now been used in variations of this procedure when the defect cannot

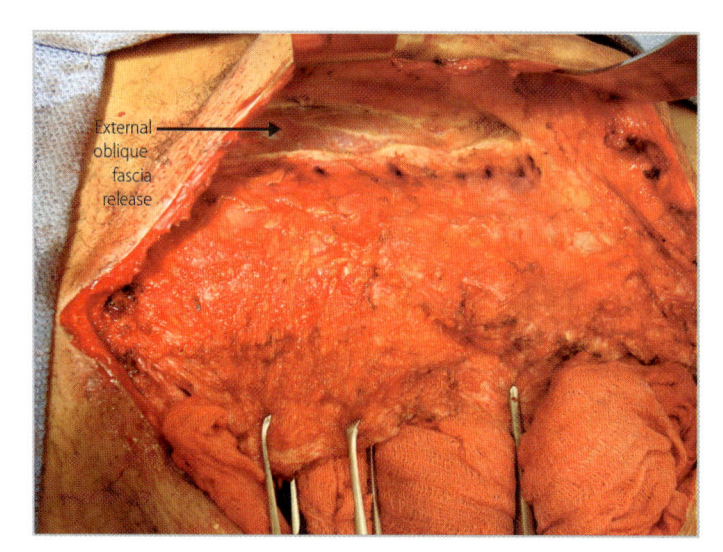

Figure 11.3 Intraoperative view of components separation with release of the external oblique fascia.

be adequately closed without undue tension after mobilization of tissues.[18] The component separation technique has been used for the treatment of large incisional hernias for complex abdominal wall reconstruction and in instances of wound contamination in order to avoid the use of prosthetic materials.

In a recent study using a component separation technique for the repair of large incisional hernias after gastric bypass, Borud et al. demonstrated a low recurrence rate (8.3%) in their patients, with the only recurrence occurring in a patient with a 15-cm hernia.[19] In their study, they did not place mesh in the fascial defect. Instead, they placed an absorbable mesh in an onlay fashion to reinforce the cut lateral edges of the external oblique musculofascial flap. The authors state that component separation provides a reliable method for closing large abdominal wall defects without the use of permanent mesh in the MWL patient. Other studies have similarly demonstrated low recurrence rates following the component separation technique.[20]

Various techniques using an assortment of autologous tissues transferred as grafts, pedicled flaps, and free flaps have been described in small case series or retrospective reviews. The simplest concept of autologous tissue use is to use de-epithelialized skin that would otherwise be discarded at surgery as a dermal autograft mesh to support hernia repair. Studies describing this technique for the closure of TRAM (transverse rectus abdominis myocutaneous) donor sites show acceptable bulge and hernia outcomes. Unfortunately, they are severely limited by inadequate power and their descriptive design.[21,22] Although such a method is appealing, especially in the bariatric population where excess skin is generally abundant, clinical data are limited and long-term resorption of the graft could be a complicating factor.

An alternate autologous graft option to bridge fascial defects is the fascia lata graft. In a review of the literature, De Vries Reilingh and colleagues[23] found moderate donor site morbidity (17%) with a hernia recurrence rate that was comparable to other methods (9%). The main drawback from this review was a rather high abdominal wound complication rate which exceeded 40% in all studies. Although not in MWL patients, the authors have performed abdominal wall reconstruction with the use of the fascia lata graft in a patient who had infected mesh after abdominal operations for cholecystectomy, pancreatitis, and loss of abdominal domain (**Figs 11.4** and **11.5**). Patients underwent explantation of the mesh, followed by multiple abdominal debridements, negative pressure wound therapy, and antibiotics. The fascia lata graft was then used for reconstruction of the abdominal wall. The wound overlying the abdomen healed, but the patient continued to gain weight and eventually required placement of a biologic prosthesis to bridge the fascial gap.

Vascularized tissue flaps, transferred on a pedicle or as free flaps, have been reported in small case series. Their use should be only as a last resort when other means have failed or the size of the fascial defect exceeds reasonable coverage with alloplastic materials and neighboring soft tissues.[24] One commonly used flap for abdominal wall reconstruction in cases where prosthetic and biologic implants have failed is the rectus femoris musculofascial flap or mutton-chop flap[25] (**Figs 11.6** and **11.7**).

THE USE OF MESH IN INCISIONAL HERNIA REPAIR

Meshes can be broadly divided into two categories: Prosthetic and biologic. With a steady stream of these products continuing to become commercially available, a comprehensive review of all materials is beyond the scope of this chapter.[26] A clear understanding of the proper-

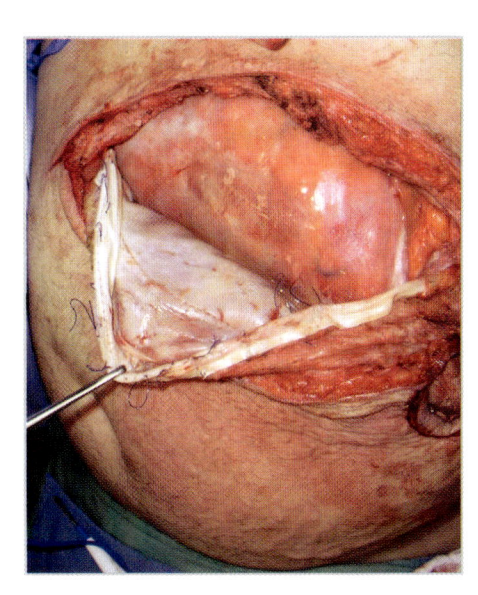

Figure 11.4 Explantation of infected mesh before using fascia lata graft.

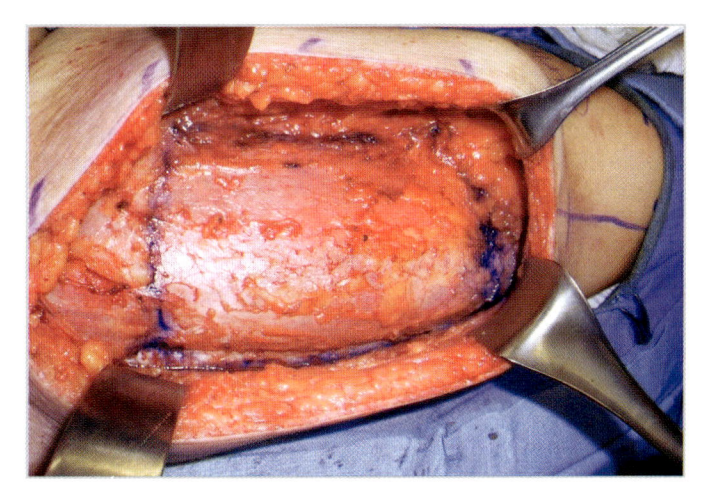

Figure 11.5 Incorporation of fascia lata graft for abdominal wall reconstruction.

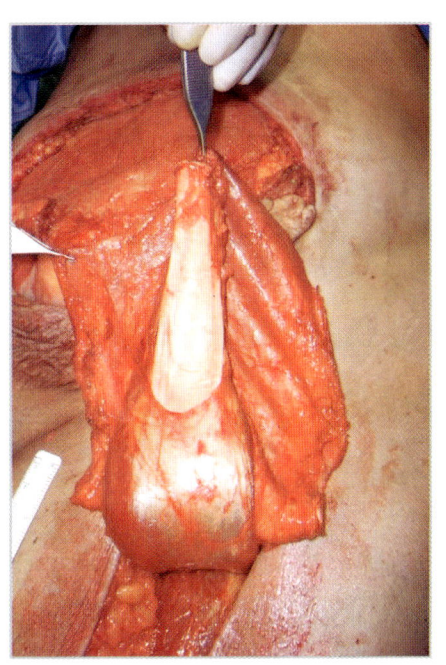

Figure 11.6 Elevation of rectus femoris flap (mutton chop flap) before placement for abdominal wall reconstruction.

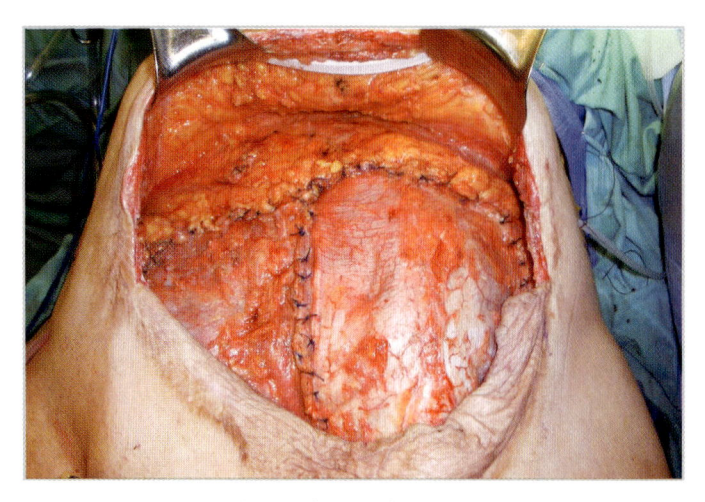

Figure 11.7 Placement of rectus femoris flap along abdominal wall.

ties specific to each and clinical settings favoring the use of one over the other, however, can guide the surgeon in selecting a mesh from the overwhelming variety of available materials.

As outlined above, there is little argument that initial incisional ventral hernia repairs should be supported by mesh. Recently, a set of guidelines published by the Ventral Hernia Working Group recommended choice of repair material for incisional ventral hernias by hernia grade.[27] Four grades were described, based on patient and hernia characteristics. Grade 1 (low risk) consisted of patients with no comorbidities and no history of wound infection or contamination near the hernia. Grade 2 included patients with comorbidities but no infection or contamination around the hernia. Grades 3 and 4 included patients with potentially or obviously infected hernias, respectively. The general conclusions of this study pointed to the use of prosthetic mesh only in grade 1 cases. For grades, the working group discouraged the use of prosthetic meshes and favored the use of biologic materials, with the strongest evidence supporting the use of biologic repairs in obviously infected cases (grade 4). The proposed theoretical advantage of biologic material is that it allows for vascular ingrowth and has the capacity to become incorporated into the surrounding tissues.

The bioprosthetic materials most commonly used for hernia repair are acellular dermal matrices (ADMs) derived from various sources including human cadavers (allogeneic) and animals (xenogeneic). The more commonly used xenogeneic products are porcine derived, making it possible to better control the conditions under which they are harvested for larger and more consistent sheets. Although allogeneic products would be expected to provoke a lower immunological response, the xenogeneic products have been chemically or enzymatically modified by various techniques to abrogate immunogenicity and make them clinically tolerable. There is ongoing debate about which processing technique (chemical cross-linkage of collagen versus non-cross-linked enzymatic removal of immunogens) leads to better immune tolerance and hernia repair results. With an overall paucity of comparative trials or high-level evidence to support their use, selection of a biologic product in cases of suspected or obvious contamination is still largely determined by surgeon preference and product familiarity. In the face of stable soft-tissue coverage, equal consideration can be given to delaying the formal hernia repair until infection is adequately treated and the patient's comorbidities are optimized. In such cases, prosthetic mesh may once again become a viable option for repair. We believe that the use of human cadaveric dermis for abdominal wall hernia repair has been shown to lead to increased hernia rates.[20]

SURGICAL PROCEDURES

Following appropriate preoperative workup and the decision to proceed with hernia repair, the surgeon must choose one of many available possible options for repair. In addition, the choices about body contouring or abdominoplasty should be discussed with the appropriate patients. In cases where mesh will be utilized, the appropriate mesh should be readily available for use, with additional sizes also available should the need arise. The approach for hernia repair can proceed laparoscopically or by an open technique, as dictated by the surgeon's experience or decision based on preoperative evaluation. In cases where higher than normal risks exist for injury to the bowel or inadvertent enterotomies due to adhesive disease, a bowel preparation should be considered. Also, in these cases, if synthetic meshes were considered preoperatively, thought must be given to alternative means of hernia repair. These may include biologic mesh or component separation. In patients undergoing cosmetic or medically indicated panniculectomy procedures, preoperative marking in the holding area is performed before the patient goes to the operating room.

The patients are placed in the supine position on the operating table, and general anesthesia is used. Preoperative antibiotics are given, and sequential compression devices are placed. A Foley catheter is usually placed, especially in laparoscopic cases and lower abdominal hernias, for full bladder decompression. Skin preparation with appropriate antimicrobial solution is then performed. Preoperative chemoprophylaxis for deep vein thrombosis (DVT) is also considered, because obese patients are more susceptible to DVTs.

Open incisional hernia repair

A midline or extended Pfannensteil incision is made over the incisional hernia. Careful dissection proceeds through the subcutaneous tissues because there may only be a thin layer of hernia sac between the skin and the abdominal viscera. The hernia sac is then entered, and a meticulous adhesiolysis is performed, separating all abdominal viscera from the overlying abdominal wall. This creates a wide intraperitoneal space for overlap between the mesh and the abdominal wall. In cases where the intraperitoneal cavity is not entered and there is little to no tension, the posterior rectus sheath can be approximated to prevent opposition of the mesh with the abdominal viscera. However, with dual layered meshes, this is not an absolute necessity. In addition, if the fascial defect is seen to be < 5 cm, consideration can be given to a primary suture repair of the hernia. If this is performed, sutures should be placed 1 cm from the fascial edges and advanced in increments of 1 cm for optimal repair.[28]

Next, wide flaps of skin and subcutaneous tissues are created bilaterally. The exposure of good and healthy fascia is obtained for incorporation of sutures and mesh. In addition, this can provide the space needed to allow the rectus muscle and fascia to cover the implanted mesh. The size of the defect is examined, and the proper size of mesh selected. This should allow an overlap of at least 4 cm on to good fascia bilaterally, as well as appropriate overlap both superiorly and inferiorly. Intra-abdominal protection devices, such as a malleable or a disposable visceral retractor (sometimes referred to as a 'fish') can be placed in the peritoneal cavity to prevent harm to the abdominal viscera. The dual layered mesh, with the peritoneal side down facing the intra-abdominal organs, is placed in the intraperitoneal cavity. Multiple options for suturing the mesh to the fascia are available. Large, permanent sutures are used and can include either Prolene or Ethibond on a large needle. These can be placed in an interrupted or running fashion, utilizing a 'U' stitch, in which the suture is passed through the fascia, into the mesh, and back through the fascia. Care is taken to ensure that there are no free spaces between sutures that would allow herniation of bowel content between the mesh and abdominal wall. This method allows significant overlap between the mesh and healthy fascia. Finally, if it can be performed without undue tension, the rectus muscles and fascia are approximated in the midline at the linea alba to cover the mesh. This will provide an improved functional and cosmetic result. Closed-suction drains are placed in the subcutaneous space, and the skin is closed. In cases of panniculectomy, staples are advised because infections and seromas can be easily drained with this closure versus a running subcuticular closure. In very obese patients we have also used negative pressure along the incision line for the first few days after surgery not only to splint the wound but also to control exudate.

Component separation technique

With the component separation technique, skin and subcutaneous tissue are mobilized as flaps bilaterally to a distance of approximately 5 cm lateral to the lateral border of the rectus muscle. The external oblique aponeurosis is then incised approximately 1–2 cm lateral to the lateral border of the rectus muscle over its entire length.[29] Utilizing the avascular plane between the external and internal oblique muscles, these muscles are separated with mobilization occurring to the midaxillary or posterior axillary line. Medially, the rectus muscles are separated from the posterior rectus sheath to create additional mobilization of the rectus muscles in the midline. Utilizing this method, the rectus can be advanced 3–5 cm in the upper abdomen (epigastric region), 7–10 cm in the midabdomen (umbilical region), and 1–3 cm in the lower abdomen (suprapubic region). This mobilization occurs bilaterally, which equates to movement of 10 cm in the epigastric region, 20 cm in the umbilical region, and 6 cm in the suprapubic region. Incision of the posterior rectus sheath can add 2 cm of mobilization.[30] Mesh can also be utilized in this repair: Most commonly, it is placed in an underlay fashion.[19] Suturing of the fascia or the mesh proceeds in a similar fashion as described in the open incisional hernia repair section. Closed-suction drains are placed in the subcutaneous space, and the skin is closed. An abdominal binder is commonly used postoperatively and the drains are kept in place for 10–14 days.

Hernia repair in combination with abdominoplasty or panniculectomy

After gastric bypass surgery, many patients succeed in achieving massive weight loss. However, they then have excessive skin with the development of a large pannus, which is now cosmetically unappealing. Adding to this may be the development of an incisional hernia from their gastric bypass procedure. The abdominoplasty incision has become an alternative open technique in the repair of an incisional hernia, utilizing an incision remote from the site of the hernia.

Not only can this procedure aid in repair of the hernia, it can also supply a means for the cosmetic correction of the overlying pannus. Concurrent hernia repair and abdominoplasty or panniculectomy has been shown to be a safe procedure, and is being used by plastic surgeons in selected patients.[31]

The combination of abdominoplasty and incisional hernia repair has many advantages, because both procedures are necessary from a functional and aesthetic standpoint. The exposure obtained from the abdominoplasty incision is superior to the standard midline incision utilized in an incisional hernia repair. After flaps are elevated, a thorough examination of the entire abdominal wall can be performed. Dissection proceeds superiorly to the xiphoid process in the midline, with limited dissection lateral to the costal margins if possible. All hernias can be identified and repaired utilizing the techniques discussed in the previous sections, including the use of the component separation technique.[32] Many patients will also have excess fascia that can be used for plication over the hernia repair, thereby reinforcing and adding strength to it. The elimination of the abdominal pannus at the time of hernia repair may lead to a decrease in the recurrence rate, because decreased tension is placed on the repair as a result of the removal of the heavy weight of the pannus. In addition, there may be a decrease in surgical time due to surgical access to the hernia.[9] The combination procedure of hernia repair and abdominoplasty also eliminates the need for a second surgery with added risks of anesthesia. Full details of the abdominoplasty procedure are discussed in Chapter 8.

COMPLICATIONS

As is the case with all surgical procedures, the repair of incisional hernias is subject to potential complications, from the surgical technique, the body's reaction to implanted materials, and infection and its sequelae. Complications occur in each type of repair, and certain complications are related to the method of repair used. As mentioned previously, primary hernia repair was historically associated with a high recurrence rate. This led to the standard use of mesh in nearly all hernia repairs. Although mesh provides the ability to eliminate tension from the closure of the hernia defect, it can be fraught with complications. There include risks of infection, mesh migration, erosion into the bowel, and the development of enterocutaneous fistula. Although it does provide static support and strength, it fails to provide dynamic support of the abdominal wall. This can lead to difficulties with abdominal wall function and, in some cases, recurrences due to stress and tension at the suture sites. The host response to the placement of a foreign body such as mesh can predispose to seroma formation, adhesions, and erosion into the bowel. Mesh infection is the most significant complication and can lead to chronic wound formation. This will require removal of the infected mesh, and will leave a large defect that will be difficult to repair and likely require some form of abdominal wall reconstruction. The most commonly encountered complications associated with the use of mesh as reported to the Food and Drug Administration include infection (42%), mechanical failure (18%), pain (9%), reaction (8%), intestinal complications (7%), adhesions (6%), seroma (4%), and erosion/migration (2%).[33] Less commonly encountered complications include no ingrowth of mesh, compromised sterility, mesh shrinkage, bleeding, and hematoma. In their review of the literature, Shell et al.[7] found seromas to be a frequent complication occurring in 16% of patients, and they found infection occurring in 7% of patients, which then required mesh excision.

The component separation technique has been shown in numerous studies to decrease the risk of recurrence. Release of the external oblique aponeurosis can lead to weakness of the abdominal wall and the formation of a hernia in this area. Skin necrosis is also a major concern in the component separation technique due to ligation of periumbilical rectus abdominis perforators, and can have a high incidence, leading to alternative methods of lateral fascial separation, including a bilateral inguinal approach described by Clarke.[34] In this so-called 'perforator preservation' technique, fascial separation is performed through separate inguinal incisions utilizing balloon dissection. By performing dissection in this manner, the periumbilical perforator vessels are preserved, and they demonstrated no postoperative episodes of skin necrosis. Mesh has also been used in this technique, and the above-listed complications can also occur when mesh is used together with the component separation technique.

When combining incisional hernia repair with abdominoplasty or panniculectomy, untoward events can arise from the performance of either procedure. Commonly encountered problems from abdominoplasty alone include wound infection, dehiscence, seroma, hematoma, and skin loss. Less common problems include DVT, pulmonary embolus, fat embolus, and umbilical necrosis.[35] In a recent retrospective review evaluating patients undergoing a combination of these procedures, Shermak found that the complications are similar to those encountered when the procedures are performed separately, with the most frequent including wound complications (20%) and seromas (12.5%).[31] This led the author to the conclusion that the combination of abdominoplasty and incisional hernia repair is a safe and effective procedure.

CONCLUSIONS

As the population continues to become increasingly obese, the need for weight loss operations will also continue to rise. Complications from these operations, including the development of an incisional hernia, will always be prevalent, and the need for surgical repair will continue to challenge surgeons. Multiple options exist for repair of these hernias, including primary suture repair, implantation of prosthetic or biologic mesh, manipulation of the anterior abdominal wall musculature in the component separation technique, and the use of autologous tissue. It is imperative that the plastic surgeon be familiar with hernias and their surgical repair in MWL patients because they will be asked to participate in the care of these individuals.

REFERENCES

1. Deitel M, Shikora SA. The development of the surgical treatment of morbid obesity. *J Am Coll Nutr* 2002;**21**:365–71.
2. Lockwood TE. Superficial fascial system (SFS) of the trunk and extremities: A new concept. *Plast Reconstr Surg* 1991;**87**:1009–18.
3. Huger WE Jr. The anatomic rationale for abdominal lipectomy. *Am Surgeon* 1979;**45**:6112–17.
4. Puzziferri N, Austrheim-Smith IT, Wolfe BM, et al. Three-year follow-up of a prospective randomized trial comparing laparoscopic versus open gastric bypass. *Ann Surg* 2006;**243**:181–8.
5. Sugerman HJ, Kellum JM, Reines D, et al. Greater risk of incisional hernia with morbidly obese than steroid-dependent patients and low recurrence with prefascial polypropylene mesh. *Am J Surg* 1996;**171**:80–4.
6. Nguyen NT, Lee SL, Anderson JT, et al. Evaluation of intraabdominal pressure after open and laparoscopic gastric bypass. *Obes Surg* 2001;**11**:40–5.
7. Shell DH 4th, de la Torre J, Andrades P, Vasconez LO. Open repair of ventral incisional hernias. *Surg Clin North Am* 2008;**88**:61–83.
8. Evans KK, Chim H, Patel KM, et al. Survey on ventral hernias: Surgeon indications, contraindications, and management of large ventral hernias. *Am Surgeon* 2012;in press.
9. Hardy JE, Salgado CJ, Chamoun G, et al. The safety of pelvic surgery in the morbidly obese with and without combined panniculectomy: A comparison of results. *Ann Plast Surg* 2008;**60**:10–13.
10. Hsu PW, Salgado CJ, Finnegan M, et al. Evaluation of porcine dermal collagen (Permacol) used in abdominal wall reconstruction. *J Plast Reconstr Aesth Surg* 2009;**62**:1484–9.
11. Luijendijk RW, Hop WC, van den Tol MP, et al. A comparison of suture repair with mesh repair for incisional hernia. *N Engl J Med* 2000;**343**:392–8.
12. Mathes SJ, Steinwald PM, Roster RD, et al. Complex abdominal wall reconstruction: A comparison of flap and mesh closure. *Ann Surg* 2000;**232**:586.
13. Bonatti H, Hoeller E, Kirchmayr W, et al. Ventral hernia repair in bariatric surgery. *Obes Surg* 2004;**14**:655–8.
14. Langer C, Schaper A, Liersch T et al. Prognosis factors in incisional hernia surgery: 25 years of experience. *Hernia* 2005;**9**:16–21.
15. Rudmik LR, Schieman C, Dixon E, et al. Laparoscopic incisional hernia repair: a review of the literature. *Hernia* 2006;**10**:110–19.
16. Ramirez OM, Ruas E, Dellon AL. 'Components separation' method for closure of abdominal-wall defects: an anatomical and clinical study. *Plast Reconstr Surg* 1990;**86**:519–26.
17. Ger R, Duboys E. The prevention and repair of large abdominal wall defects by muscle transposition: A preliminary communication. *Plast Reconstr Surg* 1983;**72**:170.
18. Hadeed JG, Walsh MD, Pappas TN, et al. Complex abdominal wall hernias: A new classification system and approach to management based on review of 133 consecutive cases. *Ann Plast Surg* 2011;**66**:497–503.
19. Borud LJ, Grunwaldt L, Janz B, et al. Components separation combined with abdominal wall placation for repair of large abdominal wall hernias following bariatric surgery. *Plast Reconstr Surg* 2007;**119**:1792–8.
20. Ko JH, Salvay DM, Paul BC, et al. Soft polypropylene mesh, but not cadaveric dermis, significantly improves outcomes in midline hernia repairs using the component separation technique. *Plast Reconstr Surg* 2009;**124**:836–47.
21. Kheradmand AA, Novin NR, Khazaeipour Z. Brief report: The use of dermal autograft for fascial repair of TRAM flap donor sites. *J Plast Reconstr Aesthetic Surg* 2011;**64**:364–8.
22. Hein KD, Morris DJ, Goldwyn RM, et al. Dermal autografts for fascial repair after TRAM flap harvest. *Plast Reconstr Surg* 1998;**102**:2287–92.
23. De Vries Reilingh TS, Bodegom ME, van Goor H, et al. Autologous tissue repair of large abdominal wall defects. *Br J Surg* 2007;**94**:791–803.
24. Wong C, Lin C, Fu B, Fang J. Reconstruction of complex abdominal wall defects with free flaps: Indications and clinical outcome. *Plast Reconstr Surg* 2009;**125**:500–9.
25. Dibbel DG Jr, Mixter RC, Dibbel DG Sr. Abdominal wall reconstruction (the 'mutton chop' flap). *Plast Reconstr Surg* 1991;**87**:60–5.
26. Shankaran V, Weber DJ, Reed RL, et al. A review of available prosthetics for ventral hernia repair. *Ann Surg* 2011;**253**:16–26.
27. Breuing K, Butler CE, Ferzoco S, et al. Incisional ventral hernias: Review of the literature and recommendations regarding the grading and technique of repair. *Surgery* 2010;**148**:544–8.
28. Millikan KW. Incisional hernia repair. *Surg Clin North Am* 2003;**83**:1223–34.
29. De Vries Reilingh TS, van Goor H, Rosman C, et al. 'Components separation technique' for the repair of large abdominal wall hernias. *J Am Coll Surg* 2003;**196**:32–7.
30. Shestak K, Edington H, Johnson R. The separation of anatomic components technique for the reconstruction of massive midline abdominal wall defects: anatomy, surgical technique, applications, and limitations revisited. *Plast Reconstr Surg* 2000;**105**:731–8.
31. Shermak MA. Hernia repair and abdominoplasty in gastric bypass patients. *Plast Reconstr Surg* 2006;**117**:1145–50.
32. Mazzocchi M, Dessy LA, Ranno R, et al. 'Component separation' technique and panniculectomy for repair of incisional hernia. *Am J Surg* 2011;**201**:776–83.
33. Robinson TN, Clarke JH, Schoen J, and Walsh MD. Major mesh-related complications following hernia repair: Events reported to the Food and Drug Administration. *Surg Endosc* 2005;**19**:1556–60.
34. Clarke JM. Incisional hernia repair by fascial component separation: results in 128 cases and evolution of technique. *Am J Surg* 2010;**200**:2–8.
35. Friedland JA and Maffi TR. Abdominoplasty. *Plast Reconstr Surg* 2008;**121**(4 suppl):1–11.

Chapter 12
Reconstruction of abdominal wall defects after bariatric surgery and simultaneous abdominal lipectomies

Mimis Cohen, Rebekah M. Zaluzec

INTRODUCTION

Obesity has become an epidemic not only in the USA but also around the world. This condition has significant implications for patients' wellbeing, secondary to the profound negative effects in daily activities, personal hygiene, work and psychology. Furthermore, morbidly obese patients present with many comorbid conditions from hypertension and diabetes to sleep apnea and joint problems which further affect patients' lives. Over 60% of Americans are currently classified as overweight, half of whom are considered to be morbidly obese.[1] For most of these individuals weight loss with diet and other conservative means is practically impossible; thus more and more patients are referred for bariatric surgery.

In 1991, a National Institute of Health (NIH) panel met to address surgical and non-surgical treatments for obesity. It stated that a particular subset of patients would benefit from bariatric surgical procedures and that these surgeries were an effective treatment for obesity.[2] As a result of this panel consensus, the number of bariatric operations started to increase steadily in the early 1990s and skyrocketed during the last decade.[3-5] With accumulated experience bariatric surgery was recognized as a safe and effective way for the management of patients who are morbidly obese. Guidelines for patient selection, team management, and preoperative, perioperative, and postoperative short- and long-term care were developed. Several procedures have evolved over the last few years to provide these unfortunate individuals with successful treatment while reducing the incidence of complications and other unfavorable results. In addition, due to the advances and advantages of minimally invasive surgery, most weight loss procedures are currently performed laparoscopically or robotically.[5] Thus, the serious wound-related complications associated with the open techniques, which may exceed a rate between 5 and 85% according to various studies, including dehiscence and incisional hernias, have been dramatically reduced.[6-12]

A number of patients are still treated with open techniques. Some present several years after the weight loss procedure with abdominal wall hernias and other abdominal wall problems.

Along with the benefit of weight loss and improvement of general health, patients develop symptomatic lipodystrophy, with skin laxity, tissue redundancy, and hanging rolls in various areas of the body and extremities, primarily the abdomen. These conditions are quite debilitating. They interfere with patients' daily activities and clothing, and affect posture, walking, and exercise. They also interfere with patients' personal hygiene, leading to intetrigo and constant skin infections from continuous rubbing of the pannus against the underlying skin of the pubic area. They can also have a negative impact on patients' psychology and self-esteem.[13]

Plastic surgeons have thus become indispensable members of the bariatric team and assist post-weight loss patients to achieve full rehabilitation with various body-contouring procedures and return to society as functional citizens. Furthermore, once wound problems of the abdominal wall or incisional hernias have developed, the plastic surgeon is often called to manage such patients, alone or jointly with the general surgeons, to undertake reconstruction of the abdominal wall and repair of the coexisting hernia, in addition to the lipectomy and body-contouring procedures.

The concept of abdominoplasty or abdominal lipectomy with simultaneous ventral hernia repair is not new. Advantages of this approach have been recognized as significant and include a more optimal hernia repair by offering the surgeon full visualization of the underlying defect, providing surgery through known planes of tissue, and moving the skin incision far from the hernia repair edge if possible,[11] reduction of hospitalization and subsequent overall cost, and decreased total convalescent time, as shown in **Fig. 12.1**. These advantages must be weighed against the necessary prolonged anesthesia and surgical time, increased blood loss, and increased rate of wound and other complications associated with lipectomies.

Initially, surgeons were reluctant to proceed with combined procedures including simultaneous repairs of the hernia and abdominal lipectomy for fear of additional complications. Grazer, in 1977, reported on 44 abdominoplasties.[14] In two-thirds of these procedures, combined operations were performed. Only two of the patients in this group underwent an intra-abdominal operation, an abdominal hysterectomy. All others simultaneously underwent a variety of cosmetic procedures or vaginal hysterectomies. Grazer stated that: 'it is not the purpose of this paper to advocate or defend the combined procedure but our complication rate appears to be similar in single or combined procedures.' In 1982, Savage[15] also reported on the topic and stated that 'this combination of procedures has been safe and effective in properly screened individuals.' He also stated that 'patients with large hernias, especially if the use of prosthetic mesh repair is required, are poor candidates for combined procedures' and concluded that 'this combination of operations is not advocated as routine.' Hester et al.[16] reported on a total of 563 patients undergoing abdominoplasty combined with other major procedures, 230 of whom had intra-abdominal or pelvic interventions. There were 16 ventral hernia repairs in their series and the complication rate was very low. Based on their experience they confirmed the basic safety of combined procedures.

In recent years, with the increase in numbers of bariatric surgery procedures, the topic of a combination of procedures has been re-evaluated extensively. Several reports with short- and long-term results have been published. Thus, with accumulated experience, it is becoming obvious

114 RECONSTRUCTION OF ABDOMINAL WALL DEFECTS

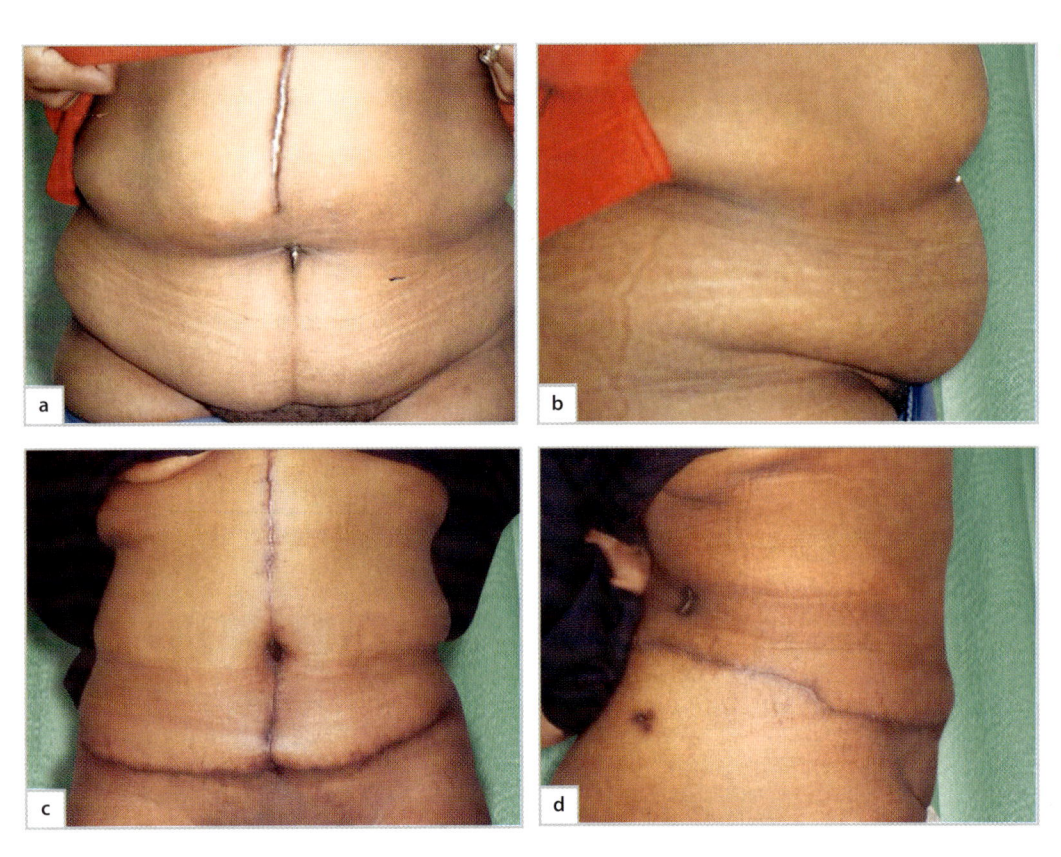

Figure 12.1 A 34-year-old woman (a) presenting 1 year of gastric bypass and weight loss of 145 lb (65.25 kg) with a large incisional hernia and abdominal lipodystrophy; (b) lateral view; (c) 14 months after repair of incisional hernia and fleur-de-lis lipectomy with stable abdominal wall and good aesthetic result; (d) lateral view.

that, for most cases, there is no contraindication in combining these procedures. The final success rate is comparable to or even better than the results obtained when the procedures are staged.[6–12,17–20]

Patient safety has, however, to be our foremost interest. Patient selection must therefore be performed very carefully and a patient's general condition optimized in preparation for the procedure. As a general rule, additional body-contouring procedures should be discouraged in this group of patients, although decisions should be individualized based on the patient's overall requirements and overall condition, and the surgeon's experience.

In this chapter, we present our experience with over 320 combined procedures for a subgroup of patients presenting with ventral hernias with or without open abdominal wall wounds which resulted from complications of weight loss surgery; preoperative evaluation protocols and the selection process are discussed in detail, short- and long-term outcomes of combined abdominal lipectomies and hernia repairs with/or without abdominal wall reconstructions analyzed, and steps taken to achieve the best possible results while reducing the number of complications/unfavorable results recommended. Lastly, recommendations are made for aggressive management of wound complications as soon as they are identified.

■ PREREQUISITES FOR SUCCESS

■ Evaluation of patients' general condition

Specific issues with bariatric patients

Patients presenting after weight loss procedures have unique problems that are different from those of other groups of patients requiring abdominal wall reconstruction, hernia repair, or abdominoplasties.[4,9,21]

As most procedures are of an elective nature, these problems must be taken into consideration, evaluated, and managed as needed, before the final planning and procedure scheduling. Initial detailed evaluation of patients' general health and psychological status, possible presence of comorbid conditions such as hypertension, diabetes, ischemic cardiac disease, respiratory problems, history of deep venous thrombosis (DVT), and smoking, among others, should be recognized and treated accordingly. As with all preoperative planning, a detailed history and physical exam are necessary to fully appreciate the bariatric procedure to be performed. The pre- and post-surgical body mass index (BMI) should be noted, as well as the time that has elapsed from the start of the onset of weight loss, the stability of current weight, and possible plans for further weight loss. The presence of significant residual intra-abdominal fat is important and needs to be recognized, because such conditions might cause undue tension to the hernia repair and possibly increase failure rate.[1,21,22]

Full nutritional and laboratory evaluation is also necessary because most of the weight loss procedures result in various malabsorption conditions, including anemia and vitamin B_{12} deficiency, which can affect healing and speedy recovery.[21,23,24] We depend and work closely with our medical colleagues to provide appropriate management of all comorbidities and optimize patients' general health in preparation for surgery.

Traditional teaching has been to defer body-contouring procedures until the patient has reached the ideal planned weight and has been able to maintain it for a minimum of 3–6 months. Patients need to show appropriate motivation, be psychologically stable, and demonstrate credible modifications in their lifestyle, including dietetic changes and exercise. They should also have realistic expectations. In our particular subgroup of patients, however, there are times when the surgeon might be forced to consider performing the procedure before appropriate planned weight loss, due to the presence of an open wound or a symptomatic hernia, as depicted in **Fig. 12.2**.

Prerequisites for success | 115

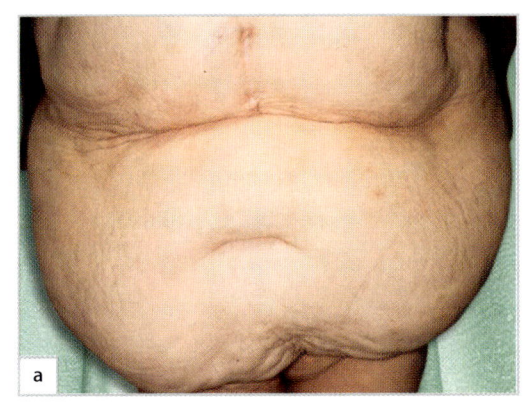

Figure 12.2 A 46-year-old woman 16 months after open bypass and 6 months after incisional hernia repair by the bariatric service. (a) Presented with large symptomatic recurrent hernia and significant symptomatic abdominal lipodystrophy; body mass index (BMI) 42. (b) Lateral view. (c) The patient presents with a stable abdominal well and good aesthetic result 13 months after hernia repair with mesh and fleur-de-lis abdominal lipectomy. (d) Lateral view.

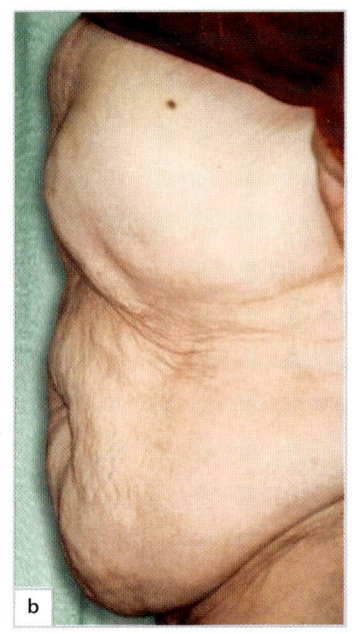

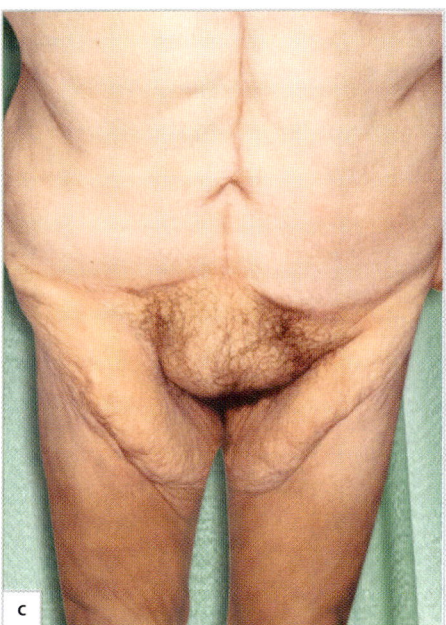

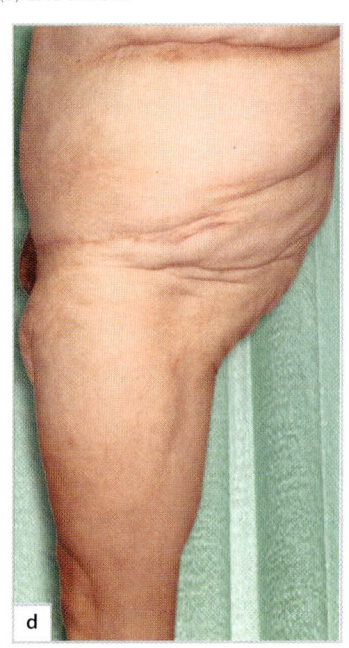

In such situations, the plastic surgeon needs to individualize the plan based on the specific case scenario. The surgeon needs to decide if the patient is truly a candidate for a combined procedure or can be better served by reconstruction of the abdominal defect/hernia, deferring the lipectomy for a future date. This is not an easy decision and should not be taken lightly. We know from experience that some form of simultaneous lipectomy is advantageous to the outcome of hernia repair, because the tension on the repair from the overlying pannus will be reduced with the lipectomy. In such situations, one might consider a suboptimal final cosmetic result with less tissue undermining and resection. This will avoid possible future wound complications and failure of the reconstructive effort.

Evaluation of the abdominal defect/hernia

The plastic surgeon needs to perform an extensive evaluation when consulted to manage patients with abdominal wall defects. In most cases after open bariatric surgery, the defect of the abdomen is due to wound dehiscence, infection, or tissue necrosis. Even minor details are important and should be taken into consideration before the planning of a reconstructive procedure including the following:
- Size and location of the defect, presence of active or chronic infection
- Possible soft-tissue losses including muscle and/or fascia from previous debridements
- Quality of the wound bed
- Quality of adjacent tissues
- Presence of mesh or other prosthetic materials
- Exposure of abdominal viscera and/or presence of fistulas.

Functional evaluation of the remaining muscles of the abdominal wall, in particular the rectus abdominis muscles, should be performed, and is done by asking the patient to sit up or strain. This information is very important not only to fully appreciate weak areas of the abdominal musculofascial system but also for the cases where a component separation technique is considered in the reconstructive plan.[25-27]

One should not forget that several patients will present with additional abdominal scars from previous intra-abdominal interventions. These scars should be taken into consideration during the general planning because parallel scars or scars at acute angles might interfere with the vascularity of the abdominal flaps and result in tissue necrosis. Examples of patients with multiple abdominal scars are shown in **Figs 12.3** and **12.4**.

When deemed appropriate, proper imaging should be obtained. This allows complete evaluation of the defect(s) of the abdominal wall and the extent of the hernia sac. In addition, the surgeon can identify pockets of possible collections, additional mesh/biomaterials or other foreign bodies and further improve the reconstructive plan. Such an example is demonstrated in **Fig. 12.5**. Review of the previous operative report(s) when available is essential in the planning and preparation of these extensive procedures.

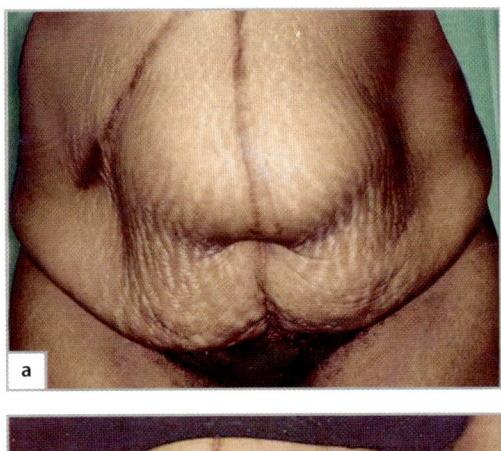

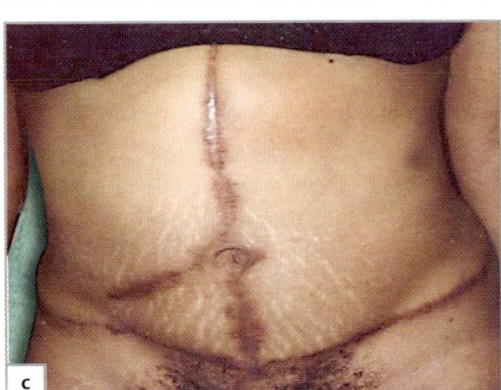

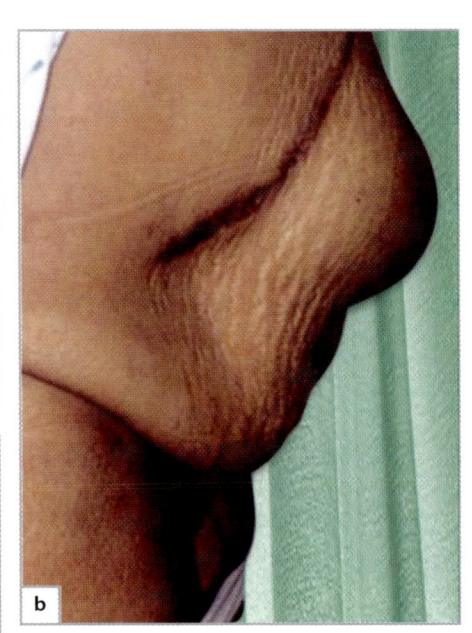

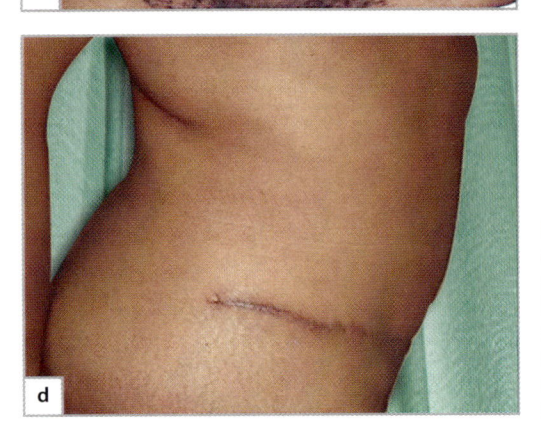

Figure 12.3 A 28-year-old woman 9 months after gastric bypass. (a) Presentation with large symptomatic incisional hernia and a right subcostal incision 8 years after cholecystectomy. (b) Lateral view. (c) patient presents with a good functional and aesthetic result 14 months after hernia repair with mesh due to the previous division of the right rectus muscle and lipectomy. (d) Lateral view

Wound preparation

Acute wounds after wound dehiscence might be clean but must be managed aggressively with debridement of all necrotic/devascularized tissues, removal of all foreign bodies, and wound care to avoid infection and further tissue loss. Exposed prosthetic material cannot be salvaged in most situations and should be removed. Ideally, every effort should be made to involve the plastic surgeon as early as possible in the care of such patients in order to establish the most appropriate coordinated plan of action (with alternatives if necessary), and provide the patient with the best possible care in a timely fashion. Unfortunately, it is often the case that the plastic surgeon is not consulted for evaluation until the wound is already infected or chronic, characterized by tissue loss, pockets of purulent collections, and possible loss of domain. As a rule, wide debridement of these wounds should be performed, including removal of all foreign bodies, meshes, etc. and drainage of all superficial or deep-seated infections. The decision will then need to be made about whether to perform immediate wound closure/reconstruction or to delay such a procedure. If immediate closure is not feasible, or desirable, then wound care should be recommended for the interval until the definitive procedure. The vacuum-assisted closure (VAC) devise has become an invaluable tool in the management of these complex wounds. Using VAC therapy, concomitant local and systemic complications are controlled: The open wound is protected and stabilized, local tissue sepsis is managed, tissue swelling reduced, and fluid and electrolyte loss controlled. The size of the wound is also gradually reduced with the use of this modality.[28] Thus VAC therapy has become an important addition in our armamentarium and has been incorporated into our treatment protocols for the management of complex wounds.

Timing of the procedures

Timing of definitive reconstruction is of utmost importance to achieve a successful outcome. Abdominal wall reconstruction should

Figure 12.4 A 38-year-old woman 10 months after open bypass. (a) Presents with large incisional hernia, symptomatic abdominal lipodystrophy, and body mass index (BMI) of 38. Note the scars from previous open bypass, cholecystectomy, appendectomy, and cesarean section. (b) Lateral view. (c) Patient presents with a stable abdominal wall 14 months after hernia repair with mesh and abdominal lipectomy; she is completely relieved from the symptoms of lipodystrophy, back to work and exercise. (d) Lateral view.

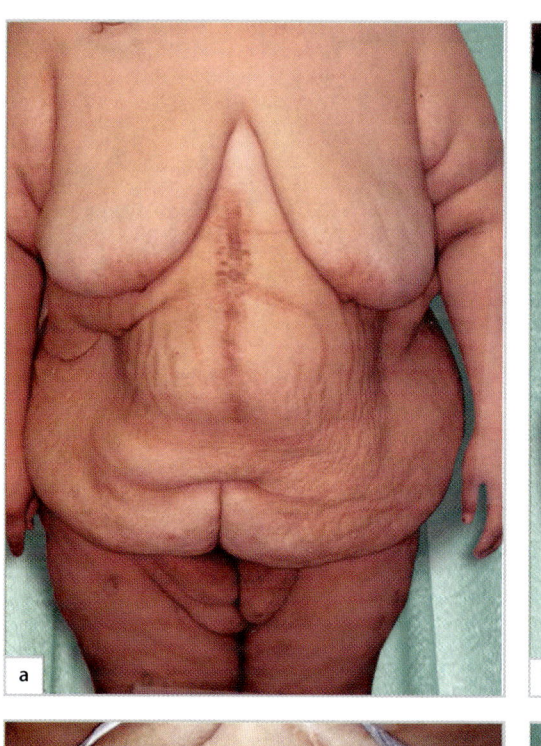

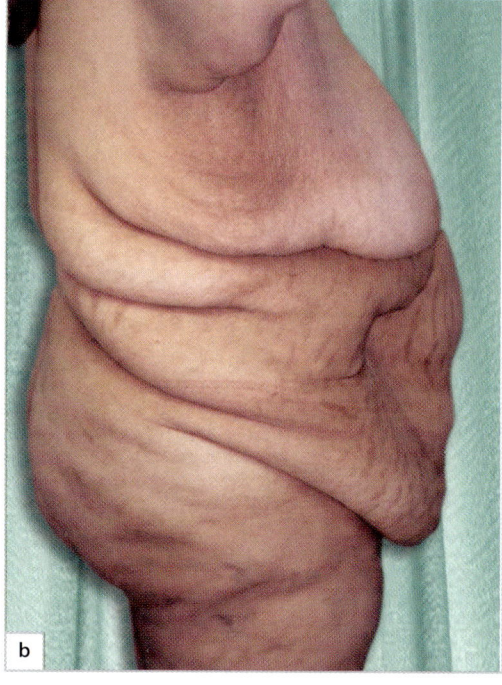

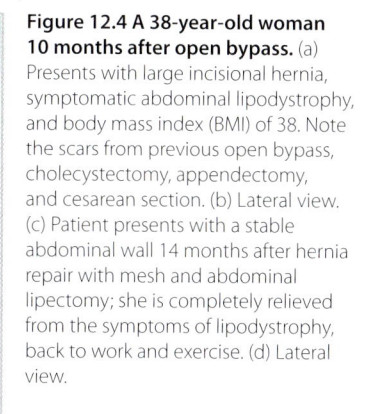

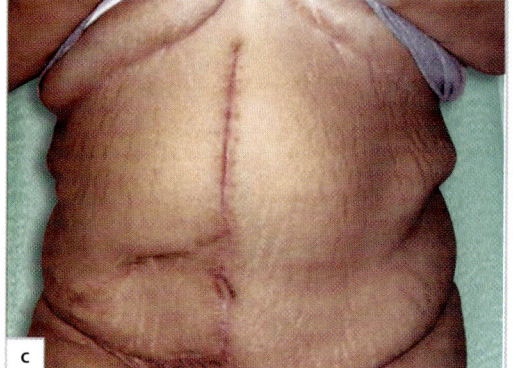

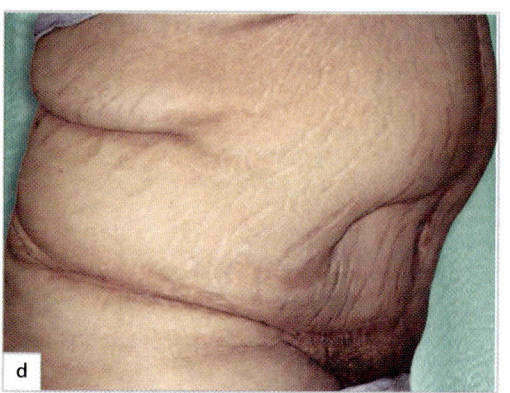

certainly *not* be combined with abdominal lipectomies in the acute setting. As mentioned above, every effort should be made to stabilize the wound and control infection. A staged protocol could be used for the group of patients when immediate reconstruction is not considered appropriate. Such patients could benefit from staged reconstruction with temporary treatment with VAC, placement of an absorbable mesh over the abdominal contents, and application of a split-thickness skin graft over the granulating bed a few days later. Thus, temporary protection is provided to the underlying viscera, loss of fluid and electrolytes is controlled, and the potential for tissue maceration, infection, and loss eliminated. In this manner, the definitive procedure can be delayed for a more optimal time.

On the other hand, chronic but stable open wounds, after wound dehiscence and without any evidence of gross infection, can be managed with concomitant reconstruction of the abdominal wall defect and lipectomy, as shown in **Figs 12.6** and **12.7**. Such procedures must, however, be individualized and used in a selected group of patients. Pros and cons should be analyzed carefully and decisions made based on each particular patient's problems, history, general condition, and local area requirements.

■ Cooperation with the bariatric surgeon

Successful management of patients presenting after weight loss procedures with abdominal wounds and/or hernias requires close cooperation between the plastic surgeon and the referring bariatric surgeon. In some instances a team approach can be highly beneficial because the talent, knowledge, and expertise of each surgeon are used to address and solve the multiple and complex surgical and systemic problems of each patient. Plastic surgeons need to fully appreciate the circumstances leading to the abdominal defect or hernia, particularly when dealing with patients presenting after major complications such as abdominal catastrophes, anastomotic leaks, fistulas, peritonitis, and systemic infections. The steps of the procedure should be planned accordingly. Each operative surgeon needs to understand the goals of the procedure, the possible limitations from previous interventions, and his or her individual role during surgery and personal responsibility for every step of the procedure. Furthermore, team management should extend beyond the operation to the immediate postoperative period. This ensures primary healing, timely identification of any surgical or medical complications, and appropriate management.

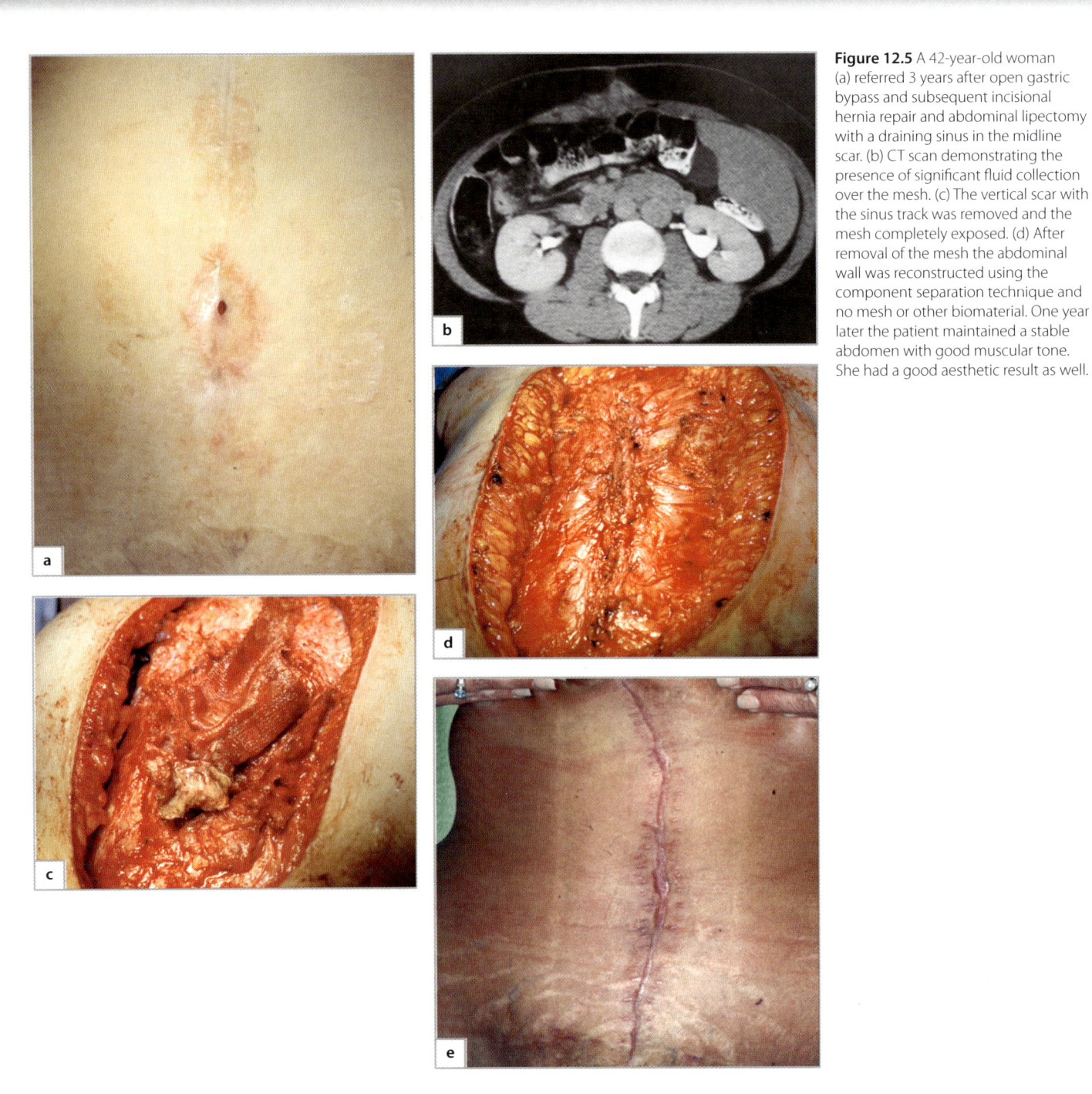

Figure 12.5 A 42-year-old woman (a) referred 3 years after open gastric bypass and subsequent incisional hernia repair and abdominal lipectomy with a draining sinus in the midline scar. (b) CT scan demonstrating the presence of significant fluid collection over the mesh. (c) The vertical scar with the sinus track was removed and the mesh completely exposed. (d) After removal of the mesh the abdominal wall was reconstructed using the component separation technique and no mesh or other biomaterial. One year later the patient maintained a stable abdomen with good muscular tone. She had a good aesthetic result as well.

RECONSTRUCTIVE PRINCIPLES

Reconstruction of open wound and panniculectomy

The purpose of abdominal wall reconstruction, hernia repair, and abdominal lipectomy is to re-establish form and function, provide strong and stable coverage to the abdominal contents, while reducing the abdominal pannus, and improve abdominal contour. Adherence to basic surgical, reconstructive, and aesthetic principles is a prerequisite for a successful outcome. As stated earlier, successful short- and long-term management of this group of patients requires close cooperation of the plastic surgeon, bariatric surgeon, and other members of the bariatric team. Infections, if present, should be controlled, all infected, necrotic, and scared tissues debrided, and all foreign bodies (e.g. previous sutures, meshes, and other prosthetic material) removed. There are three primary options for hernia repair. The decision and selection of which technique to use depend on the size and location of the defect, the quality of the surrounding muscles and fascia, any previous failures, and the surgeon's personal preference and experience. Primary fascial repair is used for relatively narrow defects. For all other cases, the hernia can be repaired using a variety of meshes/biomaterials or the component separation technique. Successful results with reconstruction using various prosthetic materials, simple direct closure, or autologous tissue reconstruction have been extensively reported.[6–12,29,30]

The authors favor using the component separation technique, when feasible, and avoid as much as possible the use of prosthetic materials.

Reconstructive principles 119

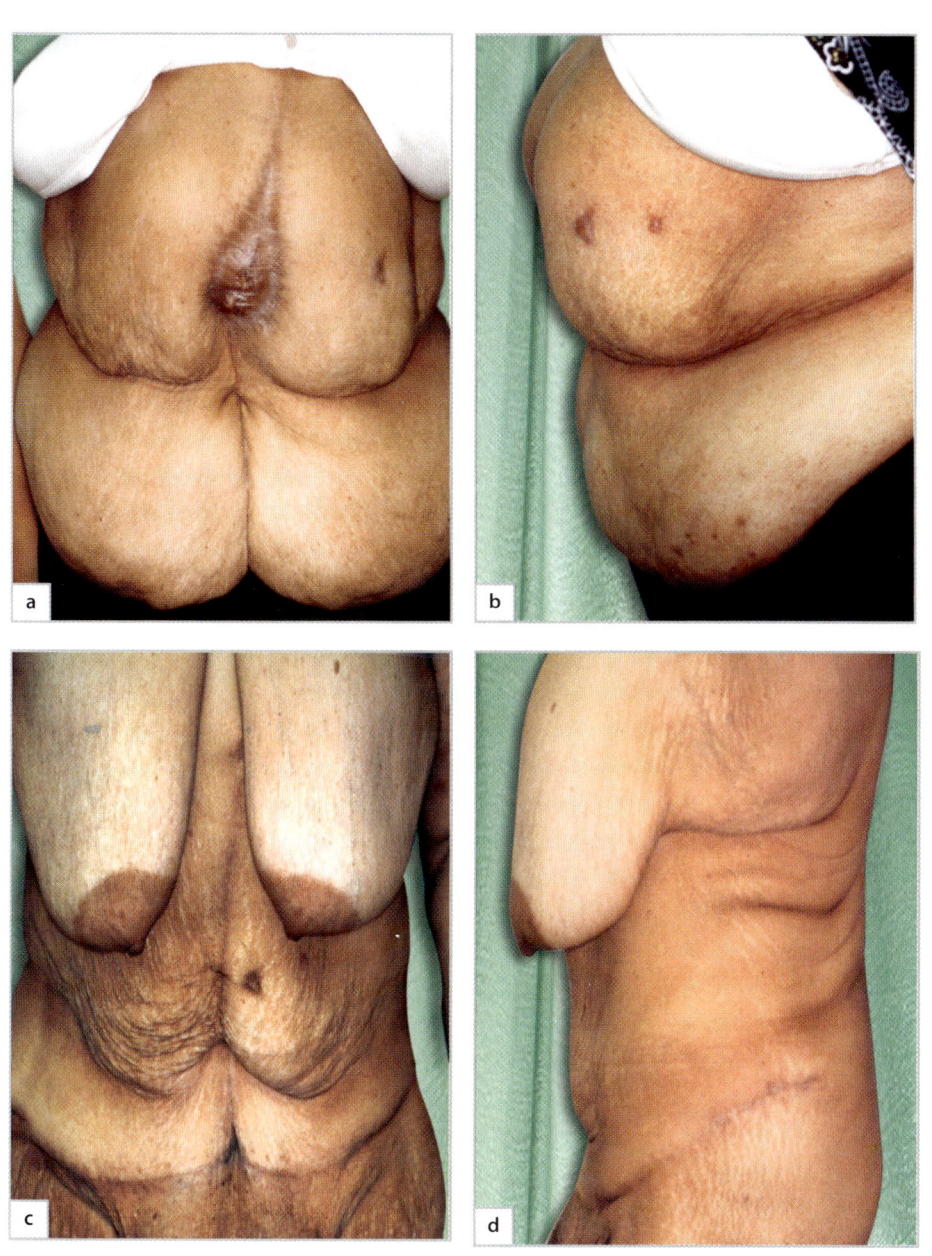

Figure 12.6 A 52-year-old woman (a) 8 months after open bypass and wound dehiscence; body mass index (BMI) 41. (b) Lateral view. (c) Sixteen months after hernia repair with component separation technique and abdominal lipectomy with very good functional and aesthetic result. (d) Lateral view.

An example is depicted in **Fig. 12.8**. The advantages and limitations of this technique have been well described.[4,20] Autologous and dynamic reconstruction is achieved with the use of this technique, with preservation of the tone, elasticity, and flexibility of the abdominal wall; the technique can be applied in infected wounds and the short- and long-term results can be consistently superior to the use of prosthetic materials with low recurrence rates.

There are limitations in the use of the technique, however, and it should not be applied in every case. It has only limited use for lateral defects and it cannot be used if the rectus muscle(s) has been divided from previous surgeries. There is also a size limitation and the separation of components should not be used for defects wider than 8 + 2 cm in the upper abdomen, 20 + 3 cm in the waist, and 6 + 2 cm in the lower abdomen.

These measurements are not absolute but merely provide a framework during the planning of the procedure. As stated earlier, the selection of each procedure should be individualized.

Attention needs to be paid to the undermining of the abdominal pannus, particularly in patients presenting with multiple scars from previous incisions. Above all, excessive tension during the hernia repair and skin closure should be avoided at all costs. Some tissue redundancy should be accepted in order to avoid closure under tension, resulting in wound dehisce and complications, prolonged hospitalization and recovery time, and possibly jeopardizing the patient's wellbeing.

■ Description of technique

The use of vertical and horizontal excision to improve appearance of the abdominal wall is not a new idea. Babcock was probably the first to describe vertical excision for panniculectomy as early as 1916 and again in 1935; Castañares[31] in 1968 presented a design very similar to the one in current use. This design was further refined by Dellon in 1985 who also coined the term 'fleur-de-lis.' This technique is successful in

120 RECONSTRUCTION OF ABDOMINAL WALL DEFECTS

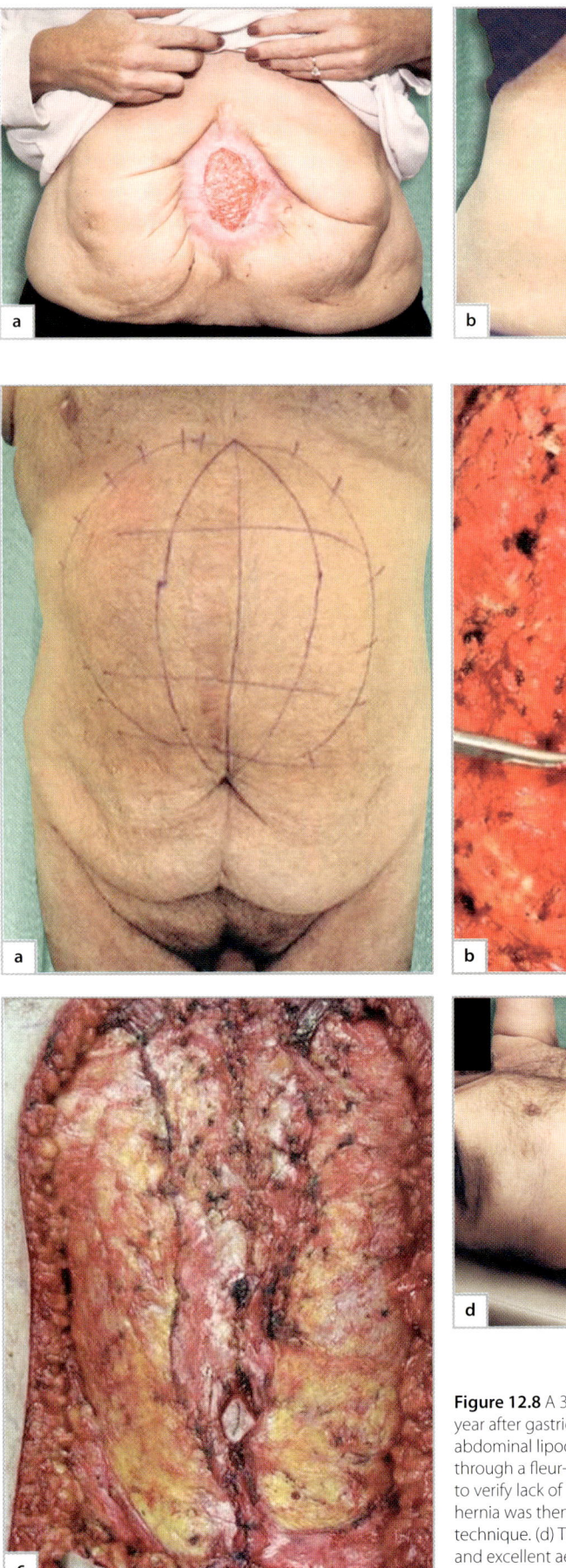

Figure 12.7 A 39-year-old woman (a) referred with an open abdominal wound 1 year after bypass and significant weight loss; body mass index (BMI) 28. (b) One year after debridement, abdominal wall reconstruction with component separation technique and lipectomy presents in excellent condition.

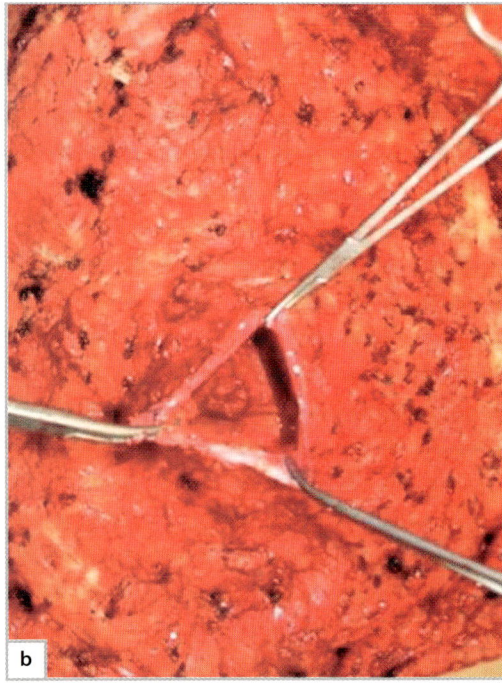

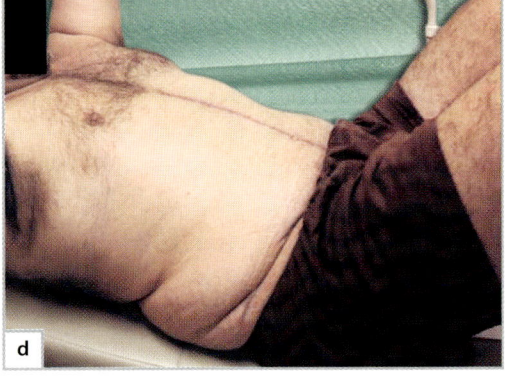

Figure 12.8 A 38-year-old man (a) presented almost 1 year after gastric bypass with a large incisional hernia and abdominal lipodystrophy. (b) The hernia was approached through a fleur-de-lis design, and the sac was opened to verify lack of adherence of bowel in the sac. (c) The hernia was then repaired using the component separation technique. (d) The patient presents with a stable abdomen and excellent aesthetic result 22 months after the reconstruction.

correcting the epigastric fullness that is not adequately managed by the traditional abdominoplasty, but never gained popularity because of the additional vertical scar and the rate of wound complications, particularly in the areas of junction between the vertical and horizontal incisions. With the increased number of body-contouring operations in patients with massive weight loss, however, the value of this procedure was recognized and several authors have reported their successful experience with the technique.[32]

The patient is marked while standing, as shown in **Fig. 12.9**, unless the abdominal pannus is too bulky. In such cases, the vertical component of the proposed incision is marked with the patient standing and the horizontal ellipse is marked with the patient lying on the operating table. Attention should be paid to the midline because the previous laparotomy scar might not be centered in the actual *anatomic midline*. After marking the actual midline, the vertical ellipse is marked, making sure, with manual evaluation and pinching, that the tissue is not over-resected. The lower transverse incision of the abdominoplasty is marked according to the specific needs. The proposed horizontal resection is also outlined. As asymmetries are common, additional stable landmarks are also marked as reference points to facilitate a symmetric outcome. Additional markings are placed vertically to the proposed incisions for better intraoperative alignment and guidance, and to further facilitate accurate closure.

If there is no open abdominal wound, dissection begins from the inferior line of the abdominoplasty incision, continuing to approximately 2 cm above the umbilicus. Excision of the vertical ellipse and full exposure of the sac and the defect are then performed, making sure that the hernia sac and the abdominal contents are not injured. At this point the surgeon is faced with three different options for the management the hernia and reconstruction of the musculofacial system. If the hernia defect is narrow, the quality of the surrounding tissues satisfactory, and a tension-free closure of the fascia can be achieved, minimal additional undermining will be required. If, on the other hand, a component separation technique is considered appropriate, the abdominal flap is undermined until about 2 cm lateral to the arcuate line, starting superiorly over the costal margin where the dissection is easier. In cases where a mesh or other prosthetic material is considered, appropriate undermining beyond the margins of the defect is also necessary to ensure suturing of the prosthetic material around healthy tissues.

The sac is then opened, the abdominal cavity explored and lysis of adhesions, if needed, is performed before repairing the hernia using one of the above-mentioned methods. In some instances, the umbilical stalk is found over the sac. In such cases, the stalk is removed with the sac.

It is beyond the scope of this chapter to discuss in detail the selection of prosthetic material or biomaterial and to describe the steps of the component separation techniques. These topics have being presented extensively in the literature. For the cases where there is no need for extensive intra-abdominal exploration and the component separation technique is selected for the reconstruction, caution should be observed. In such cases, the surgeon will still need to make sure that the abdominal contents do not adhere to the sac and the abdominal wall, and to avoid injuring them with the suture placement. Making an opening in the sac and manually evaluating the abdominal contents before proceeding with the repair is recommended.

When managing patients presenting with open abdominal wounds the surgeon should reverse the order of exploration, starting from the vertical ellipse, because, for these cases, the prime surgical goal is the management of the abdominal wall defect.

After repair of the hernia, the skin flaps are temporary approximated with staples and further adjustments in soft-tissue excisions are made, as required, to achieve the best possible aesthetic result, while closing tissues without undue tension. After copious irrigation and meticulous hemostasis, the incisions are closed in layers over suction drains.

RESULTS

Body-contouring procedures are notorious for a high rate of wound complications. Furthermore, it has been well demonstrated that the rate of complications increases with obesity and a higher rate of complications should be expected in patients with a BMI >35. The most common major abdominal complications requiring additional surgical interventions include the following:

- Tissue infection and necrosis resulting in open wounds
- Mesh extrusions
- Hernia recurrence
- Recurrent seromas.

Cellulitis, suture abscess, and minor tissue loss are in most instances treated conservatively. Wound complications from fleur-de-lis lipectomies are definitely higher than for standard abdominoplasty, but the difference is not statistically significant.[30]

The authors' short- and long-term results were presented a few years ago and are comparable to those of others. In a review of 327 patients, 211 (64.5%) were treated exclusively by our service while the remaining 116 (35.5%) were treated by a team of general and plastic surgeons. The BMI of the patients ranged from 28 to 43 with an average of 35; 254 patients presented with incisional hernias, 86 (33.5%) of which were recurrent hernias, whereas 63 presented with full-thickness defects of the abdominal wall. Of the 254 patients with hernias, 55.9% were treated by the component separation technique, 11.1% with direct closure, and 33% with the use of mesh and other biomaterials. A fleur-de-lis lipectomy was used in the vast majority of our cases at the same time as the hernia repair/abdominal wall reconstruction.

In a follow-up ranging from 14 months to 8 years, 27 patients (8.2%) who developed major wound complications requiring additional surgery were identified, including 19 patients (5.8%), who developed recurrent hernias; 24 patients (7.3%) developed seromas; 19 patients

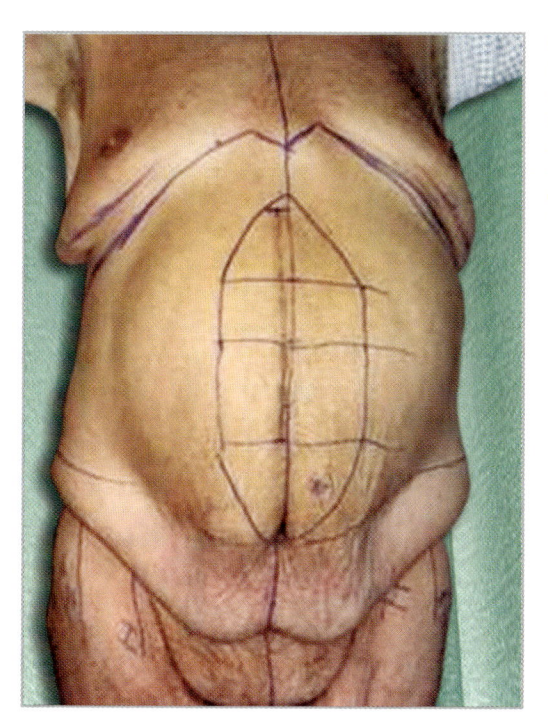

Figure 12.9 Preoperative marking of the vertical and horizontal components for a fleur-de-lis lipectomy.

(79.1%) were treated conservatively whereas 5 (20.9%) required a surgical intervention; 39 patients (16.1%) developed minor complications including wound infections, dehiscence, and suture abscesses which were managed conservatively and did not require an additional intervention.

CONCLUSIONS

Based on our experience, and that of other teams, it is believed that abdominal lipectomies can be safely combined with abdominal wall reconstruction/hernia repair procedures without a significantly higher risk of complications. Staged reconstruction should always be an option if the patient must have abdominal reconstruction/hernia repair, but is not considered to be an appropriate candidate for simultaneous lipectomy.

- Close cooperation with the bariatric surgeon and members of the bariatric team are necessary in all stages of care.
- These combined procedures should be deferred until appropriate and stable weight is achieved. Ideally, the patient's BMI should be <30 but this rule should not be so rigid and selection should be individualized for this particular subgroup of patients.
- Extensive preoperative evaluation and planning are necessary, including patient preparation, optimal general condition, appropriate cardiac and respiratory functions, and normalization of laboratory data. Patients should also be psychologically stable, motivated, and fully appreciate the possible outcomes and limitations of the surgical intervention. False expectations should be dispelled.
- Procedures should be individualized and based on specific reconstructive requirements, patients' needs, and surgeons' experience and preference. The fleur-de-lis design is very useful for a selected group of patients in particular the ones with pre-existing midline scars. This design for lipectomy affords a direct evaluation, approach, and management of the hernia, for reduction of the abdominal pannus in both vertical and horizontal dimensions, and overall better management of the epigastric pannus, if present.
- Technical considerations include strict adherence to surgical principles, avoidance of excessive undermining, judicious use of alloplastic materials or biomaterials, meticulous hemostasis, and above all *closure without tension*.
- The component separation technique represents a great alternative to prosthetic reconstruction and should be preferred for hernia repair, when possible, because it provides an autologous and dynamic reconstruction. Preservation of the tone, elasticity, and flexibility of the abdominal wall represents some important advantages for the use of this technique.
- Perioperative care with appropriate broad-spectrum antibiotics, sequential compression devices, DVT prophylaxis with heparin or low-molecular-weight heparin, abdominal binder, pain control, drain management, early ambulation, and respiratory therapy, among others, are essential.
- The margin of error is very small for these combined procedures, because even minor tissue dehiscence or loss might result in infection possible exposure, contamination, and even failure of the prosthetic alloplastic or biomaterial. Ultimately, it may result in failure of the reconstruction and hernia recurrence. Therefore, close postoperative follow-up and high level of suspicion are necessary to be able to identify and treat wound complications in a timely fashion. Complications should be managed aggressively, with early debridement and closure to prevent further tissue loss and possible failure of the reconstruction. Such an example is shown in **Fig. 12.10**.
- Hematomas should be recognized immediately and treated accordingly to prevent additional blood loss and avoid undue tension on the skin flaps.
- Seromas can be difficult to manage. Drains are left in place for a prolonged period and collections should be drained as soon as recognized, under sterile conditions. Unfortunately, in some cases, seromas continue to recur. In such situation use of sclerosing agents can be beneficial. In extreme cases, as depicted in **Fig. 12.11**, definitive treatment will require exploration and removal of the reactive capsule, and obliteration of the residual dead space with quilting sutures.
- Finally when early closure is not feasible or advisable due to the complexity of the wound or the patient's general condition, a staged reconstruction should be considered with appropriate management of the abdominal defect and postponing of the lipectomy to another time.

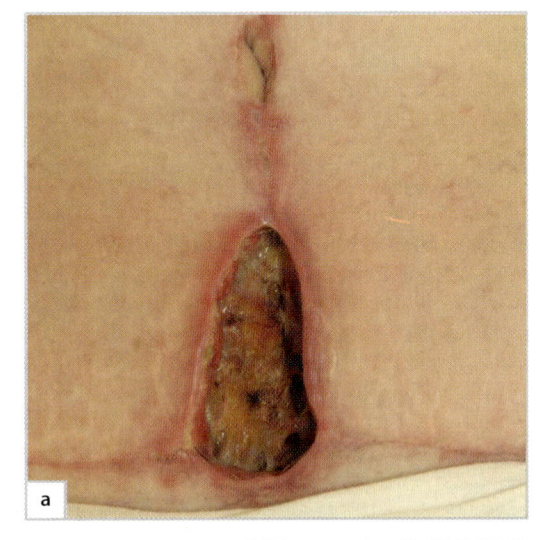

Figure 12.10 (a) Wound dehiscence and infection in the lower abdomen 5 weeks after hernia repair and lipectomy. (b) Final appearance after wide detriment and closure with readvancement of the abdominal flaps

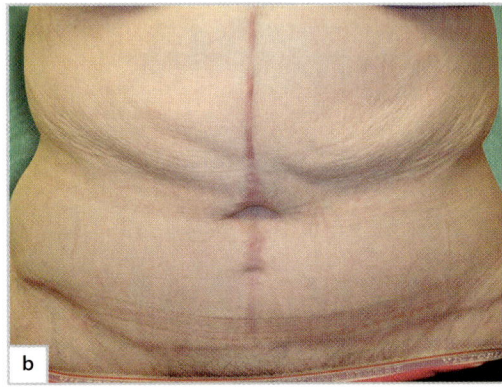

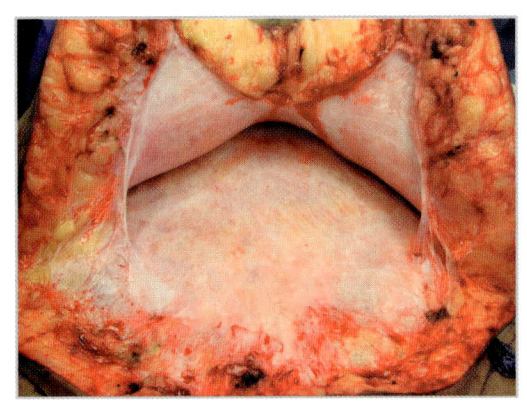

Figure 12.11 Appearance of a reactive capsule around a recurrent seroma.

REFERENCES

1. Flancbaum L, Choban PS. Surgical implications of obesity. *Annu Rev Med* 1998;**49**:215–34.
2. National Insitutes of Health. Gastrointestinal surgery for severe obesity. *NIH Consensus Statement Online* 1991;**9**(1):1–20
3. Livingston EH. Complications of bariatric surgery. *Surg Clin North Am* 2005;**85**:853–68.
4. Masoomi H, Magno CP, Nguyen XMT. Trends in use of bariatric surgery, 2003–2008. *J Am Coll Surg* 2011;**213**:261–6.
5. Nguyen NT, Root J, Zainabadi K. Accelerated growth of bariatric surgery with the introduction of minimally invasive surgery. *Arch Surg* 2005;**140**:1198–2002.
6. Berry MF, Paisley S, Low DW, Rosato EF. Repair of large complex recurrent incisional hernias with retromuscular mesh and panniculectomy. *Am J Surg* 2007;**194**:199–204.
7. Downey SE, Morales C, Kelso RL, et al. Review of technique for combined closed incisional hernia repair and panniculectomy status post-open bariatric surgery. *Surgery Obesity Rel Dis* 2005;**1**:458–61.
8. Iljin A, Szymanski D, Kruk-Jeromin J, et al. The repair of incisional hernia following Roux-en-Y gastric bypass-with or without concomitant abdominoplasty? *Obesity Surg* 2008;**18**:1387–91.
9. Ortega J, Navarro V, Cassinello N. Requirement and postoperative outcomes of abdominal panniculectomy alone or in combination with other procedures in a bariatric surgery unit. *Am J Surg* 2010;**200**:235–40.
10. Özgur F, Aksu AE, Özkan Ö, et al. The advantages of simultaneous abdominoplasty, laparoscopic cholecystectomy, and incisional hernia repair. *Eur J Plast Surg* 2002;**25**:271–4.
11. Robertson JD, De la Torre JI, Gardner PM. Abdominoplasty repair for abdominal wall hernias. *Ann Plast Surg* 2003;**51**:10–16.
12. Shermak MA. Hernia repair and abdominoplasty in gastric bypass patients. *Plast Reconstr Surg* 2005;**117**:1145–50.
13. Cintra W, Modolin ML, Gemperli R, Gobbi CIC, Faintuch J, Ferreira MC. Quality of life after abdominoplasty in women after bariatric surgery. *Obesity Surg* 2008;**18**:728–32.
14. Grazer FM. Abdominoplasty. *Plast Reconstr Surg* 1973;**51**:617–23.
15. Savage R. Abdominoplasty combined with other surgical procedures. *Plast Reconstr Surg* 1982;**70**:437–43.
16. Hester RT Jr, Baird W, Bostwick J III, et al. Abdominoplasty combined with other major surgical procedures: Safe or sorry? *Plast Reconstr Surg* 1989;**83**:997–1004.
17. Butler CR. The role of bioprosthetics in abdominal wall reconstruction. *Clin Plast Surg* 2006;**33**:213–22.
18. Gemperli R. Abdominoplasty combined with other intraabdominal procedures. *Ann Plast Surg* 1992;**29**:18–22.
19. Mazzocchi M, Dessy LA, Ranno R, Carlesimo B, Rubino C. 'Component separation' technique and panniculectomy for repair of incisional hernia. *Am J Surg* 2011;**201**:776–83.
20. Reid RR & Dumanian GA. Panniculectomy and the separation-of-parts hernia repair: a solution for the large infraumbilical hernia in the obese patient. *Plast Reconstr Surg* 2005;**116**:1006–12.
21. Baker D. Obesity-related factors in the repair and healing of recurrent incisional hernia: a summary of risk factors and perioperative strategies. *Bariatric Nursing Surg Patient Care* 2006;**1**:179–84.
22. Albino FP, Koltz PF, Gusenoff JA. A comparative analysis and systematic review of the wound-healing milieu: implications for body contouring after massive weight loss. *Plast Reconstr Surg* 2009;**124**:1675–82.
23. Kabon B, Nagele A, Reddy D. Obesity decreases perioperative tissue oxygenation. *Anesthesiology* 2004;**100**:274–80.
24. Wilson JA, Clark JJ. Obesity: impediment to postsurgical wound healing. *Adv Skin Wound Care* 2004;**17**:426–35.
25. Cohen M. Chest and abdominal wall reconstruction. In: Goldwyn R, Cohen M (eds), *Unfavorable Results in Plastic Surgery: Avoidance and treatment*. Philadelphia, PA: Lippincott, Williams & Wilkins, 2002: 674–86.
26. Cohen M. Management of abdominal wall defects resulting from complications of surgical procedures. *Clin Plast Surg* 2006;**33**:281–94.
27. Cohen M. Reconstruction of abdominal wall defects after bariatric surgery and simultaneous abdominal lipectomies. The American Association of Plastic Surgeons, 85th annual meeting, May 6–9, 2006, Abstract 18.
28. DeFrango AJ, Argenta L. Vacuum assisted closure for the treatment of abdominal wounds. *Clin Plast Surg* 2006;**33**:213–24.
29. Borud LJ, Grunwaldt L, Janz B, et al. Components separation combined with abdominal wall plication for repair of large abdominal wall hernias following bariatric surgery. *Plast Reconstr Surg* 2007;**119**:1792–8.
30. Downey SE. Approach to the abdomen after weight loss. In: Rubin PJ, Matarasso A (eds), *Aesthetic Surgery after Massive Weight Loss*. Saunders-Elsevier 2007: 49–68.
31. Castañares S, Goethel JA. Abdominal lipectomy: a modification in technique. *Plast Reconstr Surg* 1967;**40**:378–83.
32. Friedman T, Coon DO, Michaels JV. Fleur-de-lis abdominoplasty for massive weight loss patient. *Plast Reconstr Surg* 2010;**125**:1525–35.

Chapter 13 Brachioplasty

Michele A. Shermak

Brachioplasty surgery is growing in prevalence, largely due to the growing massive weight loss (MWL) population. The American Society of Plastic Surgery (ASPS) statistics demonstrate a rise in numbers of brachioplasty procedures, a 439% increase from 2000 to 2010[1] (**Fig. 13.1**). Brachioplasty is one of the more challenging body lift procedures: Presentation is variable, healing is difficult, and scars may be unforgiving. Over time, more procedure approaches have been developed to address the broad range of presentations and issues problematic to brachioplasty.

ANATOMY OF THE ARM

The relevant anatomy of the arm with respect to brachioplasty lies along the ulnar aspect[2] (**Fig. 13.2**). Skin in the arm is thin relative to the rest of the body. The subcutaneous fat is divided into superficial and deep layers, separated by a thin Scarpa fascial layer. Fat thickness needs to be considered when designing the brachioplasty markings, because it will limit the amount of skin that can be safely excised.

Under the fat, the deeper layer of well-defined fascia protects the major neurovascular structures of the arm, and envelopes the muscles. Hugging the superficial surface of the distal deep fascial layer are the cutaneous sensory nerves, which are most vulnerable to damage during brachioplasty surgery, including the medial brachial cutaneous (MBC) and medial antebrachial cutaneous (MABC) nerves. The MBC nerve originates from the medial cord of the brachial plexus and passes medially and posteriorly to the ulnar nerve. It is posterior to the basilic vein, and terminal branches are found 2–3 cm proximal to the medial epicondyle. The MABC nerve travels within the distal half to third of the arm, often together with the basilic vein. Anterior

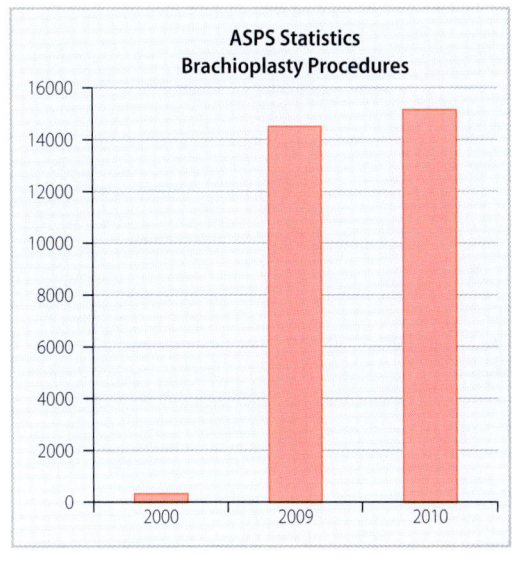

Figure 13.1 American Society of Plastic Surgery statistics on prevalence of brachioplasty procedures performed between the years 2000 and 2010.

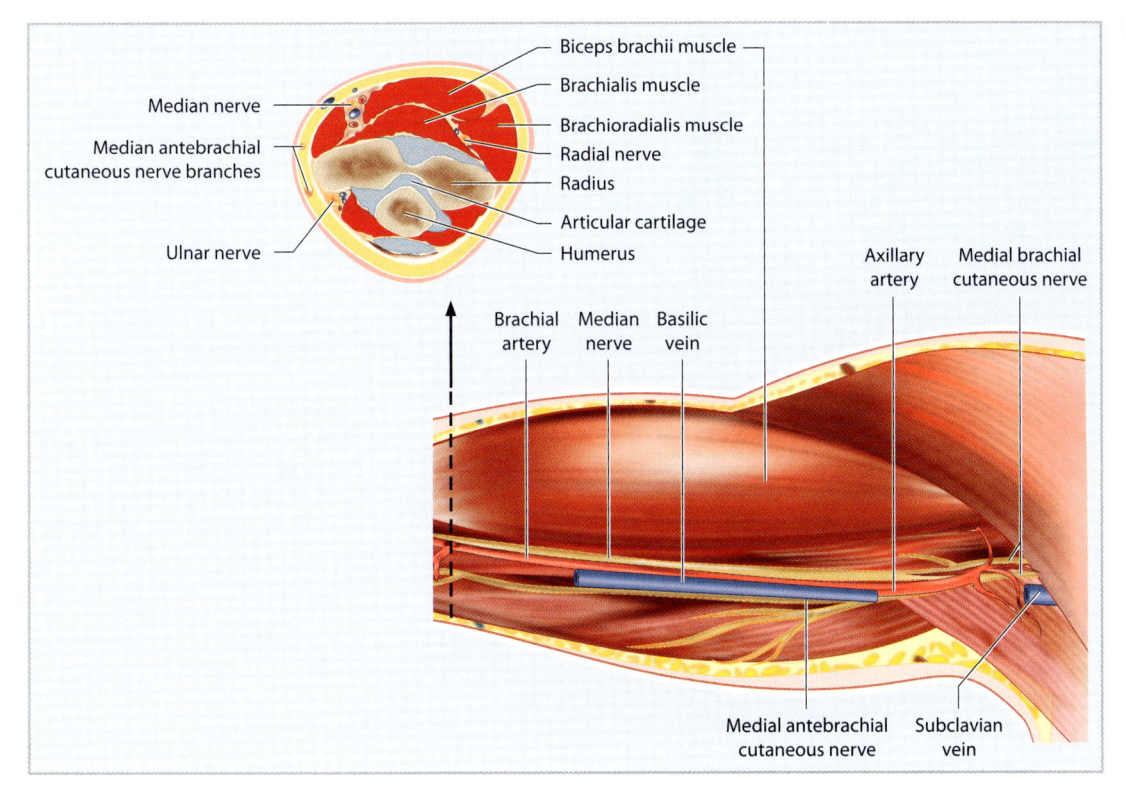

Figure 13.2 Arm anatomy.

and posterior branches of the MABC nerve originate at the medial epicondyle.[3-6] Analogous to the sensory nerves, the basilic and cephalic veins hug the deep fascia superficially. Lymphatic basins exist at the antecubital region, named the subratrochear lymph nodes, and axilla, named the axillary and deltopectoral lymph nodes, superficial to the deep fascia.[7]

Structures deep to the deep fascia include the bones and muscles of the arm, as well as the major neurovascular structures that originate from the brachial plexus and axillary artery and empty into the axillary vein.

■ HISTORY

Brachioplasty was first described 80 years ago by Thorek.[8] The literature commonly credits aesthetic brachioplasty to Correa-Iturraspe and Fernandez in 1954.[9] Since then, the procedure has evolved and undergone numerous modifications to improve on complications and outcomes, including papers by Baroudi, Pitanguy, Guerrosantos, and Lockwood.[10-13] These modifications include quadrangular flaps and T closure, Z-plasties, W-plasties, fascial suspension, and circumferential liposuction. More contemporary literature promotes axillary extensions, the use of molds, limited incisions, sinusoidal incisions, posterior incisions, and fish- and L-shaped incisions.[14-24]

■ INDICATIONS

Brachioplasty is performed for skin laxity in the arm, which may extend down to the chest wall and is not appropriate as a treatment for lipodystrophy. Traditional brachioplasty involves incisions along the length of the upper arm, tapered into the axilla.[3,13] Minimal incision brachioplasty for patients with limited or proximally localized skin excess and conservative goals requires only an axillary approach.[3,19] More extended approaches apply to MWL patients who have a bat-wing deformity, with skin redundancy continuing along the lateral chestwall.[14,23]

■ DETAILS OF THE PROCEDURE

Arms should be placed on well-padded armboards, protecting against compression injury to superficial nerves, at no more than 90° to avoid traction injury to the brachial plexus.[3,25] Breasts in women may be taped together centrally to keep them out of the field, and a bump placed under the scapula and proximal arm to aid in exposure. Arms are prepared and draped circumferentially. The blood pressure cuff should be placed on the calf, and the pulse oximeter should be moved to the nose or ear, if possible, for traditional and extended brachioplasty techniques. Intravenous catheters need to be either prepared and draped sterilely, or kept out of the sterile field altogether. Usual thromboembolic precautions should be followed, including compression hose and sequential compression devices on the calves, a pillow under the knees, and lower body warming throughout the duration of surgery.

■ Minimal incision technique

This technique applies only to those patients who have minimal laxity or an isolated panniculus of the proximal arm (**Fig. 13.3**). An ellipse is created just outside the axilla, as an incision buried within the axilla will lose significant impact in addressing laxity. Liposuction must be judicious because it may exacerbate laxity. Wound closure is layered, drainless, and reinforced with skin glue (**Fig. 13.4**).

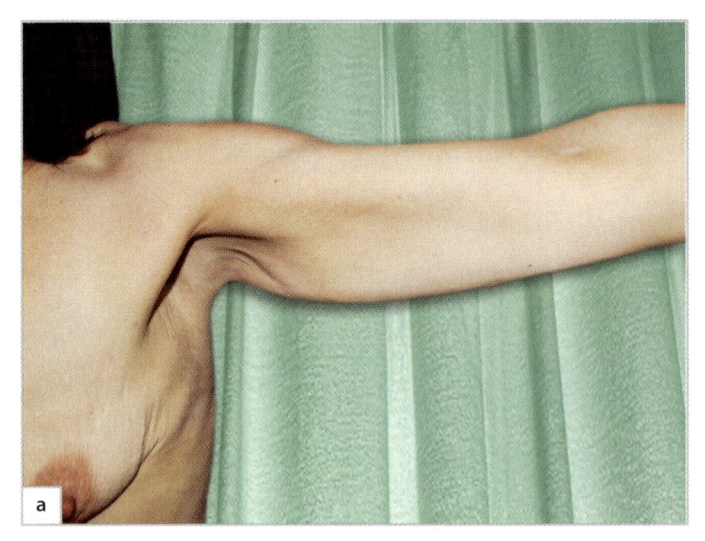

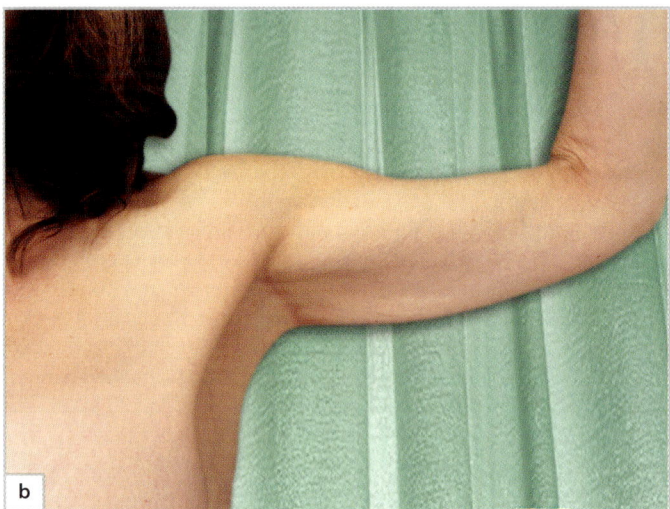

Figure 13.3 This woman in her 40s presented years after sustaining weight loss >45 kg (100 lb). (a) She had minimal laxity and ptosis of the arm and was interested in addressing this problem. (b) 6 months after minimal incision brachioplasty.

■ The traditional technique – T-incision brachioplasty

This technique is applicable to most patients presenting for brachioplasty who have arm deflation with significant skin redundancy and poor skin quality. This procedure is not a treatment for lipodystrophy (**Fig. 13.5**). This approach involves an incision in the antebrachial groove or more inferoposteriorly, with deepening of the incision to the fascia overlying muscle and neurovascular structures, and no deeper. In fact, to avoid injury to vulnerable lymphatics and superficial sensory nerves that are difficult to visualize, the deep fascia should not be skeletonized, and a pad of fatty tissue should remain on the fascia. Elevation of the skin and subcutaneous fat follows inferiorly, keeping in mind the tubular nature of the arm. Resection of the skin requires tailor tacking to avoid over-resection, and is tapered proximally to the axilla. Closure is layered, approximating the Scarpa fascia, deep and superficial dermis, and performed over a drain (**Fig. 13.6**).

Details of the procedure   127

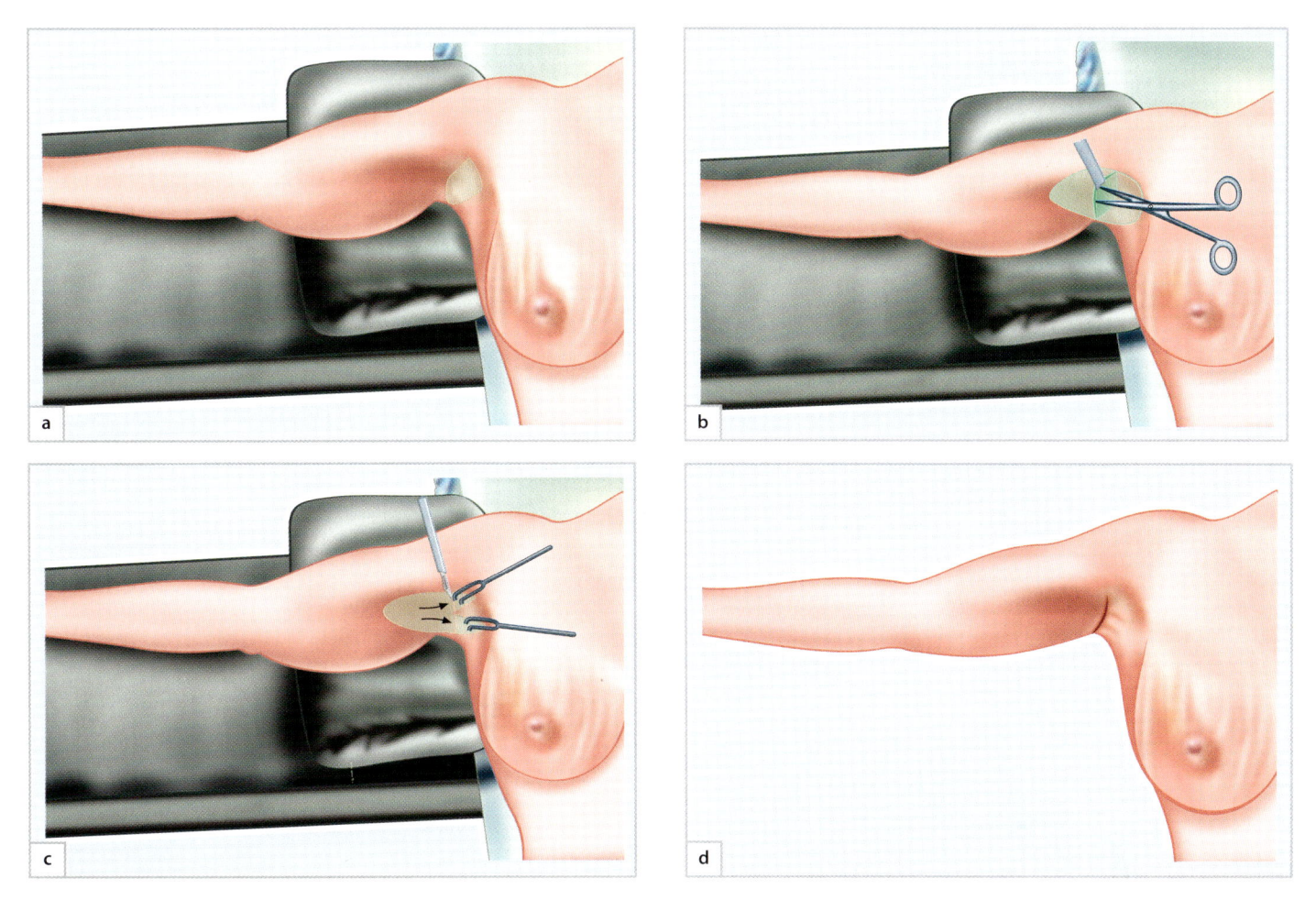

Figure 13.4 Mini-brachioplasty. (a) Markings are guided by pinch technique. The ellipse marked should be located in the distal axilla. (b) Undermining may be performed to optimize tissue removal and ease closure. (c) Tailor-tack technique may be followed to assure adequate skin removal. (d) Incision lies in the distal axilla. No drain is necessary and dressing may include only skin glue.

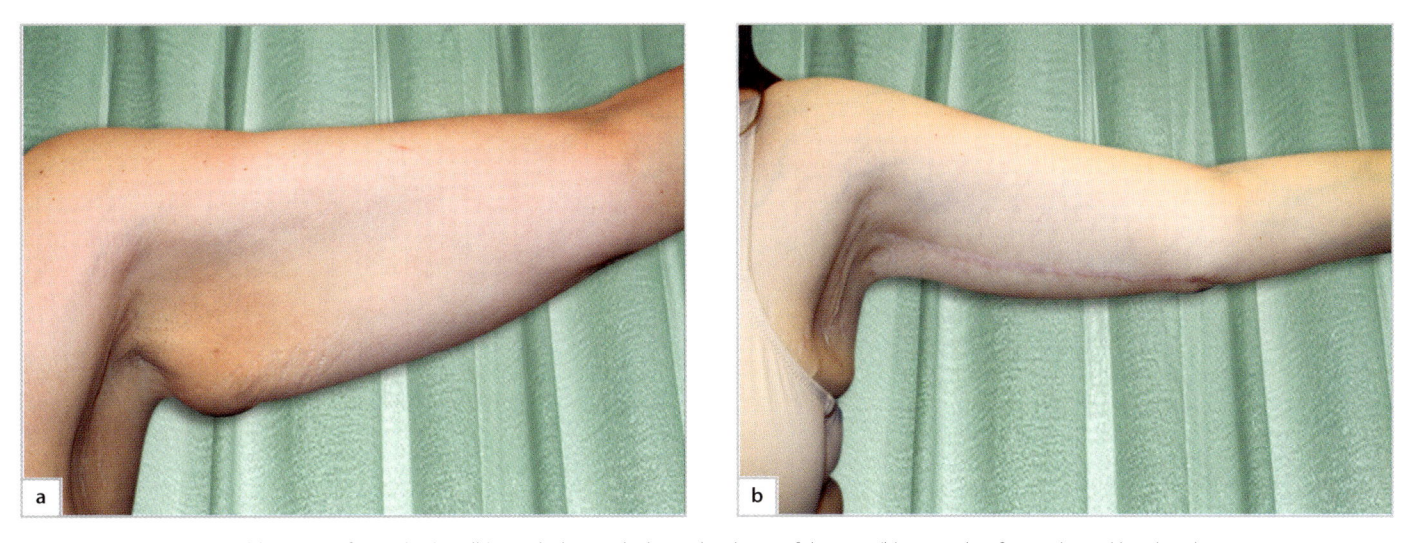

Figure 13.5 (a) A 46-year-old woman after 45 kg (100 lb) weight loss with skin redundancy of the arm. (b) 8 months after traditional brachioplasty.

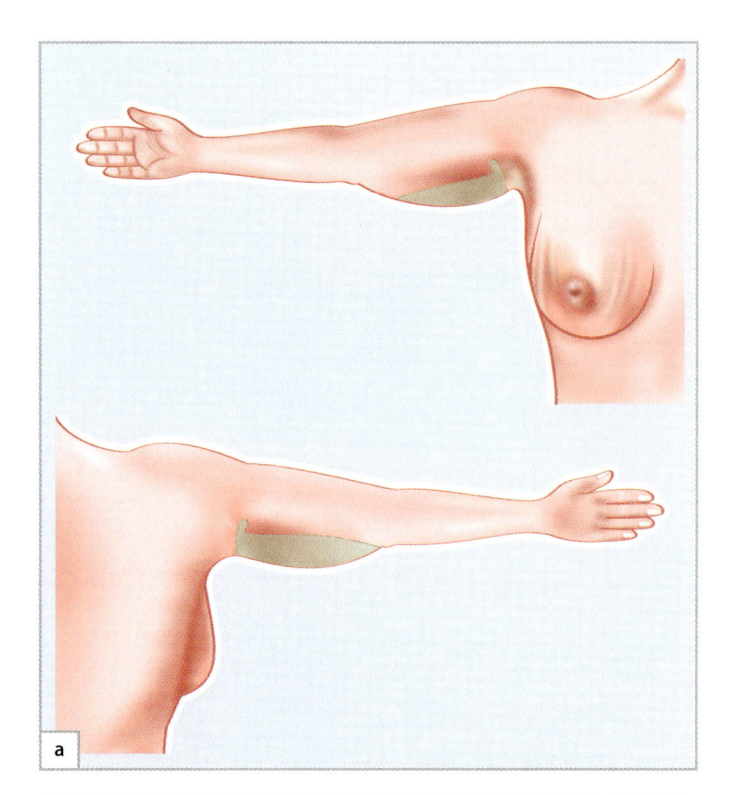

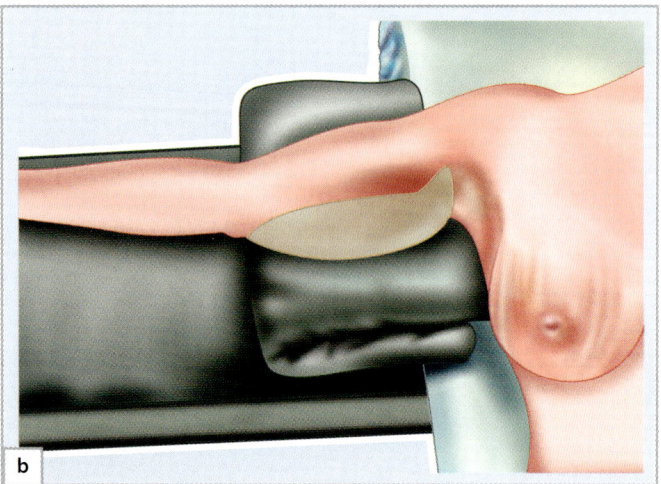

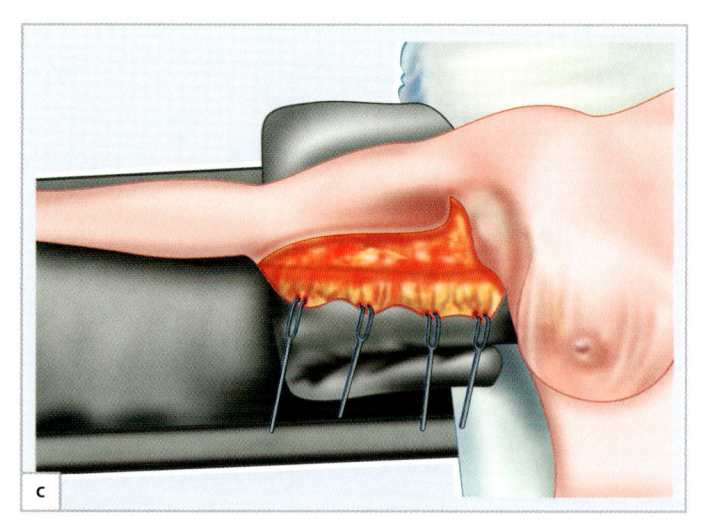

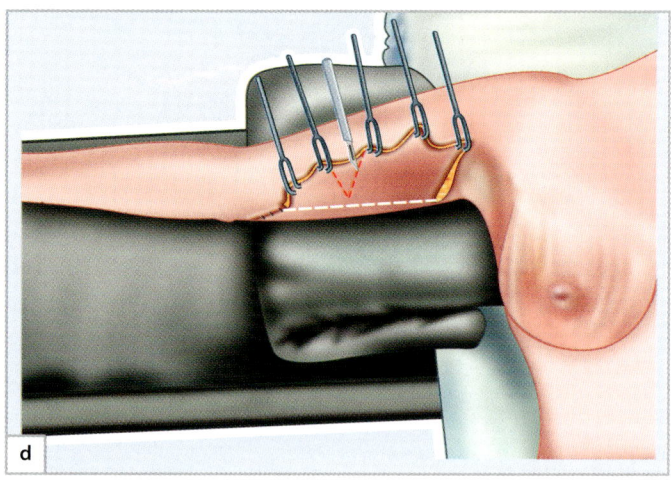

Figure 13.6 Traditional brachioplasty. *Continued opposite.*

■ The extended technique

The extended technique addresses not only redundant skin on the arm but also skin laxity and redundancy along the lateral chest wall (**Fig. 13.7**). The extended technique is analogous to the vertical thighlift, beginning skin resection in the distal arm at the elbow, with graded proximal progression and tailor-tack excision in the plane described in the traditional brachioplasty. Z-plasty of the axilla protects against contracture. After addressing the axilla, graded removal continues down the lateral chest wall to the level of the inframammary fold in the midaxillary line to avoid pulling the breast laterally. Closure of the Scarpa fascia and deep dermis, with interrupted absorbable sutures, and superficial dermis with a running subcuticular closure, is performed. A drain is placed in the potential space created, from the distal chest wall up into the axilla (**Fig. 13.8**).

■ Lipobrachioplasty

Analogous to the evolution in abdominal contouring surgery, liposuction is playing a more important role in contouring surgery of the arm. It is used as an adjunct to amplify results achieved with excisional surgery alone. Lipobrachioplasty has been reported in the literature by Nguyen and Rohrich.[21] In their technique, the area of planned excision is tumesced and suctioned. The area of excision, drawn as an ellipse on the posterior arm, is then avulsed off the underlying fascia. Closure requires neither a drain nor an approximation of the Scarpa fascia.

■ THE POSTOPERATIVE PERIOD

Immediately after surgery, patients may leave dressings in place for several days. After this, they may shower. It is recommended that

The postoperative period | 129

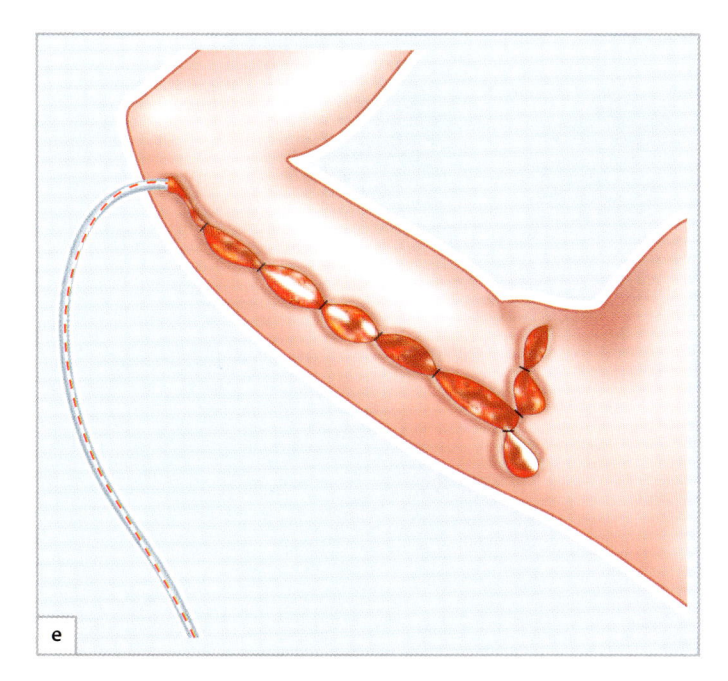

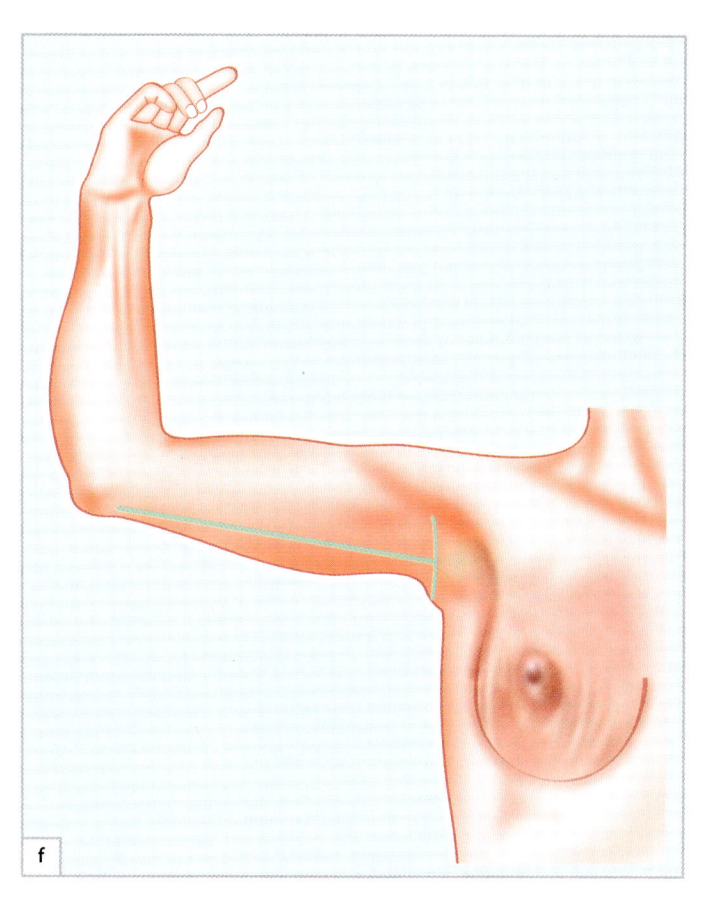

Figure 13.6 Traditional brachioplasty. (a) The arm is marked upright and in stable position, with excision proximally and along the length of the arm to allow suspension and removal of excess tissue. (b) The arm is circumferentially prepared and draped sterilely, and positioned on a padded arm board or hand table. The arm should be no more than 90° from the body. A bump can be placed under the scapula and the breasts may need to be taped in the midline to improve access to the arms. (c) The skin flap of the arm is elevated above the deep fascia to protect neurovascular structures, and the tubular geometry of the arm guides the dissection so that the skin flap is not devascularized. A layer of fat should remain on the deep fascia to help preserve lymphatics and sensory nerves, particularly in the distal third of the arm. (d) Before committing to excision of the redundant skin, tailor tacking must be performed to ensure that the tissue resected is not overly aggressive or inadequate. (e) Layered closure is performed over a drain. With significant axillary motion postoperatively, the drain protects against fluid buildup and dehiscence in this risky area. Light compressive wrap is applied as a dressing. (f) Incision is in the conformation of a 'T'.

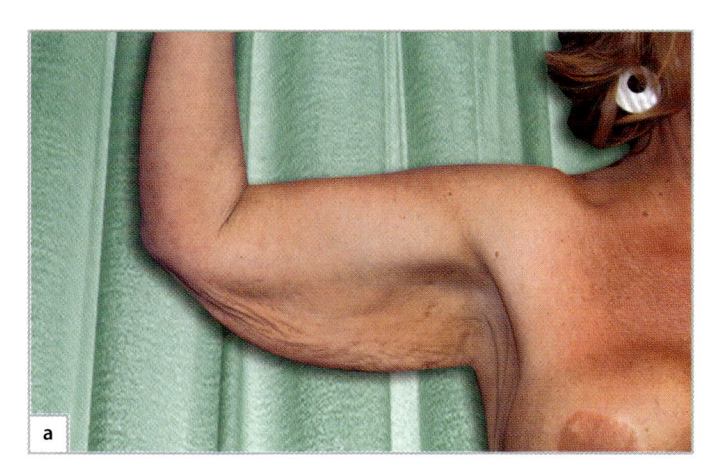

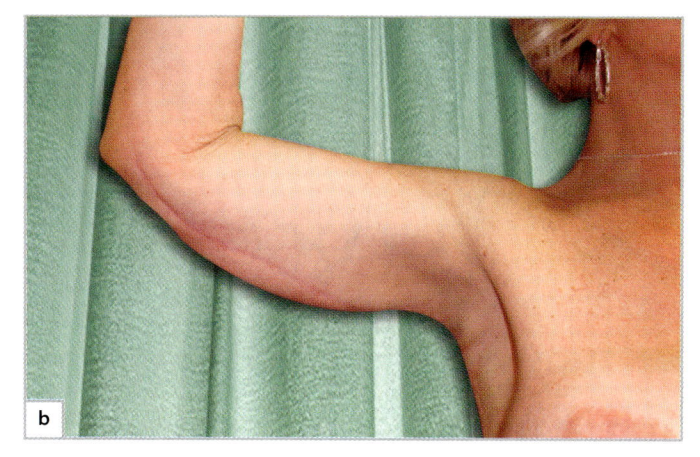

Figure 13.7 (a) A 47-year-old woman after losing >45 kg (100 lb) with skin redundancy extending from arm to lateral chest wall. (b) 2.5 years after her surgery.

BRACHIOPLASTY

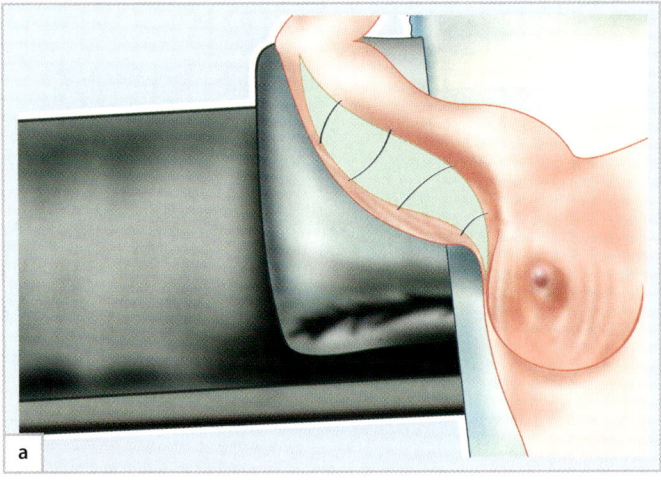

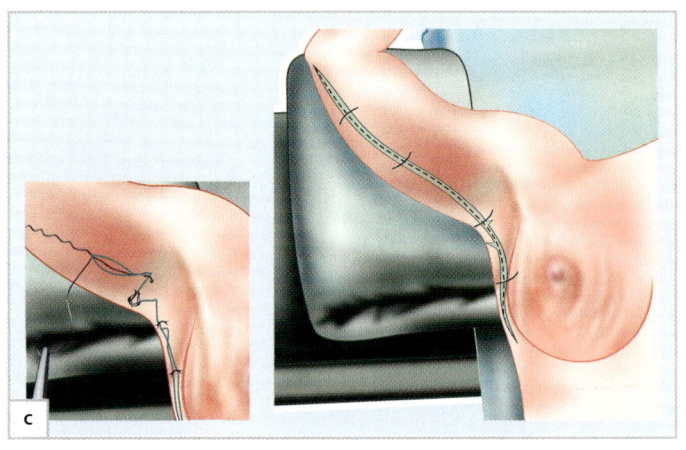

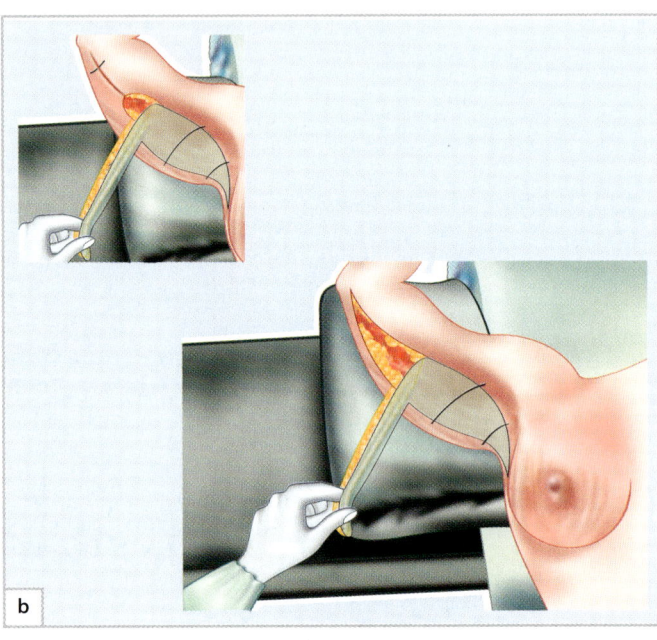

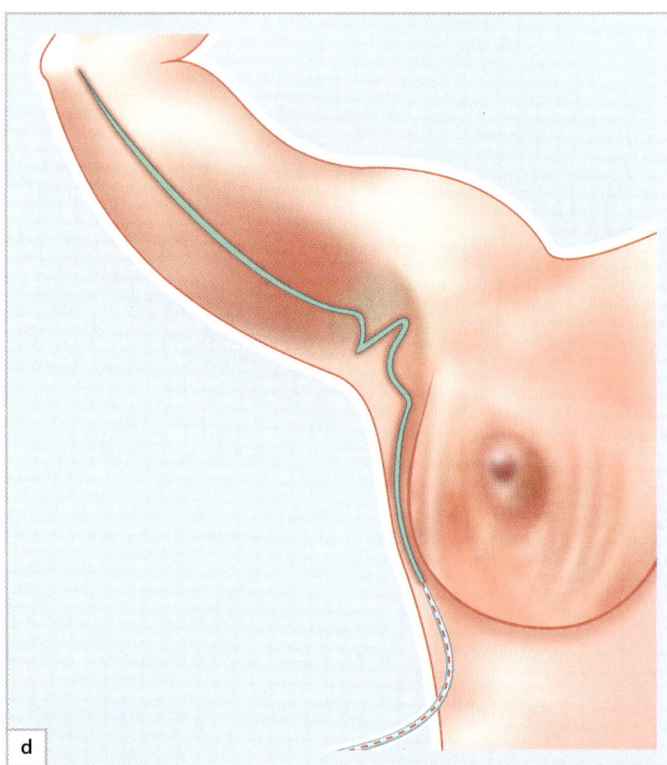

Figure 13.8 Extended brachioplasty. (a) Markings are made in the shape of a large ellipse, from the antecubital region to the axilla and progression down along the chest wall. Hash marks guide excision and closure. (b) Excision starts distally and is marched proximally in a graded fashion. Hash marks may be used as stopping points to reassess the degree of skin excision. (c) Closure is performed in three layers, and the superficial fascia and deep dermis should be closed before moving more proximally to avoid edema onset and increased tension in wound closure. A Z-plasty is performed in the axilla to prevent occurrence of a scar contracture. A drain exits the lateral chest wall at the level of the inframammary fold. (d) The closed incision.

patients elevate their arms on pillows when possible to limit swelling of the forearm and hand, with its accompanying discomfort. Non-steroidal, anti-inflammatory medications assist further in reducing inflammation and swelling.

The patient returns within a week after surgery for the first postoperative visit. With drain use, as drain outputs drop, they are removed. Limitation of physical exertion, including lifting and extreme range of motion, persists for a month. Patients may perform activities of daily living without concern.

There is no evidence-based guideline on postoperative antibiotic use after brachioplasty. In the setting of drains and concerns about infection, with seromas and lymphatic derangement from surgery, oral antibiotics are merited. If there is any evidence of infection, culture swab and treatment with oral antibiotics guided by culture are recommended.

Edema must be managed particularly after surgery on the arms. Compressive wrapping from distal to proximal and elevation may be performed by the patient. If edema is prolonged, lymphedema treatment should be assisted by a specialist.

Scar management should be discussed with patients within weeks of surgery. While incisions are fresh and healing, petrolatum ointment should be applied to the incisions. After healing is more mature, at 3 weeks or so, scar creams may be applied, including those with vitamin E. Silicone gel sheeting may be instituted at that time, or later if there is evidence of hypertrophic scar development.

Good nutrition is a priority after excisional lifting procedures. Protein and vitamin intake should be optimized, and salt and fat intake minimized. Patients should remain well hydrated. Dry mucous membranes and a wan appearance with low energy after surgery should serve as a red flag, mandating discussion with the patient about issues of concern. Patients may suffer some depression after these operations, which also may impair their appetite and nutritional status.

COMPLICATION AVOIDANCE

It is important to discuss the possibility of complications when reviewing procedures with patients and during the informed consent process, because patients are more accepting of complications if they are anticipated. Complications have been reported to occur after brachioplasty 25–40% of the time.[26-29] The most common complications seen after surgery include: Wound healing problems, encompassing seroma, dehiscence, and infection; scar problems including hypertrophic scar, placement, contracture, and widening; nerve injury comprising paraesthesiae and/or neuromas; lymphatic concerns consisting of lymphedema and lymphoceles; and technical issues including under-resection. Nerve, lymphatic and scar complications are particularly specific to brachioplasty.

Neuropathy and neuromas

Nerve injury may occur with direct laceration or through positioning which caused compression or stretch of the involved nerve. In brachioplasty surgery the nerves of particular concern include the MBC and the MABC nerves due to their superficial location and subtle visibility. The MBC nerve originates from the medial cord of the brachial plexus and passes medially and posteriorly to the ulnar nerve. It is posterior to the basilic vein, and terminal branches are found 2–3 cm proximal to the medial epicondyle. Of greater risk is injury to the MABC nerve. This nerve travels within the distal half to third of the arm, often together with the basilic vein. Anterior and posterior branches originate at the medial epicondyle.[3-6] Maintaining a layer of fatty tissue on the deep fascia of the arm and not skeletonizing this fascia protect the nerves. A more posterior scar will also take dissection further away from these nerves.

Safe positioning can prevent many neuropathies.[25,26] Arms should not be positioned at >90° at the axilla and elbow to avoid stretch. The arm board or table should be well padded to avoid compression injury to superficial nerves such as the ulnar nerve at the elbow.

Patients often experience numbness around surgical incisions due to injury to sensory nerves, but this typically improves over time. When neuropathy occurs, supportive care with massage, physical therapy, and prescription medications often results in improvement over time. If improvement does not occur, an electromyogram, nerve conduction studies, and a neurology consult may be ordered for definitive diagnosis.

If there is extreme, focal incisional tenderness and a Tinel sign after surgery, the possibility of neuroma should be considered. Initially, massage and steroid injection combined with local anesthesia may help treat this condition; however, in some cases, surgical treatment of neuroma with excision and possible nerve grafting may be necessary.[30]

Lymphatic complications

Lymphatic injury occurs through direct injury of vessels, compression, or obstruction of flow from proximal surgical scars. This presents as lymphedema of the arm or forearm, or fluid collection in the elbow. Similar to the sensory nerves of the arm, lymphatics are difficult to visualize due to their small caliber and lack of color. Leaving a layer of fatty tissue on the deep fascia assists in protecting the lymphatic vessels from injury.

With a presumed lymphocele, which more often occurs at the elbow, needle aspiration combined with compression is the first line of therapy. Surgical treatment may be necessary to ligate an unresolving lymphatic leak. Lymphazurin blue dye injection at the wrist may aid in identifying the leaking vessel during surgery.[31]

Compression therapy, massage, and physical therapy are beneficial in treating lymphedema, and usually successful outcomes will occur.[28,32] Upper extremity deep venous thrombosis (DVT) must be considered in patients with lymphedema, particularly if asymmetric, and may be ruled out with a duplex sonography study. Patients with a history of a port in the subclavian system or a venous port in the arm are more likely to be at risk for upper extremity DVT.

Scar outcome

On presenting to the plastic surgeon, many patients have concerns and misconceptions about the 'large scar' necessary to treat skin redundancy after massive weight loss. Although the scar may be long, it should be thin once it completely heals and matures. Early on, the scar may be visible, and the scar may become hypertrophic, but scar quality often improves after the first year with supportive care and scar management. Massage and vitamin E are easy to start after wounds have healed. If the scar becomes hypertrophic, silicone gel sheeting therapy may be instituted. Steroid injection also may be considered and dosage should be more dilute at first to avoid over-treatment.

Scar placement is difficult to control in the arm, because there is no fixed, stable point that can be sutured. Scars may shift and are not accurately predictable. With incision in the brachial groove, the scar should not be visible with the arms at rest. A more posterior scar ensures lack of visibility from the front at rest, but may be visible from the back.

Scar contracture is most likely to occur if the scar is a straight line across a joint surface, such as at the axilla or elbow. Early treatment of contracture includes non-invasive maneuvers to optimize the scar. If these do not work, then surgery including Z-plasty across the involved joint surface will effectively elongate the scar and alleviate the tight band.

OUTCOME STUDIES

With the prevalence in brachioplasty procedures jumping only within the past decade, there are only a small number of published outcome studies assessing an appreciable number of patients. Knoetgen and Moran looked at complication outcomes of 40 patients who underwent brachioplasty.[27] They found a 25% rate of complications, with 95% of these complications being minor and nonsurgical. Complications include seroma (10%), hypertrophic scar (10%), cellulitis (7.5%), wound dehiscence (7.5%), suture abscess (2.5%), nerve injury (5%), and the need for surgical revisions (12.5%), with additional skin removal comprising 80% of these.

Gusenoff et al. reviewed the impact of concomitant operations on brachioplasty outcome, because most brachioplasty procedures comprise a segment of a postbariatric body-contouring session addressing multiple body regions.[33] In their study looking at only MWL patients, 96% of those undergoing brachioplasty had other procedures performed. Longer operating time (>8 h) was associated with a greater risk of complications, but not arm-specific complications.

Arm-specific complications were significantly related to liposuction of the arm only at the time of excision.

Shermak et al. investigated factors impacting outcomes of brachioplasty in her study, including age, gender, race, medical comorbidities, and tobacco use.[34] They also looked at the impact on outcome of brachioplasty performed as part of a larger MWL body lift procedure versus a stand-alone procedure. Further, the impact of hospital versus ambulatory surgery center (ASC)-based surgery was assessed. Looking at 244 brachioplasty procedures, only the body mass index (BMI) was found to have a detrimental impact on brachioplasty outcome, with increased risk of infection. Brachioplasty as a stand-alone procedure fared no better than when it was performed with multiple other procedures, and there was no benefit to ASC- or hospital-based surgery.

Barbed suture is a technology that has been advocated for use in excisional body-contouring procedures to expedite closure and optimize results. Shermak et al., in their study of barbed suture closure, identified complications in wound healing and suture extrusion when using barbed suture, more so in brachioplasty than in other body regions.[35]

CONCLUSION

Brachioplasty surgery is growing in prevalence to meet the growing demands of the postbariatric population. There are multiple types of procedures available to address variable degrees of skin laxity and quality at presentation. The important tenet is the longer the scar, the more impactful the result. Despite concerns about scarring associated with brachioplasty, outcomes are uncomplicated in 75% of cases, according to the literature, with most complicated outcomes being responsive to conservative, nonsurgical therapy. Brachioplasty surgery often leads to excellent improvement in arm contour with an acceptable, necessary scar.

REFERENCES

1. American Society of Plastic Surgery. *Report of the 2010; Plastic Surgery Statistics*. Available at: www.plasticsurgery.org/Documents/news-resources/statistics/2010/-statisticss/Overall-Trends/2010/-cosmetic-plastic-surgery-minimally-invasive-statistics.pdf (accessed August 30, 2011).
2. Shermak MA, ed. *Body Contouring*. New York: McGraw-Hill, 2011.
3. Chowdhry S, Elston JB, Lefkowitz T, Wilhelmi BJ. Avoiding the medial brachial cutaneous nerve in brachioplasty: An anatomical study. *Eplasty* 2010;**10**:e 16.
4. Lowe JB 3rd, Maggi SP, Mackinnon SE. The position of crossing branches of the medial antebrachial cutaneous nerve during cubital tunnel surgery in humans. *Plast Reconstr Surg* 2004;**114**:692–6.
5. Masear VR, Meyer, RD, Pichora DR. Surgical anatomy of the medial antebrachial cutaneous nerve. *J. Hand Surg (Am)* 1989;**14**:267.
6. Race M, Saldana M. Anatomic course of the medial cutaneous nerves of the arm. *J Hand Surg (Am)* 1991;**16**:48.
7. Yu HL, Chase RA, Strauch B, eds. *Atlas of Hand Anatomy and Clinical Implications*. St Louis, MO: Mosby, 2004.
8. Thorek M. Esthetic surgery of pendulous breast, abdomen and arms in the female. *Ill Med J* 1930;**58**:48.
9. Correa-Ituraspe M, Fernandez JC. Dermolipectomia braquial. *Prensa Med Argent* 1954;**41**:2432–6.
10. Baroudi, R. Dermatolipectomy of the upper arm. *Clin Plast Surg* 1975;**2**:485.
11. Pitanguy I. Correction of lipodystrophy of the lateral thoracic aspect and inner side of the arm and elbow. *Clin Plast Surg* 1975;**2**:477.
12. Guerrosantos J. Brachioplasty. *Aesthet Plast. Surg* 1979;**3**:1.
13. Lockwood T. Brachioplasty with superficial fascial system suspension. *Plast Reconstr Surg* 1995;**96**:912.
14. Strauch B, Linetskaya D, Baum T, Greenspun D. Brachioplasty and axillary restoration. *Aesthet Surg J* 2004;**24**:486.
15. Strauch B, Greenspun D, Levine J, Baum T. A technique of brachioplasty. *Plast Reconstr Surg* 2004;**113**:1044–8.
16. deSouza Pinto EB, Erazo PJ, Matsuda CA, et al. Brachioplasty technique with the use of molds. *Plast Reconstr Surg* 2000;**105**:1854–60.
17. Vogt PA. Brachial suction-assisted lipoplasty and brachioplasty. *Aesthet Surg J* 2001;**21**:164–7.
18. Teimourian B, Malekzadeh S. Rejuvenation of the upper arm. *Plast Reconstr Surg* 1998;**102**:545–51.
19. Trussler AP, Rohrich RJ. Limited incision medial brachioplasty: technical refinements in upper arm contouring. *Plast Reconstr Surg* 2008;**121**:305.
20. Aly A, Aly A, Pace D, Cram A. Brachioplasty in the patient with massive weight loss. *Aesthet Surg J* 2006;**26**:76–84.
21. Nguyen AT, Rohrich RJ. Liposuction-assisted Posterior brachioplasty: technical refinements in upper arm contouring. *Plast Reconstr Surg* 2010;**126**:1365–9.
22. Huemer GM. Some thoughts on the posterior brachioplasty. *Plast Reconstr Surg* 2011;**127**:2516–17.
23. Hurwitz DJ, Jerrod K. The L-brachioplasty: An innovative approach to correct excess tissue of the upper arm, axilla, and lateral chest. *Plast Reconstr Surg* 2006;**117**:403.
24. Chandawarkar RY, Lewis JM. 'Fish-incision' brachioplasty. *J Plast Reconstr Aesthet Surg*. 2006;**59**:521–5.
25. Shermak MA, Shoo B, Deune EG. Prone positioning precautions in plastic surgery. *Plast Reconstr Surg* 2006;**117**:1584.
26. Davison SP, Clemens MW. Safety first: precautions for the massive weight loss patient. *Clin Plast Surg* 2008;**35**:173.
27. Knoetgen J 3rd, Moran SL. Long-term outcomes and complications associated with brachioplasty: a retrospective review and cadaveric study. *Plast Reconstr Surg* 2006;**117**:2219–23.
28. Michaels J 5th, Coon D, Rubin JP. Complications in postbariatric body contouring: strategies for assessment and prevention. *Plast Reconstr Surg* 2011;**127**:1352.
29. Symbas JD, Losken A. An outcome analysis of brachioplasty techniques following massive weight loss. *Ann Plast Surg* 2010;**64**:588–91.
30. Rosson GD, Dellon AL. Abdominal wall neuroma pain after breast reconstruction with a transverse abdominal musculocutaneous flap: cause and treatment. *Ann Plast Surg* 2005;**55**:330.
31. Taylor J, Shermak M. Body contouring following massive weight loss. *Obes Surg* 2004;**14**:1080–5.
32. Garfein ES, Borud LJ, Warren AG, Slavin SA. Learning from a lymphedema clinic: an algorithm for the management of localized swelling. *Plast Reconstr Surg* 2008;**121**:521.
33. Gusenoff JA, Coon D, Rubin JP. Brachioplasty and concomitant procedures after massive weight loss: a statistical analysis from a prospective registry. *Plast Reconstr Surg* 2008;**122**:595–603.
34. Shermak MA, Mallalieu JE, Chang D. Brachioplasty: An outcomes analysis. Scientific presentation at 22nd annual EURAPS meeting in Mykonos Greece, June 2011.
35. Shermak MA, Mallalieu JE, Chang D. Barbed suture impact on wound closure in body contouring surgery. *Plast Reconstr Surg* 2010;**126**:1735–41.

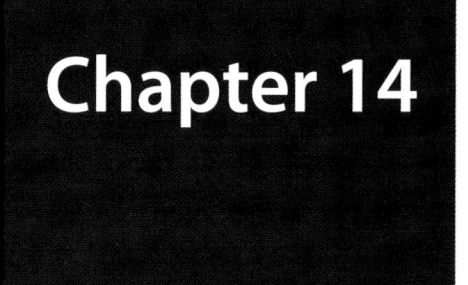

Chapter 14
Male breast surgery after massive weight loss

Brian D. Kubiak, Milton B. Armstrong

The incidence of obesity continues to rise in the USA. This has led to an increased interest in both medically supervised and surgical weight loss. As a result of significant weight loss, patients are left with lax, ptotic, redundant skin, which creates problems for the patient both medically and psychologically. There has been a recent increase in the number of both men and women seeking body-contouring procedures to deal with the redundant tissue. One particularly challenging area for reconstructive surgeons is the thoracic region in men, including the breasts.

DEFINITIONS

Male benign breast enlargement is commonly referred to as gynecomastia. This represents an enlargement of the glandular tissue in the breast. It is important to differentiate this from pseudogynecomastia or lipomastia, which is seen in men after massive weight loss (MWL). Pseudogynecomastia is an excess of skin and fat without enlargement of the breast glandular tissue.[1] On physical exam, patients with true gynecomastia will have a rubbery or firm mound of tissue that is concentric with the nipple–areola complex (NAC). No such disk of tissue will be found in pseudogynecomastia. Reconstructive challenges arise from the fact that pseudogynecomastia can be associated with ptosis, dislocation of the inframammary fold, and malposition of the NAC. In particular, the lateral inframammary fold often becomes displaced inferiorly. There are zones of adherence in the midline that prevent the overlying skin from movement during the weight loss. Laterally there is less adherence, often resulting in vertical decent and leading to a poorly defined fold laterally.[2]

CLASSIFICATION AND TREATMENT

It is the severity of a patient's pseudogynecomastia that often dictates the correct surgical treatment to achieve the optimal outcome. An adequate preoperative exam is therefore essential. To assist with this, a classification algorithm for pseudogynecomastia has been developed by Gusenoff et al.,[3] which can help with management decision-making. This scheme relies on the amount of excess skin and fat, alteration of the NAC, position of the inframammary fold, and laxity of the upper abdomen (**Table 14.1**).

Grade 1

Grade 1 pseudogynecomastia is associated with minimal excess skin and fat. The NAC is essentially normal as is the position of the inframammary fold.[3] (These patients can often be treated in a similar fashion to true gynecomastia with ultrasound-assisted liposuction.[4] The advantage of this technique is the minimal incisions and scarring that result. For this procedure, incisions should be made in the lateral inframammary fold. A super-wet technique using a 1:1 ratio of infiltrate to estimated aspirate is infiltrated subcutaneously in the intermediate fat layer. Constant passes of the liposuction cannula are then made through the intermediate fat. It is important in addition to liposuction

Table 14.1 Classification for pseudogynecomastia after massive weight loss.

Grade	Description
1	Minimal excess skin and fat, minimal alteration of the NAC, normal IMF
2	NAC and IMF below ideal IMF,[a] lateral chest roll, minimal upper abdominal laxity
3	NAC and IMF below the ideal IMF,[a] lateral chest roll, significant upper abdominal laxity

IMF, inframammary fold; NAC, nipple–areola complex.
[a]Ideal IMF defined as the inferior border of pectoralis major.
Adapted from Gusenoff et al.[1]

the subdermal layer, which is not done in traditional liposuction, to allow for maximal skin retraction. The inframammary fold also needs to be disrupted to allow for a gradual transition from the breast to the abdomen. Traditional suction lipectomy is then performed for final contouring and to evacuate the remaining loose fat resulting from the ultrasound-assisted liposuction. This should be done starting in the deep fat layer and proceeding superficially to the intermediate fat layer.[4]

When skin excess is present it may be necessary to perform skin excision alone or together with liposuction. When performed with liposuction, there is some debate about whether or not the skin excision should be performed during the same surgery. The rationale for delaying the excision is that time should be allowed for maximal tissue retraction and potentially obviating or limiting the amount of skin needing to be removed.[5] Delaying excision also allows time for sufficient revascularization of the NAC. Unfortunately, patients with MWL have typically had tension on their skin for long periods of time due to their obesity. This leads to poor skin tone and minimal retraction of this excess skin. Several techniques can be used when only minimal skin needs to be excised. One technique that provides a good aesthetic outcome with minimal surgical sequelae is the complete concentric circumareolar mastopexy. This method not only corrects skin redundancy, but can also address the areolar enlargement frequently seen in this patient population. The desired areolar size should be marked first. Traditionally this ranges between 25 mm and 30 mm in diameter, depending on the size of the patient and his chest.[6] After the inner areolar circle has been determined, the outer circle is then marked to complete the circumareolar cutaneous ring. The area is then de-epithelialized. A full-thickness incision can be made along the inferior border (from 3 o'clock to 9 o'clock) if necessary to excise any excess fat. It is then important to place an intradermal purse-string circumareolar suture before placing the cutaneous sutures to limit periareolar tension.[7] (This is important because areolar dilation and asymmetry are a known complication of concentric mastopexy. If skin excision has been delayed and blood supply to the NAC is adequate, it is possible to make the incisions through the dermis, to allow undermining and significantly reduce the bunching and pleating of the skin caused by the purse-string suture.[5]

There are important guidelines to use when performing concentric mastopexy to achieve the most predictable outcomes.[8] The first and most important principle requires that the outer concentric circle must be drawn not to exceed the original areolar diameter by more than the original exceeds the inner circle diameter. Therefore, the donut of skin between the outer and inner concentric circles should have roughly equal or less nonpigmented skin compared with pigmented skin. If this is achieved, the repaired areola should dilate back to roughly the original size. When the size of the areola needs to be reduced, a larger proportion of pigmented skin can be excised. The second principle states that the outer concentric circle diameter should not be more than twice the diameter of the inner circle. By minimizing the discrepancy of the two circles, tension can be minimized, leading to improved scarring. Finally, the last of these guidelines predicts that the final areolar diameter will be half the distance between the outer and inner circles.

When larger amounts of excess skin need to be excised or a lateral skin roll is present, a vertical component can be added to the periareolar incision. This circumvertical pattern can narrow the base diameter of the breast and excise a large amount of skin, but does add a vertical or slightly oblique scar on the breast.[5] By adding the vertical component, the diameter of the periareolar incision is reduced, which in turn reduces tension and improves scarring. During the procedure, all the excess skin is plicated together with staples until the desired lower contour has been created. When approaching the inframammary fold, the plication is curved out laterally along the fold. The plication lines are marked to delineate the extent of redundant skin. This area is then de-epithelialized followed by skin closure (**Fig. 14.1**).

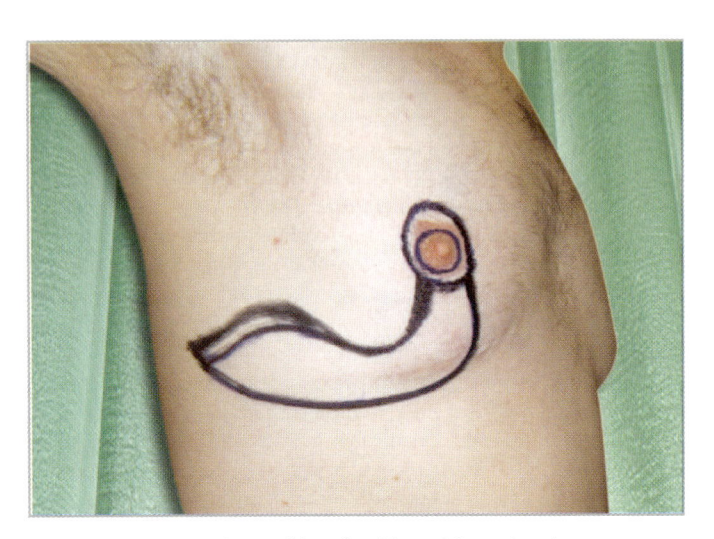

Figure 14.1 Preoperative markings for skin excision using the circumvertical technique. (With permission from Hammond,[5] p 67e).

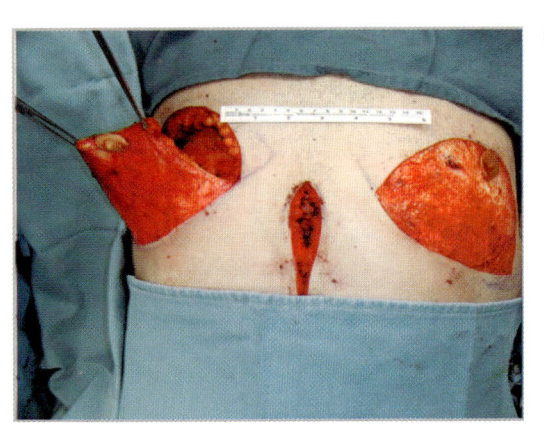

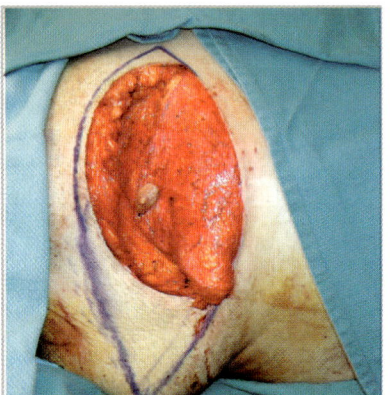

Grade 2

Grade 2 pseudogynecomastia describes excess skin and fat associated with displacement of the NAC and inframammary fold. There is typically a lateral skin roll, but minimal upper abdominal laxity.[3] Classically, an inverted-T technique has been used in these patients, but this leaves unsightly scars that are unacceptable to many patients. This technique relies on an inferiorly or superiorly based de-epithilialized pedicle similar to that used for female reduction mammoplasties. A pedicled reconstruction can also be performed using elliptical incisions of the chest wall, preserving nipple viability on a broad-based, thinned dermal pedicle.[3] The descended inframammary fold is marked, extending laterally to involve any lateral skin roll. An elliptical area of de-epithelialization is then planned extending to the superior border of the NAC. The new position of the NAC is determined and marked. The pedicle is carefully raised and delivered under the superior tissues. The incisions are closed over closed-suction drains and the skin at the position of the new NAC is excised. The NAC is brought into position and sutured (**Fig. 14.2**).

The aforementioned circumvertical technique is another viable option to treat these patients with potentially less visible scarring (see **Fig. 14.1**). New techniques have described placing incisions along the midaxillary line.[9] After making the incisions, the gland is dissected from the pectoralis fascia to allow good mobilization of the NAC. This dissection is most important along the inferior and medial borders. The new position of the NAC is determined and the gland is fixed to the pectoralis fascia with absorbable sutures to maintain that position. Excess skin and subcutaneous tissue are excised with care not to pull the NAC laterally. Ptosis recurrence may occur subsequently, which can be corrected through the original midaxillary incision (**Fig. 14.3**).

Grade 3

Grade 3 pseudogynecomastia is the most severe form that is associated with displacement of the inframammary fold and NAC in the presence of significant upper abdominal laxity.[3] These patients will require extensive skin resection and free nipple grafting is often required. Gusenoff et al. describe determining the superior incision line by placing downward traction on the chest to the desired location for the final scar. A pinch test can be used while the patient is standing to estimate the inferior margin of resection. The entire region of excess skin is resected including the lateral chest rolls and upper abdominal excess. The incisions are closed and the NAC is placed as a free nipple graft on which a bolster dressing is placed (**Fig. 14.4**).[3]

Figure 14.2 The thinned dermoglandular pedicle. (With permission from Gusenoff et al.,[3] p 1306.)

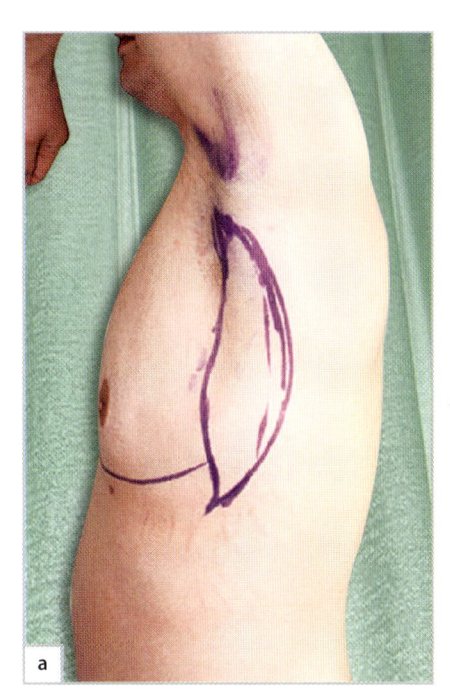

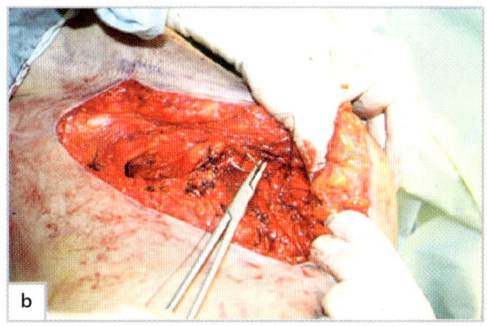

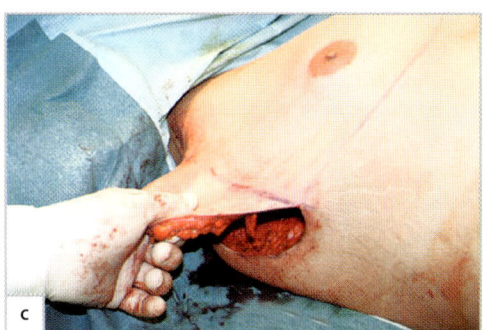

Figure 14.3 Midaxillary skin resection. (a) Preoperative markings, (b) fixation of gland to pectoralis fascia, (c) redundant skin. (From Klinger et al.[9])

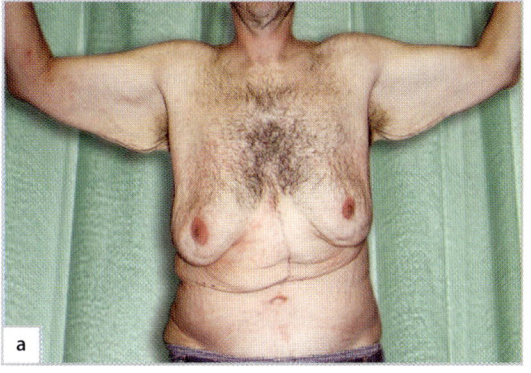

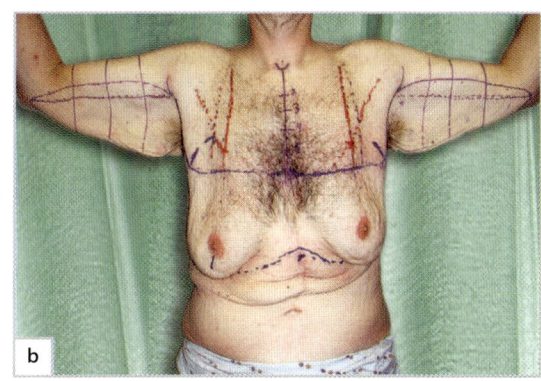

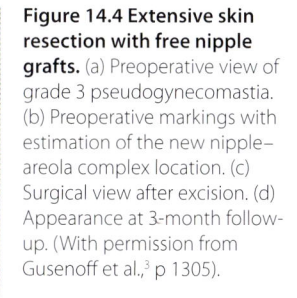

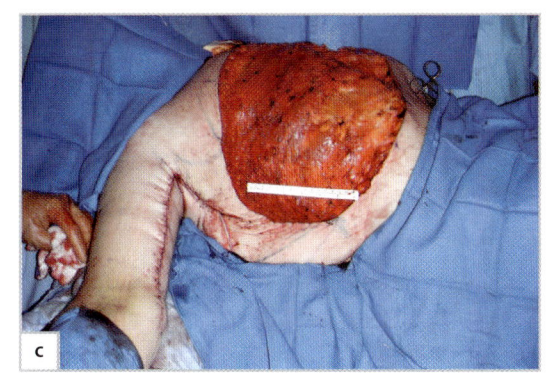

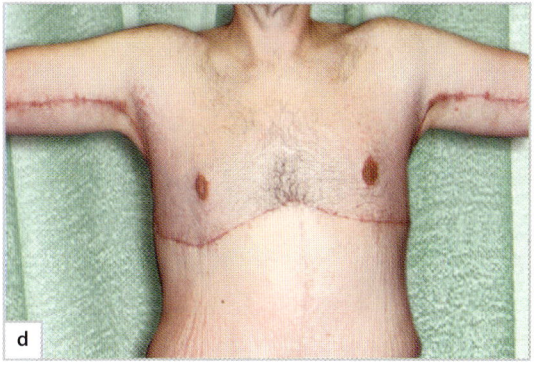

Figure 14.4 Extensive skin resection with free nipple grafts. (a) Preoperative view of grade 3 pseudogynecomastia. (b) Preoperative markings with estimation of the new nipple–areola complex location. (c) Surgical view after excision. (d) Appearance at 3-month follow-up. (With permission from Gusenoff et al.,[3] p 1305).

NIPPLE–AREOLA COMPLEX

As is seen in many of the procedures to correct pseudogynecomastia, surgical repositioning is often required due to the frequent malposition of the NAC. For aesthetic correctness, the normal anatomic position of the NAC must be understood. Multiple measurements have been proposed to determine this. An easy and accurate method has been described by Atiyeh et al.[10] This method relies on just two measurements that are related to the golden number ($\phi = 1.618$). The nipple-to-nipple distance, or horizontal coordinate, is calculated by multiplying the umbilicus-to-anterior axillary fold distance (U-AX) by the reciprocal of the golden number (0.618). This was shown to determine the internipple distance with a 95% confidence Interval. The second measurement is the umbilicus-to-sternal notch distance (U-SN). Using this measurement, two levels can be calculated between which the actual vertical position of the nipple will lie in most cases.

This is referred to as the vertical coordinates. The upper boundary is determined by subtracting the product of the U-SN and reciprocal of the golden number from the U-SN (U-SN − [0.618 × U-SN]). The lower boundary is then calculated by dividing the U-AX by 2. The vertical position of the nipple between these two boundaries depends on patient factors, such as height and torso length, as well as the surgeon's sense of aesthetic form and experience. It is important to know that internipple distance is more aesthetically important than the vertical position of the nipples and slight malposition is well tolerated (**Fig. 14.5**).[10]

MWL provides numerous benefits to patients, but can leave them with redundant and lax skin. Surgical treatment can often correct this problem and improve the patient physically and psychologically. The male breast is one area where surgical correction can be particularly challenging. It is important to carefully examine the patient's breasts to determine the severity of their enlargement and provide the appropriate surgical treatment.

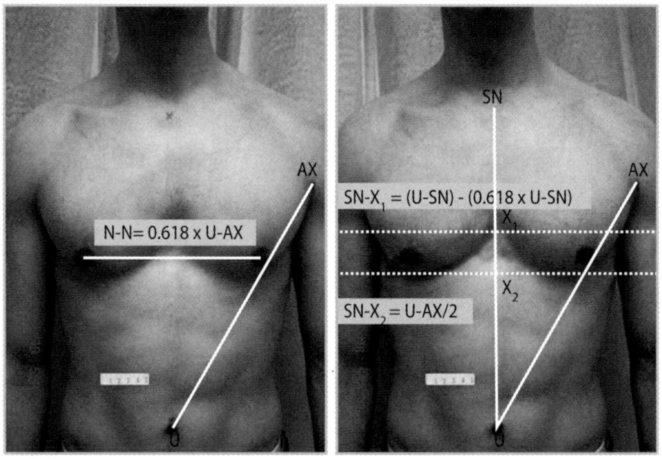

Figure 14.5 Calculations made to determine horizontal and vertical coordinates of nipples position. (With permission from Atiyeh et al.,[10] 500).

REFERENCES

1. Braunstein GD. Clinical practice. Gynecomastia. *N Engl J Med* 2007;**357**:1229–37.
2. Examination of the massive weight loss patient and staging considerations. *Plast Reconstr Surg* 2006;**117**(1 suppl):22S–30S; discussion 82S–83S.
3. Gusenoff JA, Coon D, Rubin JP. Pseudogynecomastia after massive weight loss: detectability of technique, patient satisfaction, and classification. *Plast Reconstr Surg* 2008;**122**:1301–11.
4. Rohrich RJ, Ha RY, Kenkel JM, Adams WP Jr. Classification and management of gynecomastia: defining the role of ultrasound-assisted liposuction. *Plast Reconstr Surg* 2003;**111**:909–23; discussion 924–5.
5. Hammond DC. Surgical correction of gynecomastia. *Plast Reconstr Surg* 2009;**124**(1 suppl):61e–8e.
6. Beckenstein MS, Windle BH, Stroup RT Jr. Anatomical parameters for nipple position and areolar diameter in males. *Ann Plast Surg* 1996;**36**:33–6.
7. Persichetti P, Berloco M, Casadei RM, et al. Gynecomastia and the complete circumareolar approach in the surgical management of skin redundancy. *Plast Reconstr Surg* 2001;**107**:948–54.
8. Spear SL, Kassan M, Little JW. Guidelines in concentric mastopexy. *Plast Reconstr Surg* 1990;**85**:961–6.
9. Klinger ME, Bandi V, Vinci V, et al. Innovations in the treatment of male chest deformity after weight loss: the authors' technique. *Aesthet Plast Surg* 2011;**35**:856 8.
10. Atiyeh BS, Dibo SA, El Chafic AH. Vertical and horizontal coordinates of the nipple-areola complex position in males. *Ann Plast Surg* 2009;**63**:499–502.

Chapter 15
Female breast surgery after massive weight loss

Ari S. Hoschander, Steven M. Henriques, Catherine Gordon, John C. Oeltjen

INTRODUCTION

The steady increase in bariatric surgical procedures has been associated with a concomitant increase in the number of aesthetic breast procedures. The number of mastopexy surgeries rose by 70% from 2000 to 2010.[1] Postbariatric patients seeking breast reshaping present with a unique set of challenges. These patients differ significantly from traditional patients seeking breast reshaping. More pronounced in the massive weight loss (MWL) patients is severe ptosis, deflation of the entire breast including the upper pole, loss of skin elasticity, and extension of the breast into the lateral axillary fold. In addition, patients complain of difficulty with activities of daily living due to constant rash and irritation, difficulty exercising, and compromised personal hygiene.[2]

The approach to the aesthetic reconstruction of the MWL breast has to take into consideration that there are limitations to what can be achieved. The surgeon must be familiar with the reconstructive options that are better suited for these patients because of the unique nature of the MWL breast. In planning the surgery, decisions must be made on a patient-by-patient basis depending on the volume of the breast, the degree of ptosis, and the patient's specific expectations of the procedure. Finally, just as important is appropriate and adequate counseling of the patient as to the limitations and expected outcomes of the proposed procedures.

With the continued rise in bariatric procedures and the increase in patient desire for postbariatric body-contouring procedures, plastic surgeons should be aware of the many options for reconstruction. This chapter serves as an outline of possible breast reconstruction procedures with the aim of assisting the surgeon in planning his or her approach to the MWL patient.

BREAST ANATOMY

The breasts extend from the level of the second rib to the level of the sixth rib overlying pectoralis major. The border of the breast tissue superiorly is the clavicle, medially the sternum, inferiorly the inframammary fold (IMF), and laterally the latissimus dorsi muscle. Ideally the breast is teardrop in shape with a gentle curvature of the lateral breast and a nipple–areola complex (NAC) that is centered at the apex of the breast mound just above the IMF.[3] In profile, the superior aspect of the breast is a gentle concavity ending at the NAC, with the inferior pole of the breast a convexity ending at the IMF. The IMF is a distinct entity medially, starting at the sternal edge of the breast footprint and curving laterally to blend with the lateral border of the pectoralis major.

PATIENT EVALUATION

When evaluating all patients for breast reshaping there are many anatomic landmarks to evaluate and keep in mind. In a patient with MWL there are many additional structural components to assess, each of which varies significantly between patients. Typically, as the patient loses weight, the breast mound becomes unstable and deflated. There is an excessive inelastic skin envelope that is unable to contract to conform to the remaining breast mound, medialization of the NAC, and extension of a lateral chest roll (**Fig. 15.1**).[4,5]

A careful analysis of the changes in the breast needs to be performed during the initial consultation. This evaluation will help to provide the information needed to assemble a surgical plan and allow for the best possible aesthetic outcome.

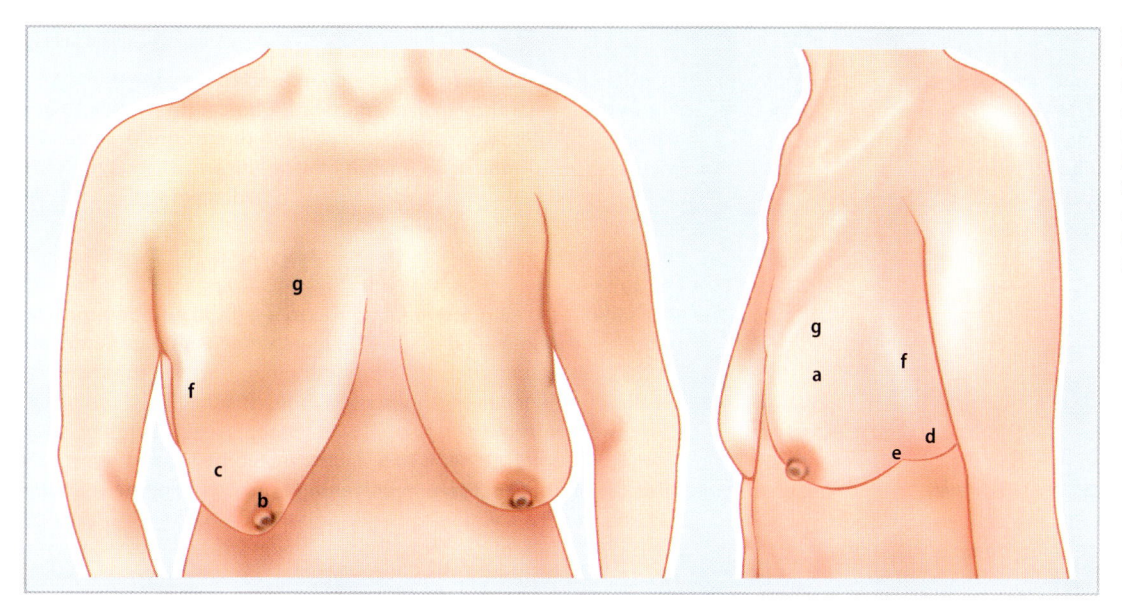

Figure 15.1 Breast anatomy after massive weight loss. (a) Severe ptosis; (b) medialization of the nipple–areola complex (NAC); (c) lateralization of the breast mound; (d) extension into the axillary fold; (e) inferiorly displaced inframammary fold (IMF); (f) skin laxity; and (g) deflated upper pole.

Degree of ptosis (Figure 15.2)

Ptosis occurs as a result of reduction in volume and projection. Almost all patients presenting for breast reshaping will present with some degree of ptosis. The increased weight of the breast associated with obesity results in descent of the breast from loss of the integrity of the Cooper ligaments and loss of skin elasticity. With the postbariatric weight loss, the volume of the breast is reduced and the skin envelope does not regain its elasticity, resulting in further descent of the breasts and exaggeration of the breast ptosis. Regnault described the degree of ptosis and graded them in his scale as follows:[6]

1. **Grade I:** Mild ptosis – the nipple is at the level of the IMF and above most of the lower breast tissue.
2. **Grade II:** Moderate ptosis – the nipple is located below the IMF but above most of the breast tissue.
3. **Grade III:** Advanced ptosis – the nipple is below the IMF and at the level of the most dependent portion of the breast.

Pseudoptosis

The nipple is located either at or above the IMF whereas the lower half of the breast sags below the fold. This is most often seen when a woman stops nursing; as her milk glands atrophy, her breast tissue begins to sag.

Parenchymal maldistribution

The lower breast tissue lacks fullness, the IMF is very high, and the nipple and areola are relatively close to the fold. This is usually a developmental deformity.

Assessment of the NAC

The principal criterion for an aesthetically pleasing NAC is symmetry regarding several parameters: Color, texture, size, and projection. It is typical for obese patients to have an NAC that is stretched, misshapen, and ill-defined.

Quantity of breast volume

Evaluation of the breast volume is critical in determining a surgical plan. It is also very important to have a frank discussion with the patient about her expectations and the breast size that she would like to achieve. The volume should be adequate for the patient, as well as the surgeon. Ultimately, it is the responsibility of the surgeon to help the patient understand what result is achievable and aesthetically pleasing.

Loss of breast volume is directly proportional to the amount of weight loss by the patient. Traditionally, this problem has been corrected with an augmentation using some variety of an implant. The use of an implant has its own risks including, but not limited to, infection, limited longevity of the implant, capsular contracture, rippling or folding, leakage or rupture, malposition, and difficulty with implant descent due to poor tissue quality inherent in MWL patients. These complications should be discussed with the patient as part of the initial consultation. As a result of the increasing awareness of these problems, there has been an increased trend for augmentation with autologous tissue. Using the patient's own native tissue avoids implant-related complications while retaining a natural feel and look of the breast.

As autologous tissue has limitations in achievable size and superior pole fullness, understanding the patient's expectations for breast size and shape are critical to achieving the desired result.

Quality of breast volume

Typically the breast tissue after MWL surgery is loose, without much structure. The breast parenchyma should be evaluated thoroughly. This is crucial to planning additional procedures that may aid in the overall shape and aesthetics of the final result of reshaping. Often the involution of the glandular tissue leaves little 'breast mound' to shape.

BMI

Before consideration for any surgical recontouring or reshaping, the patient's weight should be stable for a minimum of 3 months.[7] Having a patient with a stable weight provides a stable platform for surgical planning. If the patient continues to lose or gain weight after reshaping and contouring, the end-result could be dramatically altered, leading to a less than optimal shape or form. An additional aid to preoperative planning is information on the amount of weight loss, as well as the speed in which the weight was lost. Ideally the body mass index (BMI) should be <30 kg/m^2. If the patient's BMI is >35, consideration should be given to continued diet and exercise, possible revision of bariatric surgery, and delay of operative recontouring.

Nicotine use

As is the case with all surgical procedures, it is important to optimize the patient's ability to heal the surgical wounds, which includes nicotine use cessation. This covers cessation of the use of *any* nicotine delivery, including smoking, chewing gum or smokeless products, or wearing patches. This is a relative contraindication, because the use of nicotine causes potential vasoconstriction of the peripheral blood vessels. This vasoconstriction can result in higher incidence of flap necrosis, infection, and major wound-healing complications. The patient should be counseled on smoking cessation and the potentially devastating side effects of persistent nicotine use. Some surgeons advocate total cessation of all nicotine products before any surgical procedure. Monitoring of nicotine cessation is best achieved by measuring serum or urine *cotinine* levels, a metabolite of nicotine. The half-life of cotinine is greater than that of other metabolites, giving a longer duration of monitoring for nicotine use. Cotinine lasts up to 4 days in the human body. It is certainly within the standard of care to refuse any elective aesthetic procedure to a patient using nicotine products because, ultimately, the operating surgeon must make the

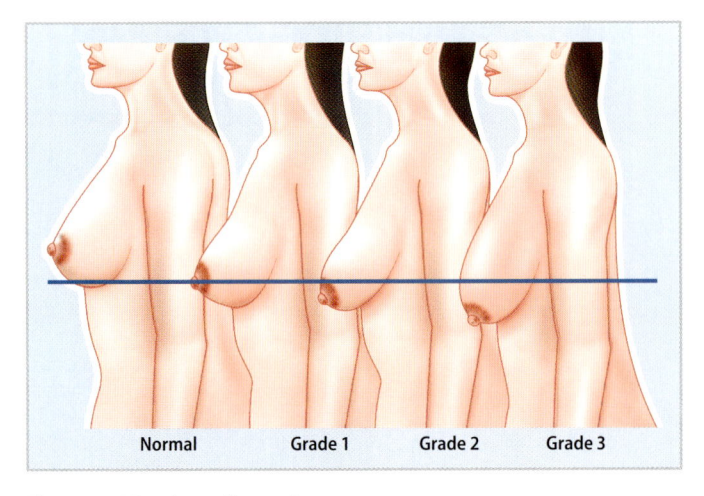

Figure 15.2 Ptosis grading scale.

final decision as to whether he or she wishes to take the additional risk associated with a patient who uses nicotine.

Inframammary fold

The IMF is the inferior border of the breast where the breast meets the chest wall. At this level, the dermis is being held by an association with, but without any direct attachments to, the confluence of the anterior and posterior breast capsule into a single superficial fascial system. The IMF is one of the major landmarks of the breast, aiding in the overall shape and position of the breast. In obese patients the skin loses its elasticity due to the weight of the breast. The arrays of collagen in the subdermal plane are loosened, allowing the IMF to descend. The inferior displacement of the IMF results in a lower position of the breast mound on the chest wall. This drop is aided by the gravitational pull on the breast tissue. After the patient loses weight, the breast volume is decreased and the IMF is left displaced, ill-defined, loose, and low. This creates a flat unaesthetic appearance. During the preoperative evaluation the position and consistency of the IMF should be noted and consideration given to repositioning if necessary. This should be incorporated into the breast recontouring procedure because it will make a significant difference to the appearance of the breast.

Surgically, this can be achieved by releasing the IMF from the chest wall and repositioning it while reshaping it. The level of the new IMF is determined and the fold is secured from the dermal superficial fascial system to the muscular fascia, ribs, and periosteum with a permanent or prolonged absorbable suture. This can provide improved contour and shape of the breast.

Nutritional status

The nutritional status of the patient is a key component in the ability of the patient to withstand the surgical insult and properly heal the surgical wounds. Whether or not the patient has undergone a surgical bariatric procedure to aid in her weight loss, she has subjected her body to a prolonged catabolic state in order to achieve the weight loss. As a result, she has nutritional deficiencies, particularly in vitamins, minerals, and trace elements, which are critical for proper wound healing. Studies to this point have shown that routine preoperative testing for vitamins and trace elements have shown no added benefit and are in fact hard to justify financially. Ordering basic nutrition labs (i.e. prealbumin, transferrin, albumin) will help the surgeon to assess nutritional status and replace basic nutritional needs as necessary.

Other surgical procedures

Complete assessment of the patient in the original consultation includes a thorough history and examination specifically including previous surgical procedures, especially those that could affect the proposed surgical plan, e.g. patients who have undergone an abdominoplasty are not candidates for abdominal autoaugmentation tissue transfers. In addition, axillary scars as continuations of brachioplasty procedures or lateral body-contouring procedures may limit the availability of autologous tissue for augmentation of the breast mound.

SURGICAL APPROACHES

The surgical planning for MWL breast surgery my often seem daunting; however, a systematic approach can lead the surgeon and patient to an optimum result.[8] One tool developed at the University of Pittsburgh is a rating scale for patients after MWL. The scale is rated 0–3 and each grade advocates a particular surgical approach (**Table 15.1**):
1. **Grade 1:** Traditional mastopexy, reduction, or augmentation techniques
2. **Grade 2:** Traditional mastopexy ± augmentation
3. **Grade 3:** Parenchymal reshaping techniques with dermal suspension; consider autoaugmentation.

Unfortunately, there is often not enough volume to reshape and produce an aesthetically pleasing breast mound. The issues of volume can be further subdivided into patients with insufficient, sufficient, or excess volume.

Mastopexy with sufficient autologous breast volume

Vertical mastopexy

The patient is marked preoperatively in the standing position. One of the most critical decisions is the new level of the nipple. The new nipple position can be determined by a variety of methods. The new nipple should be marked at a position equal with the IMF, which is 20–25 cm from the sternal notch. The NAC can be reduced in size if too large. A 4- to 5-cm NAC is commonly accepted as appropriate for a reduced breast. Estimate the amount of breast skin that can reasonably be removed without placing too much tension on the closure. This will serve as a guide to marking the vertical incision preoperatively.

Vertical mastopexy requires either a superiorly or medially based pedicle for NAC perfusion. Mastopexy is carried out in the usual fashion, bearing in mind that these patients heave significantly excess skin. Many different dissections of the vertical mastopexy have been described and each one has its own merits in individual patients. The common theme, however, is a circumareolar incision with a vertical extension toward the IMF and a repositioning of the breast parenchyma to achieve a 'lifted' breast. If lower pole tissue is used in a flap manner to create superior pole fullness or allow nipple mobility into an elevated position, the pillars on either side of the repositioned tissue should be closed with long-lasting absorbable or permanent sutures. The skin closure is performed in the usual manner with one exception; the vertical incision can be cinched, shortening the IMF to nipple length, tightening the lower breast pole, and providing more lift.

Dermal suspension

Dermal suspension can be used in combination with mastopexy for additional support and shaping of the breast. This involves fashioning a breast mound utilizing the resilience of the dermis and then suturing to and thus directly suspending the breast mound on the chest wall. This is achieved by creating skin flaps and a central mound that is then secured to the chest and can be firmly fixed to the periosteum of the underlying ribs.

Table 15.1 Pittsburg rating scale for breast deformity after MWL

Grade	Scale
0	Normal
1	Ptosis grade I/II or severe macromastia
2	Ptosis grade III or moderate volume loss or constricted breast
3	Severe lateral roll and/or severe volume loss with loose skin

From Song et al.[9]

Qiao et al. described a 'dermal bra' technique starting with a Wise pattern for the mastopexy (**Fig. 15.3**).[10]

When planning the pattern for incision for the MWL patient, it is important to keep in mind that lateral rolls can be preserved for use in autoaugmentation (**Fig. 15.4**).

The skin over the pedicle is then de-epithelialized and parenchymal flaps are elevated to the level of the clavicle; a uniform thickness of approximately 1–1.5 cm on the flaps is recommended. Flap elevation at this thickness preserves the subdermal plexus, thus ensuring skin flap viability. Flaps are raised laterally and medially, supplied by perforators of the intercostals. The central pedicle is then secured to the second rib using a permanent suture down to the periosteum. The lateral and medial flaps are secured to the third ribs in a similar fashion. The lateral dermal flap edge is secured to the lateral chest wall fascia, which allows the surgeon to control the outer contour of the breast. Using additional plication sutures within transposed dermis, now comprising the breast mound, the parenchyma can be shaped to create a central mound with improved projection. The skin is then draped over the created mound and closed in a layered fashion over drains.

It is important to pay close attention to the nipple position as well as frequent re-draping of the skin over the flaps in order to ensure proper breast shape and level of suspension. This technique suspends the breast mound to maintain long-term shape, minimize recurrent ptosis, and retain upper pole fullness.

■ Parenchymal plication

As alluded to above, parenchymal plication can be used as a sling to reduce the recurrence of ptosis (**Fig. 15.5**). This plication achieves internal support for the breast tissue, and is almost always performed together with other remodeling procedures. The plication can be performed in a variety of ways – vertically, laterally, and horizontally. This provides the surgeon with complete control to manipulate the vectors and shape of the breast tissue. Native breast parenchyma and dermis are used and long-lasting absorbable or non-absorbable sutures are placed. This redistributed breast tissue allows for the greatest aesthetic result by bringing tissue into the central location, creating a projection as well as a soft contour to the breast. The use of plication may be an additional tool to suspend the breast without having to rely on inelastic skin for support.

■ Ptosis with insufficient autologous breast volume

Insufficient breast volume available to create an adequate or desired breast mound is one of the more difficult challenges in the post-MWL patient. Autoaugmentation is being used extensively in breast aesthetic reconstruction after MWL as a way to add volume to a deflated and depleted breast envelope. There are three avenues that can be explored for patients who have insufficient volume as well as ptosis. All these patients will need a mastopexy and some form of volume augmentation. This additional volume can be achieved by using pedicled flaps or free tissue transfer, local perforator flaps or implants:

1. Augmentation mastopexy utilizing an implant in the post-MWL patient carries with it inherent issues. The primary issue is one of tissue quality. As the breast envelope is lax, the concern with placing an implant arises from the lack of support by the skin and breast tissue in a patient who has undergone MWL. Adding additional weight in the form of an implant to breast tissue that is already unable to hold shape may exacerbate the descent of the breast mound. If an implant must be used, it should be one that is small and as light as possible, in an effort to minimize the amount of stress that is placed on the skin envelope.
2. Augmentation with a local perforator flap is a method of re-distributing local redundant and excess skin and tissue to reshape the

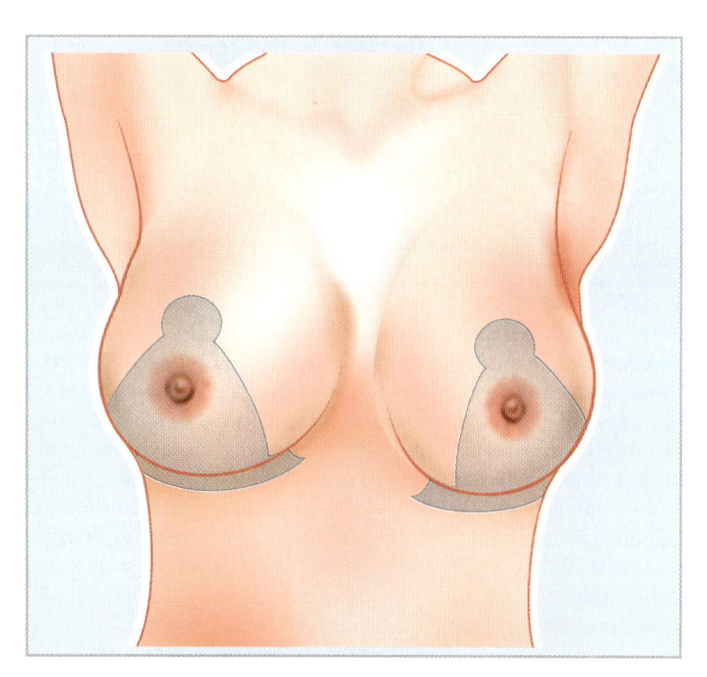

Figure 15.3 Traditional Wise-pattern incision.

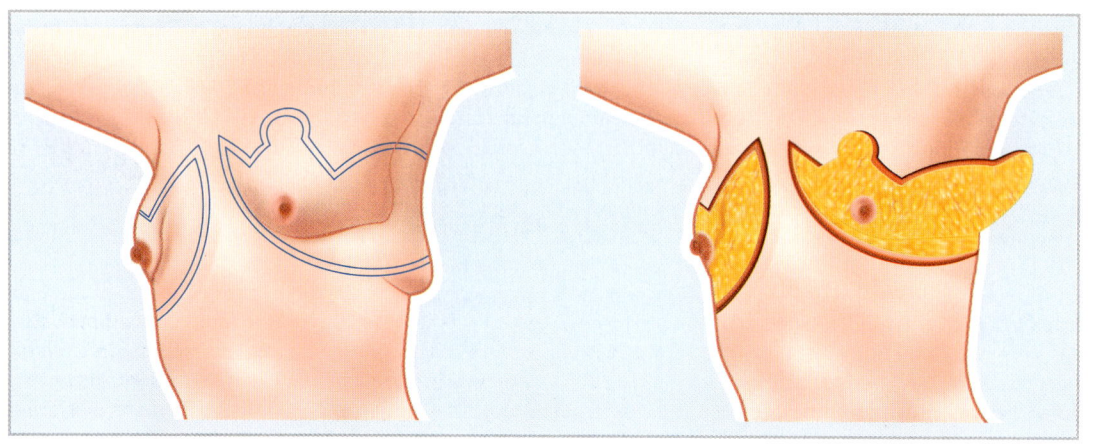

Figure 15.4 Lateral extension of the Wise-pattern Incision.

Surgical approaches

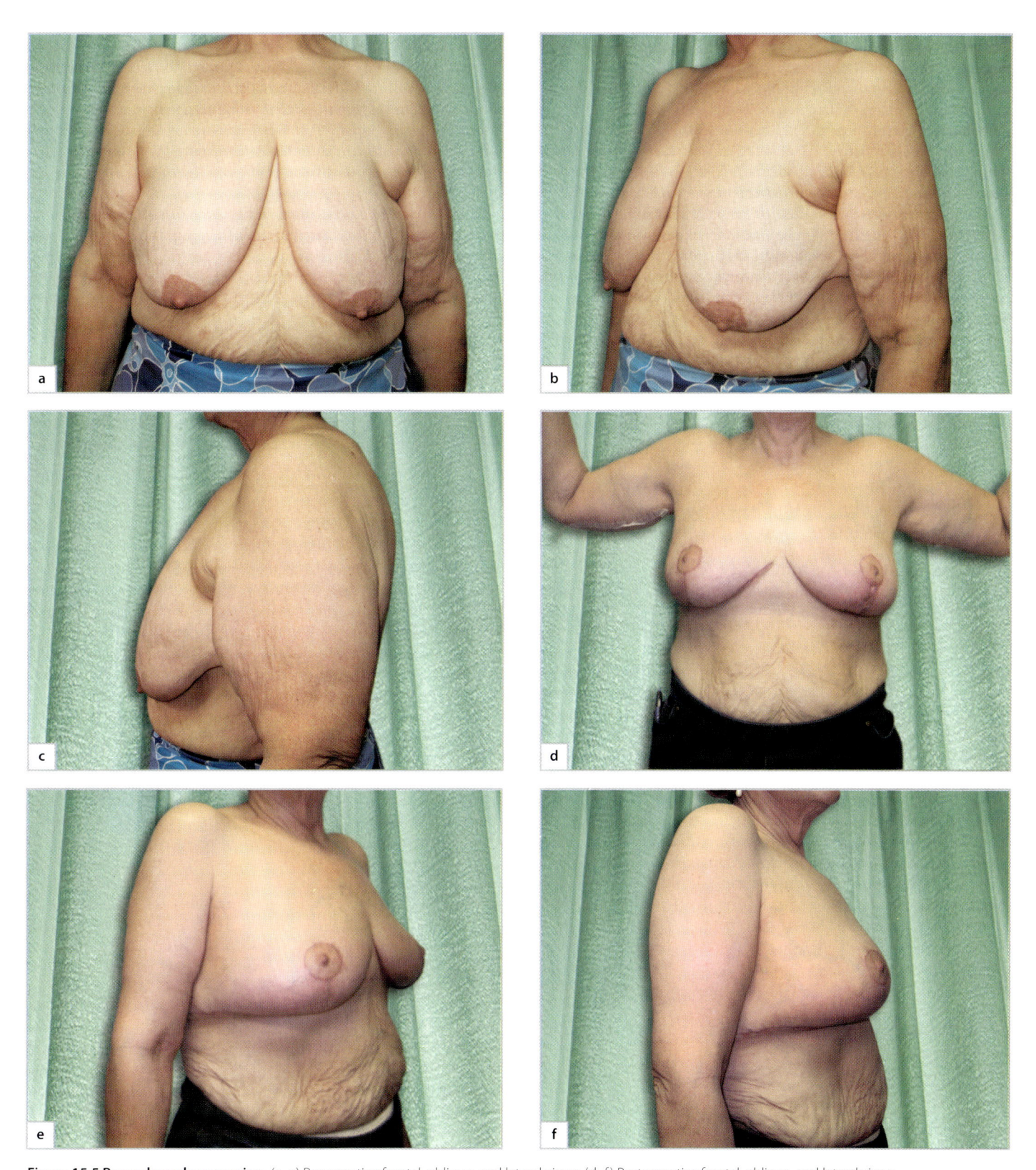

Figure 15.5 Parenchymal suspension. (a–c) Preoperative frontal, oblique, and lateral views. (d–f) Postoperative frontal, oblique, and lateral views.

breast, while maintaining adequate blood supply to these tissues. The use of local excess tissue and skin allows for the restoration of breast volume and contour. In obese patients, as the amount of fat increases, the size of the perforating vessels grows proportionately. However, as patients lose weight and the amount of adipose tissue is reduced, the size of the vessels appears to remain large in contrast to the smaller amount of tissue now being perfused by the perforator. This is often observed by the surgeon in panniculectomy and abdominoplasty surgeries, in which there are large vessels that need to be sutured or hemoclip ligated. The presence of these large perforators allows for design of local perforator-based flaps to transpose tissue to augment the breast mound.

3. Augmentation with pedicled latissimus or abdominal tissue is typically for reconstruction in patients with a defect that needs soft-tissue coverage. It could be considered as too extensive surgery for a cosmetic procedure; however, it remains a viable procedure to import extra soft tissue for breast mound formation. In addition, the abdominal tissue can be transferred as a free flap, although this procedure can be cost-prohibitive for the cosmetic patient in addition to the morbidity associated with an extensive procedure.

Implant augmentation

An implant augmentation can be used for a patient who started with small breasts before losing weight. The patient should be marked in the standard pattern in the preoperative area, with importance placed on the new position of the IMF as well as the medial edge of the breast. The style of mastopexy incision should be determined based on the patient's needs. The dissection proceeds in the standard fashion for a mastopexy; it is then carried down through subcutaneous tissue and superficial fascia on to the fascia of the serratus anterior muscle and over the fascia of the pectoralis major muscle to a level of approximately the second rib. A subpectoral pocket is created and meticulous hemostasis maintained. Once the pocket has been developed an implant is chosen that will properly fit the patient. The mastopexy is closed in the standard fashion.

Local perforator flap

Local perforator flaps offer great value to the patient who has lost a massive amount of weight. The reason for this is that they address two issues that aesthetically trouble the patient, namely the back and lateral rolls that develop from the weight loss and loss of skin elasticity. This tissue can be used to fill a depleted and unstable breast mound. The added benefits of this technique over other flaps are the speed in which it can be performed as well as the reduction in morbidity when compared with a pedicled or free latissimus or abdominal flap. It also provides some form of body sculpting and contouring, giving the patient a smooth axilla and lateral aspect of the back. In the post-MWL patient the lateral aspect of the breast is usually flattened and devoid of definition. This technique recreates the lateral border to accentuate the form of the breast.

Kwei et al. describe autologous augmentation with the use of an intercostal artery perforator (ICAP) flap.[11] This is a fasciocutaneous-based flap with perforators from the intercostal artery supplying the pedicle.

Preoperative planning of this flap starts as other procedures mentioned earlier, with marking of the patient. A Wise-pattern inferior pedicle mastopexy is drawn, adding the ICAP flap designed as a lateral extension from the mastopexy (see **Fig. 15.4**). Doppler ultrasonography is then used to mark the cutaneous perforators along the anterior axillary line. This will constitute the base of the flap and will measure anywhere from 6 cm to 8 cm. The length of the flap is dependent on the amount of redundant tissue that the patient has, typically measuring 15–20 cm.

The patient is usually rotated to prepare the lateral and posterior chest wall. The flaps are started in a posterior-to-anterior fashion. The flap is supplied by branches of the thoracodorsal artery, as well as the intercostal perforators on which the flap is ultimately based. As the flap is elevated from the muscle, the branches of the thoracodorsal bundles are ligated, with awareness not to disrupt any of the intercostal perforators until the level of serratus. The donor site is closed in a layered fashion that is tension free, achieving an upper body lift. Next, the inferior pedicle is created. Careful dissection over pectoralis up to the clavicle produces a subcutaneous pocket for the ICAP flap. The flap is then further mobilized, making sure that additional dissection is not needed. The flap is rotated 90° into position in the previously fashioned subcutaneous, suprapectoral pocket. When the ICAP flap is placed in a satisfactory position it is de-epithelialized, checking frequently for adequate perfusion. The flap is then tacked to the chest wall as well as the inferior pedicle to ensure a fixed position. The breast is closed in the typical fashion of a Wise-pattern inferior pedicle mastopexy.

The ICAP flap is a good option for the patient who lacks volume with excess ptotic lateral axillary tissue, because it provides an upper body lift and fills in a depleted breast mound to redefine the lateral edge of the breast and give the breast a gentle fullness.

Thornton et al. describe their chosen method for autoaugmentation.[12] It begins in much the same way, with a Wise-type pattern skin incision, but, instead of a pedicle that runs along the ribs in an oblique fashion, this pedicle runs vertically in the midaxillary line. The subcutaneous pedicle is based off lateral thoracic perforators. Once the pedicle is elevated and de-epithelialized, it is placed beneath the superolateral skin flap and the newly formed breast mound. The flap is then anchored to the pectoralis fascia to prevent inferior migration. The ultimate result is increased superior and lateral fullness and enhanced lateral breast margin.

Pedicled flap

Patients presenting with MWL often have a deflated breast mound. When the use of an implant or perforator-based flap is not feasible, autologous tissue may still be used in the form of a pedicled flap. The most common pedicled flaps used for breast reconstruction today are latissimus and transversus abdominis myocutaneous (TRAM) flaps.[13–15] Of these, the TRAM flaps are some of the most popular and are therefore discussed here. The post-MWL patients are some of the most ideal patients for this type of flap because they already have some redundant skin and tissue in their abdominal region. The TRAM flap is based off of a superior pedicle from the rectus muscles and the superior epigastric vessels.

The patient is evaluated preoperatively and marked in the standing position with a horizontal ellipse. The patient is then positioned in the usual fashion on the operating table. The lower incision should be performed first. This allows for the skin to be pulled down and assessed for a tension-free closure of the abdominal incision. Once the upper incision has been made, it is taken down to rectus muscle fascia, and then working laterally to medially to expose rectus abdominis fascia. At this point, the dissection of the deep inferior epigastric arteries is performed and they are ligated. The rectus muscle is then cut inferiorly. The flap can then be divided in half and bilateral tunnels formed, allowing for easy passage of the flap. In order not to compromise the blood flow, it is critical to maintain excellent hemostasis before delivering the flap through this tunnel. The flap is then placed in a proper position to add volume. The abdominal wall can be reinforced using a biologic or synthetic mesh depending upon the surgeon's preference. The abdominal skin is then closed over drains in the standard fashion.

In a patient desiring a mastopexy, who has insufficient volume, and has been determined as not a good candidate for the above augmentation approaches, it is imperative to warn her that, after the excess skin resection and lifting of the breast tissue, the breast will become significantly smaller, potentially leading to a non-existent breast mound.

Mammoplasty with excess autologous breast volume

Although rare, some women after MWL still have excess breast volume. This group of women still presents with the same types of problems as all other MWL patients: Ptosis of the breast and inelasticity of the breast skin. They have sufficient breast volume but need a lift and removal of inelastic skin. They can benefit from reduction mammoplasty, which reduces the skin envelope as well as the volume of breast tissue. These changes will ultimately add to the overall aesthetics of the breast by elevating the breast and tightening the skin envelope to give a youthful, rejuvenated look to the breast. This can be achieved with the use of a vertical or Wise-pattern reduction mammoplasty.

As is the case with most procedures, preoperative markings are critical for the eventual successful aesthetic result of the procedure. This can be made in the preoperative holding area with the surgeon's method of choice, bearing in mind any asymmetry and making corrections accordingly. As with the mastopexy, the most important marking is for the new position of the NAC. Marking and placement of the new NAC is similar to the previously described mastopexy markings.

The procedure begins by creating the new NAC, usually using a cookie cutter of an appropriate size for the patient's frame and anticipated breast size. Once the NAC as been marked and incised, de-epithelialization of the pedicle commences. Many pedicles are utilized, depending on surgeon preference and the distance that the nipple is being transposed. In any approach, the surgeon should be careful to create a pedicle that is sufficiently wide to allow for continued viability of the NAC. As with the Wise-pattern mastopexy, parenchymal long-lasting absorbable or permanent sutures can be utilized to shape and suspend the breast mound before draping the skin envelope over it.

As with any of these procedures, intraoperatively the nipple should be monitored closely and, if there is any concern that the nipple may become ischemic, a free nipple graft can be performed. Ischemia can be difficult to detect in some skin pigmentations, particularly darker complexions. The nipple can be evaluated by puncture with an 18-gauge needle. The result should be rapid return of non-congested, bright blood. The assessment can be performed multiple times throughout the case to ensure adequate blood supply to the nipple. Postoperatively, continued monitoring of the NAC for signs of congestion should be performed, and any signs of compromise addressed immediately with suture release and consideration of returning to the surgical arena.

CONCLUSION

As the 'obesity epidemic' continues and more individuals undergo MWL, the practicing plastic surgeon will be met with an ever-increasing number of difficult breast aesthetic reconstructive procedures. Although an awareness of the inherent changes in the MWL breast, including ptosis, lack of breast volume, and lack of skin elasticity, is important, it is necessary for the surgeon to approach each case individually, with an entire palette of tools to achieve the optimum cosmetic result aligned with the patient's expectations and desires. Presented here are various surgical options for the postbariatric breast, to assist in the formation of the surgeon's palette.

REFERENCES

1. American Society of Plastic Surgeons. *2010 Body Contouring After Massive Weight Loss*. ASPS Public Relations. Arlington Heights, IL: American Society of Plastic Surgeons, 14 March 2012.
2. Chandawarkar RY. Body contouring following massive weight loss resulting from bariatric surgery. *Adv Psychosom Med* 2006;**27**:61–72.
3. Colwell AS, Driscoll D, Breuing KH. Mastopexy techniques after massive weight loss: an algorithmic approach and review of the literature. *Ann Plast Surg* 2009;**63**:28–33.
4. Losken A. Breast reshaping following massive weight loss: principles and techniques [Review]. *Plast Reconstr Surg* 2010;**126**:1075–85.
5. Rubin JP, Gusenoff JA, Coon D. Dermal suspension and parenchymal reshaping mastopexy after massive weight loss: statistical analysis with concomitant procedures from a prospective registry. *Plast Reconstr Surg* 2009;**123**:782–9.
6. Regnault, P. Breast ptosis: definition and treatment. *Clin Plast Surg* 1976;**3**:193–203.
7. Colwell AS, Borud LJ. Optimization of patient safety in post-bariatric body contouring: a current review. *Aesthet Surg J* 2008;**28**:437–442.
8. Colwell AS, Driscoll D, Breuing KH. Mastopexy techniques after massive weight loss: an algorithmic approach and review of the literature. *Ann Plast Surg* 2009;**63**:28–33.
9. Song AY, Jean RD, Hurwitz D, et al. A classification of contour deformities after bariatric weight loss: The Pittsburgh Rating Scale. *Plast Reconstr Surg* 2005;**116**:1535–44.
10. Qiao Q, Sun J, Liu C, Liu Z, Zhao R. Reduction mammaplasty: and correction of ptosis: Dermal bra technique. *Plast Reconstr Surg* 2003;**111**:1122–30.
11. Kwei S, Borud LJ, Lee BT. Mastopexy with autologous augmentation after massive weight loss: the intercostal artery perforator (ICAP) flap. *Ann Plast Surg* 2006;**57**:361–5.
12. Thornton DJ, Fourie le R. Autologous augmentation-mastopexy after bariatric surgery: waste not want not! *Aesthet Plast Surg* 2010;**34**:519–24.
13. Jensen JA. TRAM flap delay: new data addressing old questions. *Plast Reconstr Surg* 2009;**123**:1883–5.
14. Erdmann D, Sundin BM, Moquin KJ, et al. Delay in unipedicled TRAM flap reconstruction of the breast: a review of 76 consecutive cases. *Plast Reconstr Surg* 2002;**110**:762–7.
15. Hudson DA. The surgically delayed unipedicled TRAM flap for breast reconstruction. *Ann Plast Surg* 1996;**36**:238–42; discussion 242–5.

Chapter 16
Gluteal contouring after massive weight loss

Morad Askari, Haaris S. Mir

The specific development of the gluteal area has been a particular trait of *Homo sapiens*, separating humans from primates. The muscles of the pelvis and gluteal region contribute to the evolution of the erect posture of humans and play a critical role in balancing the trunk over the lower extremities. In addition, the large deposits of fat over gluteal muscles play an important role in cushioning when in a seated position, as noted by Montagu.[1] Yet, throughout history, this region of the body has been recognized as a component of sexual appeal and beauty in many communities. As a result, the aesthetics of gluteal area and the effect of weight change on its morphology have been studied and reported.[2,3]

Today, there is an increasing demand for gluteal contouring operations to enhance the aesthetics of the buttocks. These procedures range from buttock augmentation using various reshaping techniques with autologous tissue or flaps to use of synthetic implants. After anatomic changes that follow massive weight loss, gluteal contouring operations are especially sought after in the bariatric surgery population. However, they pose a challenge to plastic surgeons. Although traditional body-contouring procedures such as lower body lifts or belt lipectomy address removal of excess skin and subcutaneous tissue, these operations commonly fail to restore the projection and aesthetic characteristics of the buttocks.

In this chapter, we review the anatomy of the gluteal region and the effect of extensive weight loss on this area. Classification of buttock ptosis is discussed, and important points in evaluating the gluteal area are described to facilitate the treatment strategy. Finally, several surgical techniques are described in approaching gluteal contouring in massive weight loss (MWL) patients.

ANATOMY

Understanding of specific topical anatomic landmarks is helpful in evaluation and surgical treatment of gluteal deformity. These landmarks reflect aesthetic features of this part of the body and guide the surgical planning (**Fig. 16.1**). The landmarks include the following:[4]
- The iliac crest,
- The posterosuperior iliac spine (PSIS)
- The coccyx
- The lateral trochanteric depression
- The infragluteal fold.

The iliac crest marks the superior border of the buttocks whereas the PSIS corresponds to two distinct areas of depression in the sacrum. The PSIS is formed from the confluence of the insertion of gluteus maximus and the lumbosacral aponeurosis. The topical tissue depression at the PSIS is characteristic of the aesthetic buttock. The coccyx can be palpated in the superior portion of the gluteal crease and forms the inferior corner of the 'sacral triangle.'[2] The superior borders of the triangle are the two PSIS points (**Fig. 16.2**). Enhancement of this triangle contributes to the attractive appearance of the gluteal region. The lateral trochanteric depression is shaped by the insertion of buttock and lower extremity muscles into the greater trochanter. The inferior gluteal fold is the inferior border of the buttocks and is formed by fascia connecting the skin in this region to the underlying bony skeleton of the pelvis and femur. Although a short infragluteal fold implies younger and fuller-appearing buttocks, a longer fold suggests older, ptotic, and more deflated buttocks.[3]

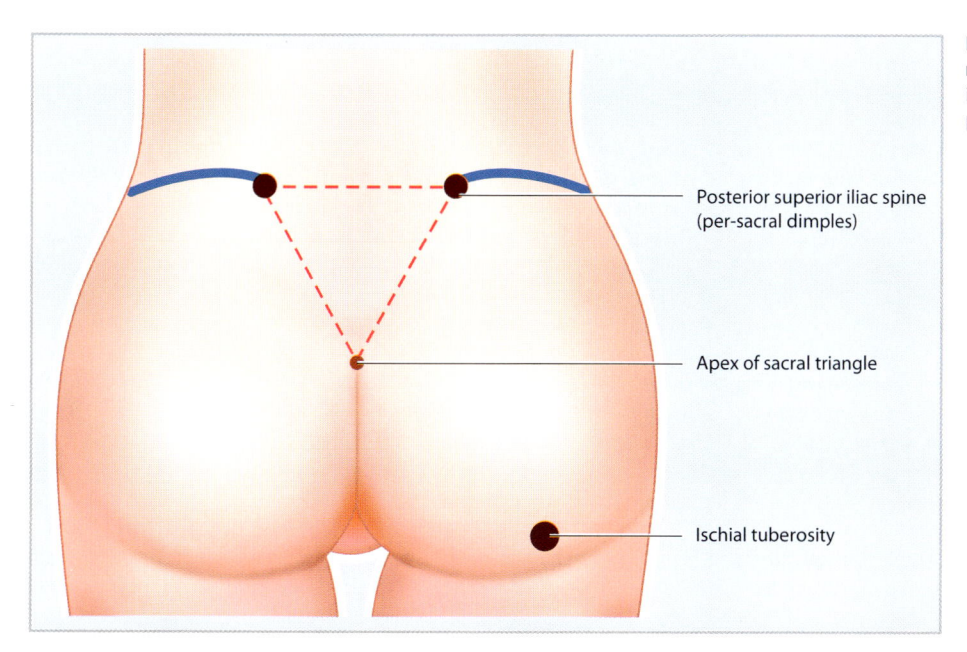

Figure 16.1 **Superficial landmark of the gluteal region.** The iliac crest, the posterosuperior iliac spine, and coccyx/sacrum. (Redrawn with permission from Conteno and Young.[4])

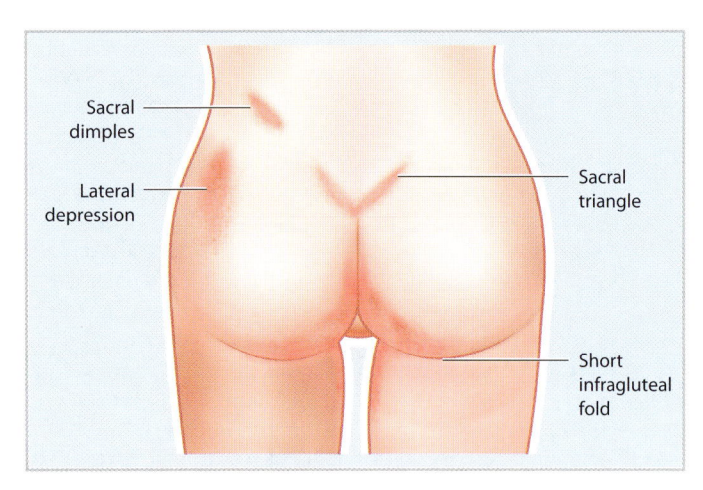

Figure 16.2 Topical aesthetic features of the buttock. Enhancement of the sacral triangle, as well as sacral and lateral depression and a short infragluteal fold, contribute to the aesthetic appearance of the buttocks. ((Redrawn with permission from Conteno and Young.[4])

Projection of the buttocks is the result of several components including the subcutaneous fat deposits, gluteus maximus muscle mass, and lumbar lordosis of the spine. Although the a greater part of the projection is likely due to the muscle mass, the fat distribution provides the round appearance of the buttock and an attractive infragluteal fold. The distribution of this fat is affected by gender, age, and ethnicity.[1] Similar to the abdominal fat, the gluteal fat is structured in an analogous superficial fascial system (SFS).[5] Analogous to the Scarpa fascia, a superficial fascial 'apron' separates deep and superficial layers of the fat. Laxity of this layer can contribute to ptosis and drooping of the buttock. This superficial layer inferiorly joins the investing fascia of gluteus maximus to form the infragluteal fold.[6]

Among the muscles of the gluteal region, gluteus maximus is most relevant to the discussion of buttock aesthetics and contouring surgery. This muscle serves as a powerful extensor of the flexed femur and stabilizes the hip laterally. It originates from the posterior aspect of the ilium, the dorsal surface of the sacrum, coccyx, and sacrotuberous ligament, and inserts on the gluteal tuberosity of the femur, as well as the iliotibial tract. Innervation of gluteus maximus is through the inferior gluteal nerve.

An understanding of the superficial neurovascular anatomy of the gluteal region is imperative to minimizing surgical complications. Gluteal skin is perfused through perforators from the superior and inferior gluteal arteries, both of which are branches of the internal iliac artery. The superior portion of the buttock is additionally perfused by lumbar perforators.[7] For the most part, sacrificing several of these branches – a necessary part of many gluteal contouring techniques – will not compromise the robust vascular supply to this region. Yet careful ligation of these branches is an important part of these operations. Sensation to the gluteal skin and lateral trunk originates from dorsal rami of S3 and S4 as well as the cutaneous branch of the iliohypogastric (L1) and superior cluneal (L1–3) nerves. There is a great likelihood of transient loss of sensation over this distribution after gluteal contouring surgery, and thus it is best if it is included in the preoperative discussion with the patient and with appropriate precautions postoperatively.

Anatomic changes with weight loss

Obesity tends to result in a more centralized fat distribution, thus causing an android body type in both sexes. It has been shown that weight gain results in an increase in the height and width of the buttock. This results in a longer intergluteal crease, while shortening and lowering the infragluteal fold.[8] In contrast, weight loss generally results in excess skin between the perceived superior margin of the buttocks and the iliac crest, and drooping of the intergluteal crease and infragluteal fold.[9] Anatomic changes in the buttocks due to weight loss are to some degree an exaggeration of changes experienced with normal aging: Loss of adipose volume within the buttocks, lengthening of the infragluteal fold, increased hip width, general laxity of the skin, and buttock ptosis.[3,6] MWL further exacerbates these changes and contributes to *platypygia* or flattening of the buttocks. Platypygia can be made worse by a circumferential body lift without addressing gluteal projection. In addition, the changes that occur after weight loss due to bariatric surgery tend to be in an uneven manner, with a greater loss of volume in the buttock compared with some other locations in the body.[8] Similarly, obese patients who undergo weight loss surgery may, over time, have developed skeletal changes that, after MWL, may further exaggerate soft-tissue changes in the buttocks. These changes include increased kyphosis of the thoracic spine resulting in an anterior inclination of the pelvis. In addition, hypocalcemia, vitamin D deficiency, hypothyroidism, or sex hormone imbalance after gastric bypass surgery will worsen these skeletal changes, thus further enhancing the primary platypygia caused by soft-tissue changes.[10,11]

■ EVALUATION OF THE GLUTEAL REGION

The shape of the buttock is influenced by four main components:[12]
1. Underlying bony skeleton
2. Gluteus maximus
3. Topography of the fat deposits superficial to the muscle
4. The skin.

Among these components, the skin and subcutaneous fat are the easiest components to modify in order to achieve the aesthetic goals of the operation.

Mendieta defines the gluteal 'frame' as the above components, less gluteus maximus. By evaluating gluteal muscle separately from the frame, the evaluation of the buttocks is simplified. Three points have been defined in evaluation of the frame type of the buttock: point A, the most protruding point on the upper lateral hip; point B, the most protruding point on the upper lateral thigh; and point C, the midpoint between points A and B (**Fig. 16.3**).[12] The combination of these three points allows classification of buttocks into four groups: A shape, V shape, square shape, and round shape with attention to the degree of depression in the lateral hip (**Fig. 16.4**). The appearance of the gluteal frame is also affected by the sacral height which should be less than a third of the length of the intergluteal crease. If this relation is not adequate, the crease could be elevated through a lift or by adding volume to the upper medial buttock, while it can be shortened if required by modification of the incision design.

In evaluating gluteus maximus, the ratio of the height of the muscle to the width is important. A tall ratio (2:1) will require different a differently shape implant or flap versus a short muscle (1:1). The muscle is further evaluated by dividing it into four quadrants. Each quadrant is assessed for volume sufficiency to determine if more volume is needed.

The junction between the frame and the muscle is crucial to the aesthetic appearance of the buttocks. The sacral triangle represents the connection between the medial upper portion of gluteus maximus

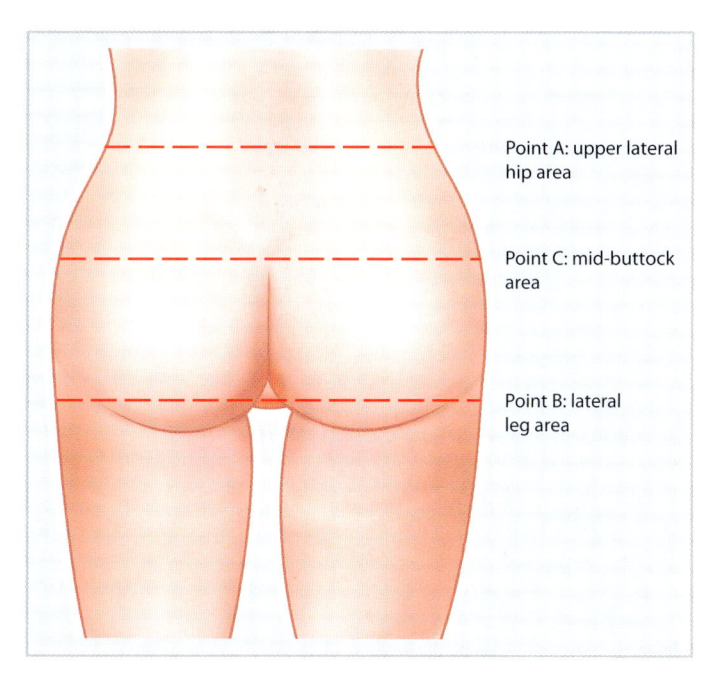

Figure 16.3 Evaluation of the 'frame.' The three points are considered in determining the type of the gluteal frame. (Redrawn with permission from Mendieta.[12])

Point A: upper lateral hip area
Point C: mid-buttock area
Point B: lateral leg area

and the sacrum. This area should have some of degree of definition. A flat and blunt appearance will benefit from fat grafting whereas an excess protuberance here will improve with liposuction. Inferiorly, the junction between, the intergluteal crease should ideally have a 'diamond shape' with 45° slant from the inferior-most point of the crease to the medial thigh. Frequently excess skin or subcutaneous tissue may be obscuring the area for which direct excision or liposuction may be considered. Finally, the junction between the lateral gluteal area and the lateral thigh should be smooth with no excessive protuberance or demarcation.

Ptosis

All MWL patients will have some degree of ptosis. The adipose tissue in the gluteal region is encased in a dense matrix of suspensory connective tissue, which connects to the dermis above and the muscle fascia below, as well as to the bony skeleton of the pelvis. As the adipose tissue decreases in volume due to the weight loss, the previously full envelope droops. In addition, both weight loss and aging contribute to loss of firmness of the suspensory connective tissue. Gonzalez defines ptosis as sagging of lax redundant gluteal tissue inferior to the infragluteal fold at the mid-posterior thigh.[13] This process happens from medial to lateral. As the buttock tissue becomes lax and ptotic the infragluteal fold becomes longer and defined. In defining the classification of gluteal ptosis, two sagittal lines – one crossing through the ischial tuberosity (line T) and one through the midpoint of posterior thigh (line M) - are used (**Fig. 16.5**). As the degree of ptosis increases (0–5), the infragluteal fold surpasses line T and M, respectively, whereas the amount of ptotic tissue increases from medial to lateral. *Pseudoptosis* refers to the descent of the infragluteal fold secondary to excessive laxity and failure of the suspensory connective tissue of the buttocks, and should be differentiated from gluteal ptosis. Not surprisingly, massive weight results in an element of psuedoptosis superimposed on a high degree of gluteal ptosis.

Determining the degree of ptosis will be helpful in choosing the appropriate surgical strategy. The choice between an implant versus upper buttock lift requires attention to gluteal ptosis. Yet, the absence of ptosis alone does not obviate the need for tissue augmentation. Lateral evaluation and overall assessment of all of the components described above will allow development of an appropriate surgical plan on a case-by-case basis.

TREATMENT APPROACHES

There are three basic options for patients seeking gluteal augmentation and contouring. When deciding whether placement of gluteal implants, liposuction, or augmentation with fat injections is appropriate, or a combination of the different modalities , the preoperative consultation must be geared to understanding what the patient's goals and wishes are.[14] Currently, the most common surgical techniques performed for gluteal augmentation make use of implants, as well as a combination of liposuction/lipoinjection procedures.[15]

Gluteal augmentation with implants

Interest in implant-based gluteal augmentation has increased over the last few decades. Patients who have experienced MWL may not be the best candidates for primary gluteal augmentation for platypygia. A common finding in these patients is lack of sufficient fat or tissue volume to pad an implant. Thin skin may makes the implant more visible and more susceptible to palpability, extrusion, or even implant migration.[11] Even though implant-based gluteal augmentation may enhance the gluteal aesthetics, complications are not uncommon. Currently the implants are limited to silicone elastomers; placement of these implants must be made in carefully selected and well-informed patients.[16]

Submuscular implant placement

Implant placement in the submuscular plane is relatively straightforward. Implant visibility is reduced by providing total muscle coverage with gluteus maximus. The position of the sciatic nerve dictates the level at which the implant is placed. The sciatic nerves passes from under the pirformis muscles at the level of the greater trochanters. Submuscular dissection must be stopped once the level has been reached.[16]

Disadvantages to placing a submuscular implant include incorrect implant placement as well as seromas (most common), wound dehiscence (second most common), implant migration, capsular contracture, implant extrusion, infection, compartment syndrome, or even sciatica. Overdissection of the implant pocket and placement of the implant too low may cause sciatic nerve irritation or compression. This may also be responsible for the increased postoperative pain in patients with submuscular implant placement.[11,16]

In men, the point of maximal projection is slightly higher than in women due to the short anthropometric shape of the male pelvis. It is considered more favorable to have a more superiorly placed implant in a male with a short buttock or a female with volume deficiency in the superior third of the buttocks. An implant placed too high may result in a 'shelf butt' or cause the potential 'double bubble' effect.[11,16]

Intramuscular implant placement

The techniques that have the most aesthetically pleasing results with the least irregularities are those where the implant is placed intramuscularly.[17,18] The advantage of intramuscular placement of an implant is that the anatomy of the sciatic nerve does not limit implant placement

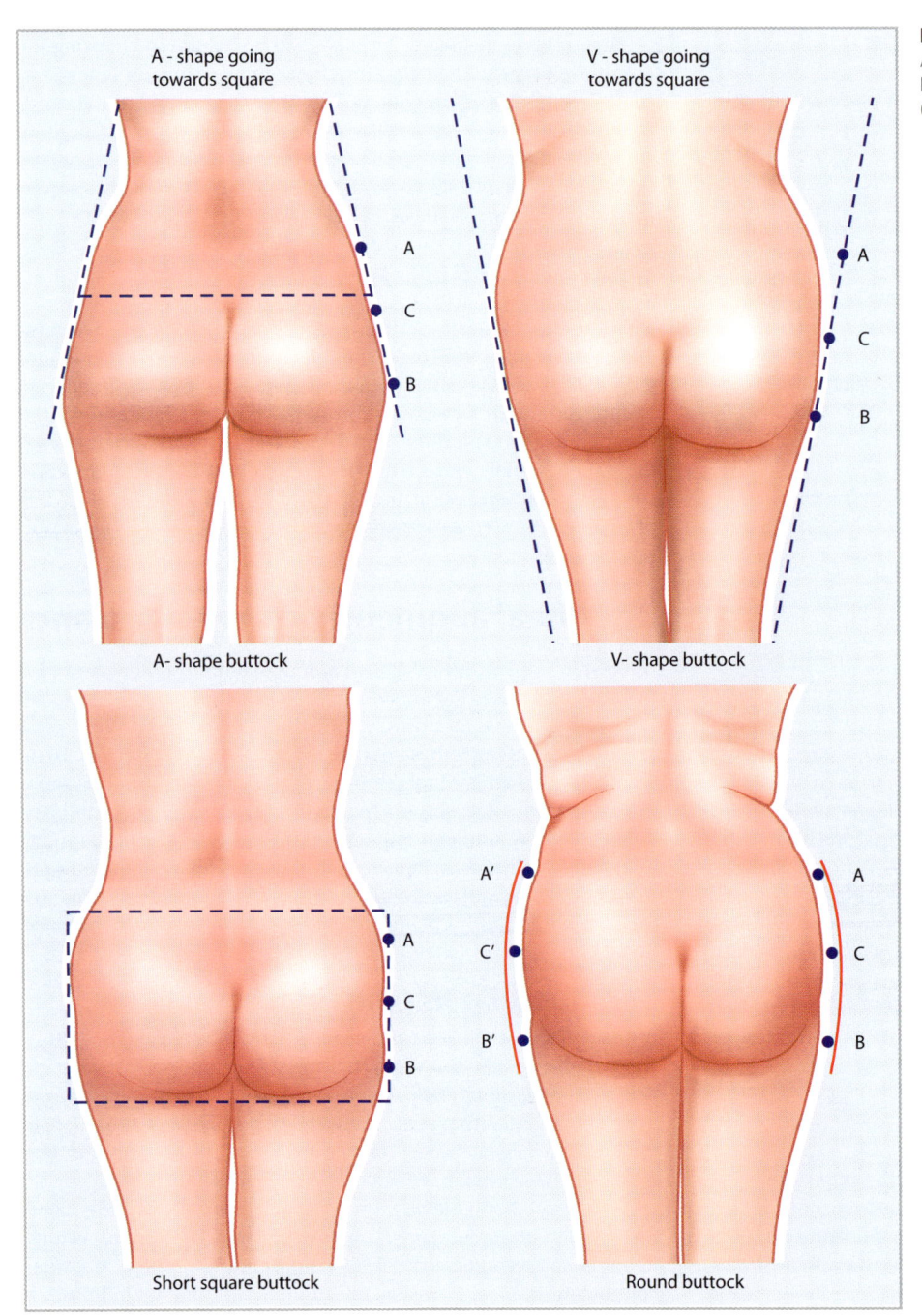

Figure 16.4 Different frame types. Based on points A, B, and C, four different frame types are defined. Point C determines the degree of gluteal depression. (Redrawn with permission from Mendieta.[12])

(**Fig. 16.6b**); however, there is certainly a risk of shredding the muscle. Care must be taken on the lateral dissection in the intramuscular plane because this is where the implant may be come subcutaneous. Aesthetically, an implant placed in the intramuscular pocket does keep the implant in the middle of the buttock. In the event that a superior or inferior third augmentation is needed, the intramuscular implant may give the buttock a peculiar appearance on a lateral view.[11]

In 2003 Vergara and Amezcua[20] showed a complication rate of 10% in 160 patients. The complications included seromas (10%), asymmetry (2.6%), capsular contracture (2%), over-correction (0.66%), and implant rupture (0.66%). Mendieta[17] had a 30% wound dehiscence rate in 2003 before switching to a different incision. Overall, if done correctly, the intramuscular approach results in the most satisfactory results.

Subfascial implant placement

The subfascial approach was described by De la Pena in 2004.[2] It was developed as a solution to the complications caused by other methods of implant placement. In the subfascial approach, the subfascial plane is undermined to raise the gluteal aponeurosis covering the anterior two-thirds of gluteus medius and gluteus maximus. With the muscles being uninterrupted, a platform is established on which to place the implant. The aponeurosis provides contouring and anatomic coverage of the implant once it is in place. This technique is relatively straightforward, the results are reproducible, and the subfascial implant placement produces good aesthetic outcomes, particularly when lower pole volume is desired.

Treatment approaches

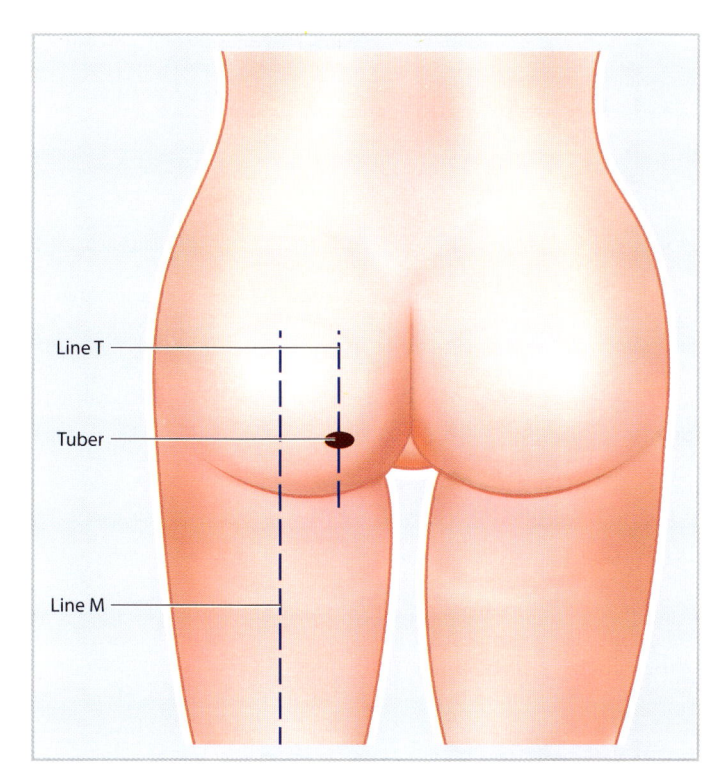

Figure 16.5 Evaluation of gluteal ptosis. Relative position of infragluteal fold to two sagittal lines through the ischial tuberosity (line T) and the midpoint of posterior thigh (line M) are used to determine the degree of gluteal ptosis.

The limitations to this technique are anatomy and implant visibility. Palpability remains a problem[21] (see **Fig. 16.6**).

Autologous gluteal augmentation

Reports on gluteal augmentation with de-epithelialized flaps have been published.[21-23] In addition, others have reported using autologous tissue to prevent gluteal deformities in patients undergoing circumferential body lifts. These reports were lacking in detail and did not substantiate any potential augmentation.[24,25] However, muscle flaps named according to their blood supply (superior and inferior gluteal arteries) and transverse lumbosacral flaps have been described and used for gluteal volume enhancement.[26]

In patients who undergo circumferential body lifts, autologous tissue that would normally be discarded in the posterior region can be molded to replicate an implant. This is set beneath the circumferential body lift flaps. The autologous gluteal augmentation flap was the first flap described. It simulated the round, non-anatomic design of submuscular gluteal implants (**Fig. 16.7**).

Aesthetic results with island flaps are for the most part suboptimal. The amount of volume that is provided is insufficient to overcome the gluteal flattening seen in MWL patients who have undergone circumferential body lifts.[27] With experience gained from autologous guteal augmentation flaps, the moustache autologus gluteal augmentation flap was designed (**Fig. 16.8**). The moustache flap uses lower back and lateral flank tissue as a partial transposition flap based on perforators from the superior gluteal artery and lumbar peforators.[7] No major complications have been associated with autologus gluteal augmentation except for epidermolysis, delayed wound healing, or skin necrosis. Despite this, Conteno[27] preferred using the moustache flap when significant, long-lasting esthetic augmentation is desired in patients who have experienced MWL.

Combination of autologous and implant gluteal augmentation

Three options are available for patients seeking augmentation or recontouring of the gluteal region: Gluteal implants, liposuction, and augmentation with fat injections. There is frequently a necessity to use all three modalities in MWL patients. This is done to achieve attractively shaped buttocks with proper proportions and good projection. The patient's goals must be understood before surgical intervention, as well as risks and benefits including need for further surgery/augmentation. All areas of excess and deficiencies may be addressed in a combined multimodality approach.[14]

A thorough understanding of the patient's goals must be made before embarking on gluteal contouring in a MWL patient. Oftentimes, gluteal contouring may be done at the time of circumferential body lift. A multimodal approach to augmentation and contouring results in the most desirable outcomes.

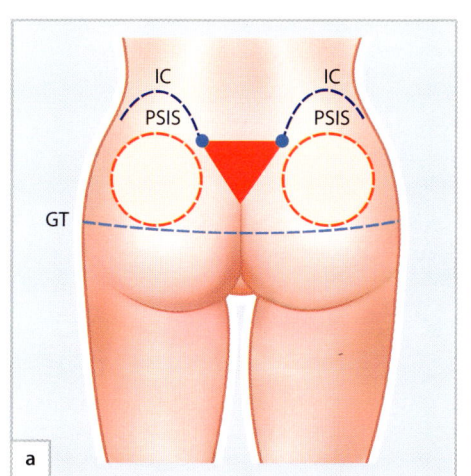

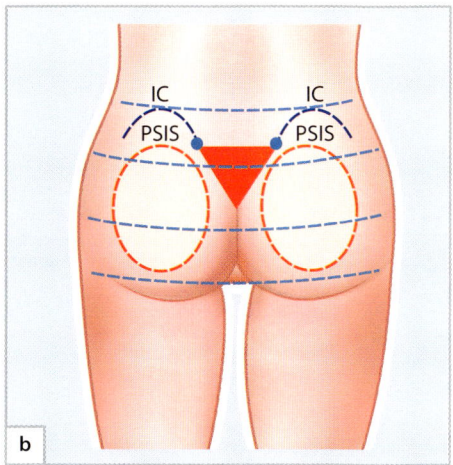

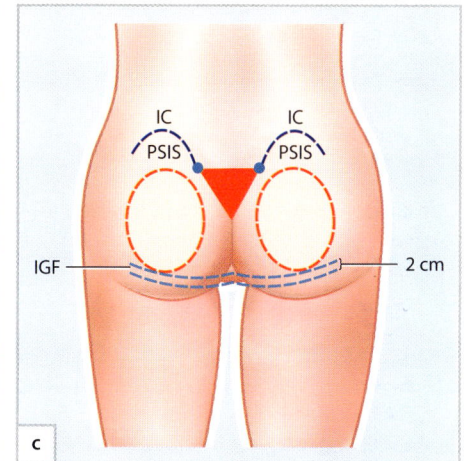

Figure 16.6 Gluteal implant locations for (a) submuscular, (b) intramuscular, and (c) subfascial procedures. GT, greater trochanter; IC, iliac crest; IGF, infragluteal fold; PSIS, posterosuperior iliac spine.

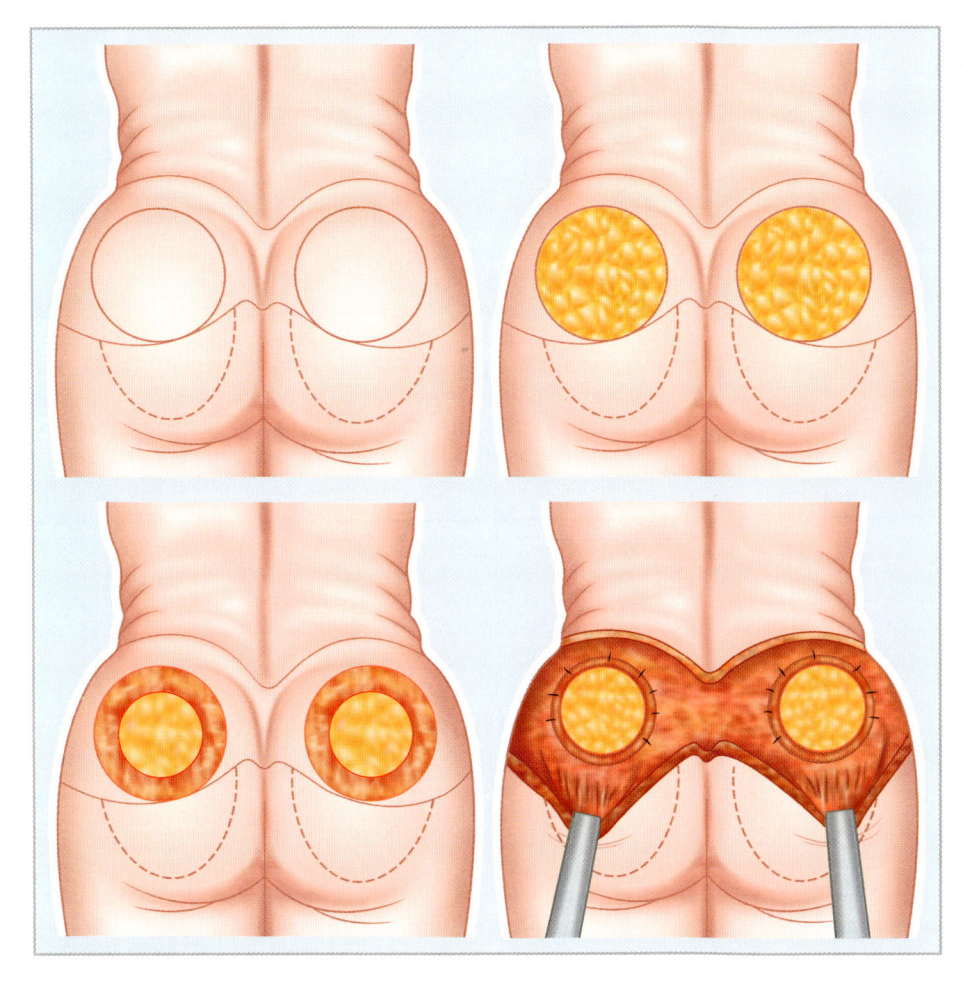

Figure 16.7 Island autologus gluteal augmentation flap design. (a,b) The island flap is outlined and de-epithelialized. (c) The flap dissection is beveled down through the superficial fascial system (SFS) and lumbosacral gluteal fascia, and surrounding excess tissue is removed down to the level of the lumbosacral fascia. This creates the two dermal 'islands' of tissue. (d) The superior half of each island is imbricated (dermis to SFS), and the islands are anchored to the gluteal fascia at the desired level. As the inferior circumferential body lift (CBL) skin flap is elevated and advanced over the autologous gluteal augmentation (AGA) flap, the overlying CBL and underlying AGA flaps are attached together with no. 1 Vicryl Plus quilting sutures to reduce dead space. (Redrawn with permission from Conteno.[27])

REFERENCES

1. Montagu A. The buttocks and natural selection. *JAMA* 1966;**198**:169.
2. De la Pena JA. Subfascial technique for gluteal augmentation. *Aesthet Surg J* 2004;**24**:265–73.
3. Babuccu O, Gozil R, Ozman S, et al. Gluteal region morphology: the effect of the weight gain and aging. Aesthetic Plast Surg 2002;**26**:130–3.
4. Conteno RF, Young VL. Clinical anatomy in aesthetic gluteal body contouring surgery. *Clin Plast* Surg 2006;**33**:347–358.
5. Lockwood TE. Superficial fascial system (SFS) of the trunk and extremities: a new concept. *Plast Recontr Surg* 1991;**87**:1019–27.
6. Da Rocha RP. Surgical anatomy of the gluteal region's subcutaneous screen and its use in the plastic surgery. *Aesthet Plast Surg* 2001;**25**:140–4.
7. Taylor GI. The angiosomes of the body and their supply to perforator flaps. *Clin Plast Surg* 2003;**30**:331–42.
8. Kopelman PG. The effects of weight loss treatments on upper and lower body fat. *Int J Obes* 1997;**21**:619–25.
9. Colwell AS, Borud LJ. Autologous gluteal augmentation after massive weight loss: aesthetic analysis and role of the superior gluteal artery perforator flap. *Plast Recontr Surg* 2007;**119**:345–6.
10. Fabris de Souza SA, Faintuch J, Valezi AC, et al. Postural changes in morbidly obese patients. *Obes Surg* 2005;**15**:1013–16.
11. Conteno RF, Mendieta CG, Young LV. Gluteal contouring surgery in the massive weight loss patient. *Clin Plast Surg* 2008;**35**:73–91.
12. Mendieta CG. Classification system for gluteal evaluation. *Clin Plast Surg* 2006;**33**:333–45.
13. Gonzalez, R. Etiology, definition, and classification of gluteal ptosis. *Aesth Plast Surg* 2006;**30**:320–6.
14. Aiache AE. Gluteal recontouring with combination treatments: Implants, liposuction, and fat transfer. *Clin Plast Surg* 2006;**33**:395–403.
15. Harrison D, Selvaggi G. Gluteal augmentation surgery: indications and surgical management: *J Plast Reconstr Aesthet Surg* 2007;**60**:922–8.
16. Bruner TW, Roberts TL III, Nguyen K. Complications of buttocks augmentation: diagnosis, management and prevention. *Clin Plast Surg* 2006;**33**:449–66.
17. Mendieta CG. Gluteoplasty. *Aesthet Surg J* 2003;**23**:441–55.
18. Mendieta CG. Intramuscular gluteal augmentation technique. *Clin Plast Surg* 2006;**33**:423–34.
19. Vergara R, Amezcua H. Intramusclar gluteal implants: fifteen years' experience. *Aesthet Surg J* 2003;**23**:86–91.
20. De la Pena JA, Rubio OV, Cano JP, et al. Subfascial gluteal augmentation. *Clin Plast Surg* 2006;**33**:405–22.
21. Gonzalez M, Guerrerosantos J. Deep planed torso-abdominoplasty combined with buttocks pexy. *Aesthet Plast Surg* 1997;**21**:245–53.
22. Guerrerosantos J. Secondary hip-buttock-thigh plasty. *Clin Plast Surg* 1984;**11**:491–503.
23. Pitanguy I. Surgical reduction of the abdomen, thighs and buttocks. *Surg Clin North Am* 1971;**51**:479–89.
24. Pascal JF, Le Louarn C. Remodeling Body lift with high lateral tension. *Aesthet Plast Surg* 2002;**26**:223–30.
25. Regnault P, Daniel R. Secondary thigh-buttock deformities after classical techniques: prevention and treatment. *Clin Plast Surg* 1984;**11**:505–16
26. Strauch B, Vasconez LO, Hall-Findlay EJ. *Grabb's Encyclopedia of Flaps*, 2nd edn. Philadelphia, PA: Lippincott-Raven, 1988.
27. Conteno RF. Autologous gluteal augmentation with circumferential body lift in the massive weight loss and aesthetic patient. *Clin Plast Surg* 2006;**33**:479–96.

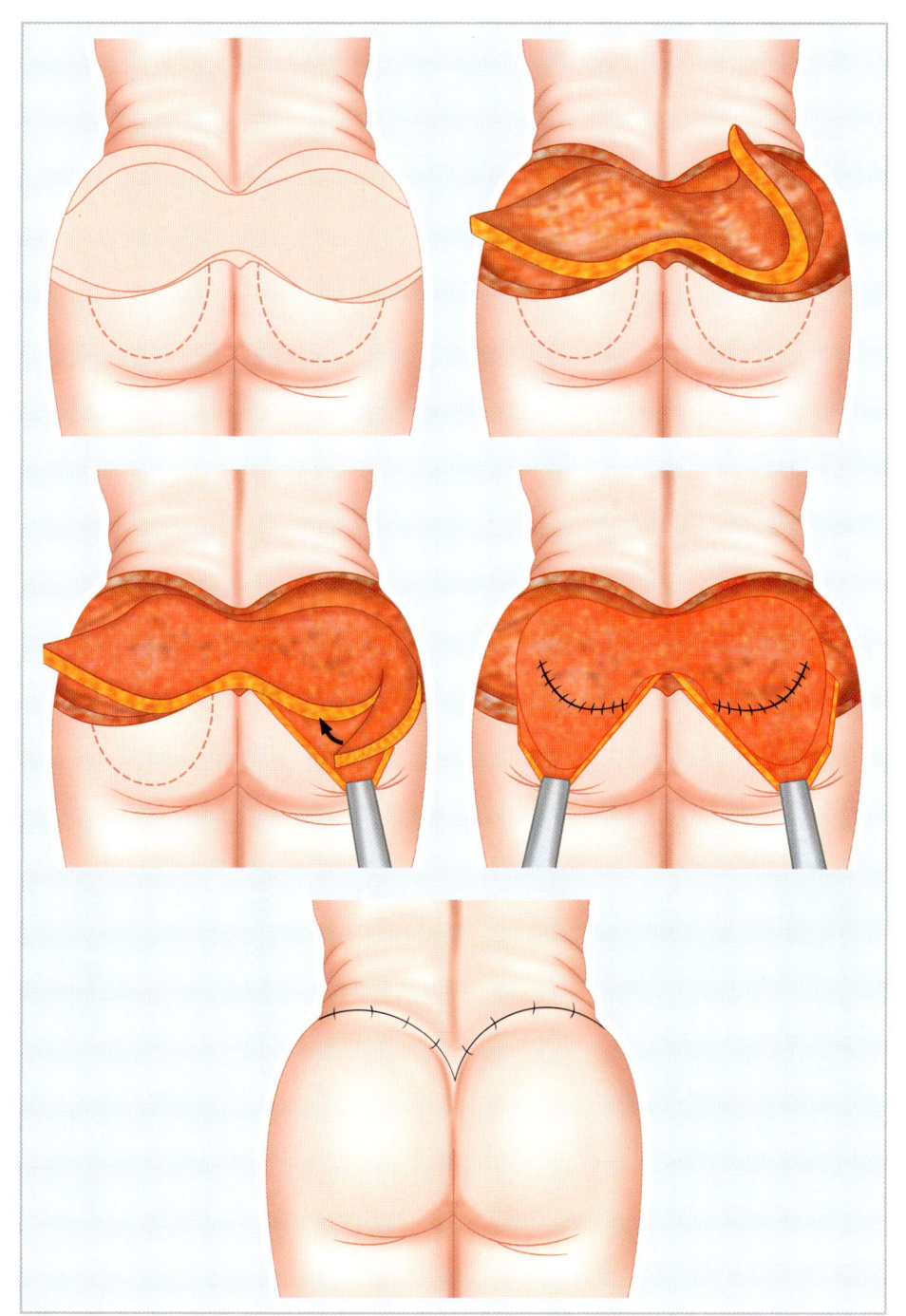

Figure 16.8 Moustache flap design. (a) Outline of the moustache flap shows placement of the central bridge of tissue and lateral flap extensions, or handlebars. (b) The flap is de-epithelialized, and the moustache handlebars are elevated from the fascia. (c) The handlebars are rotated medially, any excess lateral tissue is trimmed off, and the flap is imbricated to itself laterally to prevent trochanteric fullness. (d) The rotated flaps are fixed centrally to the gluteal fascia with no. 1 Vicryl Plus and imbricated to create an anatomic mound of tissue. (e) A closed moustache flap with sparse stapling. (Redrawn with permission from Conteno.[27])

Chapter 17

Medial and lateral thigh surgery after massive weight loss

Susan E. Downey

The thigh of the post-massive weight (MWL) loss patient continues to be one of the most challenging areas for both the patient and the plastic surgeon. After MWL, the thigh probably has the poorest cosmetic improvement as well as the highest complication rate. As with all other areas of the MWL body there are wide variations in presentation. A few MWL patients who carried their weight primarily in the truncal area will have only a slight upper medial thigh laxity. At the other end of the spectrum, there are patients who despite MWL continue to have disproportionately large non-deflated legs. The full range and every variation in between can be seen.

EVALUATION OF THE PATIENT

As with any MWL patient no one surgical plan will fit all patients. The first step is evaluation of the patient. Borud[1] has classified post-MWL into three types. Type 1 has near or complete deflation of the medial thigh with no fatty excess. The skin excess is limited to the upper third of the thigh. Type 2 also has little or no fatty excess but has significant skin excess extending down the length of the thigh.' Type 3 has significant residual fat excess without complete deflation. Strauch and Herman[2] have further classified the post-MWL thighs in two types: Cone or cylindrical in shape. They describe the cone shape as superior or proximal excess with little or no distal excess. Cylindrically shaped thighs have significant horizontal and vertical excess skin, with ptosis that extends down to the knee.

HISTORY

Medial thigh lift was first introduced by John Lewis in 1957.[3] In 1971 Pitanguay[4] described a horizontal incision designed to lie under the bathing suit line. As he did with the lower body lift, Lockwood[5] advanced the treatment of the thigh with his description in 1988 of the superficial fascial system and a superficial anchoring technique that led to a decrease in complications. There were, however, very few advances or even interest in thighplasties until the late 1990s. This corresponded with the increase in obesity and concurrent rise in bariatric procedures. This then led to a large number of MWL patients entering plastic surgeons' offices. The American Society for Aesthetic Plastic Surgery, in their annual statistics report,[6] show an increase in the number of thighplasties performed increasing from 2895 in 1997 to 15 366 in 2010.

CRESCENT MEDIAL THIGH LIFT

For patients who fall into the Borud type 1 with skin excess limited to the upper third of the thigh, a crescent-shaped medial thighplasty can be considered. Care must be taken in appropriately choosing patients for this procedure, because it removes tissue only in one direction vertically. Any excess in the horizontal dimension will not be addressed. If the patient has excess in this dimension as well, he or she may be disappointed with the outcome. Markings are made with the patient in the standing position, with the proposed incision line in the groin crease. The excess to be removed is then grasped and the markings for the proposed excision are drawn. These markings are just an estimate of the tissue to be removed and, before cutting away the excess in the operating room, the ability to close the wound should be confirmed and the resection adjusted as needed. As this excision is an elliptical one, the upper line is shorter than the lower line. This can lead to bunching or pleating of the incision line which may take months to resolve. The patient should therefore be forewarned about this. The major drawbacks to this procedure are (1) inadequate resection, (2) pulling down or distortion of the labia, and (3) inferior migration of the scar. All these are serious complications or sequelae, and all attempts should be made to avoid their occurrence. Inadequate resection is avoided by careful patient selection. Patients with vertical and horizontal excess would be better treated with a vertical as well as a horizontal excision. Distortion of the labia can be avoided or lessened by use of the superficial anchoring technique, as described by Lockwood, or by placing the scar and therefore more of the tension lower on the thigh. This can, however, lead to a more visible scar and also result in inferior migration of the scar over time (**Fig. 17.1**). Patients need to know that the scar may migrate and will most likely be visible in a bathing suit no matter where it is placed in the groin area.

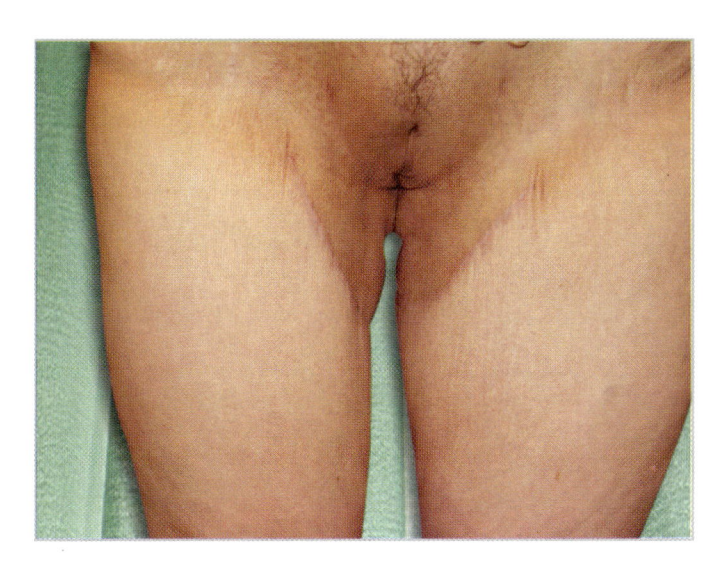

Figure 17.1 Inferior descent of medial thigh scar.

First-stage debulking

For patients who fit into the Borud type 2 classification with residual excess fat, a primary thigh lift will not give an adequate improvement in contour. Usually a first-stage aggressive liposuction of the fat excess is necessary. Following deflation then the patient can if they wish undergo an extended thigh lift. A minimum waiting period should elapse between the deflation and the thighplasty, but most patients are so pleased with the improvement in contour and the new proportions of their body that this is not usually an inconvenience (**Figs 17.2** and **17.3**).

EXTENDED MEDIAL THIGH LIFT

For patients who fall into the Borud type 2 classification, little or no fatty excess, but significant skin excess extending in the circumferential dimension all the way down the thigh, an extended thighplasty is the recommended procedure. This involves a scar extending down the medial aspect of the thigh from the groin crease to the knee. In a few patients the scar can be shortened to midthigh, not going all the way to the knee, but this is not the case for most patients. Extension all the way to the knee is necessary to remove the excess skin. As with most procedures after MWL the tradeoff of the scar for the improvement in contour should be considered. For patients with minimal excess skin, the scar may not be acceptable. For patients with a lot of excess skin the scar will be a very acceptable alternative (**Figs 17.4** and **17.5**; **17.6–17.11**).

Initial approaches to this area involved a horizontal and vertical scar meeting in a T at the highest point of the incision. This led to high rates of complications with a lot of tension on the T juncture, especially when sitting, and consequent wound breakdown in this area. Although the scar may be more visible in the slightly more anterior position, placing the scar slightly more anteriorly takes the tension off the scar when the patient is sitting. This reduces the risk of wound breakdown. Another advance that decreases the risk of wound breakdown is to avoid the T juncture and instead make the incision line a gentle curve, extending from the knee and sliding slightly forward as it curves into the groin crease.

Cram and Aly describe a technique that involves extensive liposuction of the area to be excised before skin removal.[7] In their technique, after marking the patient in the standing position, extensive liposuction is carried out of the elliptical area to be excised. As the skin of this area

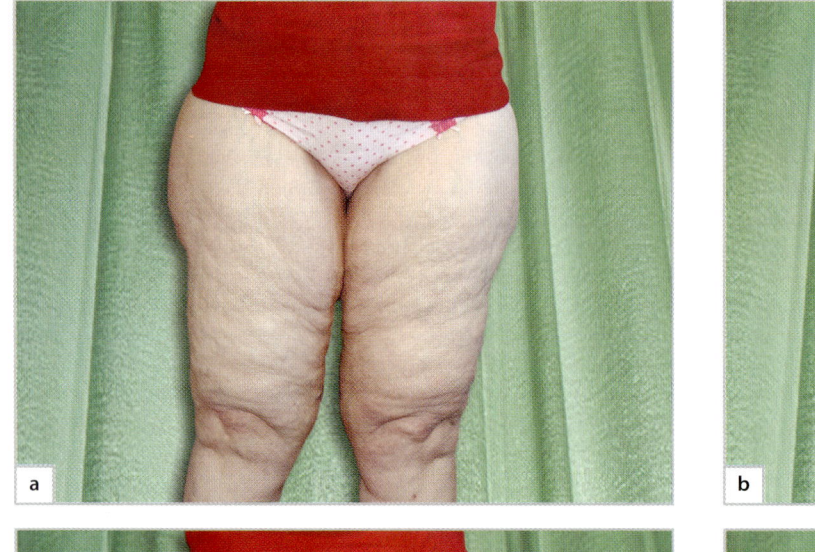

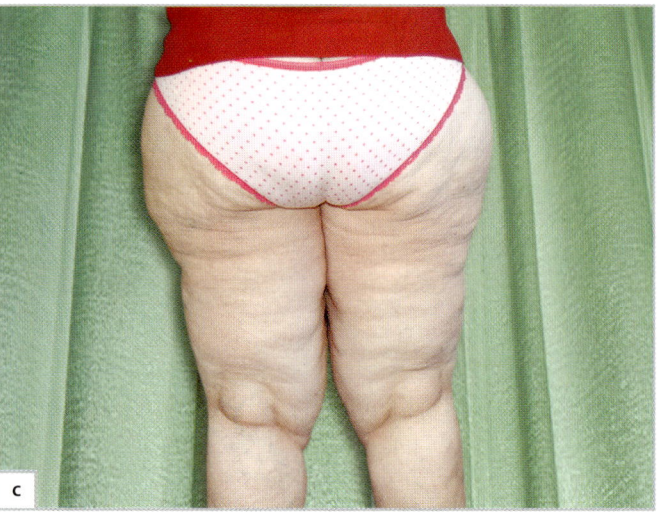

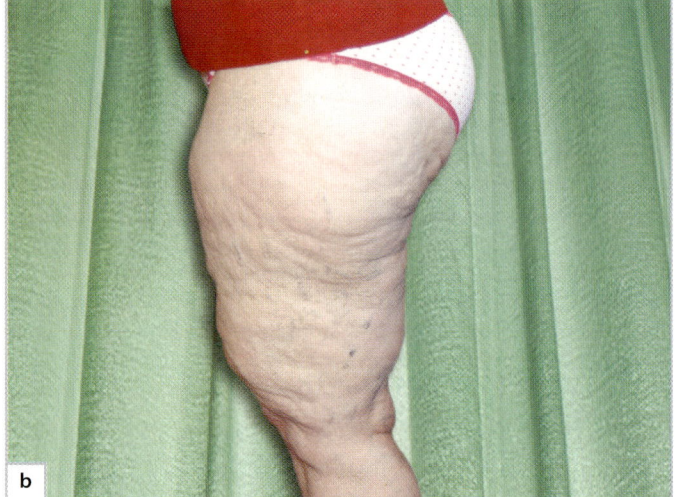

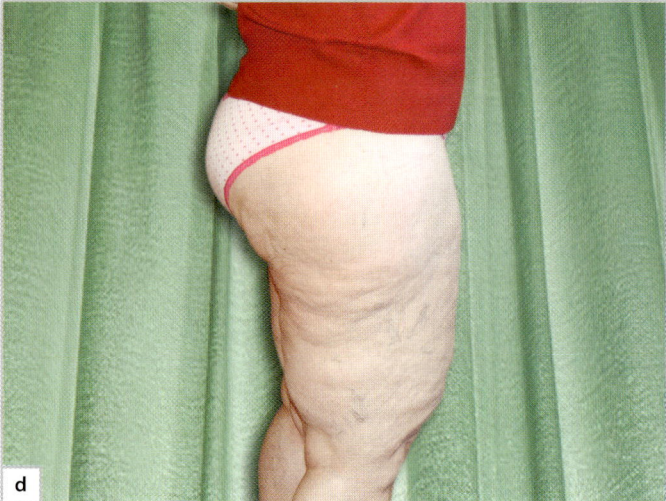

Figure 17.2 A 55-year-old after 72 kg (160 lb) weight loss with minimal deflation of thighs.

Extended medial thigh lift 155

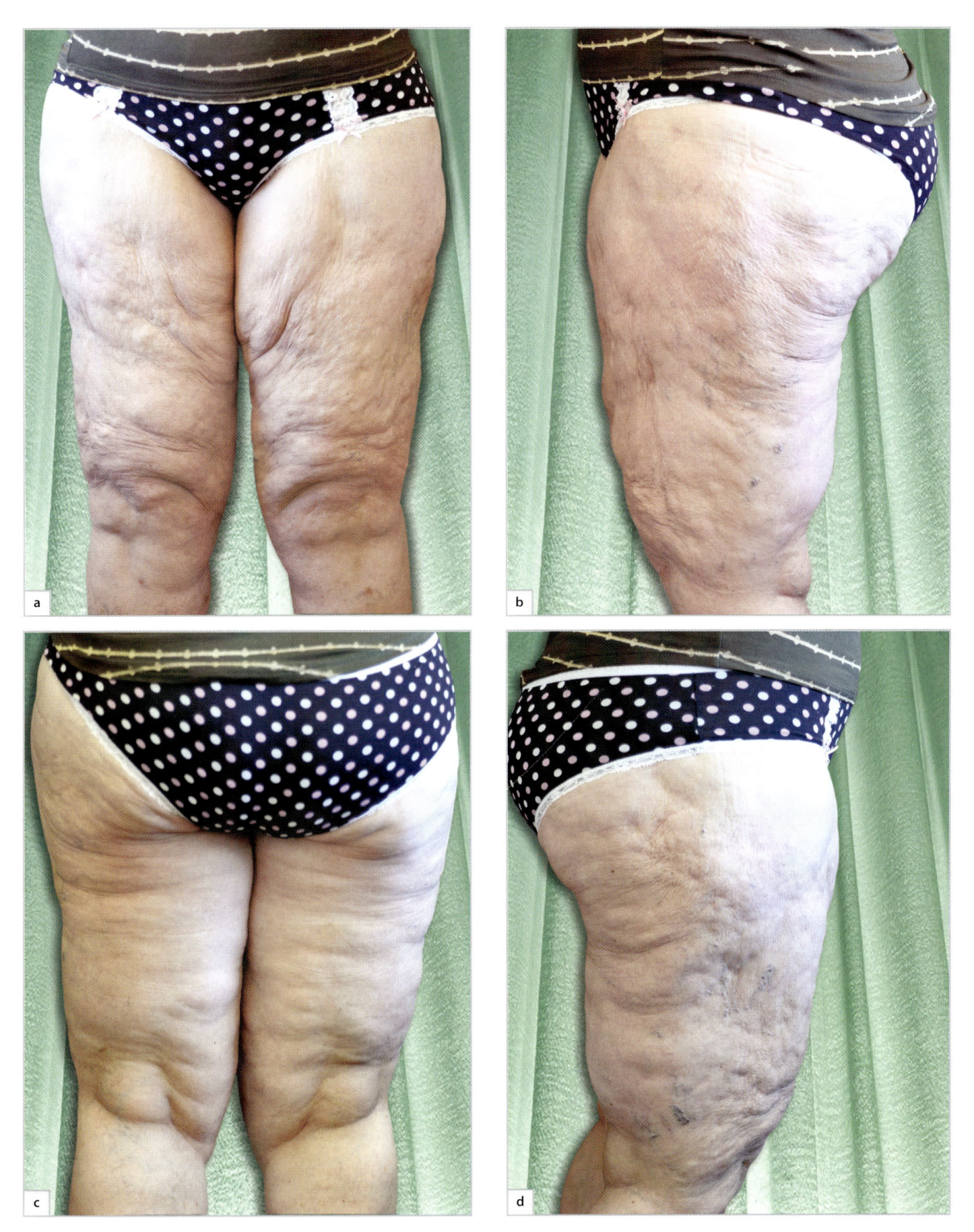

Figures 17.3 Same patient as Fig. 17.2: one year postoperatively after 2025 ml lipoaspirate from left thigh and 2160 ml lipoaspirate from right leg.

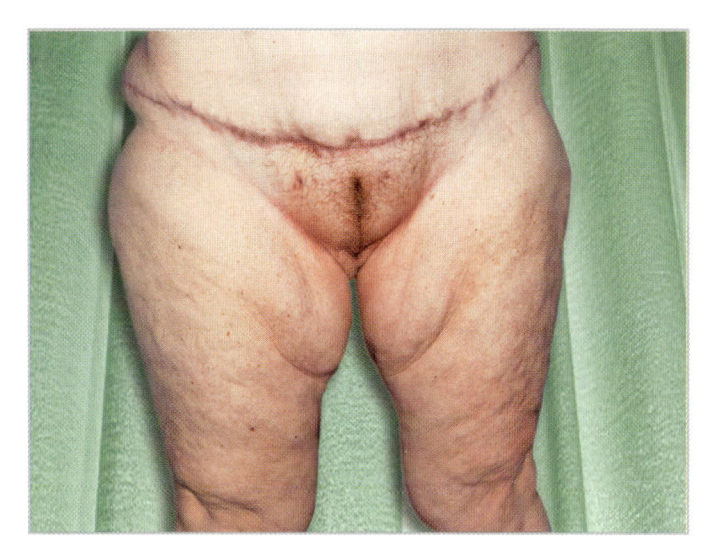

Figure 17.4 A 51-year-old after 45 kg (100 lb) weight loss.

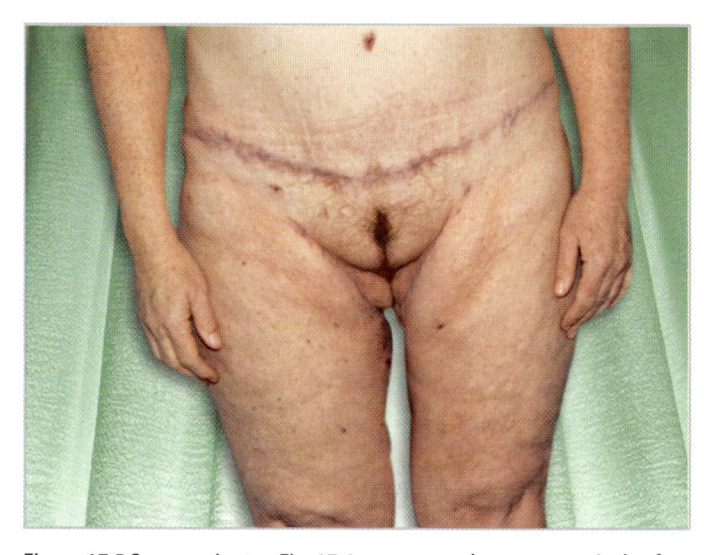

Figure 17.5 Same patient as Fig. 17.4: seven months postoperatively after extended medial thighplasty.

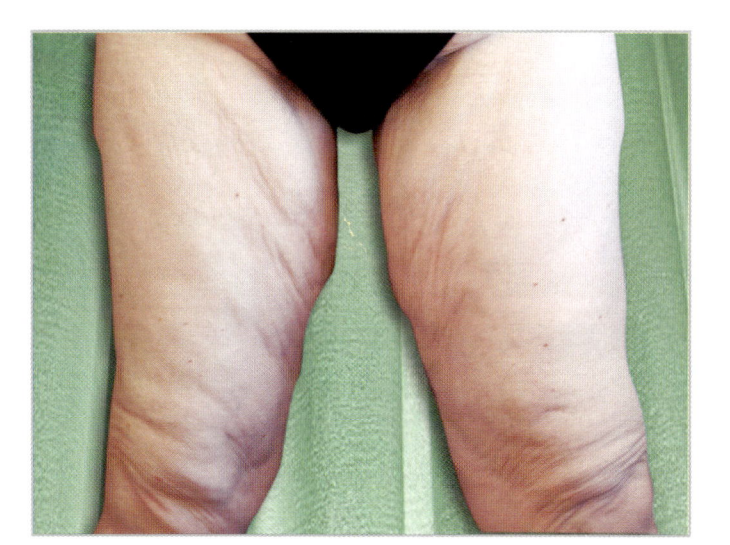

Figure 17.6 A 53-year-old after 48.6 kg (108 lb) weight loss.

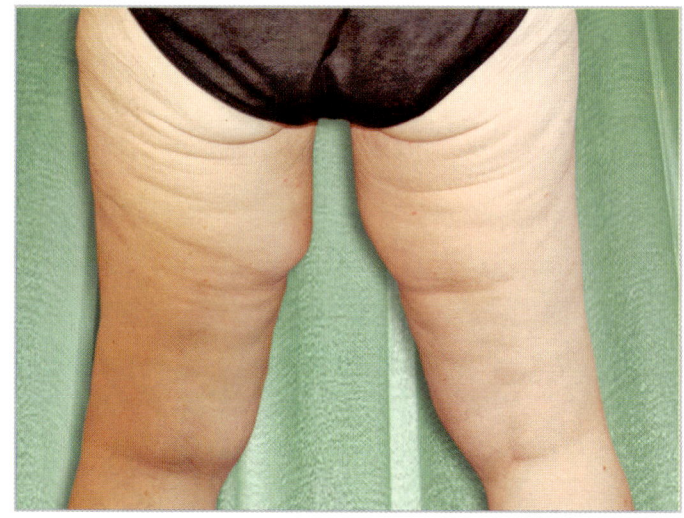

Figure 17.7 Same patient as Fig. 17.6: preoperative posterior view.

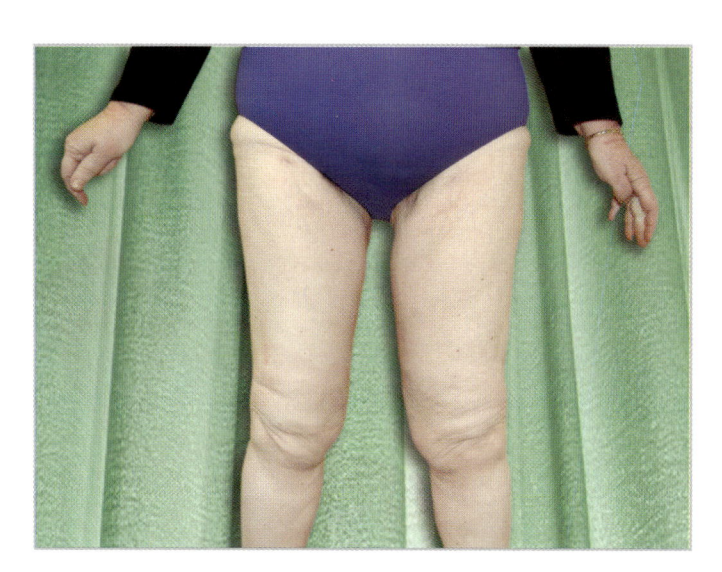

Figure 17.8 Same patient as Fig. 17.6: three months postoperatively after extended medial thighplasty.

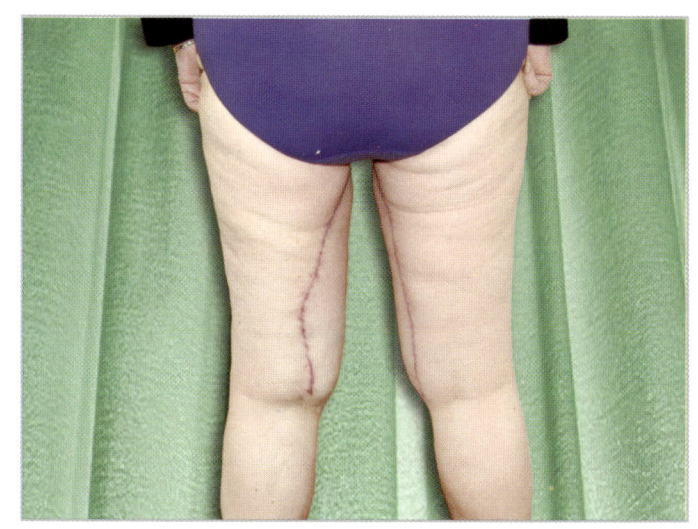

Figure 17.9 Same patient as Fig. 17.6: posterior view 3 months after extended medial thighplasty.

Extended medial thigh lift 157

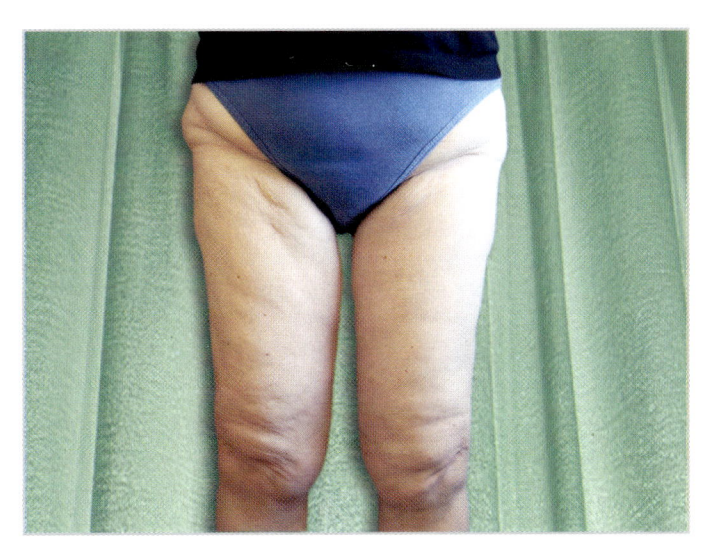

Figure 17.10 Same patient as Fig. 17.6: fifteen months postoperatively after extended medial thighplasty.

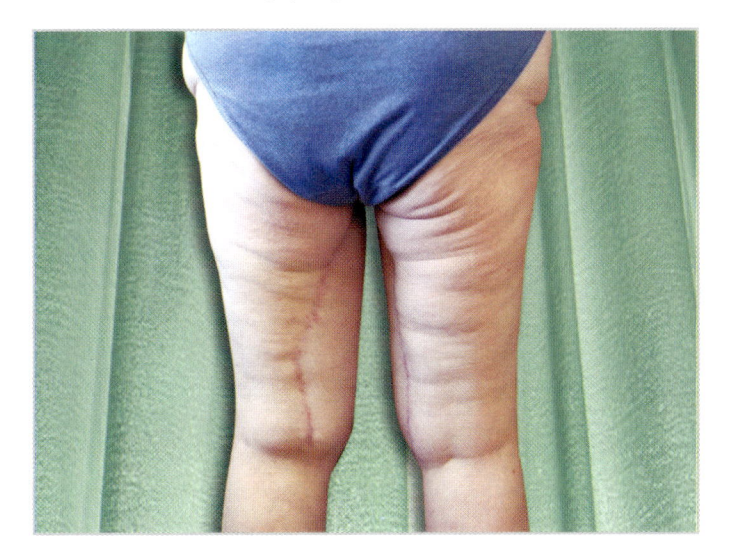

Figure 17.11 Same patient as Fig. 17.6: posterior view 15 months after extended medial thighplasty.

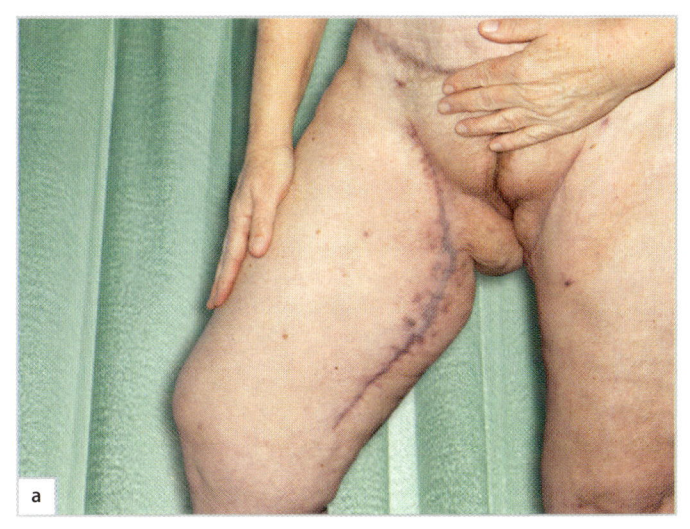

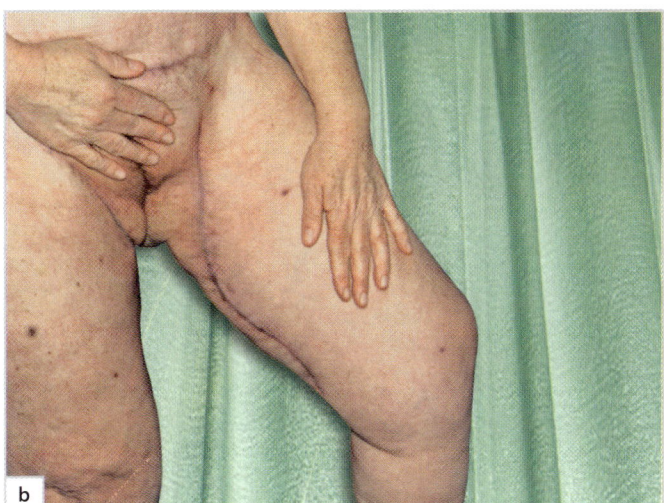

Figures 17.12 Medial thighplasty scars demonstrating gentle C curve of incision.

is to be excised the liposuction can be aggressive. At the end of the liposuction the remaining skin should be quite thin. The thin skin is then excised in an elliptical manner. This technique removes skin only in one dimension. Any resultant dog ear is then worked out posteriorly into the perineal crease mark which becomes the inferior buttock crease.

An alternative method that avoids a posterior extension of the incision is the gentle C excision mentioned above (**Fig. 17.12**). The patient is again marked in the standing erect position with a vertical incision then gently curving into an anterior incision in the groin crease. Markings are again done in the standing position. The loose medial thigh skin is pulled forward and a vertical line is drawn, which will be the final incision line. The excess skin is then pinched and the area to be excised marked. In this technique, liposuction is not done but direct excision of both skin and fat is carried out. Incision should first be done on the posterior line, which will eventually be the final scar position. The anterior line can then be adjusted if the original marking of the amount of tissue to be excised turns out to have been overly optimistic.

As with all other procedures for the post-MWL patient, the scar is a tradeoff for the improvement in contour. Patients may not want a scar down to their knees, but if their excess skin extends this far they will not have the improvement in contour that they also wish for if they do not have an extended scar. Patients will often demonstrate the improvement that they wish for by pulling up on the skin and fat and asking: 'Why can't you just do this?' The explanation is that the excess is in two dimensions, not just one, and without two-dimensional excision, the excess skin and fat will not be adequately addressed. A minority of patients can have a limited vertical resection because their excess truly does not extend to the knees. Even for these patients, it should be pointed out that the medial thigh scar may be visible in skirts, because skirts rise when a woman sits and more of the leg becomes visible even if the skirt is knee-length when standing.

Surgical procedure

The critical markings must be done as with all MWL patients when the patient is in the standing position before going to the operating room (**Fig. 17.13**). In patients who have lost extensive amounts of weight, in particular, the laxity of the skin makes marking while the patient is

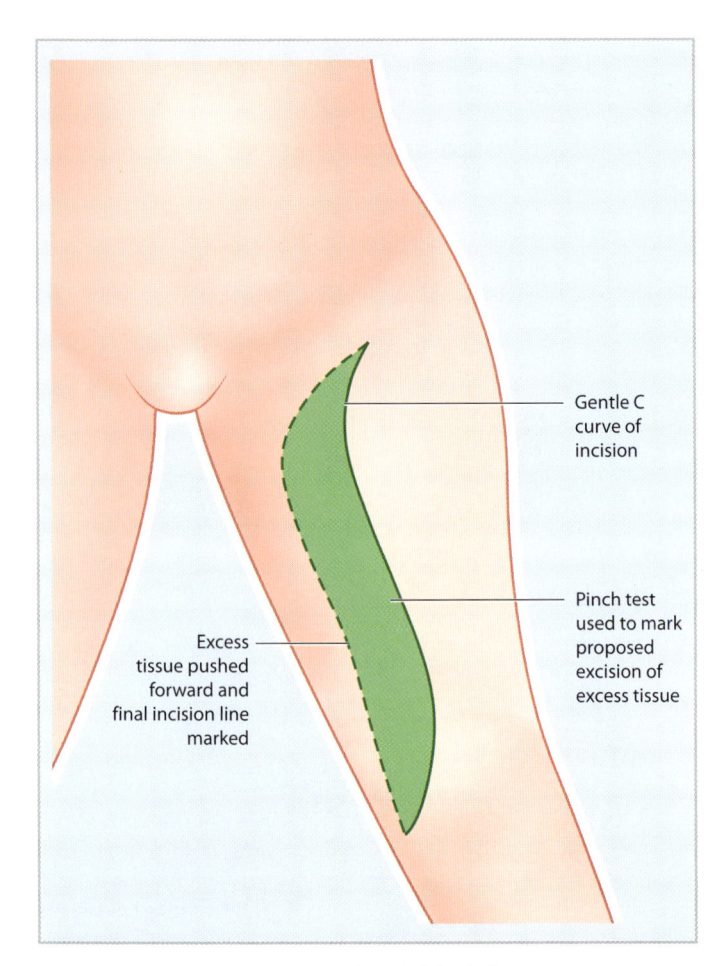

Figure 17.13 Markings for extended medial thighplasty.

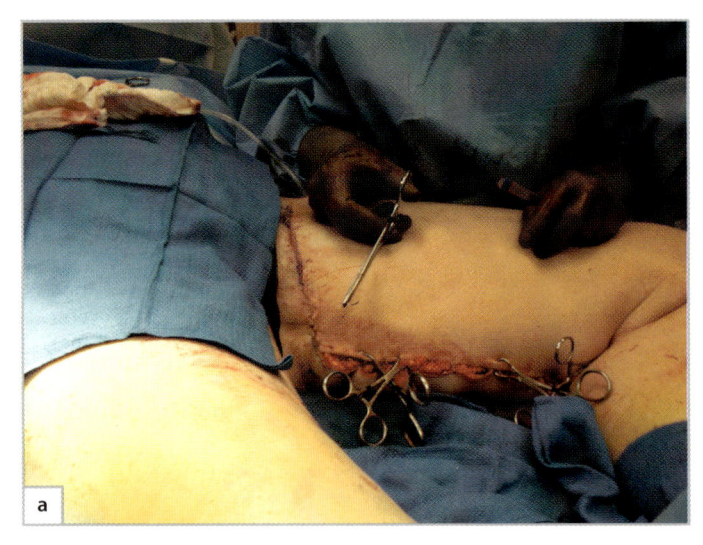

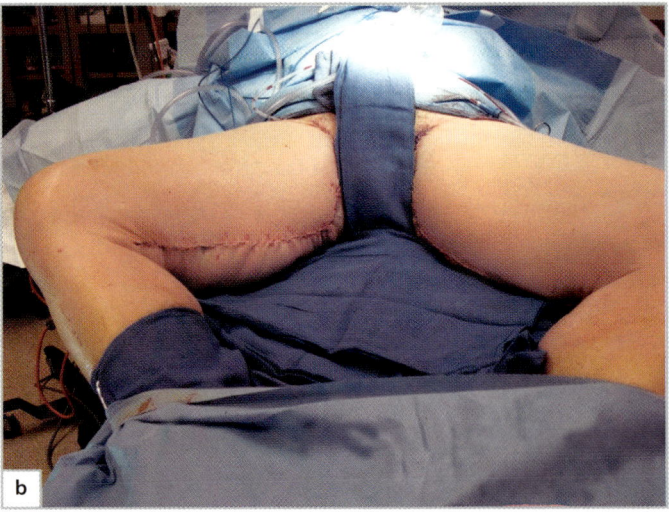

Figures 17.14 Frog-leg position of patient in operating room for medial thighplasty.

asleep extremely difficult. With the patient in the standing position and the legs slightly separated, the loose skin of the medial thigh is pulled forward and a vertical line is drawn from the groin area down the middle of the thigh to the knee. This line represents the final position of the scar. The incision is then marked to curve lightly anterior and up into the groin crease. Placing the scar slightly more anteriorly will decrease the risk of wound breakdown and takes some tension off the incision line when the patient is seated, especially on a toilet. The loose skin is then pulled back and an estimate of the amount to be resected is drawn. The actual amount to be resected is determined in the operating room but a close estimate can be done with this method. Asymmetries, which are the rule rather than the exception, can be reviewed again in the operating room.

Positioning in the operating room continues to be a problem. Supine and frog-legged is probably the most common approach (**Fig. 17.14**), but many different devices and supports such as gynecologist's or orthopedic stirrups have been tried. Once the patient has been positioned on the operating table, the posterior (or final scar position) incision is made. Dissection is carried down to the fascia overlying the thigh muscles, and the anterior skin and fat are then mobilized. During the resection care should be taken to preserve the saphenous vein if encountered. The skin and fat are then draped over the final incision line and the excess is resected in a tailor-tack method. This method avoids the potential to over-resect. Once the excess has been excised, the wound can be closed over a drain. The drain may be less uncomfortable if it exits through the uppermost end of the incision. Several recent advances have made closure easier on the surgeon. First the use of barbed sutures can greatly reduce the closure time.[8] Second the use of surgical glue protects by sealing the wound, especially in an easily contaminated area.

Garments are not generally used if a fully extended thighplasty is done because it can pinch vulnerable skin, roll up, or otherwise make it difficult to examine the wound. The drain is left in until the drainage has decreased to a reasonable amount. Sitting for long periods during the immediate postoperative period is discouraged. Patients should be encouraged to either stand or recline but avoid sitting on a hard surface unless on the toilet or at the dinner table.

LATERAL THIGH

Many patients who have lost a large amount of weight present with residual lateral excess often referred to as 'saddlebags.' These may be small in nature or extensive. These fat deposits can be addressed at the same time as the medial thigh or separately. Certainly this area needs to be assessed on its own, because, for some patients, the excess fat in this area can make them look heavier than they are or, in the case of some male patients, large saddlebags may feminize their contour (**Fig 17.15a**).

Small areas of fat deposits can be treated with liposuction as in the non-MWL patient. Significant lipodystrophies or large saddlebags may be addressed as direct excisions (**Fig. 17.15b**). These can be done as a stand-alone procedure or together with a lateral excision along the entire torso. If the procedure is done as a stand-alone procedure, the lateral excision can also be incorporated into the thigh excision at a later time.

Direct excision of the lateral thigh area is done in a wedge-shaped manner. Markings are made in the standing position before going to the operating room. The procedure is most easily carried out with the patient in the lateral position. If this area of lipodystrophy is large, there may be a component of lymphedema. A drain may therefore be needed, because leaving the wound undrained could lead to wound disruption.

■ COMPLICATIONS

Thighplasties probably have the highest number of complications of all the procedures done on MWL patients. Complication rates have been reported to be as high as 29%.[9] Hematomas can occur frequently in thighplasties. Bruschi et al. reported a hematoma complication rate of 14%.[10] This may be related to the position of the incision line and stress on the area when the patient sits. As with other body-contouring procedures for the MWL population, a hematoma may become quite large due to the extreme stretchability of the skin. Large hematomas will require a return to the operating room for evacuation. Careful monitoring will allow a hematoma to be addressed early, which will minimize the sequela.

Seroma rates have also been reported to be as high as 4%,[11] and lymphoceles as a complication of thighplasty.[12] Both of these are difficult problems. Serial aspiration and possibly injection of a sclerosing substance such as doxycycline are the first-line defense. If the seroma or lymphocele persists, a return to the operating room, excision of the capsule, and closure over a drain may be necessary. In persistent cases, injection of lymhazurin and inspection of the wound for a lymphatic leak that can then be oversewn may be required.

Wound breakdown is also a common problem (**Fig. 17.16**). This is most likely due to the location of the incision line near to the genital area, as well as to tension on the incision when the patient sits. Placing the incision in a more anterior location will help minimize the risk of wound breakdown. If wound breakdown occurs this is

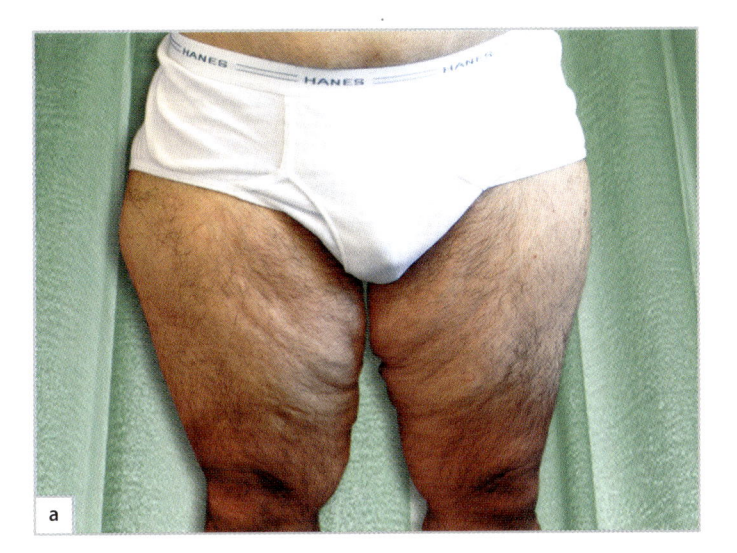

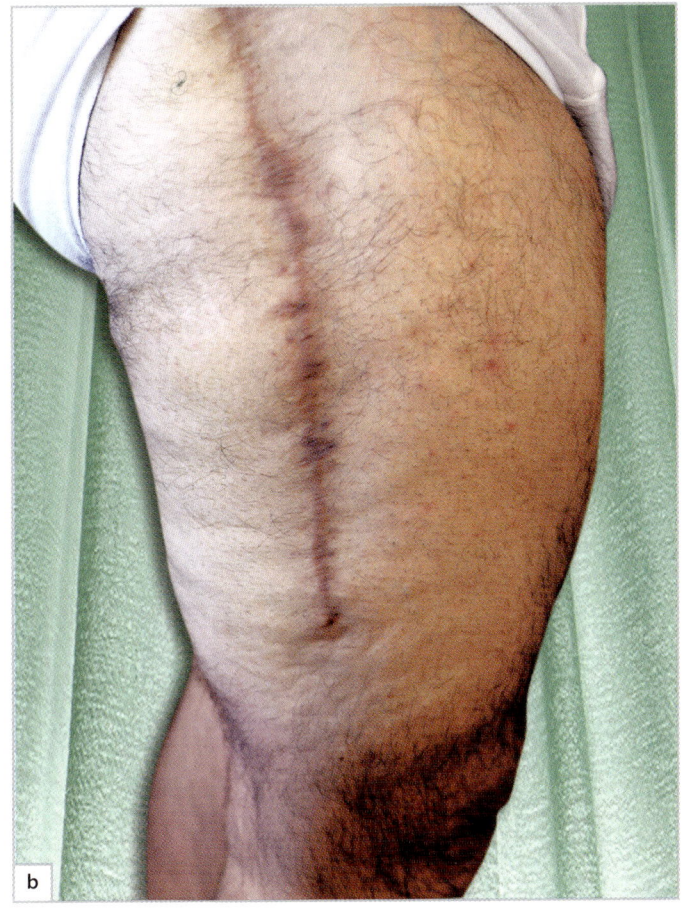

Figure 17.15 (a) A 41-year-old man after 76.5 kg (170 lb) weight loss. (b) A 3-month follow-up after lateral thigh direct excisions.

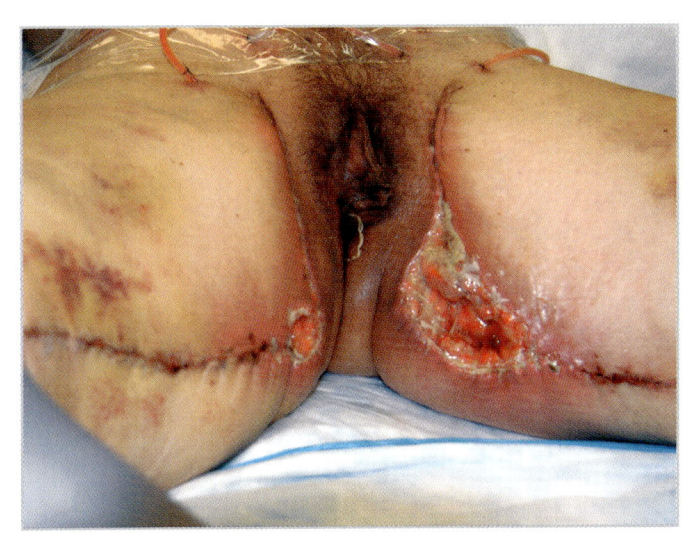

Figure 17.16 Wound dehiscence after extended medial thighplasty.

most commonly at the highest point of the incision. Making both a vertical and a horizontal incision greatly increases the risk of breakdown in this area. A gentle curved incision, which is placed slightly lower than the groin crease, is less prone to breakdown. If wound breakdown does occur there may be an extended period of healing and a return trip to the operating room for reclosure or, in severe cases, skin grafting may be required (**Figs 17.17** and **17.18**).

Labial spreading is a significant concern with thighplasties. It can occur due to excess tension on the groin closure. Lockwood's technique of anchoring to Colles fascia in the aging patient diminishes this complication. In the MWL patient, placing the scar slightly inferior to the actual groin crease will avoid tension on the labia and minimize the risk of tension pulling the labia inferiorly.

Some patients after thighplasties are not satisfied with their aesthetic improvement. Cellulite is a common problem in the thighs and probably contributes to this issue. Preoperatively patients may pull their thigh skin tight and believe that this is how their skin will look after surgery. Preoperative counseling needs to address this issue and give the patients a more realistic idea of the outcome.

CONCLUSION

Improvements in techniques have led to a decrease in the complications for thighplasties. Careful patient selection is necessary to achieve the best possible cosmetic outcome as well as a satisfied patient. The medial as well as the lateral aspects of the thigh need to be evaluated and possibly treated. Some patients may benefit from extensive liposuction if their thighs are not adequately deflated despite MWL. Careful evaluation and surgical planning will result in the best surgical outcome for both the surgeon and the patient.

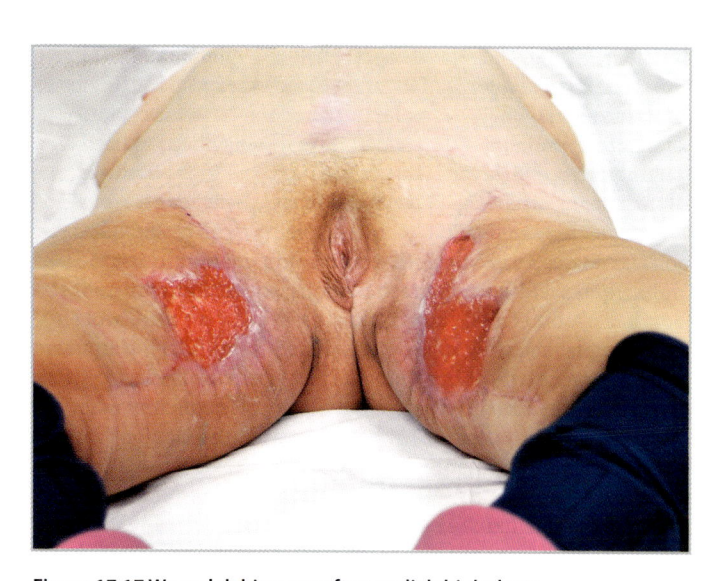

Figure 17.17 Wound dehiscence after medial thighplasty.

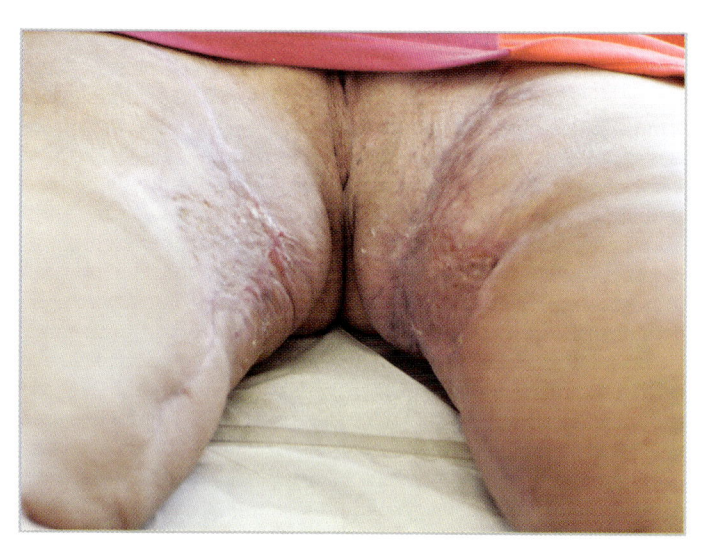

Figure 17.18 Skin grafting of medial thigh dehiscence.

REFERENCES

1. Borud I, ed. Thigh Lift. In: *Atlas of Body Contouring After Weight Loss*. Woodbury: Cine-Med Publishing, 2008, pp.144–87.
2. Strauch B, Herman CK, eds. Medial thigh contouring: Cones and cylinders. In: *Encyclopedia of Body Sculpting after Massive Weight Loss*. New York: Thième, 2011, pp.265–71.
3. Lewis JR Jr. The thigh lift. *J Int Coll Surg* 1957;**27**:330–4.
4. Pitanguy I. Surgical reduction of the abdomen, thigh and buttocks. *Surg Clin North Am* 1971;**51**:479–89
5. Lockwood TE. Fascial anchoring technique in medial thigh lifts. *Plast Reconstr Surg* 1988;**82**:299–304.
6. American Society of Aesthetic Plastic Surgery. *Cosmetic Surgery National Data Bank Statistics*. ASAPS, 2010. Available at: www.surgery.org/media/statistics (accessed June 11, 2012).
7. Cram A, Aly A. Lower extremity body contouring after massive weight loss. In: Aly A (ed.), *Body Contouring after Massive Weight Loss*. St Louis, MO: Quality Medical Publishing, 2006, pp.213–36.
8. Hurwitz DJ, Reuben B. Quill barbed sutures in body contouring surgery: a six year comparison study with running absorbable braided sutures, *Plast Reconstr Surg* 2011;**128**(4 suppl):62–3.
9. Ellaban MG, Hart NB. Body Contouring by combined abdominoplasty and medial vertical thigh reduction: experience of 14 cases. *Br J Plast Surg* 2004;**28**:20–3.
10. Bruschi S, Datta G, Bocchiotti MA, Boriani F, Obbialero FD, Fraccalvieri M. Limb contouring after massive weight loss: Functional rather than aesthetic improvement. *Obes Surg* 2009;**19**:407–11.
11. Shermak MA, Rotellini-Coltvet LA, Chang D Seroma development following body contouring surgery for massive weight loss : patient risk factors and treatment strategies. *Plast Reconstr Surg* 2008;**122**:280–8.
12. Leitner DW, Sherwood RC. Inguinal lymhocele as a complication of thighplasty. *Plast Reconstr Surg* 1983;**72**:878–81.

Chapter 18
Facial contouring after bariatric surgery

Kenneth L. Fan, Benjamin T. Lemelman, Seth R. Thaller

INTRODUCTION

American obesity is an epidemic.[1] With low morbidity and mortality rates, bariatric surgery has been demonstrated to dramatically reduce medical comorbidities related to obesity, ever increasing the demand for the operation.[2,3] In 2007, 250 000 weight loss operations were performed. As a consequence, body-contouring procedures have been rising.[4] Massive weight loss (MWL), defined as deliberately loosing more than 100 lb (45 kg), leaves patients loose, ptotic skin envelopes and associated contour irregularities from residual adipose deposits.[5] These deformities result in functional difficulties in the form of intertriginous rash, compromised hygiene, skin breakdown, exacerbation of joint and back pain, and mobility issues. When MWL is characterized by a poor aesthetic outcome, psychological issues may develop. Surgical body contouring results in improved quality of life, self-perception, and body image, with reduction of anxiety and sexual dysfunction.[5,6] A study examining 70 gastric bypass patients found that around half underwent body-contouring procedures.[7] Most desired areas for contouring were unsurprisingly waist/abdomen, rear/buttock, upper arms, and chest/breast. These issues are addressed with abdominoplasty, belt lipectomy, brachioplasty, and mastopexy.

However, 20% of MWL patients also desire facial contouring.[7] Postbariatric face/neck requires specialized surgical management. Weight loss leaves significant skin laxity and soft-tissue malposition, giving the appearance of accelerated aging. The mechanics and physiology of remnant tissue differ from those of the 'normal' aged face.[8] Skin from MWL tends to be thicker, but less elastic and pliable.[9] Extracellular matrix is damaged, marked by poorly organized collagen structure, elastin degradation, and scar formation, all of which correlate poorly with actual age.[10,11] Special attention needs to be paid with to the MWL patient who desires facial contouring. This chapter attempts to address these issues.

PREOPERATIVE EVALUATION OF THE BODY-CONTOURING PATIENT

Body weight should remain stable for 2 months until a body-contouring procedure is considered, corresponding to 12–18 months after gastric bypass.[12] Surgical complications have been shown to be decreased with less pre-panniculectomy body mass index (BMI).[13] Most recommend against body contouring in patients with a BMI > 32.[14,15] Nutritional and metabolic homeostasis are also achieved in the delay period. Extra time also affords skin contraction. Along with histological changes in tissue composition, this contraction process contributes to the decreased elasticity of postbariatric skin compared with similarly aged patients.[8,10,11] Improved aesthetic outcomes are achieved as operations are performed around the ideal body weight. Patients with a BMI around 28–32 have been shown to achieve better contouring outcome than those with a higher BMI.[15]

When evaluating a patient, medical morbidities must be examined. Benefits of bariatric surgery have been established. Even modest weight loss translates into improved glycemic control, reduced blood pressure, hemostatic factors, and serum lipids, as well as reduced cardiac events, cardiac mortality, and total mortality.[16,17] Reduction in sleep apnea, arthritis, and infertility is also seen. For diabetes mellitus, type 2 resistant to medical therapy, bariatric surgery has been proven to be the most effective in gaining complete control.[2] Obesity leads to increased incidence of heart failure, myocardial infarction, and other cardiovascular events. With MWL, regression in cardiac events, cardiac morbidity, and overall morbidity is observed.[16] Despite improvement in these disorders, complete resolution may not occur. Inherently, MWL patients are still overweight. This subjects patients to increased risk of postoperative complications.[13] Screening for certain morbidities associated with MWL is mandatory.

An increased incidence in depression and use of antidepressants has been noted.[12] Psychological screening, with consultation if necessary, should be performed. Up to 20% of patients may have unresolved type 2 diabetes after bariatric surgery. Serum glucose levels should be checked.[2] Oral hypoglycemics should be discontinued before surgery. Nicotine use has been associated with increased incidence of flap necrosis, infection, and wound-healing complications.[15] Through impaired wound healing, increased vasoconstriction, and deficient oxygen transport, smoking complicates rhytidectomy, among other elective procedures.[18–20] Postbariatric patients are subject to malabsorptive procedures, increasing the incidence of anemia, particularly in who still women menstruate.[15] Multiple procedures can lead to increased blood loss, worsening anemia, and risk of transfusion.[21] Iron and vitamin supplementation is encouraged. Adherence to the postbariatric nutritional program should also be recommended preoperatively to ensure vitamin, protein, and mineral supplementation for adequate wound healing.[14]

Facial contouring can be combined with other procedures at the plastic surgeon's discretion. To the best of our knowledge, there is a paucity of literature detailing the incidence of complications of combining facial contouring with other body-contouring procedures. However, performing three or more body-contouring procedures is associated with increased risk of blood transfusion and greater length of hospital stay.[21] Anecdotally, some authors recommended total surgical time limited to 6–7 hours, waiting 3 months between staged procedures.[14,22]

VENOUS THROMBOEMBOLISM PROPHYLAXIS

Venous thromboembolism (VTE) and its sequela threaten bariatric patients as the most common cause of mortality after body-contouring procedures.[21] The risk of deep vein thrombosis (DVT) is highest in the first and second weeks after surgery.[14] In a survey combining a total of 9937 rhytidectomies, 35 DVTs (0.35 %) and 14 pulmonary embolisms

(PEs; 0.14%) were recorded.[23] Among DVTs, 83.7% occurred under general anesthesia. However, this study did not exclusively examine MWL patients.

Most MWL patients would be classified as high risk (proximal DVT Incidence: 4–8%; clinical PE incidence: 2–4%) according to the American College of Chest Physician (ACCP) classification. This is related to risk factors, such as major surgery, age > 40 years, obesity (BMI > 30), and varicose veins.[24] These patients should receive low-dose unfractionated heparin (LUDH) every 8 h, low-molecular-weight heparin (LMWH) > 3400 U daily, and/or intermittent pneumatic compression. With multiple additional risk factors, intermittent compression devices or graded compression stockings are added.

Recently, the American Society of Plastic Surgery (ASPS) issued VTE prophylaxis guidelines tailored to plastic surgery patients.[25] The guidelines, based off data validating the Caprini Risk Assessment Model in plastic surgery[26], provide risk stratification and VTE prophylaxis recommendations. Most MWL patients have more than three points (obesity, > 40 years, surgery planned). Patients with three points or more undergoing major surgery (> 60 min, e.g. body contouring, abdominoplasty), should consider postoperative LMWH or unfractionated heparin. Due to increased incidence of VTE events despite compliance with recognized VTE guidelines, particularly in obese individuals, special recommendations are made in body-contouring, abdominoplasty, major breast reconstruction, major lower extremity reconstruction, and major head/neck cancer procedures.[27]

POSTBARIATRIC FACE AND NECK

The ideal neck has several components.[28] A sharp mandibular angle provides a distinct shadow below the jaw line. The cervicomental angle approaches 90°. A visible sternocleidomastoid muscle (SCM) begins at the angle of the mandible, transitioning into a visible sternal notch. The submental triangle is taut, without convexity. A strong, well-contoured chin provides youthful definition and distinction between the face and the neck. With weight gain, these landmarks are distorted or camouflaged. Instead, a round face and full, prominent neck result from increased adipose tissue. During MWL, the expanded skin envelop drapes giving the appearance of a 'droopy' face with 'turkey neck'.[8] This can be distressing to postbariatric patients. They may perceive these features as premature aging. Although redundant tissue in chest, abdomen, and arms may be disguised in clothing, the face is much more difficult to conceal.

Areas of excess skin need to be denoted on preoperative evaluation.[8] Typically, the submental area has more surplus integument than the jowls. Pre- and subplatysmal fat accumulation leads to stretching of the skin. Subsequent fat loss leaves behind redundant, thick skin in the platysmal areas which poorly conforms to the contours of the neck. This skin is characterized by its lack of elastin, collagen depletion, damaged extracellular matrix (ECM), and thick dermis.[9–11] Remaining lipodeposits may obscure underlying structures.[28] Various regions of the neck, such as the submental and submandibular triangles, are left with bulging fat deposits. Along with laxity of the platysma, these deposits disguise the cervicomental angle. Jowling and submandibular fat blur transition between face and neck. A lack of chin projection alone can also give the impression of a short neck. It lessens the transition between the face and neck.[28] Laxity in the platysma may result in vertical neck banding. Weight loss and excess skin give the appearance of integument stretching in the downward vector. Generally, this skin laxity exceeds that of the superficial musculoaponeurotic system (SMAS). The perioral area is generally subject to accelerated atrophy and nasolabial folding.

SURGERY

Due to efficient elevation, SMAS manipulation and/or lateral platysmal tacking to the mastoid periosteum has been largely successful in eliminating the need for direct platysmal manipulation.[30–32] However, in the postbariatric patient, the remaining platysmal fat and laxity may overwhelm and contribute to an unsatisfactory appearance of the heavy neck.[28] A 2- to 3-cm incision posterior to the submental crease allows exposure of the platysma, evaluation, and introduction of liposuction cannula for remaining lipodeposit removal (**Fig. 18.1**). Dissection with a cannula also allows a way of undermining anterior and midportions of the cervical region. Additional fat can be removed from the lateral neck around the inferior border of the mandible.

This is followed by wide undermining in the subcutaneous plane via scissor dissection, which extends from the mandible to the cricoid, thereby releasing any skin attachments that interfere with smooth redraping. Skin flaps need to be left uniformly moderately thick to avoid an unnatural contour.[33] Unnatural contour may be seen in superficial suctioning and can be avoided by facing the suction cannula aperture adjacent to deeper preplatysmal fat.

Postbariatric patients may not have readily discernable platysmal banding. Upon lipectomy, midline platysma muscle redundancy or laxities may become easily apparent.[28,33] Several management options exist. Plication usually extends from the mentum to the thyroid cartilage. Some advocate taking 1-cm bites which include the deeper fascia for greater hold and avoidance of pull through.[28] A conservative platysmal resection can be performed. Surgeons must be careful to avoid tension on reapproximation. Wedge excision usually occurs below the level of the thyroid cartilage for improved contour.[31] As an alternative, corset platysmaplasty, described by Feldman, utilizes continuous sutures running up and down the midline until a desired contour has been achieved.[34] Criticisms of this technique include platysmal bunching.

Ptosis, excess, and laxity of the skin are key issues in the postbariatric face, exceeding SMAS looseness.[8] Therefore, modifications to basic SMAS procedures are necessary (**Fig. 18.2**). Postbariatric patients are typically younger than the traditional patient presenting

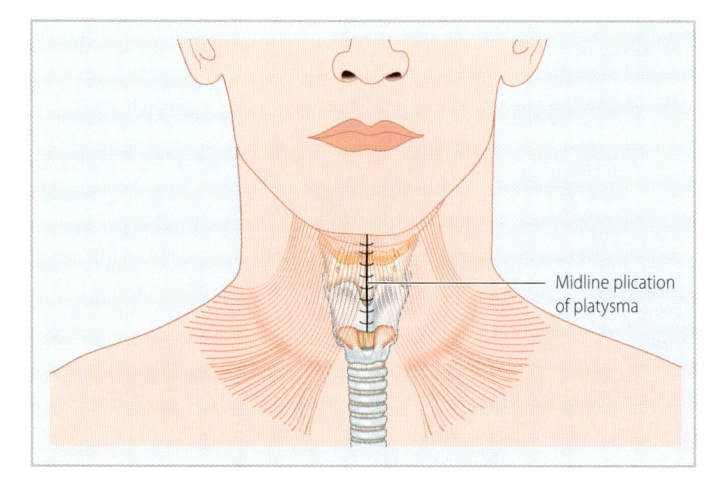

Figure 18.1 Platysmaplasty in the postbariatric patient. Large laxities in weight loss patients may contribute to unsatisfactory appearance of the heavy neck. Removal of lipodeposit, redraping skin, and platysma plication may be necessary.

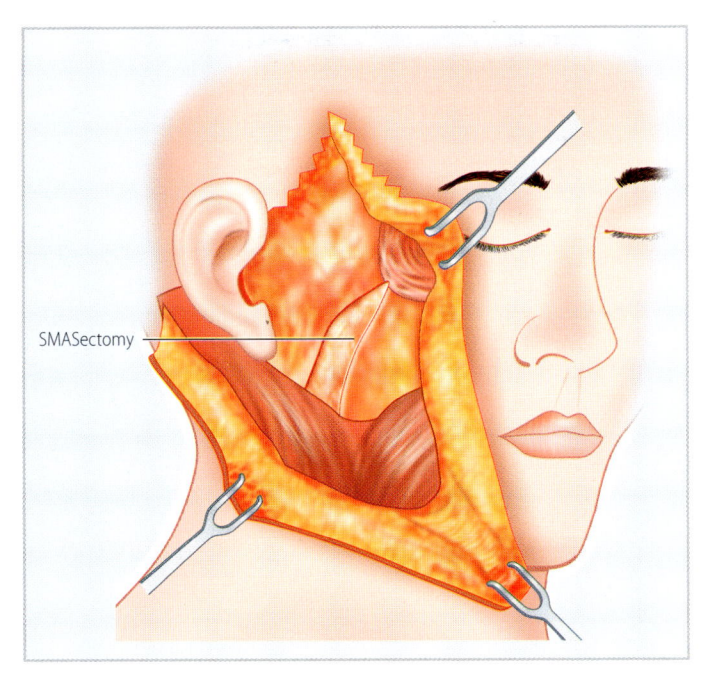

Figure 18.2 Superficial musculoaponeurotic system (SMAS) facelift in the postbariatric patient. Less SMAS manipulation is required in the postbariatric patient. Patients are typically younger. Ptosis, excess, and laxity of skin are key issues exceeding SMAS looseness.

for rhytidectomy. Younger patients are unable to commit to specific hairstyles; incisions need be camouflaged. Some authors assert the benefits of deep-plane rhytidectomy techniques[35]; others question its benefit.[36] Regardless of technique, usually less overall SMAS manipulation (imbrication, excision, or elevation) is necessary. Instead, due to the inelasticity of the skin, significantly more skin undermining is required to afford smooth redraping.[9–11]

POSTOPERATIVE CARE

Common postoperative body-contouring sequelae include seroma, hematoma, wound breakdown, infection, and VTE complications.[29] Pre-panniculectomy BMI has independently predicted postoperative complications.[13] Patients with a BMI >25 have nearly three times the risk of postoperative wound complications. With a 9% PE rate in postbariatric patients undergoing abdominoplasty, early ambulation is essential.[37] Postbariatric patients are typically nutritionally challenged. To avoid wound-healing impairments, regular diet should be instituted as soon as possible. Having bariatric surgery is not in itself a risk factor for wound dehiscence, infection, seroma, or hematoma.[38] Instead, preoperative BMI predicts perioperative complications better. Further, male gender, hypothyroidism, and Ehlers–Danlos syndrome have been associated with wound dehiscence and healing issues in body-contouring patients.[21]

Due to the inelasticity of the skin, careful inspection of bunching and dimpling should be performed during the first and second postoperative visits.[8] These areas need to be massaged. Skin may bunch at the lateral ends of the submental incision, particularly if a significant superior pull occurs. If massaging does not alleviate this issue, revision can occur in a few weeks time. It is important to indicate that revision is a reflection of the quality of the skin, not of the surgery.

CONCLUSION

Postbariatric patients experience rapid weight loss. In many cases, the facial disfigurement is more distressing than that of the body, due to difficulties in hiding the effects. Patients seek rhytidectomy as a means of rejuvenating their facial appearance to match that of their body. However, due to the unique pathology, careful and specialized preoperative evaluation, surgery, and postoperative care need be undertaken. With these unique processes explained in this chapter, great results can still be obtained, with increased harmony, body perception, and self-esteem.

REFERENCES

1. Division of Nutrition PA, and Obesity, National Center for Chronic Disease Prevention and Health Promotion. Obesity and Overweight for Professionals. *Data and Statistics: U.S. Obesity Trends 1985–2010.* Available at: www.cdc.gov/obesity/data/trends.html (accessed January 12, 2012).
2. Pories WJ, Swanson MS, MacDonald KG, et al. Who would have thought it? An operation proves to be the most effective therapy for adult-onset diabetes mellitus. *Ann Surg.* 1995;**222**:339–50; discussion 350–2.
3. Benotti PN, Wood GC, Rodriguez H, Carnevale N, Liriano E. Perioperative outcomes and risk factors in gastric surgery for morbid obesity: a 9-year experience. *Surgery* 2006;**139**:340–6.
4. Gusenoff JA, Rubin JP. Plastic surgery after weight loss: current concepts in massive weight loss surgery. *Aesthet Surg J* 2008;**28**:452–5.
5. Song AY, Rubin JP, Thomas V, Dudas JR, Marra KG, Fernstrom MH. Body image and quality of life in post massive weight loss body contouring patients. *Obesity (Silver Spring)* 2006;**14**:1626–36.
6. Bolton MA, Pruzinsky T, Cash TF, Persing JA. Measuring outcomes in plastic surgery: body image and quality of life in abdominoplasty patients. *Plast Reconstr Surg* 2003;**112**:619–25; discussion 626–7.
7. Mitchell JE, Crosby RD, Ertelt TW, et al. The desire for body contouring surgery after bariatric surgery. *Obes Surg* 2008;**18**:1308–12.
8. Sclafani AP. Restoration of the jawline and the neck after bariatric surgery. *Facial Plast Surg* 2005;**21**:28–32.
9. Choo S, Marti G, Nastai M, Mallalieu J, Shermak MA. Biomechanical properties of skin in massive weight loss patients. *Obes Surg* 2010;**20**:1422–8.
10. Light D, Arvanitis GM, Abramson D, Glasberg SB. Effect of weight loss after bariatric surgery on skin and the extracellular matrix. *Plast Reconstr Surg* 2010;**125**:343–51.
11. Orpheu SC, Coltro PS, Scopel GP, et al. Collagen and elastic content of abdominal skin after surgical weight loss. *Obes Surg* 2010;**20**:480–6.
12. Rubin JP, Nguyen V, Schwentker A. Perioperative management of the post-gastric-bypass patient presenting for body contour surgery. *Clin Plast Surg.* Oct 2004;**31**:601–10, vi.
13. Arthurs ZM, Cuadrado D, Sohn V, et al. Post-bariatric panniculectomy: pre-panniculectomy body mass index impacts the complication profile. *Am J Surg* 2007;**193**:567–70; discussion 570.
14. Colwell AS, Borud LJ. Optimization of patient safety in postbariatric body contouring: a current review. *Aesthet Surg J* 2008;**28**:437–42.
15. Nemerofsky RB, Oliak DA, Capella JF. Body lift: an account of 200 consecutive cases in the massive weight loss patient. *Plast Reconstr Surg* 2006;**117**:414–30.
16. Van Gaal LF, Wauters MA, De Leeuw IH. The beneficial effects of modest weight loss on cardiovascular risk factors. *Int J Obes Relat Metab Disord* 1997;**21**(suppl 1):S5–9.

17. Goldstein DJ. Beneficial health effects of modest weight loss. *Int J Obes Relat Metab Disord* 1992;**16**:397–415.
18. Rees TD, Liverett DM, Guy CL. The effect of cigarette smoking on skin-flap survival in the face lift patient. *Plast Reconstr Surg* 1984;**73**:911–15.
19. Rohrich RJ. Cosmetic surgery and patients who smoke: should we operate? *Plast Reconstr Surg* 2000;**106**:137–8.
20. Silverstein P. Smoking and wound healing. *Am J Med* 1992;**93**(1A):22S–4S.
21. Shermak MA, Chang D, Magnuson TH, Schweitzer MA. An outcomes analysis of patients undergoing body contouring surgery after massive weight loss. *Plast Reconstr Surg* 2006;**118**:1026–31.
22. Aly A, Downey SE, Eaves FFI, Kenkel JM. Panel Discussion – Evolution of body contouring after massive weight loss [Abstract]. *Plast Reconstr Surg* 2006;**118**(suppl):55.
23. Reinisch JF, Bresnick SD, Walker JW, Rosso RF. Deep venous thrombosis and pulmonary embolus after face lift: a study of incidence and prophylaxis. *Plast Reconstr Surg* 2001;**107**:1570–5; discussion 1576–7.
24. Geerts WH, Pineo GF, Heit JA, et al. Prevention of venous thromboembolism: the Seventh ACCP Conference on Antithrombotic and Thrombolytic Therapy. *Chest* 2004;**126**(3 suppl):338S–400S.
25. American Society of Plastic Surgeons. ASPS Campaign for VTE Awareness, 2011. Available at: www.plasticsurgery.org/for-medical-professionals/legislation-and-advocacy/key-issues-in-plastic-surgery/venous-thromboembolism.html (accessed June 11, 2012).
26. Pannucci CJ, Bailey SH, Dreszer G, et al. Validation of the Caprini risk assessment model in plastic and reconstructive surgery patients. *J Am Coll Surg* 2011;**212**:105–12.
27. Murphy RX, Jr., Peterson EA, Adkinson JM, Reed JF 3rd. Plastic surgeon compliance with national safety initiatives: clinical outcomes and 'never events'. *Plast Reconstr Surg* 2010;**126**:653–6.
28. Wachholz JH. Surgical treatment of the heavy face and neck. *Facial Plast Surg Clin North Am* 2009;**17**:603–11, vii.
29. Taylor J, Shermak M. Body contouring following massive weight loss. *Obes Surg* 2004;**14**:1080–5.
30. Baker DC. Lateral SMASectomy. *Plast Reconstr Surg* 1997;**100**:509–13.
31. Thorne C. Facelift. In: Thorne C, Grabb WC, Smith JW, eds. *Grabb and Smith's Plastic Surgery*. Philadelphia: Wolters Kluwer Health/Lippincott Williams & Wilkins; 2007: 498–508.
32. Baker DC. Minimal incision rhytidectomy (short scar face lift) with lateral SMASectomy: evolution and application. *Aesthet Surg J* 2001;**21**:14–26.
33. Wolfe SA, Fusi S. Treatment of the particularly fatty neck and the short-interval secondary facelift. *Aesthet Plast Surg* 1991;**15**:195–201.
34. Feldman JJ. Corset platysmaplasty. *Plast Reconstr Surg* 1990;**85**:333–43.
35. Litner JA, Adamson PA. Limited vs extended face-lift techniques: objective analysis of intraoperative results. *Arch Facial Plast Surg* 2006;**8**:186–90.
36. Ivy EJ, Lorenc ZP, Aston SJ. Is there a difference? A prospective study comparing lateral and standard SMAS face lifts with extended SMAS and composite rhytidectomies. *Plast Reconstr Surg* 1996;**98**:1135–43; discussion 1144–37.
37. Aly AS, Cram AE, Chao M, Pang J, McKeon M. Belt lipectomy for circumferential truncal excess: the University of Iowa experience. *Plast Reconstr Surg* 2003;**111**:398–413.
38. Vastine VL, Morgan RF, Williams GS, et al. Wound complications of abdominoplasty in obese patients. *Ann Plast Surg* 1999;**42**:34–9.

Chapter 19
Role of suction-assisted lipectomy

Joseph F. Capella

INTRODUCTION

Suction-assisted lipectomy (SAL) has played an integral role in body contouring for several decades and has proven to be an important component of our postbariatric body-contouring practice for >10 years. The traditional ideal candidate for SAL is an individual with good skin tone who has isolated pockets of fat refractory to weight loss. A significant aesthetic improvement can often be achieved in this patient population with limited adverse sequelae (**Fig. 19.1**). When SAL is applied as a sole modality to patients who are less than ideal candidates, those with redundant soft tissue with diminished elasticity, the results can be unsatisfactory. Poor candidates are often postpartum women and individuals after weight loss (**Fig. 19.2**). SAL as an adjunctive modality in this patient population, however, particularly when used in combination with soft-tissue excisional body-contouring procedures, can improve aesthetic outcome. In addition, SAL will often facilitate the performance of soft-tissue excisional procedures and broaden the range of patients who are acceptable candidates for body contouring. SAL as an adjunctive modality is an essential component of our postbariatric body-contouring practice, particularly with regard to the upper and lower extremities.

BACKGROUND

Morbidly obese individuals have characteristic areas of fat deposition that vary slightly between men and women. The most prominent areas include the neck, posterior arm, axilla, subaxillary region, breasts, lower abdomen, mons pubis, hips, medial and lateral thighs, and medial leg. After weight loss, these same areas will have varying amounts of residual fat, some degree of soft-tissue excess and likely some compromise to the elastic qualities of these tissues (**Fig. 19.3**). The extent of redundancy and elastic qualities of the soft tissue depend on many variables including the duration of time that the patient remained overweight, age at weight loss, degree of obesity, sex, complexion, tobacco consumption, and exposure to ultraviolet light.[1,2] Despite significant advances in plastic surgery, the body-contouring techniques available to us today consist primarily of the removal or transfer of soft tissue or the placement of prostheses. No substantial gains have been made in the way of improving soft-tissue quality and elasticity. These limitations apply to the management of the body contour concerns of the weight loss patient as well.[3]

UPPER EXTREMITY CONTOURING

Contour deformities of the axilla, arm, and forearm after weight loss are often of great concern for many individuals. This is largely due to the ready visibility of the upper extremity in everyday activities. Patients will frequently complain of a 'bat-winged' appearance, stretch marks along their arms, large size of the arm relative to the forearm, excess skin and fat at the axilla and lateral thoracic region, and, for some individuals, loose skin along the proximal forearm (**Fig. 19.3**). Patients will often present with a request that their arms

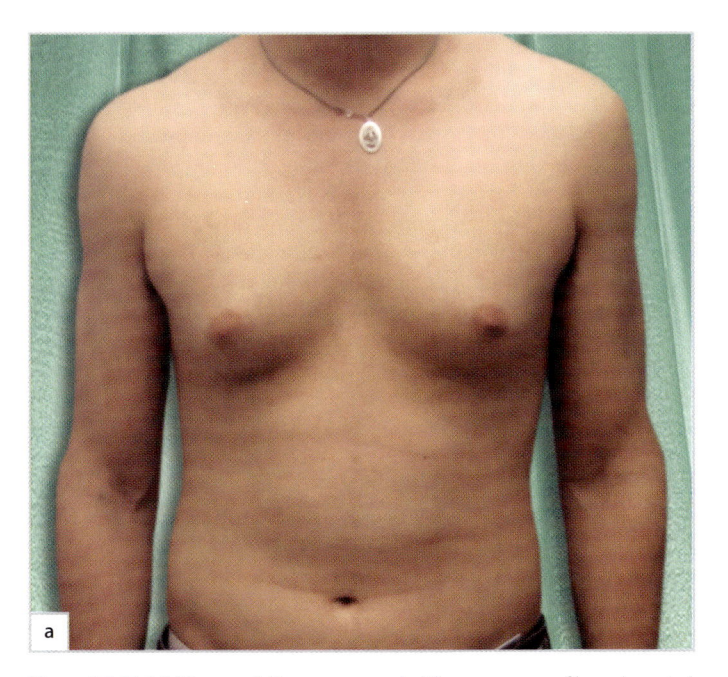

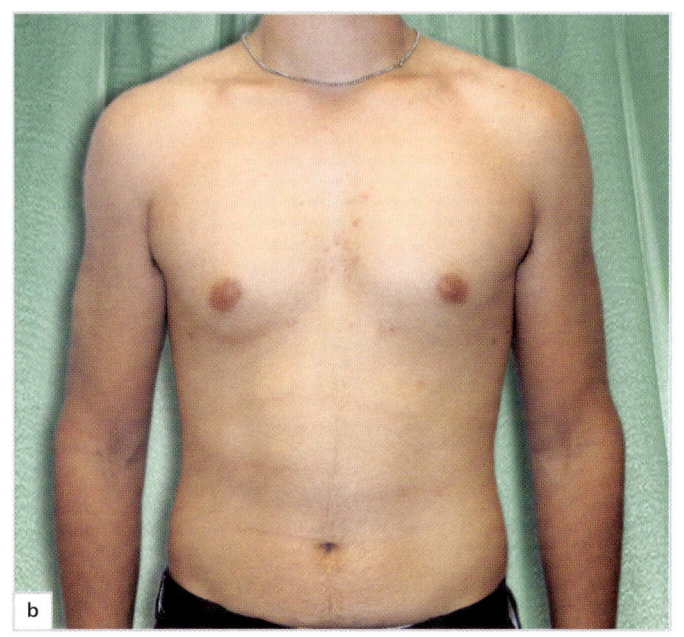

Figure 19.1 (a) A 16-year-old boy concerned with appearance of large breasts (gynecomastia). (b) 1 year after liposuction of chest.

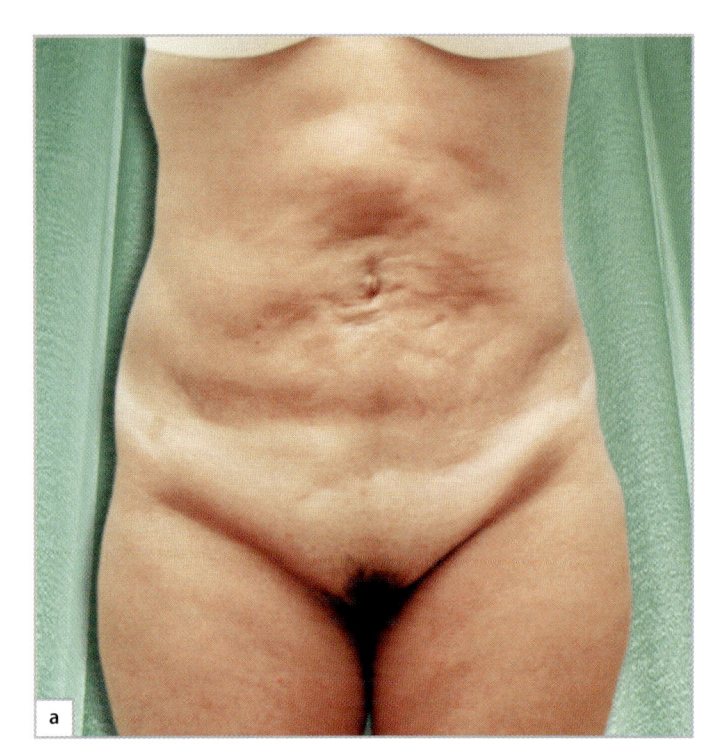

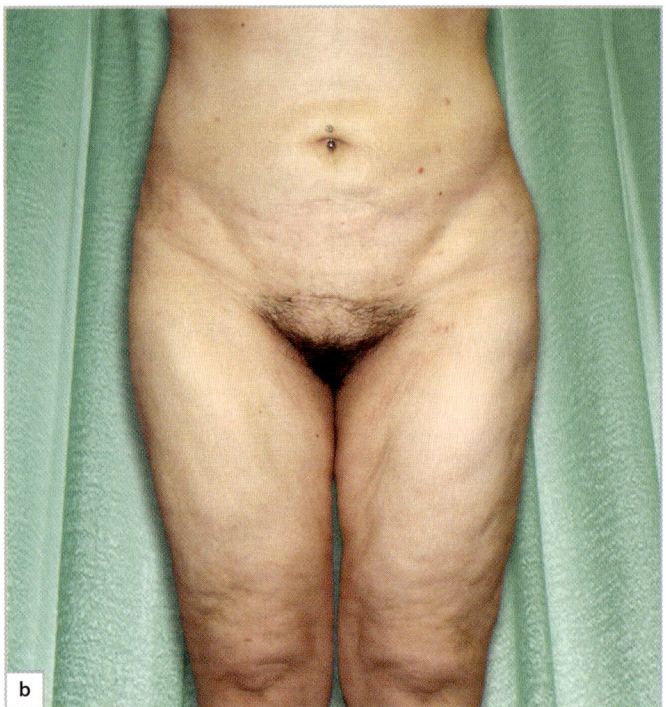

Figure 19.2 (a) A 35-year-old postpartum woman disappointed with appearance of abdomen after liposuction performed by another surgeon. (b) A 40-year-old postbariatric woman disappointed with appearance of abdomen and thighs after liposuction performed by another surgeon.

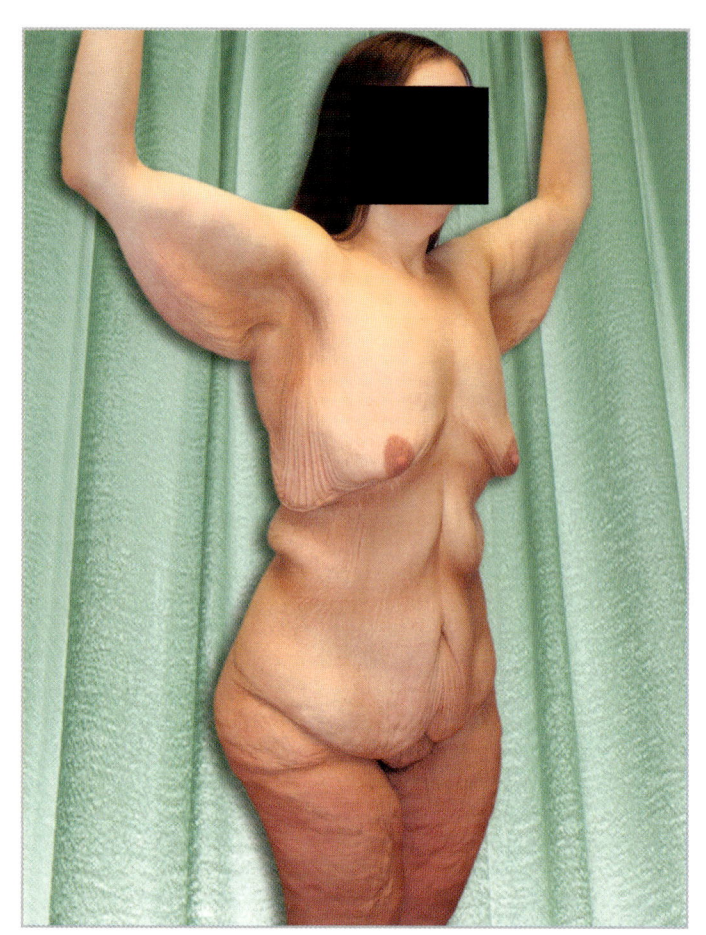

Figure 19.3 A 28-year-old woman after 84.6 kg (188 lb) weight loss through lifestyle changes. Areas of soft-tissue excess reflect characteristic regions of fat deposition in the obese woman.

be made smaller. The size of a postbariatric patient's arms is largely a function of the amount of residual fat and subcutaneous tissues. Patients presenting at or near a normal body mass index (BMI) usually have less residual fat and a more 'deflated' appearance, and are generally thought of as better candidates for brachioplasty than those with larger amounts of residual fat. Descriptions of brachioplasty procedures for the most part have been geared toward these lower BMI individuals.[4,5]

Brachioplasty was first described in the 1930s. Most publications on this topic since that time have been technique oriented and included a relatively small series of patients. Technical variations have mostly related to scar location and design, and modifications for transitioning from the arm to the axilla and lateral thoracic region. Liposuction in the brachioplasty literature has been limited almost entirely to short scar techniques, procedures that for the most part have not been considered applicable to most postbariatric patients. The potential benefits of liposuction in postbariatric patients have been recognized for some time as a modality for 'debulking' the arms. Concerns about swelling and a compromise to the circulation to the skin have led some surgeons to suggest performing liposuction as a staged procedure, several months before a brachioplasty. Others have advocated liposuction at the time of brachioplasty, limited only, however, to the predetermined area of soft tissue to be removed.[6-32]

For more than 10 years, liposuction has played a critical role in our technique for brachioplasty. Our preference is to perform liposuction immediately before the excisional component of a brachioplasty procedure. We have noted several benefits from concomitant liposuction. The first has been to allow for a broad range of patients, those with normal, near normal, and higher BMI values to have a significant improvement in contour. Many plastic surgeons will discourage patients with a BMI

>32 from having brachioplasty, noting that the results are likely to be unsatisfactory. Liposuction at the time of brachioplasty can offer higher BMI patients the possibility of marked improvement. The removal of excess fat with liposuction can decrease the diameter of the arm and proximal forearm to a degree that could not otherwise be achieved with an excisional procedure alone. We have also found that liposuction at the time of brachioplasty provides certain technical advantages. A readily identifiable plane of dissection below the superficial fascial system is created by liposuction which allows for the procedure to be executed more efficiently and safely. Deep fascia can be preserved, as can the superficial sensory nerves. In addition, the removal of excess fat allows for more accurate removal of excess soft tissue. An attempt to reshape and significantly reduce the diameter of the arm by skin removal alone will likely lead to wound-healing problems. Removing excess fat before measuring excess skin and subcutaneous tissues will produce more predictable outcomes with fewer complications.

Our technique for brachioplasty has been described.[4,24] Briefly, the arm and axilla are marked with the patient standing, the arm abducted to 90°, and the elbow flexed and rotated to be in a plane parallel with the body (**Fig. 19.4**). Markings are placed with the goal of the excess tissue at both the axilla and arm to be addressed, and for the scar along the arm to ultimately lie along its posteromedial aspect. In addition, this marking produces a form of Z-plasty to prevent scar contracture along the axilla. Tumescent fluid (50 ml 1% lidocaine and 1 ml 1/1000 epinephrine in 1 liter saline) is injected into the subcutaneous tissues of the medial, posterior, and later aspects of the arm, and superficially into the subcutaneous tissues of the axilla. Tumescent fluid is injected into the anterior arm and proximal medial forearm if excess fat is noted in these regions as well. The volume of tumescent fluid injected into the various regions should be approximately equivalent to the amount of effluent expected. Greater amounts of tumescent fluid may make an accurate assessment of excess soft tissue more difficult. The excess skin previously marked at the axilla is excised first. No liposuction is performed at the axilla. Tumescent fluid at the axilla assists with hemostasis and analgesia. Standard suction lipectomy is then performed along the medial, posterior, and lateral arm and anterior arm or proximal medial forearm as needed. Upon completion of the suction lipectomy, via an incision along the previously placed marks along the medial arm, a plane of dissection immediately deep to the superficial fascial system is created to the posterolateral aspect of the arm. With the tissue edges at the axilla approximated, a Pitanguy long skin demarcator is used to mark the excess soft tissue along the arm that is to be removed (**Fig. 19.5**). The tissue edges are approximated with interrupted 2/0 Vicryl suture and a running 3/0 Moncryl suture. No drain is placed. Sterile dressings are removed after 48 hours and no special garments are prescribed thereafter.

Outcomes

After our technique for brachioplasty the vast majority of patients are pleased with their results. Patients most likely to achieve or approach an aesthetic ideal and to have a very high level of satisfaction are those with presenting with a BMI < 28 and who have had significant weight loss before surgery, a BMI change > 20 (**Fig. 19.6**). Patients presenting at a higher BMI, > 28, and who have also experienced very substantial weight loss before surgery are also very likely to be satisfied but are less likely to achieve an aesthetic ideal (**Fig. 19.7**). Liposuction plays a critical role in producing a substantial aesthetic improvement in this patient group. Candidates for surgery presenting at a higher BMI, > 32, and who have had relatively little weight loss before surgery, a BMI change < 5, are usually the least satisfied and have the smallest

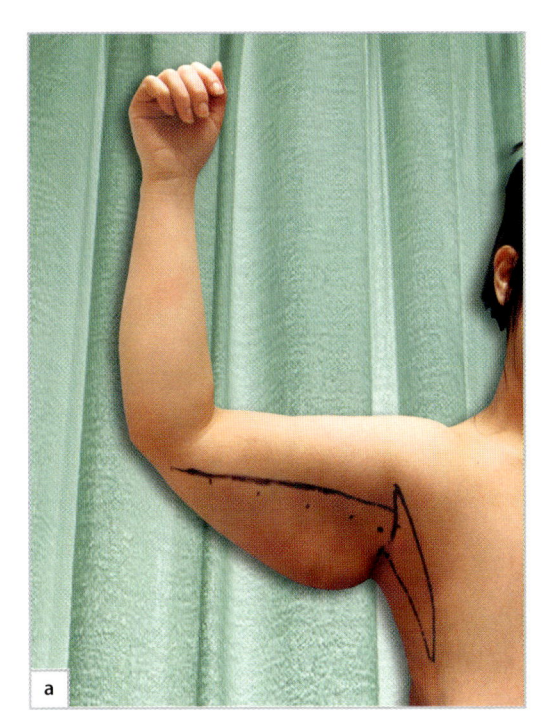

Figure 19.4 (a) Markings for brachioplasty. (b) Illustration to accompany marking.

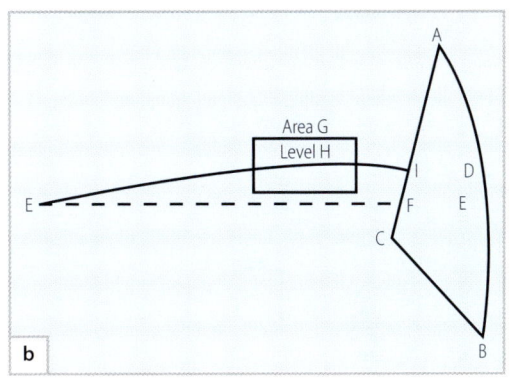

aesthetic improvement (**Fig. 19.8**). Critical to achieving the best results with arm-contouring surgery is addressing the upper body as a whole. Patients are unlikely to be satisfied with their arms if their forearms, axilla, or lateral thoracic has not been addressed and contributes to their upper body concerns.

Major complications after brachioplasty are few (**Table 19.1**).[4] In our review of 350 brachioplasty cases (700 arms), skin dehiscence was the most frequent complication at 25%. Few of the dehiscences occurred acutely, i.e. within the first 24–48 hours after the procedure, but rather began to become evident approximately 2 weeks after the procedure. Nearly all, 95%, occurred at the Z-plasty closure in the axilla. Most skin dehiscences are < 2 cm in size. Avoiding this complication is challenging because some form of Z-plasty must be present for the closure to extend from the axilla to the arm and prevent scar contracture. Although advising the patient to limit extension of the arm may be helpful, it is unlikely to entirely prevent this problem. Dehiscence is treated with dressing changes. In some instances, hypergranulation tissue may arise in the area of skin dehiscence. Nitrate application is very effective. Seromas are the second most frequent problem at 10%. The vast majority, approximately 90%, occur along the distal medial third of the arm, immediately beneath the scar. Most become evident at about 3 weeks postoperatively and range in diameter from 1 cm to 4 cm. Initially we manage them by needle aspiration.

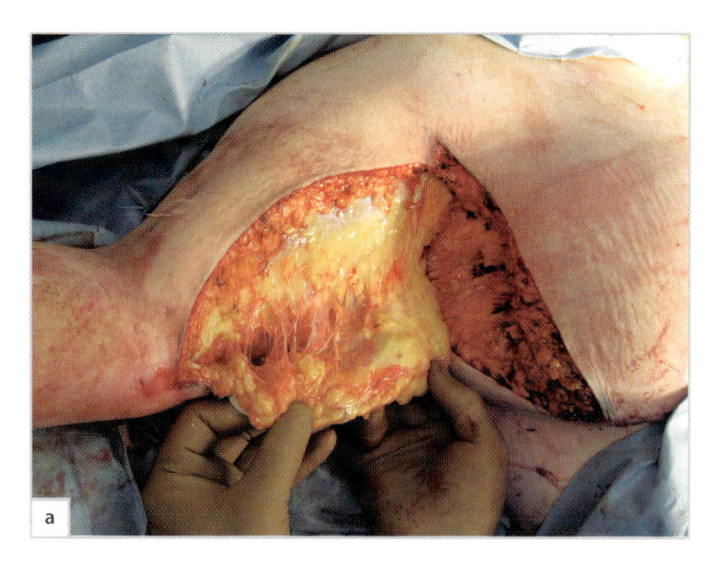

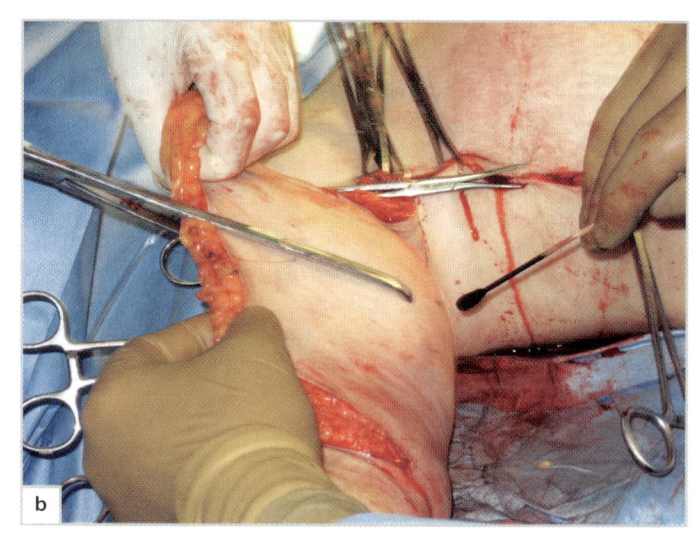

Figure 19.5 (a) Appearance of subcutaneous tissues after liposuction to medial and posterior arm. Plane of dissection readily visible. (b) Use of Pitanguy large skin demarcator to determine amount of soft-tissue excess

This technique unfortunately has a very high recurrence rate. The technique of 'marsupialization,' incising the skin over the seroma, draining the seroma, and suturing the seroma cavity to the skin, is 100% effective but results in a scar that may be wider than the adjoining scar and prolong the healing of the wound. Our preference at this time is to drain the seroma via the scar and place a secured Penrose-type drain into the seroma cavity. This technique has also proven to be very effective. Patients are maintained on antibiotics while the Penrose is in place. Overall in our series, infections have been very infrequent, as have bleeding and hematomas. Complaints of dysaesthesia beyond 3 months have been few and rare beyond 6 months. Skin necrosis has also been very infrequent despite liposuction being performed in virtually all cases. We have only one documented instance of deep vein thrombosis (DVT) in a patient undergoing brachioplasty. The patient presented with a palpable cord extending from the forearm to the arm, suggestive of superficial thrombophlebitis. An upper extremity venous Doppler ultrasonography study, revealed involvement of the deep system of the arm. There have been no instances of pulmonary embolism.

LOWER EXTREMITY CONTOURING

In our practice, SAL has played an equally important role in the management of the lower extremity as the upper extremity in the weight loss patient. The thighs, and in particular the medial thighs, are often of great concern to both men and women after weight loss. For some women, the legs may be of concern as well. Despite the frequency of requests for correction of lower extremity deformities, many plastic surgeons have been reluctant to embrace thighplasty procedures because of the risk of significant complications, relatively poor results, and the potential for readily visible scars.[33–35] Contour deformity of the lower extremity in the weight loss patient, similar to the upper extremity, is primarily the result of redundant soft tissue and poor tissue elasticity. Effective correction of the lower extremity deformity requires that the lower body and extremities be addressed as a unit. At consultation, we explain to prospective weight loss patients that thigh contour deformities cannot be corrected if the deformities of the lower abdomen, hips, and buttocks are not corrected first. All patients are asked to stand in front of a mirror and apply upward traction to the lower abdomen while the examiner applies traction to the hips and buttocks (**Fig. 19.9**). This maneuver highlights the contribution of the lower body to the thigh deformity or what can be described as the vertical vector component. Grasping the soft tissue of the medial thighs illustrates the horizontal vector component of the thigh deformity (**Fig. 19.10**). In our practice, the vast majority of patients seeking correction of their lower extremities are advised to undergo a body lift or simultaneous abdominoplasty, or thigh and buttock lift before considering other thighplasty surgery. Our technique for body lift, which has been described, effectively addresses the vertical vector component of the thigh deformity.[1,37,38] For some patients, a body lift alone satisfactorily contours the lower extremities (**Fig. 19.11**). For others, a medial thigh lift with a vertical component may be necessary to address the horizontal vector of the deformity and achieve a satisfactory result (**Fig. 19.12**).

SAL is an integral component of our technique for medial thigh lift and is used in certain cases of body lift as well. Women after weight loss with residual lipodystrophy along the lateral thighs may benefit from liposuction in this region when undergoing a body lift. Liposuction will improve the contour of the lateral thighs and may facilitate elevation of the soft tissues of the distal lateral thighs in an attempt to eliminate cellulite. Traction of the lateral thigh soft tissues provided by the body lift will help minimize the possibilities of contour deformities resulting from SAL (**Fig. 19.13**). We avoid liposuction along the anterior thigh because this may lead to contour deformities despite the body lift. In the past, as a 'debulking' procedure, we would perform SAL along the medial thighs in higher BMI individuals who planned to have a medial thigh lift at a later date. We soon abandoned this approach for several reasons. First, if the patient, for whatever reason, did not proceed with a medial thigh lift, liposuction alone along the medial thighs would worsen their medial thigh deformity. Second, we found that the scar tissue resulting from prior liposuction would make a medial thigh lift technically more difficult to perform.

Our technique for medial thigh lift has been described.[36] Briefly, the goal of the technique is to have the scars lie along the thigh perineal crease, proximal gluteal crease, and medial aspect of the thigh. The patient is evaluated for marking while standing and facing the surgeon. The lower extremities should be parallel and several centimeters apart. A vertical line is drawn along the medial thighs from the thigh perineal crease to the medial aspect of the knees. The line should terminate at a point just distal to the deformity to be treated, typically the junction of the knee with the leg. The line should not be visible when evaluating

Lower extremity contouring 169

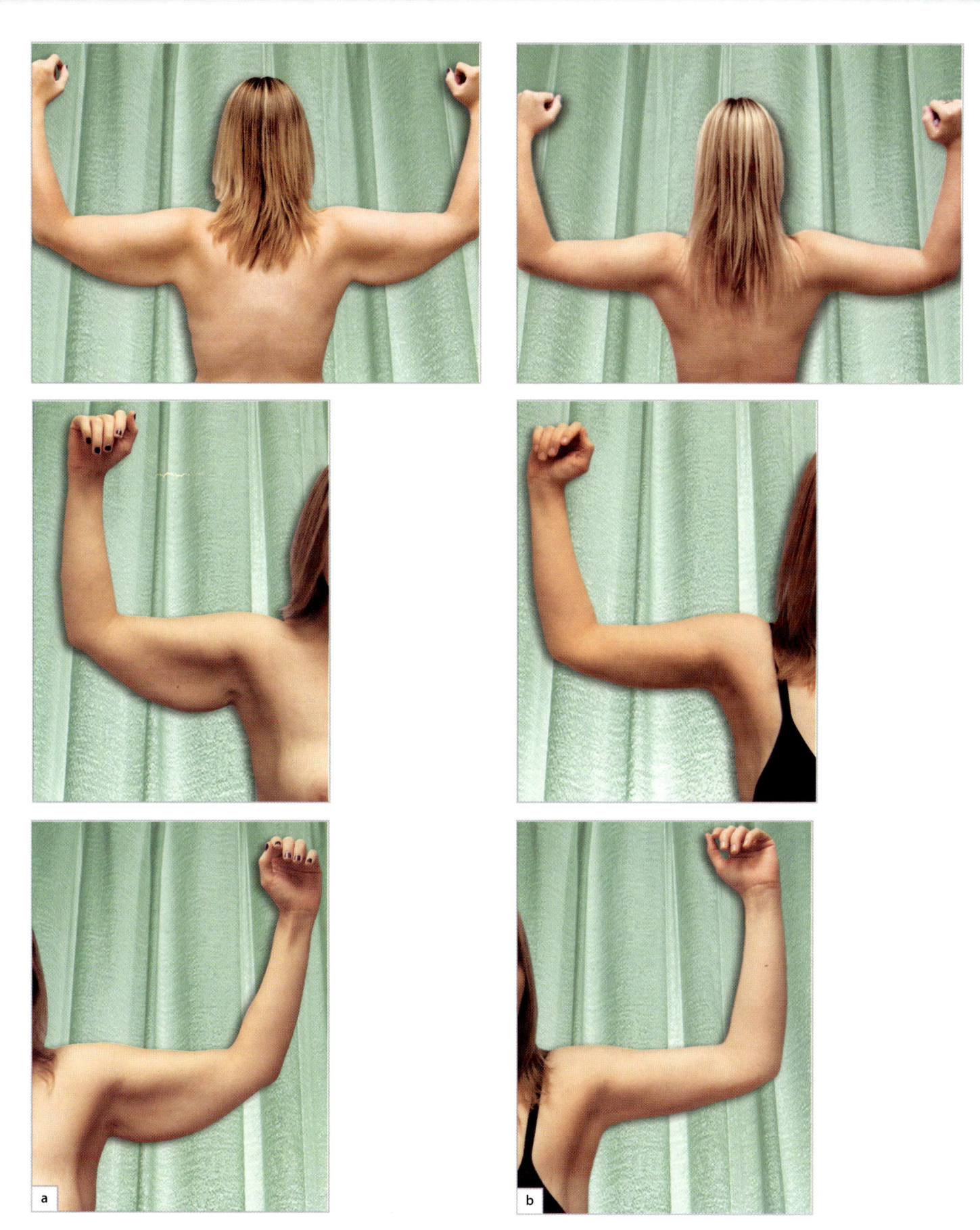

Figure 19.6 (a) A 25-year-old woman 4 years after bariatric surgery and weight loss of 58 kg (128 lb). Current weight and body mass index (BMI): 62 kg (137 lb), 25 respectively. Highest weight and BMI: 120 kg (265 lb), 48. (b) Six months after brachioplasty with concomitant liposuction.

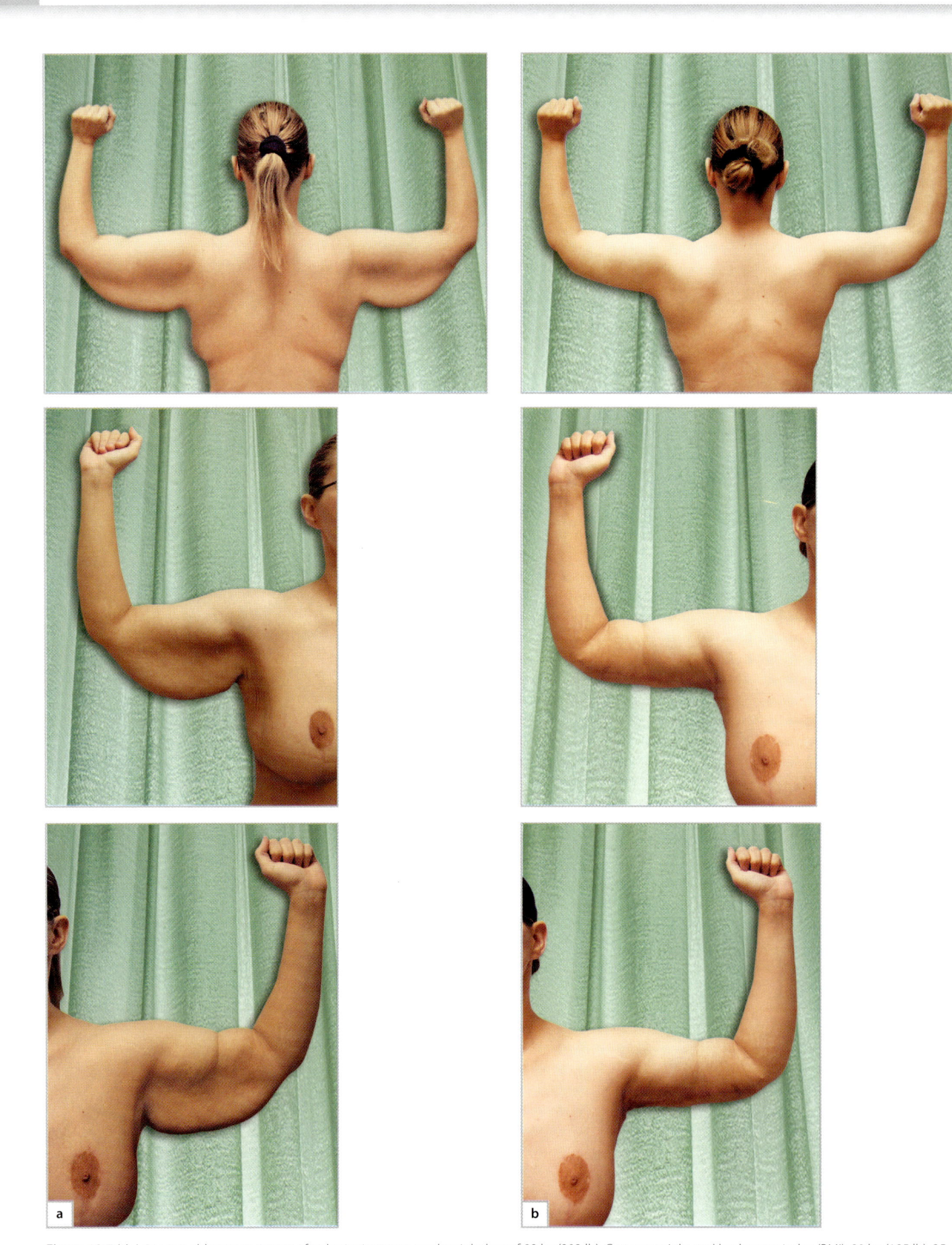

Figure 19.7 (a) A 31-year-old woman 4 years after bariatric surgery and weight loss of 92 kg (203 lb). Current weight and body mass index (BMI): 89 kg (195 lb), 35 respectively. Highest weight and BMI: 181 kg (398 lb), 71. (b) Three months after brachioplasty with concomitant liposuction.

Lower extremity contouring 171

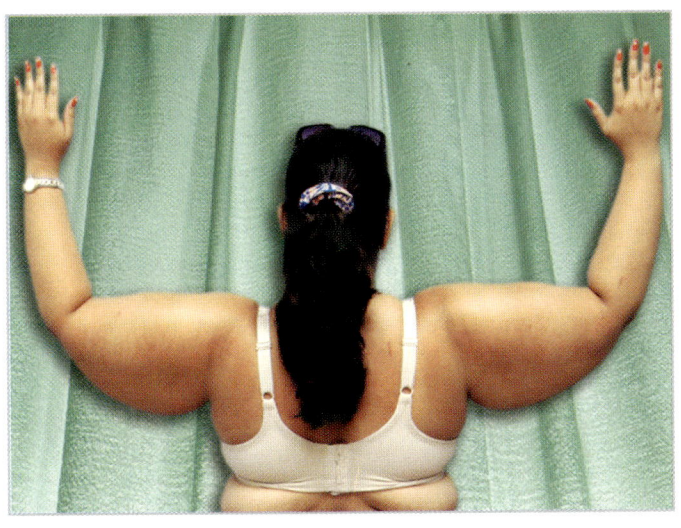

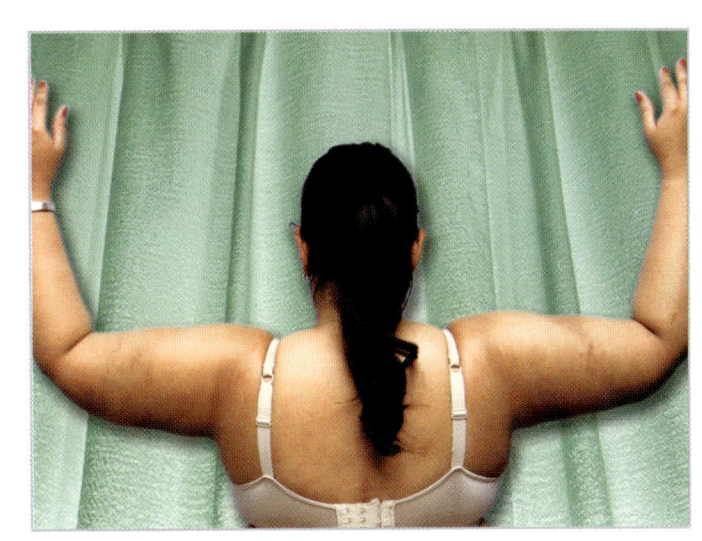

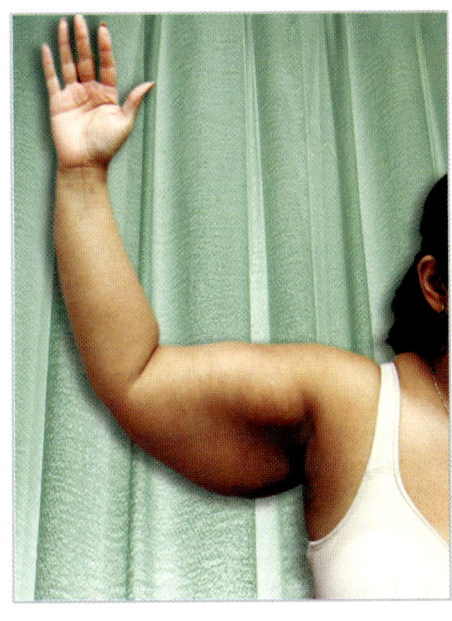

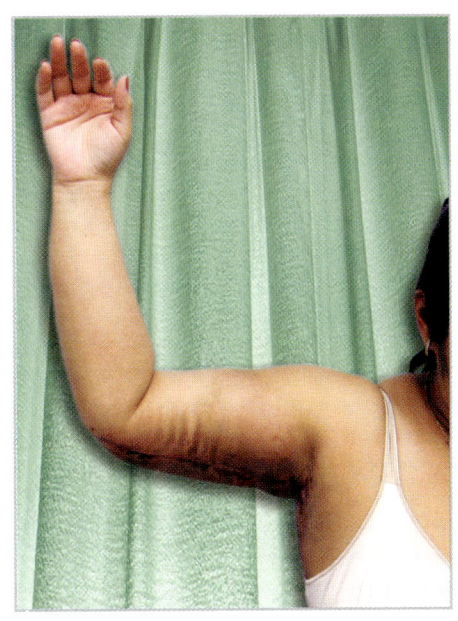

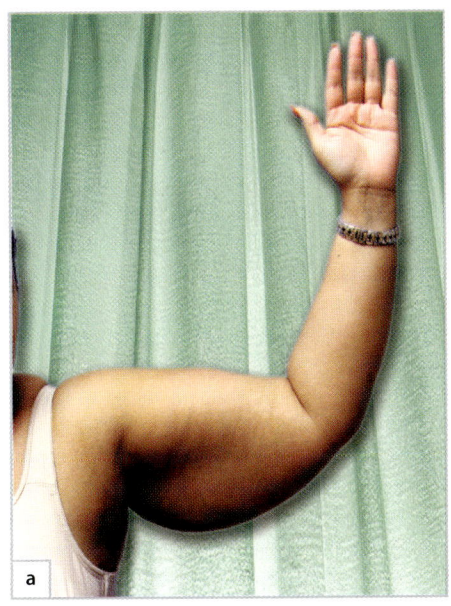

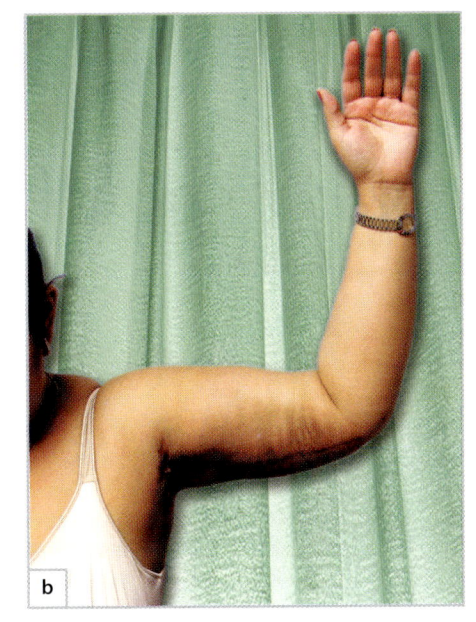

Figure 19.8 (a) A 37-year-old woman 7 years after weight loss of 20 kg (45 lb). Current weight and body mass index (BMI): 100 kg (220 lb), 37 respectively. Highest weight and BMI: 120 kg (265 lb), 44. (b) Six months after brachioplasty with concomitant liposuction.

ROLE OF SUCTION-ASSISTED LIPECTOMY

Table 19.1 Complication rates associated with brachioplasty – 350 cases (700 arms).

Complication	Complication rates (%)
Skin dehiscence	35
Seroma	7
Infection	3
Hematoma	0.6
Skin necrosis	0.6
Deep vein thrombosis	0.3

the standing patient from either an anterior or a posterior perspective. The remaining marks are made with the patient supine after anesthesia.

After induction and with the patient under general anesthesia, a cotton swab soaked in methylene blue is used to delineate a line extending from just inferior to the pre-existing scar from a circumferential body lift or abdominoplasty to the thigh perineal crease on either side of the mons pubis (**Fig. 19.14**). Marking should then transition from the thigh perineal crease to the proximal gluteal crease. The marking should stop several centimeters before the gluteal crease makes contact with the operating table. This will ensure that the proximal medial thigh scar will not be visible along the lower

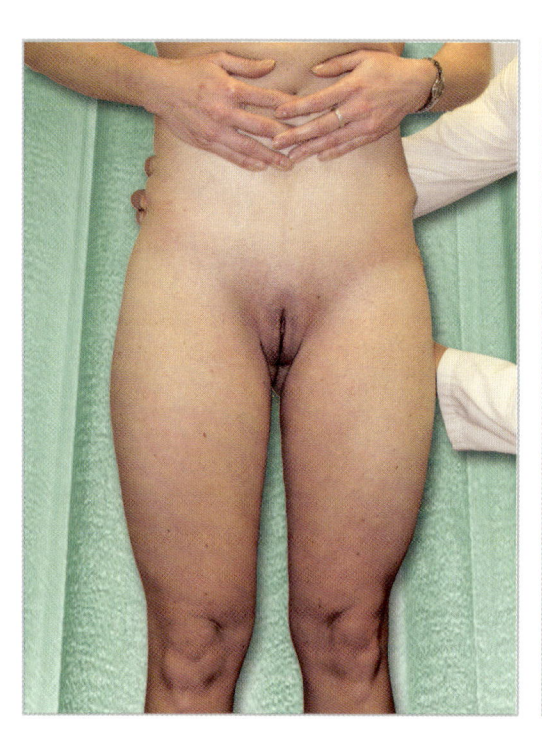

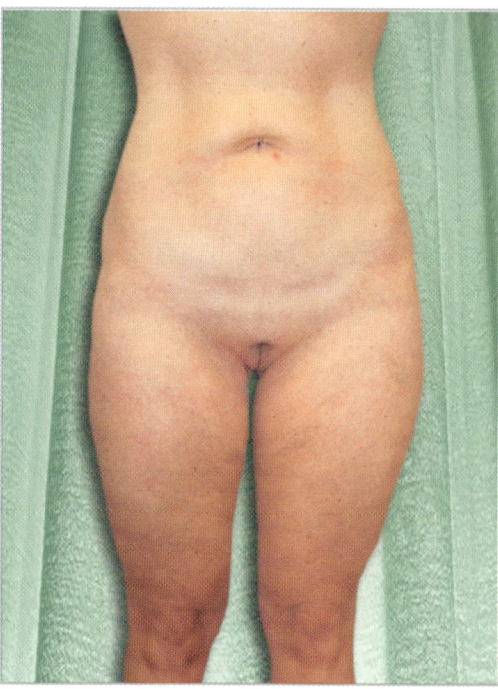

Figure 19.9 This maneuver, the application of upward traction to the lower abdomen by the patient and the lateral thighs by the examiner, helps eliminate the variables outside of the medial thighs contributing to the medial thigh deformity. It also serves to illustrate for patients the function of circumferential body lifting procedures.

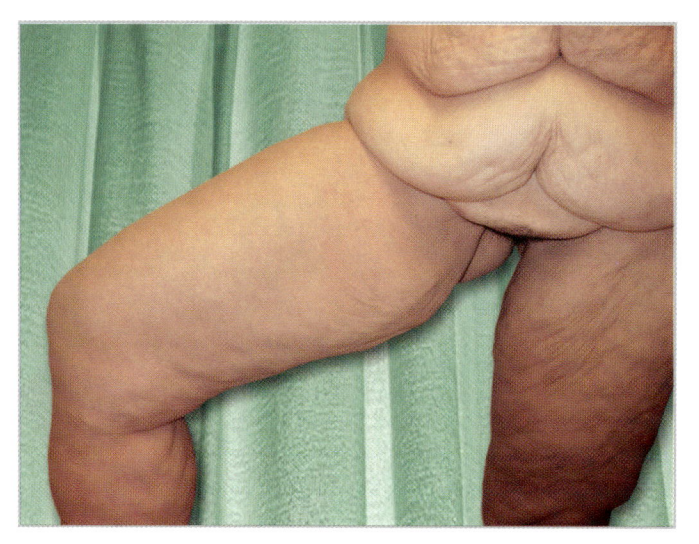

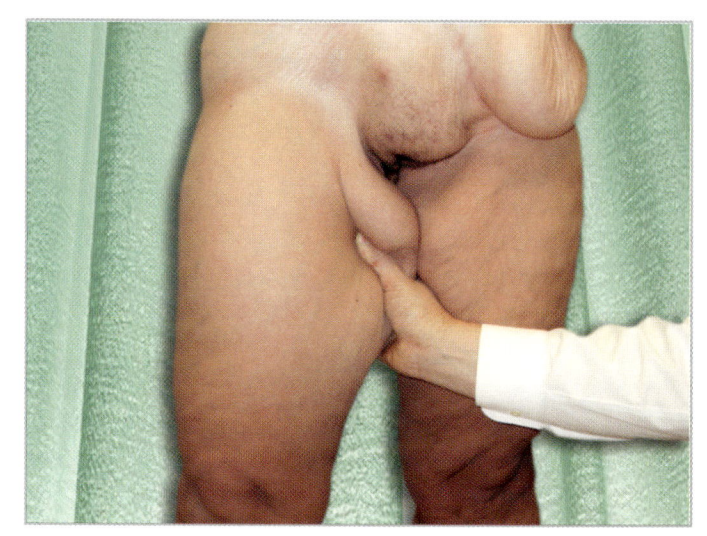

Figure 19.10 Traction on the soft tissues of the medial thigh with the patient standing and abducting a lower extremity highlights soft tissue excess in the horizontal vector and illustrates the function of the vertical medial thigh lift.

Lower extremity contouring

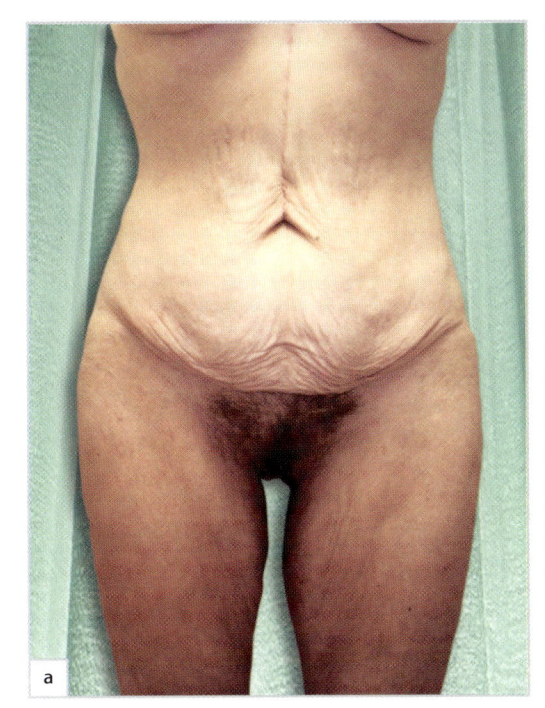

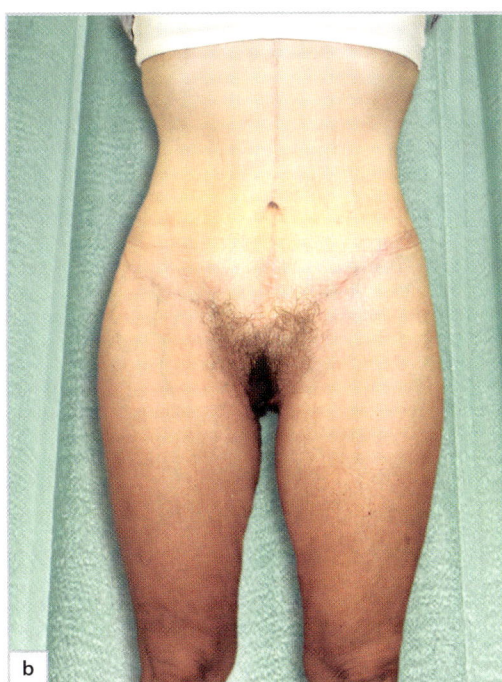

Figure 19.11 (a) A 36-year-old woman 23 months after gastric bypass surgery and weight loss of 73 kg (161 lb). Current weight and body mass index (BMI): 55 kg (121 lb), 20 respectively. Highest weight and BMI ever achieved: 128 kg (282 lb), 47. The medial thigh deformity was one of her primary concerns. (b) Eighteen months after body lift. The body lift provided sufficient improvement of her medial thighs for her to forgo any further surgery to her medial thighs.

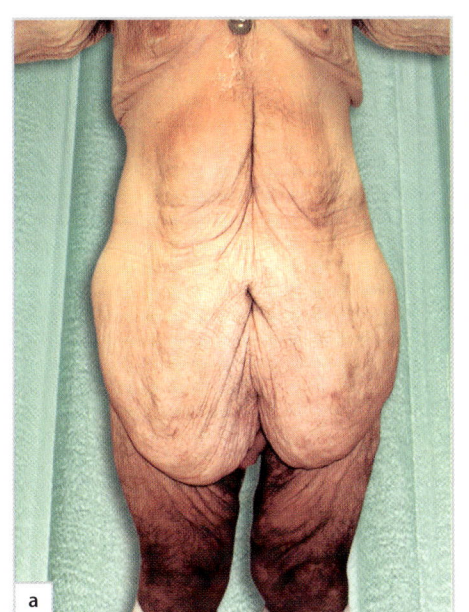

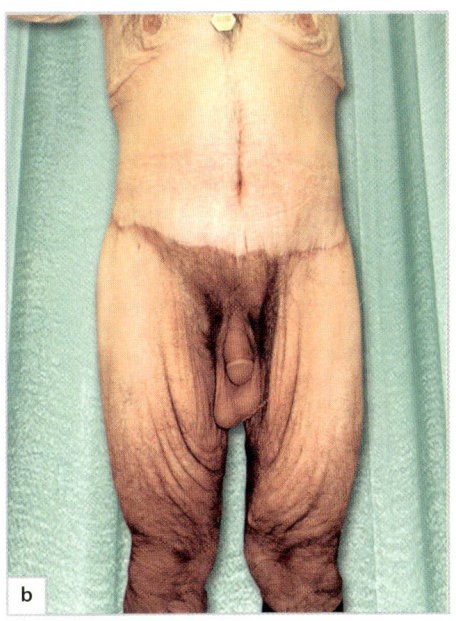

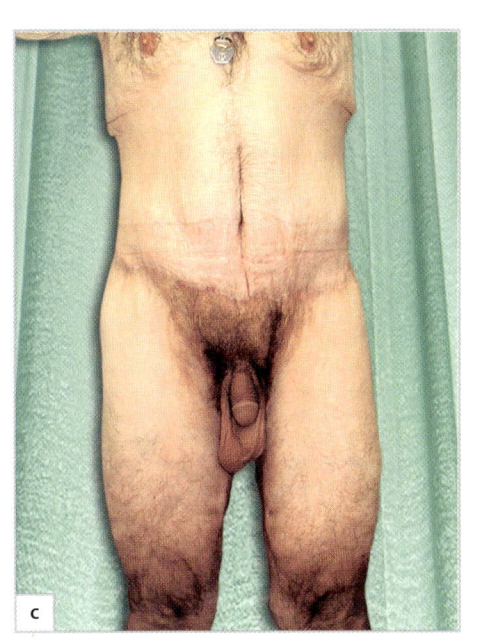

Figure 19.12 (a) A 40-year-old man 21 months after gastric bypass surgery and weight loss of 75 kg (165 lb). Current weight and body mass index (BMI): 90 kg (198 lb), 32 respectively. Highest weight and BMI ever achieved: 166 kg (366 lb), 59. (b) Seven months after body lift. (c) Three months after medial thigh lift with a vertical component extending to junction of knee with leg.

buttocks from a posterior perspective. Tumescent fluid (50 ml 1% lidocaine and 1 ml 1/1000 epinephrine in 1 liter of 0.9% saline) is then injected into the soft tissues of the right medial thigh and knee. While the effects of the tumescent fluid are taking place, the skin along the marking at the right thigh perineal and gluteal crease is incised. Liposuction is usually not performed on individuals with a BMI < 21. Less benefit is seen in this patient population. Liposuction is then performed along the medial knee and thigh areas, deep to the superficial fascial system. In many instances more effluent can be removed than tumescent volume injected. The 'pinch' technique is then utilized by the surgeon to estimate the excess skin and soft tissue to be removed (**Fig. 19.15**).

This technique maintains the final closure centered over least perceptible location. The first 'pinch' is usually over the area of greatest soft-tissue excess, often the middle third of the medial thigh. The assistant then uses Adair or towel clamps to maintain the position of the estimated tissue to be removed. Methylene blue dots are marked on either skin edge, all along the medial thigh and knee region where the clamps are in place. The clamps are then all released and removed. The series of dots along the medial thigh and knee delineate the pattern

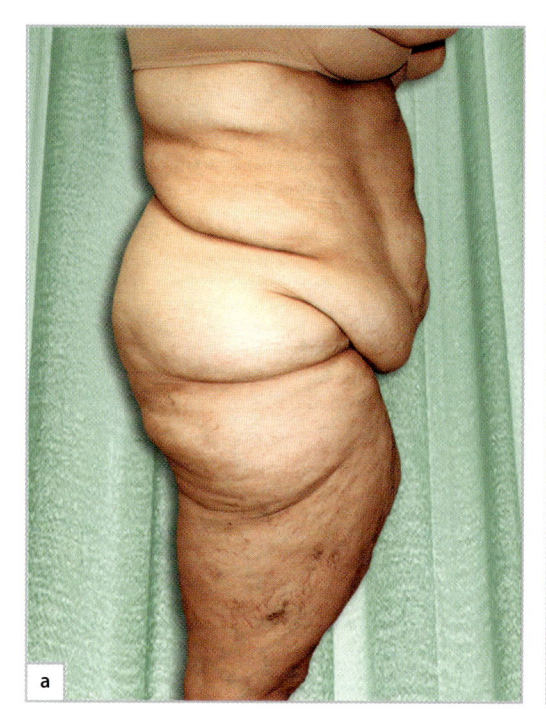

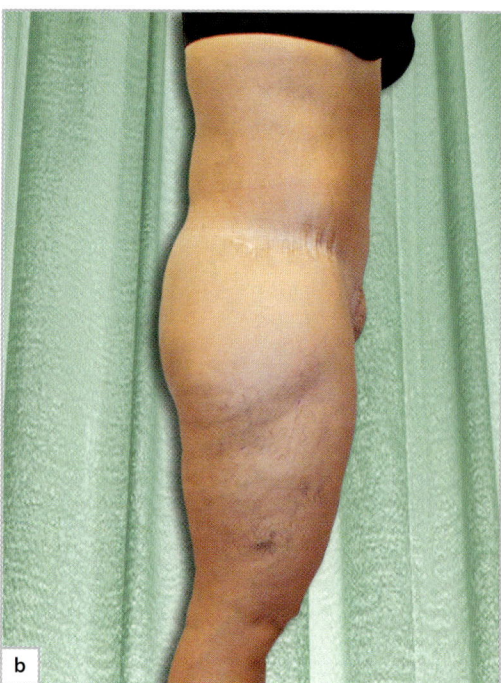

Figure 19.13 (a) A 41-year-old woman 17 months after gastric bypass surgery and weight loss of 36 kg (79 lb). Current weight and body mass index (BMI): 75 kg (165 lb), 31 respectively. Highest weight and BMI: 11 kg (24 lb), 46. (b) Seven months after body lift. Liposuction at the time of the body lift facilitated correction of the lateral thigh deformity in this patient.

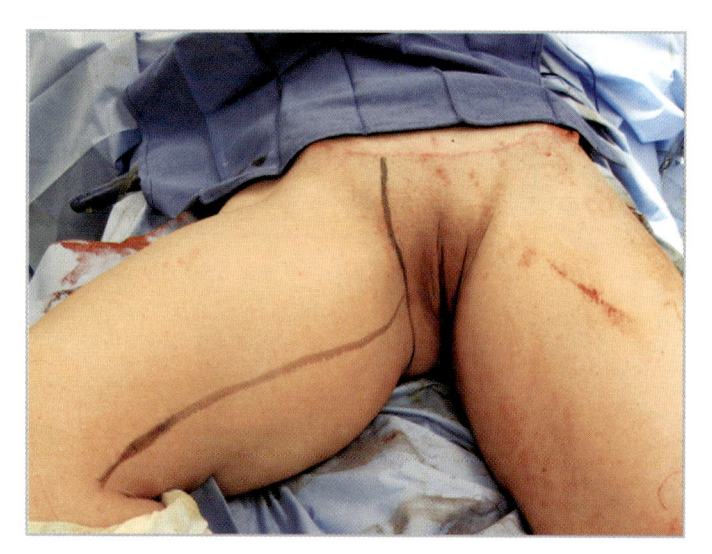

Figure 19.14 A cotton swab soaked in methylene blue is used to delineate a line extending from just inferior to the pre-existing scar from a circumferential body lift or abdominoplasty to the thigh perineal and gluteal crease on either side of the mons pubis.

of the skin and soft tissue to be removed. The cotton swab is used to connect the dots. Some of the dots my not correspond exactly to the overall pattern being produced and these are not followed (**Fig. 19.16**). In this way, a smooth contour is maintained along the medial thighs. Having completely demarcated an area of skin and soft tissue to be removed, along both the proximal and medial thighs and knee areas, the skin along the marking is incised completely. Beginning just distal to the knee, the flap is elevated under moderate tension. Previously performed liposuction creates a readily identifiable plane of dissection with a characteristic 'honeycomb' appearance (**Fig. 19.17**). Closure along the medial thigh is performed with interrupted 2/0 Vicryl sutures placed through the superficial fascial system (SFS) and deep dermis approximately 1 cm from the skin edge. The vertical closure is completed with a continuous, intracuticular 3/0 Monocryl suture. Tissue edges in the gluteal crease region are approximated initially with a no. 1 Vicryl suture placed through the SFS and deep dermis approximately 1 cm from the tissue edge (**Fig. 19.18**). Closure continues into the thigh perineal and mons pubis areas in a similar fashion. No. 0 Vicryl sutures are placed along the wound at a deep dermal level to further reinforce the closure; intracuticular 3/0 Monocryl sutures complete the closure. The same procedure is then performed on the left thigh. Sterile dressings are applied followed by elastic wraps.

■ Outcomes

Similar to brachioplasty, after our technique for medial thigh lift the vast majority of patients are pleased with their results. A circumferential body lift before the medial thigh lift is critical, however, to providing an optimum outcome after a medial thigh lift. Similar to brachioplasty, patients most likely to achieve or approach an aesthetic ideal and to have a very high level of satisfaction are those with a presenting BMI < 28 who have had significant weight loss before surgery, a BMI change of > 20 (**Fig. 19.19**). Patients presenting at a higher BMI, > 28, and who have also experienced very substantial weight loss before a surgery, are also very likely to be satisfied but are less likely to achieve an aesthetic ideal (**Fig. 19.20**). Liposuction plays a critical role in producing a substantial aesthetic improvement in this patient group. Candidates for surgery presenting at a higher BMI, > 32 and who have had relatively little weight loss before surgery, BMI change < 5, are usually the least satisfied and have the smallest aesthetic improvement.

Complications after medial thigh lift procedures are usually minor and very similar in frequency and management to those after brachioplasty (**Table 19.2**).[36]

Lower extremity contouring 175

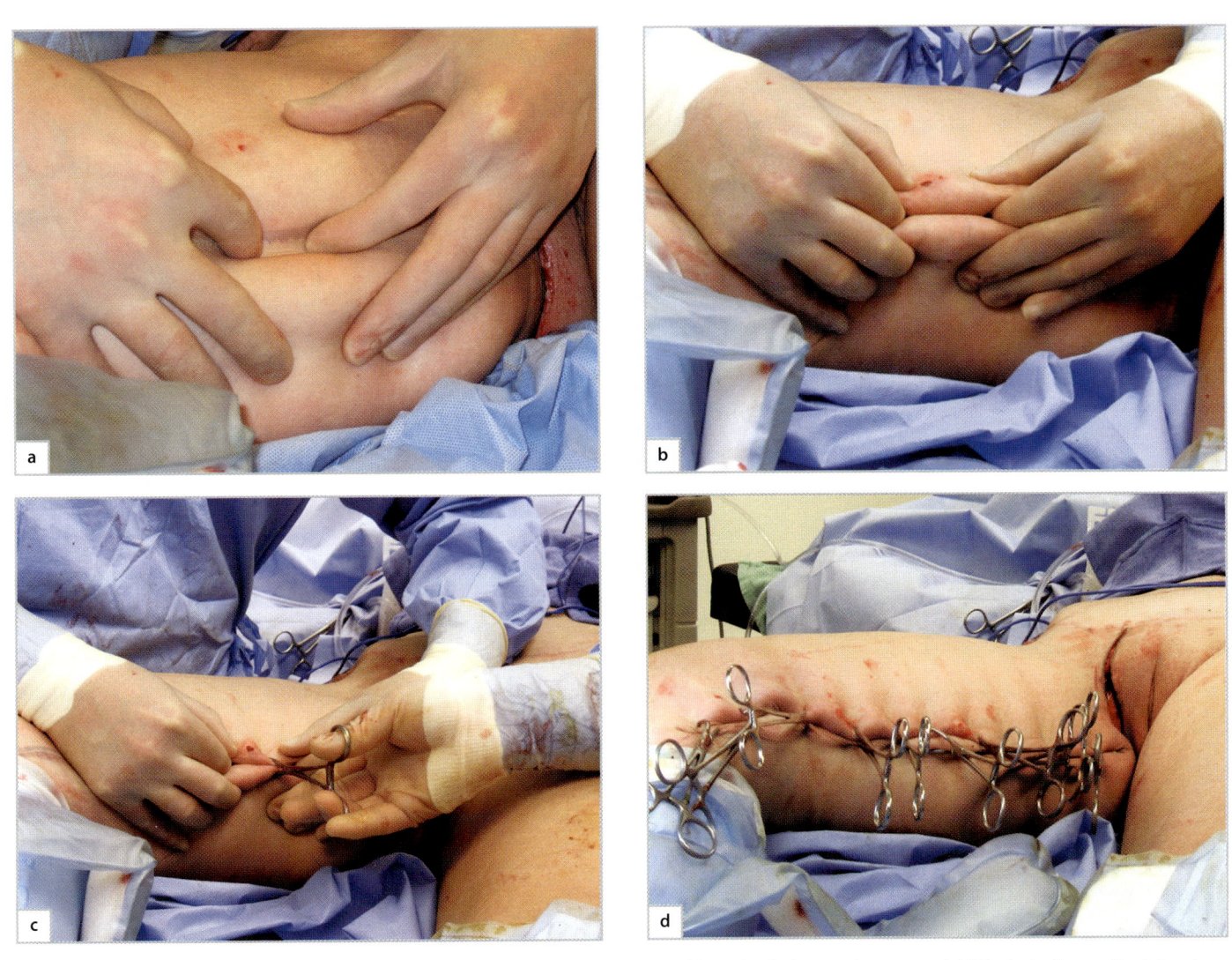

Figure 19.15. The 'pinch' technique is utilized by the surgeon to estimate the excess skin and soft tissue to be removed. (a) The index finger of both hands depresses the previously made marking along the medial thigh and knee. This technique maintains the final closure centered over least perceptible location. (b) The first 'pinch' is usually over the area of greatest soft-tissue excess, often the middle third of the medial thigh. (c,d) The assistant then uses Adair or towel clamps to maintain the position of the estimated tissue to be removed.

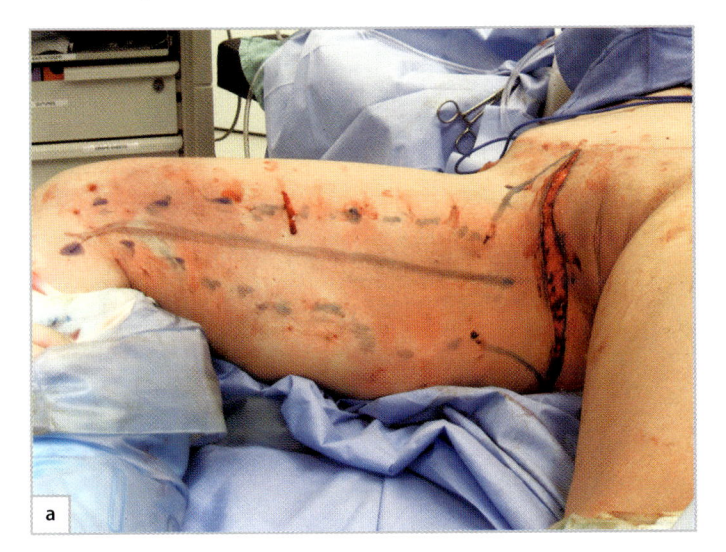

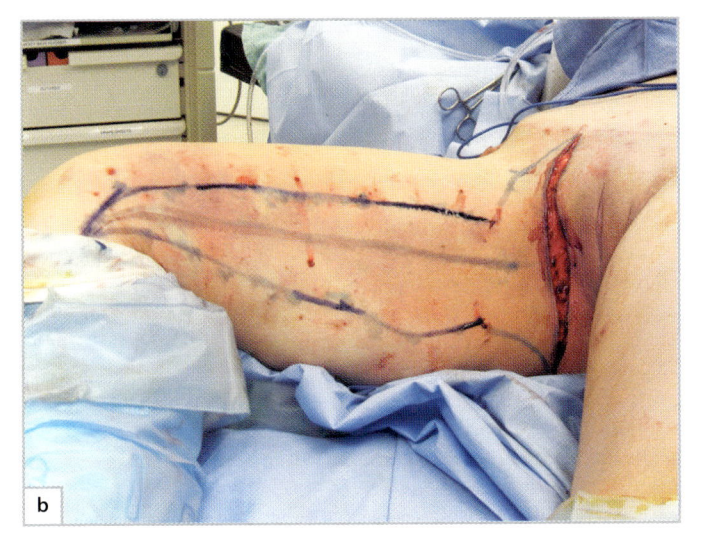

Figure 19.16 (a) The methylene blue swab is used to place dots on either skin edge along the medial thigh and knee region while the clamps are in place. The clamps are all released and removed. The series of dots along the medial thigh and knee delineate the pattern of the skin and soft tissue to be removed. (b) The cotton swab is used to connect the dots. Some of the dots may not correspond exactly to the overall pattern being produced and these are not followed. In this way, a smooth contour is maintained along the medial thighs.

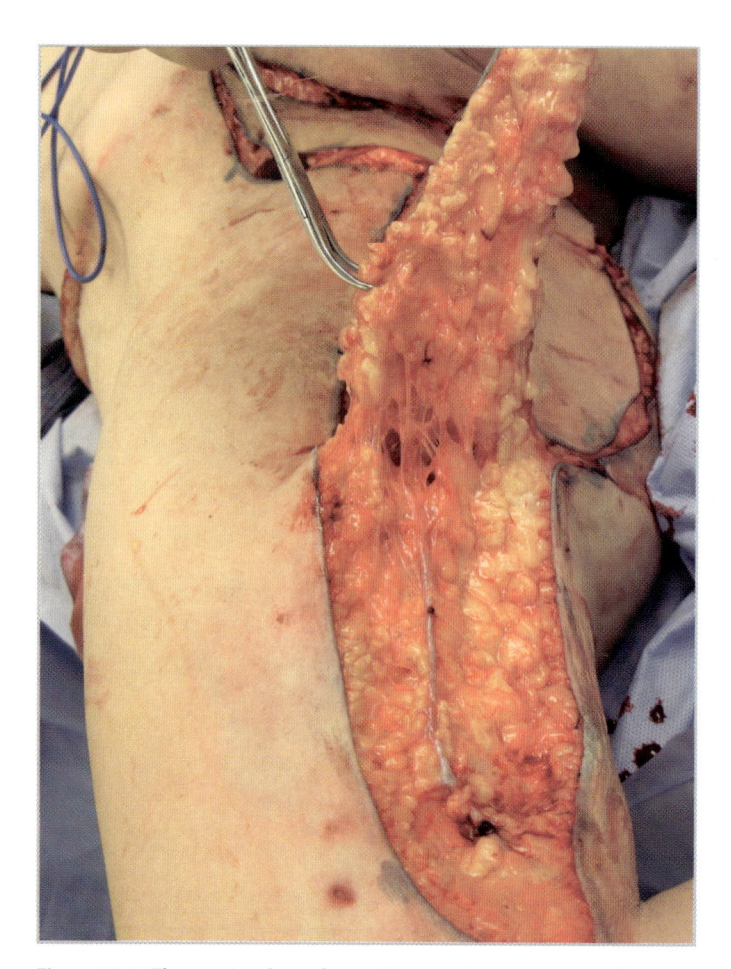

Figure 19.17 The previously performed liposuction creates a readily identifiable plane of dissection with a characteristic 'honeycomb' appearance. An effort is made to preserve the greater saphenous vein and its tributaries, although this is not always possible.

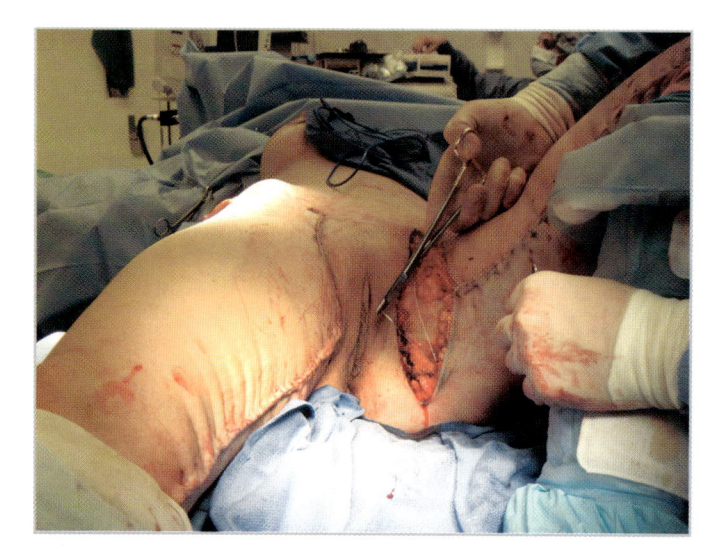

Figure 19.18 The cephalad tissue edge along the most posterior extent of the gluteal crease wound is approximated to the caudal tissue edge in a manner that does not produce a standing cone or 'dog ear' on the buttocks. Avoidance of this problem is facilitated by flexing the right hip and knees to 90° with slight hip abduction and having an assistant align the tissue edges.

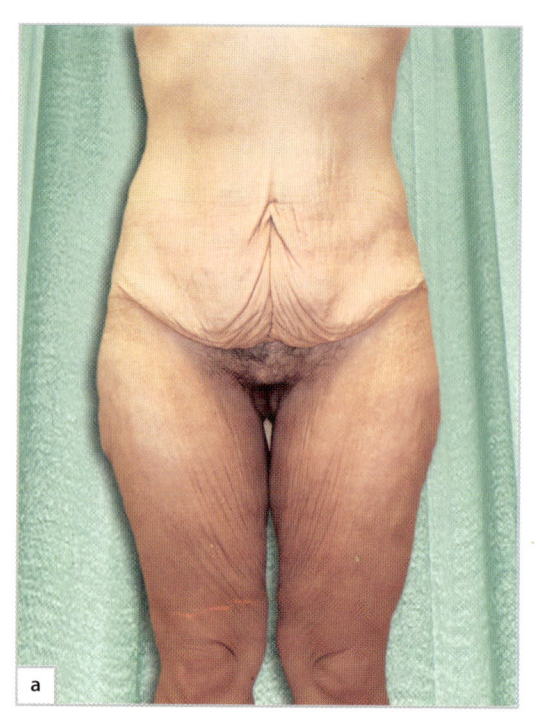

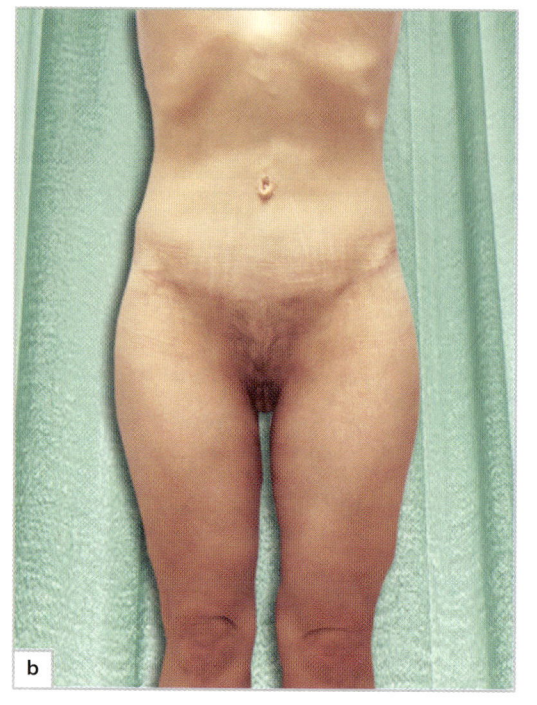

Figure 19.19 (a) A 46-year-old woman 13 months after gastric bypass surgery and weight loss of 70 kg (153 lb). Current weight and body mass index (BMI): 50 kg (109 lb), 20 respectively. Highest weight and BMI ever achieved: 119 kg (262 lb), 48. (b) Seventeen months after body lift and 4 months after medial thigh lift with a vertical component and revision lateral thigh lift.

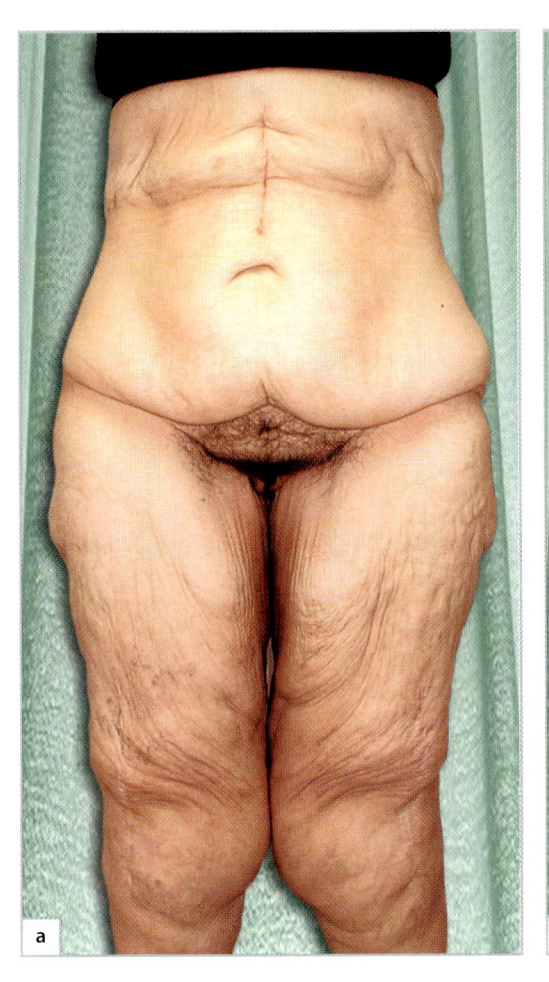

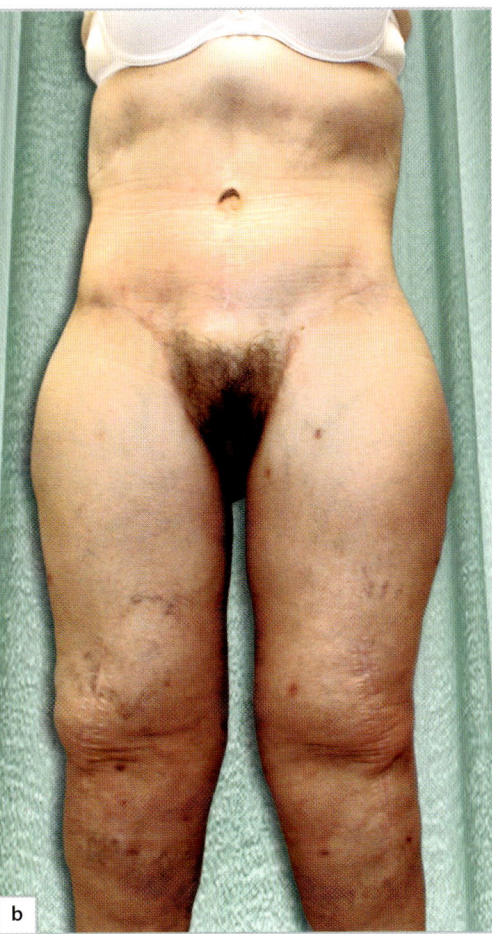

Figure 19.20 (a) A 55-year-old woman 13 months after gastric bypass surgery and weight loss of 52 kg (115 lb). Current weight and body mass index (BMI): 71 kg (156 lb), 30 respectively. Highest weight and BMI ever achieved: 123 kg (271 lb), 53. (b) Twenty-two months after body lift and 10 months following medial thigh lift with a vertical component extending onto leg. Liposuction was an important component of the medial thigh lift procedure.

Table 19.2 Complication rates associated with vertical medial thigh lift brachioplasty – 250 cases (500 thighs).

Complication	Complication rates (%)
Skin dehiscence	28.4
Seroma	19.8
Infection	1.2
Hematoma	0.4
Skin necrosis	0.4
Deep vein thrombosis	0.4
Pulmonary embolism	0.0

CONCLUSION

SAL has played a critical role in the management of the upper and lower extremities in our postbariatric body-contouring practice. Although SAL as a sole modality may have a deleterious effect on the body contour of a postbariatric patient, in combination with soft-tissue excisional procedures, liposuction can significantly improve outcomes. The use of SAL in our surgical approach to brachioplasty, medial thigh lift, and body lift has allowed for higher BMI individuals to have a significant improvement in contour and for the techniques to be performed more safely and efficiently.

REFERENCES

1. Capella JF, Oliak DA, Nemerofsky RB. Body lift: an account of 200 consecutive cases in the massive weight loss patient. *Plast Reconstr Surg* 2006;**117**:414.
2. Capella JF, Travato M, Woehrle S. Screening and safety issues in the massive-weight loss patient. In: Nahai F (ed.), *Art of Aesthetic Surgery: Principles and technique*, 2nd edn St. Louis. Quality Medical Publishing, 2010, pp. 2797–817.
3. Capella JF. Special problems in re-operative body contouring. In: Nahai F (ed.), *Art of Aesthetic Surgery: Principles and technique*, 2nd edn St. Louis. Quality Medical Publishing, 2010, pp. 3169-80.
4. Capella JF, Travato M, Woehrle S. Brachioplasty. In: Nahai F (ed.), *Art of Aesthetic Surgery: Principles and technique*, 2nd edn St. Louis. Quality Medical Publishing, 2010, pp. 2819–52.
5. Capella JF, Travato M, Woehrle S. Upper limb contouring. In: Warren R (ed.), *Plastic Surgery*, 3rd edn. New York: Elsevier, 2012: in press,=.
6. Thorek, M. esthetic surgery of the pendulous breast, abdomen and arms in the female. *Ill Med J* 1930;**58**:48.
7. Posse RP. *Cirugia Estetica*. Buenos Aires, Argentina, 1946.
8. Correa-Iturraspe M, Fernandez JC. Dermolipectomia braquial. *Prensa Med Argent* 1954;**34**:2432.

9. Baroudi R. Dermatolipectomy of the upper arm. *Clin Plast Surg* 1975;**2**:485.
10. Guerrero-Santos J. Brachioplasty. *Aesthet Plast Surg* 1979;**3**:1.
11. Juri J, Juri C, Elias JC. Arm dermolipectomy with a quadrangular flap and T closure. *Plast Reconstr Surg* 1979;**64**:521.
12. Pitanguy, I. Correction of lipodystrophy of the lateral thoracic aspect and inner side of the arm and elbow dermosenescence. *Clin Plast Surg* 1975;**2**:477.
13. McCraw, L. H., Jr. Surgical rehabilitation after massive weight: Case report. *Plast Reconstr Surg* 1974;**53**:349.
14. Hallock, G.G. and Altobelli, J.A. Simultaneous brachioplasty, thoracoplasty and mammoplasty. Aesthetic Plast Surg 9: 233, 1985.
15. Hauben DJ, Benmier P, Charuzi I. One-stage body contouring. *Ann Plast Surg* 1988;**21**:472.
16. Goddio AS. A new technique for brachioplasty. *Plast Reconstr Surg* 1989;**84**:85.
17. Lockwood T. Brachioplasty with superficial fascial system suspension. *Plast Reconstr Surg* 1995;**96** 912.
18. Temourian B, Malekzadeh S. Rejuvination of the upper arm. *Plast Reconstr Surg* 1998;**102**:545.
19. Richards MA. Minimal incision brachioplasty: a first choice option in arm reduction surgery. *Aesthet Surg J* 2001;**21**:301.
20. Vogt PA. Brachial suction-assisted lipoplasty and brachioplasty. *Aesthet Surg J* 2001;**21**:164–7.
21. Abramson DL. Minibrachioplasty: Minimizing scars while maximizing results. *Plast Reconstr Surg* 2004;**114**:1631.
22. Strauch B, Greenspun D, Levine J, et al. A technique of brachioplasty. *Plast Reconstr Surg* 2004;**113**:1044.
23. Taylor J, Shermak M. Body contouring following massive weight loss. *Obes Surg* 2004;**14**:1080.
24. Capella JF. Brachioplasty. Baker, Gordon Symposium. February 1, 2005.
25. Pascal JP, Le Louarn C. Brachioplasty. *Aesthet Plast Surg* 2005;**29** 423.
26. Knoetgen, J, III, and Moran, S. L. Long term outcomes and complications associated with brachioplasty: A retrospective review and cadaveric study. *Plast Reconstr Surg* 2006;**117**:2219.
27. Aly A, Cram AE, Pace D. Brachioplasty in the patient with massive weight loss. *Aesthet Surg J* 2006;**26**:76.
28. Hurwitz DJ, Holland SW. The L brachioplasty: An innovative approach to correct excess tissue of the upper arm, axilla, and lateral chest. *Plast Reconstr Surg* 2006;**117**:403.
29. Cannistra C, Valero R, Benelli C, et al. Brachioplasty after massive weight loss: A simple algorithm for surgical plane. *Aesthet Plast Surg* 2007;**31**:6.
30. El Khatib HA. Classification of brachial ptosis: Strategy for treatment. *Plast Reconstr Surg* 2007;**119**:1337.
31. Gusenoff JA, Coon D, Rubin JP. Brachioplasty and concomitant procedures after massive weight loss: a statistical analysis from a prospective registry. *Plast Reconstr Surg* 2008;**122**:595.
32. Bruschi S, Datta G, Bocchiotti MA, et al. Limb contouring after massive weight loss: functional rather than aesthetic improvement. *Obes Surg* 2009;**19**:407.
33. Leitner DW, Sherwood RC. Inguinal lymphocele as a complication of thighplasty. *Plast Reconstr Surg* 1983;**72**:878.
34. Moreno CH, Neto HJ, Junior AH, Malheiros CA. Thighplasty after bariatric surgery: evaluation of lymphatic drainage in lower extremities. *Obes Surg* 2008;**18**:1160.
35. Lockwood T. Fascial anchoring technique in medial thigh lifts. *Plast Reconstr Surg* 1988;**82**:299.
36. Capella JF. Vertical medial thigh lift with liposuction. In: Rubin PJ, Richter DF, Jewell M, Uebel C (eds), *Body Contouring and Liposuction*. Philadelphia: Elsevier, 2012: in press.
37. Capella JF. Body lift. *Clin Plast Surg* 2008;**35**:27.
38. Capella JF. An approach to the lower body after weight loss. In: Matarasso A, Rubin P (eds), *Aesthetic Surgery in the Massive Weight Loss Patient*. New York: Elsevier, 2007, pp. 69-99.

Chapter 20

Unfavorable results: identification and avoidance

Michael S. Golinko, Albert Losken

INTRODUCTION

Over one in three adults (33.8%)[1] in the USA is classified as obese, defined by a body mass index (BMI) ≥ 30 kg/m². Of these, approximately 2% will undergo bariatric surgery. However, with the number of bariatric surgeons doubling every 6 years,[2] the number undergoing this surgery is likely to increase. Approximately three-quarters of patients having gastric bypass surgery desire some form of body contouring,[3] and the number of patients undergoing a body-contouring procedure is also likely to increase. Body contouring may involve any part of the body with the goal of removing excess skin that formerly contained adipose tissue. According to the 2010 American Society of Plastic Surgery (ASPS), over 52 000 procedures including abdominoplasty, breast contouring, body lifting, brachioplasty, and thigh lift were performed by ASPS members alone, representing an overall 6% increase from 2009.[4] The most prevalent procedure performed was abdominoplasty/panniculectomy (35%). The postbariatric patient represents a unique challenge to the plastic surgeon, both in terms of achieving a desirable result and minimizing perioperative complications. This chapter seeks to systematically identify, report, and discuss the unfavorable results and complications with each of the procedures most commonly performed after weight loss surgery.

ABDOMINOPLASTY AND PANNICULECTOMY

Abdominal contouring procedures constitute the most common plastic surgery procedure after weight loss surgery.[4] To achieve favorable results after abdominal procedures, patients need to be satisfied, wounds healed, contours improved, and symptoms addressed. These procedures often involve long incisions, wide undermining, and thick flaps. The risk of complications such as seromas, hematomas, and wound dehiscence is not uncommon (**Table 20.1**). It is possible to minimize these complications with appropriate patient selection, technique and risk stratification in this often high-risk group of patients.

Dehiscence

The mean dehiscence rate in the literature is approximately 14% (**Table 20.1**). Authors who reported a low dehiscence rate attributed this to selecting patients who are non-smokers and have a low maximum and current body mass index (BMI). Skin dehiscence was most commonly observed in body lifts at the buttock cleft and hips, which are areas prone to more tension.[15] Few authors had to make return trips to the operating room to repair the wound (6% in one study[13]), and most cases of dehiscence are managed at the bedside with local wound care or reinforced suture. Other than patient selection geared toward ensuring optimal weight loss and ensuring at least 6 weeks of smoking cessation, technical modifications such as horizontal mattress sutures or some type of retention suture may mitigate this complication. One study found that the risk of wound dehiscence increased over threefold when multiple procedures were performed, i.e. panniculectomy, plus another procedure.[7] Other technique modifications include minimizing tension on the skin closure and layered closure to prevent other complications such as seroma or skin necrosis, which contribute to wound dehiscence (**Fig. 20.1**).

Seroma

Seroma formation was also commonly reported, in approximately 12.9% of patients. Standard of care includes placing a closed-suction drain, closure in layers to minimize dead space, and minimizing undermining if possible. Authors who reported the lowest rates stated that they removed drains when the output was ≤ 20 ml[10] and used abdominal binders for 6 weeks postoperatively.[10] Authors experienced higher than average seroma rates without a protocol in place to remove drains. In most cases an abdominal binder is placed for a minimum of 3 weeks. Seromas can be aspirated at the bedside or under ultrasound guidance. Some authors advocate placing patients on 1 week of prophylactic antibiotics.[9] Early recognition of fluid collections can prevent secondary infection, wound dehiscence, and even necrosis. Appropriate and adequate drainage of fluid, in addition to compression therapy, appear to be the best way to minimize seromas; in addition, there may be some evidence that use of cautery as opposed to a scalpel may decrease fluid collections.[9] Although not specifically mentioned in this subgroup of abdominoplasty patients, the use of progressive tension or quilting sutures has been shown by several authors to decrease seromas.[16,17] The use of sealants such as fibrin glue has not shown as much promise and even been shown to increase seroma formation compared with controls in one study.[18]

Surgical site infection

The mean surgical site infection was 9.3%. Arthurs et al.[13] state that a pre-panniculectomy BMI [3]37 correlated with a postoperative cellulitis or hematoma; 81% had ASA (American Society of Anesthesiologists) class 2–3 but this was not a statistically significant predictor of surgical site infection (SSI) or hematoma. Two additional studies also found current BMI to be the single strongest predictor of encountering a complication.[7,12] Authors cited that, the less change in BMI from pre- to postbariatric surgery, the less chance of infection, the current BMI being the strongest weight-based predictor of infection. Appropriate use of perioperative antibiotics should be employed. Re-dosing of antibiotics is indicated for procedures lasting more than 4 h or with massive blood loss, and should be re-dosed every one to two half-lives of the antibiotic. Decreased surgical time has been shown in one study to lower infection rate to 5.3%.[7] There has been no proven role for additional dosing after skin closure in a non-contaminated setting.[19] Smoking has felt to be a risk factor for infection; however, Araco et al. demonstrated that 14 infections still occurred even after patients had quit smoking 4 weeks before the procedure, indicating that more objective evidence

Table 20.1 Summary of abdominal contouring procedures.

Reference	No.	SSI (%)	D (%)	VTE (%)	H (%)	S (%)	Avoidance complications
Ortega et al.[5]	34	–	–	0	12	35	↓ wt of specimen removed (<4.8 kg) ↓ current BMI (<34)
Zuelzer et al.[6]	122	13	0	0	12.3	16	↓ current BMI (<30)
Coon et al.[7]	171	5.3	9.5	0	4.7	4.1	Decrease operating room time, single procedure, current BMI D, SSI, max. BMI and Δ BMI (both were not significant for hematoma rate)
Vico et al.[8]	23	4		8.7	4	4	Routine DVT prophylaxis
Araco et al.[9]	137	20.4	NR	1.6	5.1	5.1	Use of cautery for flap dissection (H, RR 11.6) over scalpel Minimize hematoma (SSI 43% infection hematoma vs non)
De Kerviler et al.[10,a]	62	2.4	20	0.8	4.2	7.7	Lower BMI pre-body contouring ↓ weight of tissue resected
Greco et al.[11]	139	14	13	–	7	17	BMI <25 (wound complication, ASA class) or 2.37, surgical time 1.01 hr
Au et al.[12]	129	14.7	2.3	–	6.2	6.2	↓ current BMI <40 all complications
Arthurs et al.[13]	126	17	11	–	13	17	↓ current BMI (<25 or 3.3 postop complication)
Acarturk et al.[14]	102	16	13	1	2	–	↓ current BMI
Body lifts							
Nemerofsky et al.[15]	200	3.5	32.5	1.7	3.5	16.5	A/c not used perioperatively, ↓ maximum BMI, current BMI, **former and current smokers** (69% vs 46%), buttock cleft, and hip dehiscence, avoid BMI >35
Means		9.3	14.0	1.7	6.7	12.9	

[a]Combines data from body contouring after bariatric surgery (59.6) and the remainder diet/exercise (40.04%).
Bold text = reached statistical significance (p <0.05).
ASA, American Society of Anesthesiologists; BMI, body mass index; D, dehiscence; H, hematoma; RR, relative risk; S, seroma; SSI, surgical site infection; VTE, venothromboembolic event.

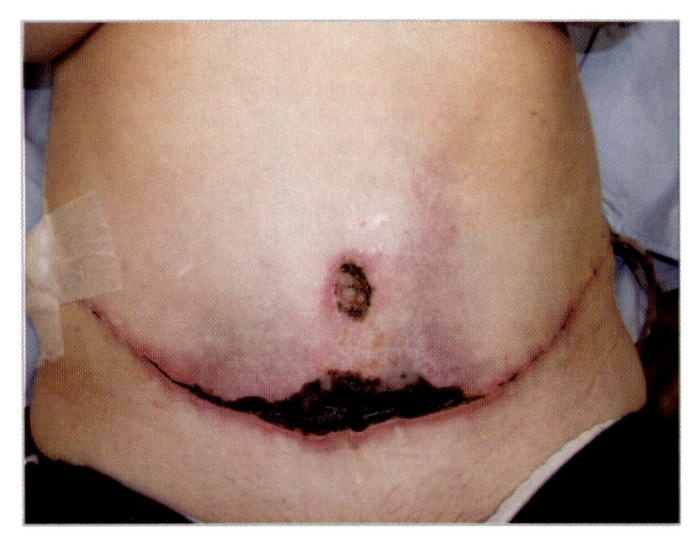

Figure 20.1 Full-thickness skin necrosis beneath the umbilicus following **abdominoplasty** is often due to over aggressive thinning of abdominal skin flaps, tight closure, and/or wide undermining.

of cessation or a larger period of abstinence is needed.[9] Although there is no level 1 evidence for antibiotic prophylaxis in the setting of a drain, one series that did leave patients on antibiotics until drains were removed (up to a maximum of 5 weeks) had an infection rate of only 3.5%.[15] Interestingly, several authors cited decreased surgical time as a significant factor in minimizing any complication.[7,11]

Although *Staphylococcus aureus* remains the predominant isolate from a surgical site, there is increasing prevalence of methicillin-resistant *S. aureus* (MRSA) cultured from wounds. Therefore, there is some evidence to support preoperative nasal swabs of patients and antibiotic prophylaxis, with 5 days of nasal mupirocin (Bactroban), and preoperative vancomycin or equivalent if testing positive. Prophylaxis without pre-screening is not advised because the same study found a *higher* rate of SSI with vancomycin prophylaxis in the group who tested negative for MRSA.[20] Preoperative skin prep has not been shown to significantly reduce SSI with any preparation, although there has been a clear benefit in reduction of SSI[21] using chlorhexidine- versus iodine-based prep, 9.5% versus 16%.[22] Skin necrosis can be avoided by appropriately placing incisions, avoiding excessive undermining, not thinning out the flaps, and avoiding patients who smoke. Caution should be taken when liposuction is performed on flaps that will need to be undermined. Finally, as with any surgical procedure, it has been shown that prolonged procedures, trauma, shock, blood transfusions, hypothermia, hypoxia, and hyperglycemia can increase the risk of infection.[23]

■ Hematoma

Although the incidence of hematomas is relatively low (6.7%, range 2–13%), this complication most often requires a return trip to the operating room for evacuation.[5,13] Very few patients will require a blood transfusion. Most authors felt that the risk of venous thromboembolism (VTE) outweighed the risk of hematoma in this patient population, and chemical deep venous thrombosis (DVT) prophylaxis should not be stopped or delayed because of risk of hematoma formation.[24] Moreover, when statistically analyzed, change in BMI from pre- to postbariatric surgery most strongly correlated with increased hematomas (odds ratio 1.08). This correlation was stronger in patients with multiple procedures than those with a single procedure.[7] One study did not find any statistical difference in major bleeding complications of patient with a different BMI; however, those patients who were heavier did experience more minor complications.[6] The use of cautery was clearly shown to decrease the hematoma rate from 1.1% with cautery to 12.8% with a scalpel (relative risk 11.6). In addition, a higher rate of wound infection was found in patients with hematomas. Almost half the patients with hematomas (43%) developed a surgical site infection, versus 5.3% patients without a hematoma.[9]

Venous thromboembolism

The mean prevalence of VTE in the literature is 1.7%. This number is not much different from patients undergoing their weight loss procedure as well, up to 1.54% as demonstrated in the Bariatric Outcomes Longitudinal Database, which examined surgical outcomes of over 73 000 patients up to 90 days after surgery.[25] Authors reporting a higher than average rate,[8] did not routinely give prophylaxis to patients and thus admittedly started to modify their practice after looking at their data. There is a well-established risk of VTE disease and BMI; one study of over 1000 patients found the risk of VTE associated with BMI was 12.03 (95% confidence interval 1·53–94·29) and ≥ 30 kg/m², respectively, after adjustment for age and estrogen use.[26] Abdominoplasty patients are particularly at risk because of the length of the procedures, preoperative BMI, possible immobilization, and often combination with other procedures increasing surgical time. Most centers before performing bariatric surgery administer 5000 U heparin just before induction; this same practice may be warranted in the body-contouring population, along with prophylaxis until discharge. The American College of Chest Physicians (AACP) cites level 1 evidence for three times daily dosing of chemical prophylaxis for obese patients undergoing bariatric surgery,[27] and, although many patients have undergone significant weight loss by the time that they present to the plastic surgeon, this population may still be at risk.

BREAST CONTOURING

After significant weight loss, the breast in both males and females may undergo significant change and require surgical improvement. Once the skin envelope has been reshaped to better fit the new BMI, additional procedures are often necessary, such as parenchymal plication, dermal suspension, and autoaugmentation to reshape the breast mound. In contrast to other cosmetic breast patients, bariatric patients have an ill-defined breast mound, with an inelastic skin envelope that may merge with other anatomic areas, making an aesthetically pleasing result a challenge.[28,32] The Pittsburgh rating scale takes into account the component of nipple and glandular ptosis that occurs in massive weight loss patient, and this must be considered in surgical planning.[29]

Fewer complications were observed in patients undergoing reduction mammoplasty, mastopexy, or augmentation compared with abdominal body contouring. Frank skin necrosis was observed only in 1% of the patients, with cellulitis, and seroma also being rarely observed, 1.5% and 2.7%, respectively (**Table 20.2**). The most common complications in breast contouring were dehiscence 4.8% and hematoma 4.3%. The breast is not as prone to infection as the abdominal operations and therefore these numbers are understandably less. There is some evidence that broader coverage of antibiotics during breast surgery with potential nipple and ductal contamination may be warranted.[33] Rubin et al.[30] do report a lower rate of hematoma and wound dehiscence when the skin was closed in two layers, closed suction drains and a compressive dressing was applied. Combined studies that looked at body contouring along with a breast procedure also reported fewer complications with patient selection,[5,7] although no discrimination was made on complications between breast procedures apart from the abdominal operation.

Table 20.2 Summary of breast contouring studies.

Reference	No.	SSI (%)	D (%)	H (%)	S (%)
Rubin et al.[30]	108	0	2.7	0	2.7
Migliori et al.[31]	195	–	3.1	8.7	–
Losken and Holtz[32]	35	2.9	8.5		
Mean		1.5	4.8	4.3	2.7

D, dehiscence; H, hematoma; S, seroma; SSI, surgical site infection; VTE, venothromboembolic event.

Table 20.3 Extremity contouring procedures.

	No.	C (%)	D (%)	VTE (%)	H (%)	S/L (%)
Brachioplasty						
Symbas and Losken[34]	31	6.5	–	–	6.5	6.5
Gusenoff et al.[35]	101	2.9	8.9	–	0	23.7
Bruschi et al.[36]	13	0	23	7.6	7.6	7.6
Mean		3.1	15.9	7.6	4.7	12.6
Thigh lift						
Bruschi et al.[36]	35	0	8.5	0	14.3	12.5
Shermak et al.[37]	97	7.2	–	0	1	3.1

C, cellulitis; D, dehiscence; H, hematoma; L, lymphocele; N, necrosis; S, seroma; VTE, venothromboembolic event.

Extremity contouring

Extremity contouring procedures are not without complications, given the difficulties inherent to the anatomic locations (**Table 20.3**). Aly et al.[38] reported a 13.5% dehiscence rate in brachioplasty for massive weight loss patients, although a third of these patients were smokers.[36,37] Gusenoff et al.[35] found that surgical site infection was significantly reduced in patients who had experienced less dramatic change in BMI – the mean in their study was 29. Moreover they found that surgical times > 8 hours related to increased complications although not to any one complication in particular. Seromas and lymphoceles are also not uncommon and were reported in over 12% of patients. This could be avoided by minimal undermining, closure of the dead space, compression garments, and occasionally drainage tubes. Any surgery on the upper extremity is prone to lymphatic disruption, particularly near the axilla. Use of quilting sutures, as in abdominoplasty, may decrease this rate. Injury to the medial antebrachial cutaneous nerve can also occur after brachioplasty, with resultant sensory loss on either side the of the brachioplasty incision, although few have been reported.[34,35] Based on the position of entry of this nerve, a more posterior scar, such as with the double-ellipse technique described by Aly et al.,[38] can minimize this complication. Scarring can often be unfavorable in the extremities, which needs to be discussed with the patient preoperatively (**Fig. 20.2**). If tension is not constant along the length of the incision, irregularities in contour can occur (**Fig. 20.3**).

In inner thigh lift or thighplasty, the largest studies report a seroma rate of between 4 and 13%. In Shermak's study of 71 patients, drains were not routinely placed for the thigh lift.[37] The group developed a seroma algorithm, which began with simple aspiration and, if unresolved, placement of a catheter, with or without the addition of antibiotic sclerosis. Their group developed a modification of the original procedure described by Lockwood,[39] called the anterior proximal extended thighlift (APEX). In their statistical analysis, they found that a BMI > 35 correlated with a high risk of infection, but a lower risk of lymphedema, which the authors attribute to a difficulty in diagnosis in larger patients. In addition, each year in age correlated to a 9% increase risk of a wound-healing complication.

Facial contouring

Facial contouring is less common in the weight loss patient when compared with breast and body contouring.[40] Although there is a classification system for body contour deformities for virtually every other area of the body, none has been reported for the face.[41] There is a paucity of data on facial contouring; however, it is known that loss of abdominal fat correlates well with loss of buccal and malar fat pad volume as measured by computed tomography (CT).[42] Facial aging tends to be accelerated with weight loss and correction revolves around re-suspension and volume replacement. Skin is often very thin, inelastic, and excessive. Complications are similar to facial rejuvenation in the non-weight loss patients, however, which requires strict attention to skin quality for maximal results. It is not yet known to what degree the SMAS (superficial musculoaponeurotic system) layer may be affected by dramatic weight loss.

GENERAL CONSIDERATIONS FOR OPTIMAL OUTCOMES

The discussion that follows synthesizes evidence and experience on various aspects of the care of the postbariatric weight loss patient. A summary of the main points is provided in **Table 20.4**.

Initial weight loss operation

According to Michaels et al.[43] patient selection may be the single most reliable method to prevent complications. All initial consultations begin with a history. The timing of the weight loss surgery and what type, i.e. roux-en-Y gastric bypass (RYGB) or laparoscopic band (LB), may change the timing and staging of various body-contouring procedures. Several factors about the initial operation must be considered by the plastic surgeon. First, the presence of abdominal scars, either laparoscopic or open, and the potential position of an adjustable gastric band port must all be considered in designing a panniculectomy or abdominoplasty. Certainly if the patient has sought an adjustment of the band recently, contouring may need to be deferred. Moreover, a finite number of patients have had removal of their laparoscopic bands or a band over an RYGB in which the pouch was made too large. These pieces of history are important because they may change the optimal window for the plastic surgeon to intervene. The timing of surgery is also an important factor. Although it has not been studied rigorously, experts recommend a minimum of 3–4 months of weight stability before operating, which usually occurs at least a year after the weight loss procedure.[44] Studies reporting timing of surgery after bariatric surgery were Ortega et al.:[5] 29 months, Acarturk et al.:[14] 17 months, Arthurs et al.:[13] minimum 12 months, de Kerviler et al.:[10] stable weight at 12 months. Generally, a weight stability, demonstrated over a 6-month period, for a minimum of a year after the bariatric procedure is advised.[39]

The theoretical basis of wound-healing complications has been discussed in some detail by Albino et al.[45] They cite obesity as a known chronic inflammatory condition, where levels of the matrix metalloproteinase MMP9 and the tissue inhibitor of metalloproteinase TIMP-1 (inflammatory mediators) were found in higher levels of obese children. Moreover, preoperative levels of interleukin (IL)-6

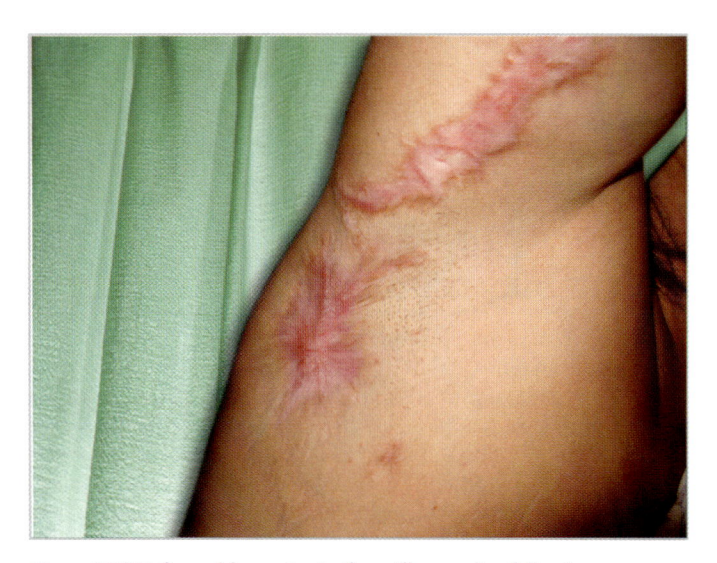

Figure 20.2 Unfavorable scaring in the axillary region following brachioplasty.

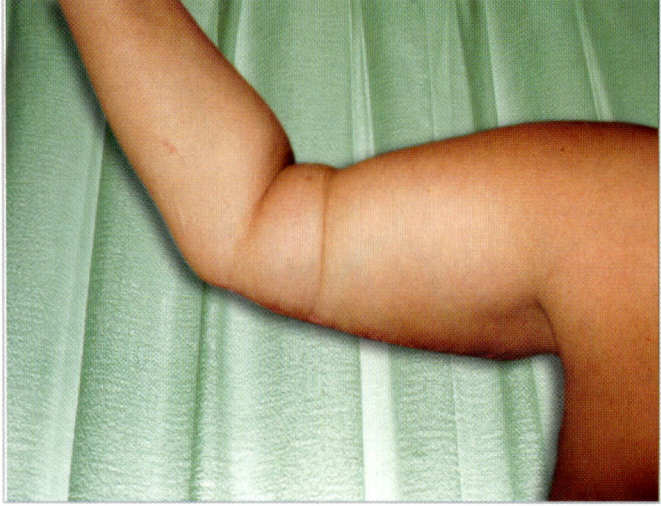

Figure 20.3 A tight contracture band distal in the upper arm where tension distribution was uneven.

Table 20.4 Summary of modifiable risk factors to reduce complications in body-contouring procedures.

All procedures
↓ current body mass index (BMI) ↓ Δ BMI
Optimize protein/vitamin deficiencies
Chemical deep vein thrombosis prophylaxis starting at induction
Smoking cessation ≥6 weeks
Chlorhexidine prep
Stable weight ≥ 3–4 months
OR time < 8 hours
Appropriate antibiotic prophylaxis, MRSA nasal swab in select patients
↓ ASA class
Use of cautery for flap dissection

were higher in obese patients than not. More convincingly, levels of IL-8, transforming growth factor b, and TIMP-1 were all reduced in patients who underwent gastric bypass surgery with concomitant weight loss.[45] All these clinical and theoretical data point to the emphasis on stabilization of weight loss, and the argument to perform a body-contouring procedure when the bariatric patient is as close to the ideal body weight as possible.

Prevention of VTE disease

Perhaps the most life-threatening complication of operating on a massive weight loss (MWL) patient is the risk of pulmonary embolism. The risk to patients undergoing plastic surgery procedures cannot be overemphasized. Particularly in light of a recent survey of ASPS member surgeons performing breast reconstruction, only 38% gave their patients prophylaxis in accordance with ACCP's guidelines.[46] Regardless, however, administration of 5000 U heparin at induction of general anesthesia may be advised and poses little bleeding risk to the patient. Young and Watson performed a detailed literature review of plastic surgery patients, and emphasized the role of preoperative prophylaxis, chemical, or sequential compression devices (SCDs), for procedures >1 hour or for patients receiving general anesthesia.[47] The vast majority of patients undergoing body contouring procedures after MWL fall into the moderate-risk category – defined as any procedure on a patient aged 40–60 years undergoing general anesthesia for ≥ 30 min.[48] It is important to garner from the history whether the patient had a perioperative deep vein thrombosis/pulmonary embolism at their weight loss procedure because this places them in a high-risk category, and they should have chemical prophylaxis as well as pneumatic compression. Other steps that maximize venous return are having the patient walk from the preop area to the operating table, placing above- and below-knee SCD boots and early ambulation. Continuation of perioperative prophylactic doses of low-molecular-weight heparin until the patient is ambulatory is advised.

Nutritional status

Optimal nutrition is important to minimize complications in any surgical patient. Nutritional deficiencies in the weight loss patient are a well-known occurrence, as documented with most deficiencies occurring the first year after bariatric surgery.[49,50] Plastic surgeons should have the patient appropriately screened for common deficiencies such as iron deficiency anemia, vitamins B_{12} and B_6, folate, vitamin C, vitamin E, selenium, zinc, and copper, because all of these are salient deficiencies in the bariatric patient and affect wound healing. Moreover in a study of 90 body-contouring patients (53% of whom had bariatric surgery), 38% had abnormally low albumin, 28% had low transferrin, 33% had a vitamin A deficiency, 16.3% iron deficiency, and 9.5% vitamin B_{12} deficiency.[51] Another study of 100 body-contouring patients at a stable weight showed that approximately 14% of patients had low albumin, almost 40% had iron deficiency, and nearly 15% had vitamin B_{12} deficiency.[52] Although largely studied in chronic wounds,[53-55] poor nutritional status, i.e. low albumin, is known to delay wound healing, which can be problematic in MWL patients in whom incisions are often long and wound-healing complications are not uncommon. Before undergoing a body-contouring procedure, the patient should have an albumin level in the normal range for the testing laboratory and a normal prealbumin, indicating adequate intake in the last 7–10 days. Moreover, a complete blood count, coagulation panel, and vitamin B_{12} level should all be assessed and corrected before surgery. Consultation with a nutritionist is appropriate.

Exercise

A study by Koltz et al.[56] and others found that, in 133 bariatric patients presenting for body contouring, exercise more than five times a week correlated with a larger change in BMI and lower current BMI. Although it is clear that a lower BMI at the time of body contouring is associated with improved outcomes across all procedures, more exercise to produce a larger change in BMI may be deleterious in certain cases of either abdominoplasty or panniculectomy.[11,44]

Smoking

Greco also looked at smoking and diabetes in a multiple logistic regression model and found that smoking did affect the chance of having a wound complication. Gravante et al.[57] looked at 60 prospectively enrolled patients who underwent gastric banding, and then abdominoplasty, and they found the infection rate to be 25%, with all but one infection occurring in a non-smoker. In addition to dietary modification, the most important lifestyle modification that a patient can make is to stop smoking. The effect of smoking on wound dehiscence has been shown[58] and, more specifically, the greater number of complications in patients undergoing panniculectomy.[59] Moreover there is good theoretical evidence for cessation of any nicotine product for 4 weeks before surgery due to vasoconstrictive effects.[56,60] Elective procedures involving long incisions and undermining should be avoided on patients who are actively smoking.

Medical comorbidities

Morbidly obese patients have an increased prevalence of medical comorbidities which should be optimized before surgery. Although it has been shown that many of the common issues such as diabetes, hypertension, or sleep apnea can improve or remit,[61] the plastic surgeon should inquire as to the current management or resolution of these issues. Routine stress testing before surgery has been recommended for some patients.[62] Pulmonary disease is one of the medical conditions most correlated with surgical site infection and wound dehiscence.[62] Therefore, every effort to obtain a careful history, and physical review of systems with regard to asthma, tuberculosis, pneumonia, emphysema, smoking, pulmonary blebs, even allergies should be made. This will help plan a more aggressive postoperative regimen, including early ambulation, aggressive use of the incentive spirometery, bronchodilators, chest physical therapy, and pulmonary toilet in an attempt to minimize these complications.

MANAGING PATIENT EXPECTATIONS

A recent study demonstrated that bariatric patients between 2 and 10 years after surgery were more interested in waist and abdominal contouring. The only significant predictor of lower patient satisfaction was higher BMI at the time of the body-contouring procedure.[63] In another study surveying 70 postbariatric patients, approximately half of whom had undergone body contouring, patients were most dissatisfied with waist/abdomen and upper arms. Patients were most satisfied with the appearance of their face. The majority of patients (75%) wanted surgery on their abdominal area, whereas only 38.8% wanted facial contouring. An even smaller percentage wanted upper back contouring – 23.9%.[40] A large part of identifying unfavorable outcomes involves having careful initial consultation with the patient beforehand. Song et al.[64] found that, in a small sample of patients undergoing bariatric surgery and subsequent abdominoplasty and panniculectomy, the three areas of most distress were abdomen (69% of patients), flanks (56%), and hips/outer thighs (44%). It is prudent, as in all procedures of this nature, to have a frank and realistic discussion with the patient about what the goals are for a particular operation, what the goals may be in the long term, and what is the safest way to proceed.

Moreover, knowledge of the expected complications in this group will help the surgeon and patient come through the operation better informed, and hopefully more satisfied with the end-result even when complications occur. Skin quality after weight loss is often poor and inelastic. Patients need to be aware that despite skin tightening at the initial procedure, re-excision can be required due to recurrent laxity (**Fig. 20.4**). It is also important that the patient maintain the weight loss, because gaining it back will potentially undo the benefits of the body-contouring procedures (**Fig. 20.5**).

■ CONCLUSION

Body-contouring after weight loss surgery is expected to increase in the coming years. Abdominoplasty and panniculectomy are likely to remain the most commonly requested procedure. Reconstructive surgeons need to be cognizant of the safest approaches and ways to minimize complications. MWL patients and procedures are at risk of complications. Risk stratification is important and appropriate patient and technique selection will help minimize morbidity. Postoperative management is equally important because potential morbidity could be avoided with knowledge of possible complications. Seromas, for example, should be drained because stasis could lead to a cellulitis and wound infection. Surgical site infection, if untreated, could result in wound dehiscence. Appropriate preoperative planning, patient selection, managing expectations, surgical technique, and postoperative care are all equally important in maximizing safety and patient satisfaction.

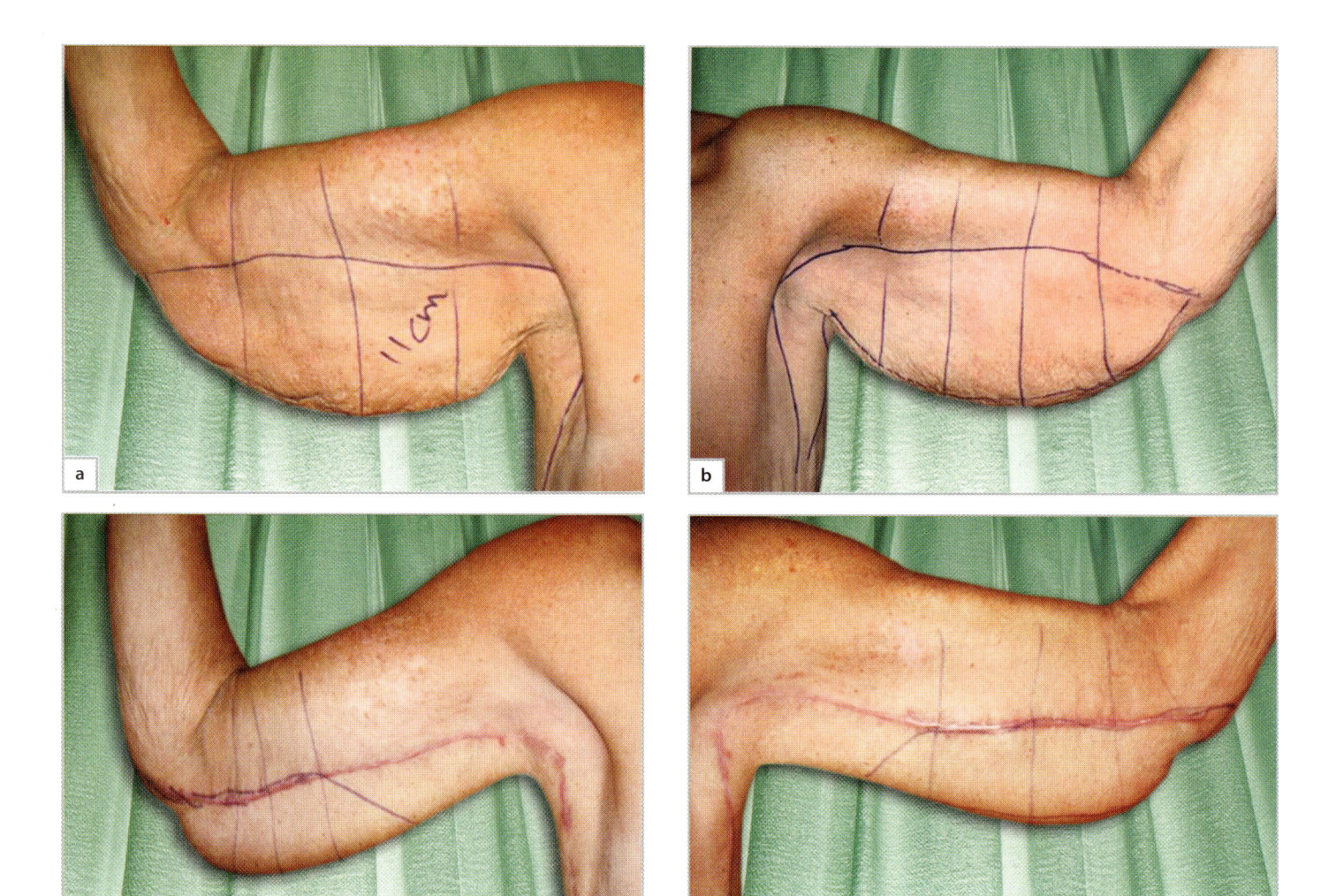

Figure 20.4a–d Markings are shown of extensive brachioplasty for arm lipodystrophy. *Continued opposite.*

Conclusion 185

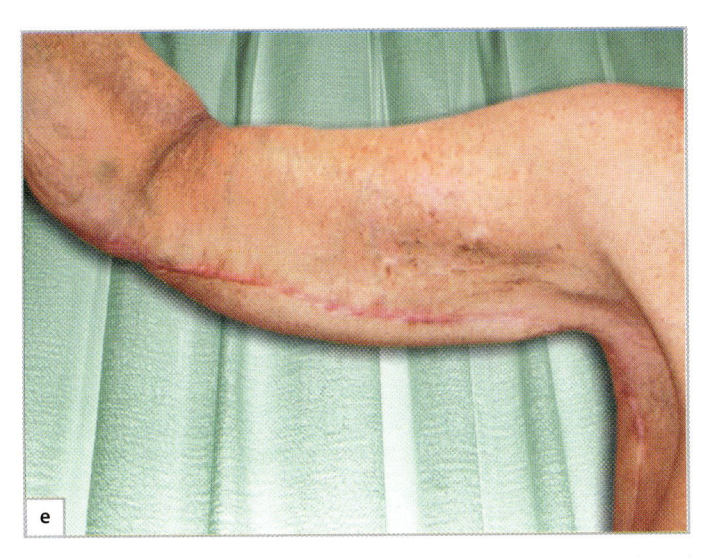

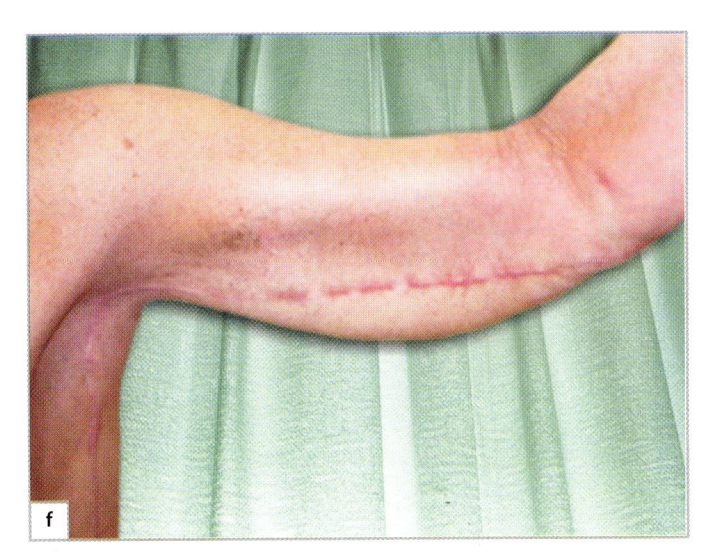

Figure 20.4e–f 18 months later, the patient had significant redundancy due to loss of elasticity and required re-excision. Her final result is shown 1 year after a second operation.

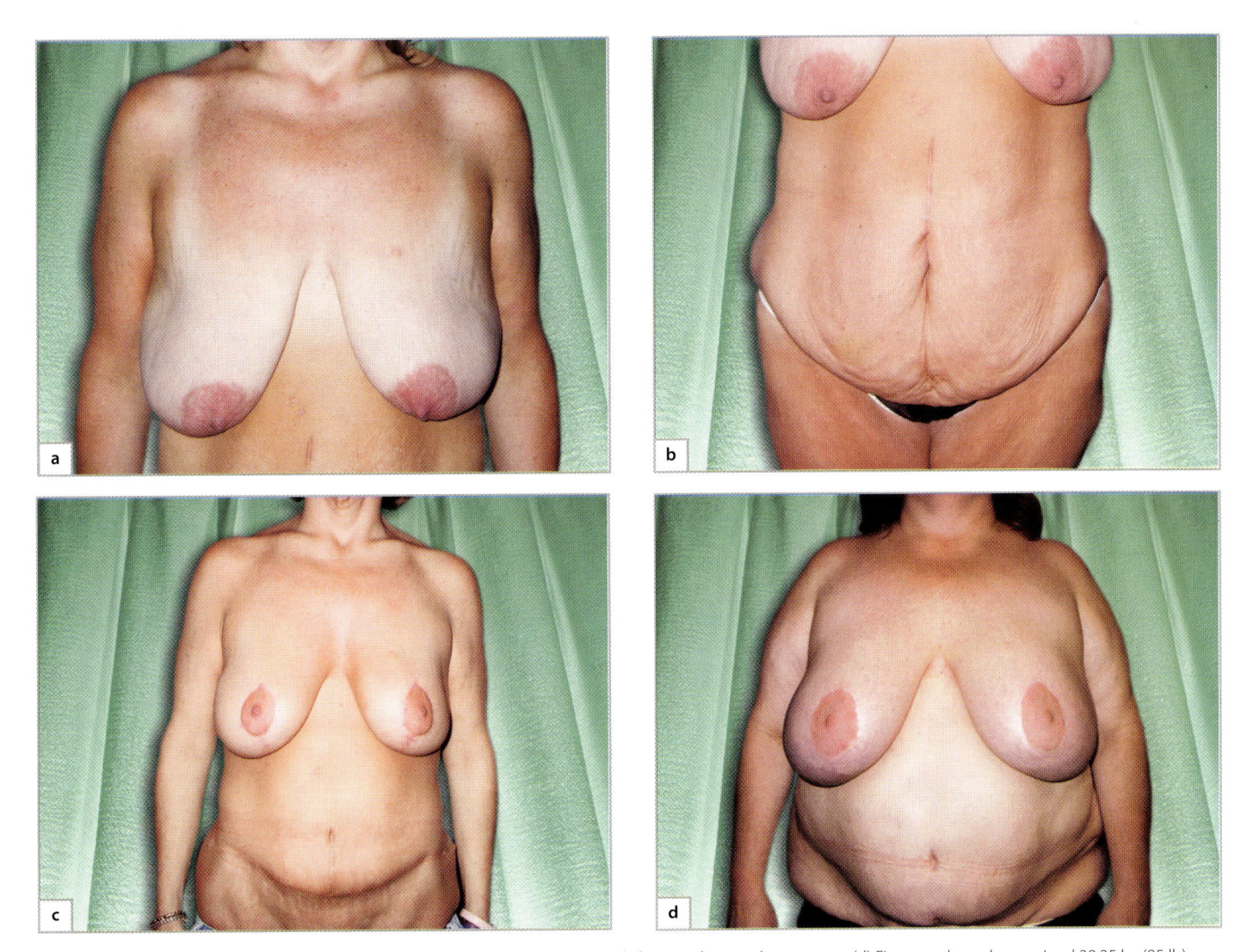

Figure 20.5 (a,b) This 42-year-old woman lost 45 kg (100 lb). (c) She underwent abdominoplasty and mastopexy. (d) Five years later she regained 38.25 kg (85 lb) with loss of the beneficial effects of body contouring.

REFERENCES

1. Flegal KM, Carroll MD, Ogden CL, Curtin LR. Prevalence and trends in obesity among US adults, 1999–2008. JAMA 2010;**303**:235–41.
2. Nguyen NT, Masoomi H, Magno CP, Nguyen XM, Laugenour K, Lane J. Trends in use of bariatric surgery, 2003–2008. *J Am Coll Surg* 2011;**213**:261–6.
3. Kitzinger HB, Abayev S, Pittermann A, et al. The prevalence of body contouring surgery after gastric bypass surgery. *Obes Surg* 2012;**22**:8–12.
4. American Society of Plastic Surgeons. Procedural Statistics. Available at: www.plasticsurgery.org/news-and-resources/statistics.html (accessed Nov 1, 2011).
5. Ortega J, Navarro V, Cassinello N, Lledo S. Requirement and postoperative outcomes of abdominal panniculectomy alone or in combination with other procedures in a bariatric surgery unit. *Am J Surg* 2010;**200**:235–40.
6. Zuelzer HB, Ratliff CR, Drake DB. Complications of abdominal contouring surgery in obese patients: current status. *Ann Plast Surg* 2010;**64**:598–604.
7. Coon D, Gusenoff JA, Kannan N, El Khoudary SR, Naghshineh N, Rubin JP. Body mass and surgical complications in the postbariatric reconstructive patient: analysis of 511 cases. *Ann Surg* 2009;**249**:397–401.
8. Vico PG, De Vooght A, Nokerman B. Circumferential body contouring in bariatric and non-bariatric patient. *J Plast Reconstr Aesthet Surg* 2009;**63**:814–19.
9. Araco A, Sorge R, Overton J, Araco F, Gravante G. Postbariatric patients undergoing body-contouring abdominoplasty: two techniques to raise the flap and their influence on postoperative complications. *Ann Plast Surg* 2009;**62**:613–17.
10. de Kerviler S, Husler R, Banic A, Constantinescu MA. Body contouring surgery following bariatric surgery and dietetically induced massive weight reduction: a risk analysis. *Obes Surg* 2009;**19**:553–9.
11. Greco JA, 3rd, Castaldo ET, Nanney LB, et al. The effect of weight loss surgery and body mass index on wound complications after abdominal contouring operations. *Ann Plast Surg* 2008;**61**:235–42.
12. Au K, Hazard SW 3rd, Dyer AM, Boustred AM, Mackay DR, Miraliakbari R. Correlation of complications of body contouring surgery with increasing body mass index. *Aesthet Surg J* 2008;**28**:425–9.
13. Arthurs ZM, Cuadrado D, Sohn V, et al. Post-bariatric panniculectomy: pre-panniculectomy body mass index impacts the complication profile. *Am J Surg* 2007;**193**:567–70; discussion 570.
14. Acarturk TO, Wachtman G, Heil B, Landecker A, Courcoulas AP, Manders EK. Panniculectomy as an adjuvant to bariatric surgery. *Ann Plast Surg* 2004;**53**:360–6; discussion 367.
15. Nemerofsky RB, Oliak DA, Capella JF. Body lift: an account of 200 consecutive cases in the massive weight loss patient. *Plast Reconstr Surg* 2006;**117**:414–30.
16. Khan UD. Risk of seroma with simultaneous liposuction and abdominoplasty and the role of progressive tension sutures. *Aesthetic Plast Surg* 2008;**32**:93–9; discussion 100.
17. Di Martino M, Nahas FX, Barbosa MV, et al. Seroma in lipoabdominoplasty and abdominoplasty: a comparative study using ultrasound. *Plast Reconstr Surg* 2010;**126**:1742–51.
18. Bercial ME, Sabino Neto M, Calil JA, Rossetto LA, Ferreira LM. Suction drains, quilting sutures, and fibrin sealant in the prevention of seroma formation in abdominoplasty: which is the best strategy? *Aesthet Plast Surg* 2012;**36**:370–3.
19. McDonald M, Grabsch E, Marshall C, Forbes A. Single- versus multiple-dose antimicrobial prophylaxis for major surgery: a systematic review. *Aust N Z J Surg* 1998;**68**:388–96.
20. Gupta K, Strymish J, Abi-Haidar Y, Williams SA, Itani KM. Preoperative nasal methicillin-resistant Staphylococcus aureus status, surgical prophylaxis, and risk-adjusted postoperative outcomes in veterans. *Infect Control Hosp Epidemiol* 2011;**32**:791–6.
21. Webster J, Osborne S. Preoperative bathing or showering with skin antiseptics to prevent surgical site infection. *Cochrane Database Syst Rev* 2006;(**2**):CD004985.
22. Darouiche RO, Wall MJ, Jr, Itani KM, et al. Chlorhexidine-Alcohol versus Povidone-Iodine for Surgical-Site Antisepsis. *N Engl J Med* 2010;**362**:18–26.
23. Cheadle WG. Risk factors for surgical site infection. *Surg Infect (Larchmt)* 2006;**7**(suppl 1):S7–11.
24. Pannucci CJ, Wachtman CF, Dreszer G, et al. The effect of post-operative enoxaparin on risk for re-operative hematoma. *Plast Reconstr Surg* 2011.
25. Winegar DA, Sherif B, Pate V, DeMaria EJ. Venous thromboembolism after bariatric surgery performed by Bariatric Surgery Center of Excellence participants: Analysis of the Bariatric Outcomes Longitudinal Database. *Surg Obes Relat Dis* 2011;**7**:181–8.
26. Delluc A, Le Moigne E, Tromeur C, et al. Site of venous thromboembolism and prothrombotic mutations according to body mass index. Results from the EDITH study. *Br J Haematol* 2011;**154**:486–91.
27. Geerts WH, Bergqvist D, Pineo GF, et al. Prevention of venous thromboembolism: American College of Chest Physicians Evidence-Based Clinical Practice Guidelines (8th Edition). *Chest* 2008;**133**(6 suppl):381S–453S.
28. Losken A. Breast reshaping following massive weight loss: principles and techniques. *Plast Reconstr Surg* 2010;**126**:1075–85.
29. Song AY, Jean RD, Hurwitz DJ, Fernstrom MH, Scott JA, Rubin JP. A classification of contour deformities after bariatric weight loss: the Pittsburgh Rating Scale. *Plast Reconstr Surg* 2005;**116**:1535–44; discussion 1545–6.
30. Rubin JP, Gusenoff JA, Coon D. Dermal suspension and parenchymal reshaping mastopexy after massive weight loss: statistical analysis with concomitant procedures from a prospective registry. *Plast Reconstr Surg* 2009;**123**:782–9.
31. Migliori FC, Gabrielli A, Rizzo R, Serra Cervetti GG. Breast contouring in postbariatric patients: a technique selection algorithm. *Obes Surg* 2010;**20**:651–6.
32. Losken A, Holtz DJ. Versatility of the superomedial pedicle in managing the massive weight loss breast: the rotation-advancement technique. *Plast Reconstr Surg* 2007;**120**:1060–8.
33. Bartsich S, Ascherman JA, Whittier S, Yao CA, Rohde C. The breast: a clean-contaminated surgical site. *Aesthet Surg J* 2011;**31**:802–6.
34. Symbas JD, Losken A. An outcome analysis of brachioplasty techniques following massive weight loss. *Ann Plast Surg* 2010;**64**:588–91.
35. Gusenoff JA, Coon D, Rubin JP. Brachioplasty and concomitant procedures after massive weight loss: a statistical analysis from a prospective registry. *Plast Reconstr Surg* 2008;**122**:595–603.
36. Bruschi S, Datta G, Bocchiotti MA, Boriani F, Obbialero FD, Fraccalvieri M. Limb contouring after massive weight loss: functional rather than aesthetic improvement. *Obes Surg* 2009;**19**:407–11.
37. Shermak MA, Rotellini-Coltvet LA, Chang D. Seroma development following body contouring surgery for massive weight loss: patient risk factors and treatment strategies. *Plast Reconstr Surg* 2008;**122**:280–8.
38. Aly A, Soliman S, Cram A. Brachioplasty in the massive weight loss patient. *Clin Plast Surg* 2008;**35**:141–7; discussion 149.
39. Lockwood T. Lower body lift with superficial fascial system suspension. *Plast Reconstr Surg* 1993;**92**:1112–22; discussion 1123–5.
40. Mitchell JE, Crosby RD, Ertelt TW, et al. The desire for body contouring surgery after bariatric surgery. *Obes Surg* 2008;**18**:1308–12.
41. Iglesias M, Butron P, Abarca L, Perez-Monzo MF, de Rienzo-Madero B. An anthropometric classification of body contour deformities after massive weight loss. *Ann Plast Surg* 2010;**65**:129–34.
42. Sutherland K, Lee RW, Phillips CL, et al. Effect of weight loss on upper airway size and facial fat in men with obstructive sleep apnoea. *Thorax* 2011;**66**:797–803.
43. Michaels J, Coon D, Rubin JP. Complications in postbariatric body contouring: postoperative management and treatment. *Plast Reconstr Surg* 2011;**127**:1693–700.
44. Gusenoff JA, Rubin JP. Plastic surgery after weight loss: current concepts in massive weight loss surgery. *Aesthet Surg J* 2008;**28**:452–5.
45. Albino FP, Koltz PF, Gusenoff JA. A comparative analysis and systematic review of the wound-healing milieu: implications for body contouring after massive weight loss. *Plast Reconstr Surg* 2009;**124**:1675–82.
46. Pannucci CJ, Oppenheimer AJ, Wilkins EG. Practice patterns in venous thromboembolism prophylaxis: a survey of 606 reconstructive breast surgeons. *Ann Plast Surg* 2010;**64**:732–7.
47. Young VL, Watson ME. The need for venous thromboembolism (VTE) prophylaxis in plastic surgery. *Aesthet Surg J* 2006;**26**:157–75.
48. Geerts WH, Pineo GF, Heit JA, et al. Prevention of venous thromboembolism: the Seventh ACCP Conference on Antithrombotic and Thrombolytic Therapy. *Chest* 2004;**126**(3 suppl):338S–400S.

49. Agha-Mohammadi S, Hurwitz DJ. Potential impacts of nutritional deficiency of postbariatric patients on body contouring surgery. *Plast Reconstr Surg* 2008;**122**:1901–14.
50. Brolin RE, Gorman RC, Milgrim LM, Kenler HA. Multivitamin prophylaxis in prevention of post-gastric bypass vitamin and mineral deficiencies. *Int J Obes* 1991;**15**:661–7.
51. Agha-Mohammadi S, Hurwitz DJ. Enhanced recovery after body-contouring surgery: reducing surgical complication rates by optimizing nutrition. *Aesthet Plast Surg* 2010;**34**:617–25.
52. Naghshineh N, O'Brien Coon D, McTigue K, Courcoulas AP, Fernstrom M, Rubin JP. Nutritional assessment of bariatric surgery patients presenting for plastic surgery: a prospective analysis. *Plast Reconstr Surg* 2010;**126**:602–10.
53. Legendre C, Debure C, Meaume S, Lok C, Golmard JL, Senet P. Impact of protein deficiency on venous ulcer healing. *J Vasc Surg* 2008;**48**:688–93.
54. Keys KA, Daniali LN, Warner KJ, Mathes DW. Multivariate predictors of failure after flap coverage of pressure ulcers. *Plast Reconstr Surg* 2010;**125**:1725–34.
55. Ohura T, Nakajo T, Okada S, Omura K, Adachi K. Evaluation of effects of nutrition intervention on healing of pressure ulcers and nutritional states (randomized controlled trial). *Wound Repair Regen* 2011;**19**:330–6.
56. Koltz PF, Chen R, Messing S, Gusenoff JA. Prospective assessment of nutrition and exercise parameters before body contouring surgery: optimizing attainability in the massive weight loss population. *Plast Reconstr Surg* 2010;**125**:1242–7.
57. Gravante G, Araco A, Sorge R, Araco F, Delogu D, Cervelli V. Wound infections in post-bariatric patients undergoing body contouring abdominoplasty: the role of smoking. *Obes Surg* 2007;**17**:1325–31.
58. Manassa EH, Hertl CH, Olbrisch RR. Wound healing problems in smokers and nonsmokers after 132 abdominoplasties. *Plast Reconstr Surg* 2003;**111**:2082–7; discussion 2088–9.
59. Zannis J, Wood BC, Griffin LP, Knipper E, Marks MW, David LR. Outcome study of the surgical management of panniculitis. *Ann Plast Surg* 2011.
60. Krueger JK, Rohrich RJ. Clearing the smoke: the scientific rationale for tobacco abstention with plastic surgery. *Plast Reconstr Surg* 2001;**108**:1063–73; discussion 1074–7.
61. Picot J, Jones J, Colquitt JL, et al. The clinical effectiveness and cost-effectiveness of bariatric (weight loss) surgery for obesity: a systematic review and economic evaluation. *Health Technol Assess* 2009;**13**:1–190, 215–357, iii–iv.
62. Webster C, Neumayer L, Smout R, et al. Prognostic models of abdominal wound dehiscence after laparotomy. J Surg Res 2003;**109**:130–7.
63. Steffen KJ, Sarwer DB, Thompson JK, Mueller A, Baker AW, Mitchell JE. Predictors of satisfaction with excess skin and desire for body contouring after bariatric surgery. *Surg Obes Relat Dis*.
64. Song AY, Rubin JP, Thomas V, Dudas JR, Marra KG, Fernstrom MH. Body image and quality of life in post massive weight loss body contouring patients. *Obesity (Silver Spring)* 2006;**14**:1626–36.

Chapter 21

Tissue transfer for cancer reconstruction in the massive weight loss patient

Deniz Dayicioglu

INTRODUCTION

With ever-increasing worldwide obesity and resultant numbers of patients undergoing bariatric surgery, plastic surgeons may encounter more patients in their practice requiring reconstructive surgery after cancer. Following postbariatric massive weight loss (MWL), this special population presents with a deflated skin envelope, redundancy of skin, and subcutaneous tissues in areas that could, if used appropriately, be advantageous in reconstructive surgery. Yet this could be challenging for three-dimensional planning, due to poor wound healing and unique problems associated with this population.

Multiple epidemiological studies have outlined the correlations of obesity with cancer. However, there is limited literature on this group of patients who have undergone MWL and have been diagnosed with cancers that require reconstruction. For better functional and aesthetic outcomes with fewer complications, lessons learned from body-contouring literature should be integrated into reconstructive efforts.

PREOPERATIVE WORKUP

Similar to body-contouring surgeries for MWL patients, patients who will have reconstruction secondary to cancer should have a detailed workup. This will decrease complications. Overall complication rates for postbariatric body-contouring procedures are as high as 45%. Nutritional status plays a key role in wound healing and should be addressed in any MWL patient because failure to follow up or patient noncompliance after bariatric surgery is as high as 25%. Below is a summary of the preoperative tests that are widely used for MWL patients. These can be translated to reconstructive surgery after cancer (**Table 21.1**).

HISTORY

During history taking of a MWL patient, some additional points should be elucidated (**Table 21.1**).

PHYSICAL EXAMINATION AND PREOPERATIVE SURGICAL PLANNING

Location and the proximity of the excess tissue and the proposed location of the defect will determine whether a local flap, skin graft, or free flap is appropriate. Planning and design of flaps are different in this population. This is directly related to the quality of the skin, subcutaneous fat, and location of excess lax tissue. Body-contouring literature describes markings that can guide the reconstructive surgeon (**Table 21.3** and **Figs 21.1** and **21.2**).[2]

Table 21.1 Preoperative workup lab tests for a postbariatric massive weight loss (MWL) patients undergoing cancer-related reconstruction.[1]

Routine tests	Additional tests FOR MWL patients
Complete blood cell count	Iron
Total lymphocyte count	Vitamin B_{12}
Electrolytes	Folate
Prothrombin/partial thromboplastin time	Calcium
	Vitamin A
12-lead EKG	Vitamin D
Chest radiograph	Zinc
	Thiamine
	Protein
	Total protein
	Albumin
	Prealbumin
	Ferritin

Table 21.2 Important points to include when taking the history of a patient after massive weight loss, all of which may adversely affect wound healing.

- Weight loss method
- History of liposuction
- Total weight loss
- Balanced diet
- Current body mass index
- Psychiatric history and clearance if necessary
- Previous history of deep vein thrombosis
- Other medical problems such as diabetes mellitus, hypertension, sleep apnea
- Long-term follow-up compliance after bariatric surgery
- Time of stabile weight
- Smoking
- Skin infections and rash

Assessment of excess skin

Excess skin after bariatric surgery can lead to exercise impairment and affect overall functionality. It can further contribute to other problems including rash, inflammation, cellulitis, and mycoses. Therefore these procedures are considered functional rather than aesthetic.[3] Hiding the scars, consideration of aesthetic units, and zones of adherence should all be taken into account when dealing with any reconstructive need in the MWL patient.

Before using abdominal tissues, the patient should be examined in a supine position, and the abdominal wall contour evaluated. The shape of the abdomen – whether scaphoid or convex – will help to elucidate the intra-abdominal fat content, which should be noted in the medical record. 'Translation of pull' to evaluate extent of tissue

Table 21.3 The rationale for skin excess and their uses for reconstructive surgery.

Anatomic location of skin excess	Cosmetic procedure	Reconstructive procedure
Legs	Thighplasty	Perineal and lower extremity reconstruction
Abdomen	Abdominoplasty	TRAM, DIEP breast reconstruction
Breast	Mastopexy/Augmentation	Breast reconstruction, oncoplastic breast reduction
Back	Body lift	Posterior trunk reconstruction
Buttock	Buttock lift	IGAP, SGAP breast Reconstruction
Abdomen and flank	Total body lift	TRAM, DIEP, IGAP, SGAP flaps Breast reconstruction Posterior and anterior trunk reconstruction, perineal reconstruction
Lateral chest, lateral abdomen	Lateral thoracic excisions	TAP, IGAP, ICAP, LAP flaps Lateral trunk reconstruction
Upper arm, lateral chest and axilla	Brachioplasty	Medial arm flap Lateral arm flap

DIEP, deep inferior epigastric artery perforator; IGAP, inferior gluteal artery perforator; LAP, lumbar artery perforator; SGAP, superior gluteal artery perforator; TAP, thoracodorsal artery perforator; TRAM, transverse rectus abdominis.

movement, by pinching the truncal tissues and determining how far away it is from the proposed area of resection, should be done. The 'dive test' helps to determine the extent of abdominal wall laxity and whether the amount of intra-abdominal content is excessive. This test helps in visualization of the excessive skin on the superior trunk as well.[4]

Hernias and previous incisions

Depending on the type of bariatric surgery, patients may have different abdominal incision patterns. These scars must be considered when planning skin incisions. Gastric banding procedures, for example, might have a pump located under the abdominal skin. This area should not be violated at the time of surgery. Occult abdominal wall hernias can be hidden in this population and should always be kept in mind through surgery, because physical examination might be inadequate to identify them through excess skin and abdominal tissue.

Patient education

Patients must understand the cancer treatment plan, location and extent of resection, the proposed reconstructive options, and alternatives. Patients should be notified of presenting deformities and realistic goals should be established and documented. Preoperative discussion should include assessment of the most probable postoperative course, potential risks, and complications.

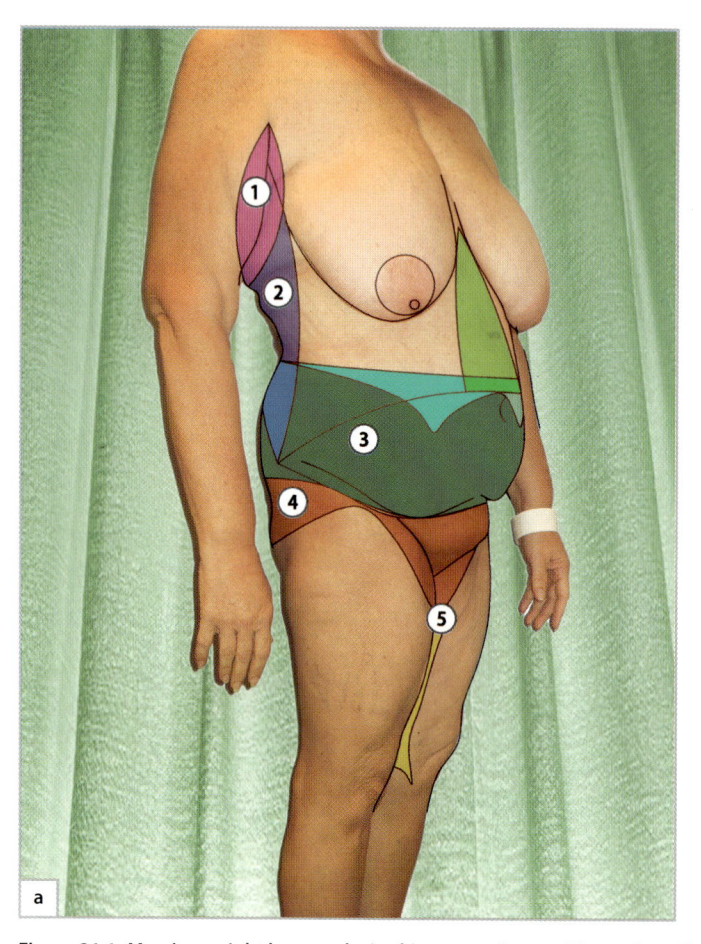

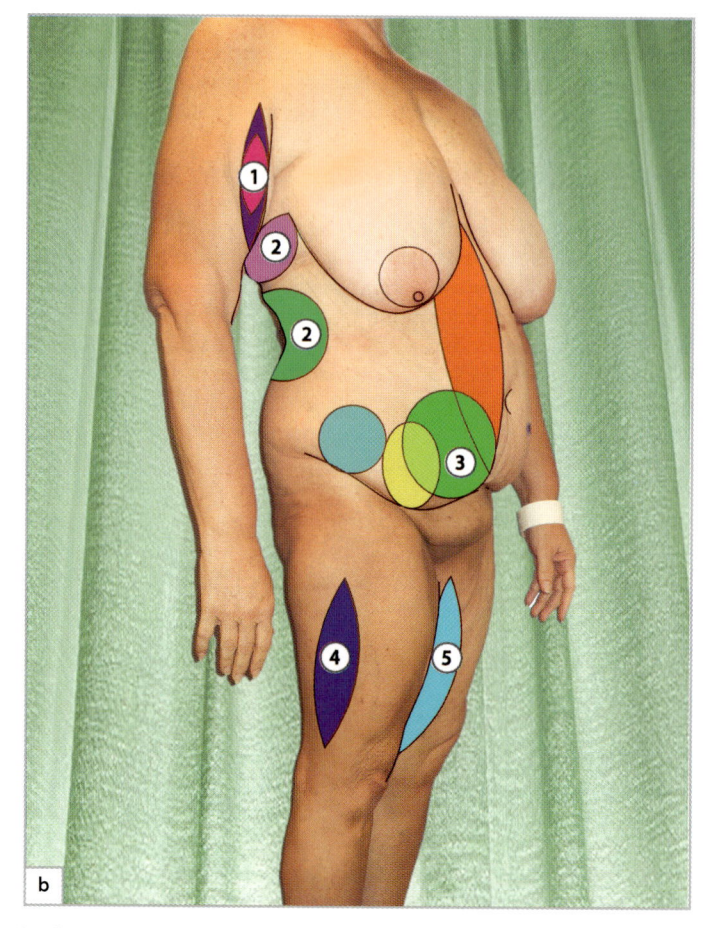

Figure 21.1 Massive weight loss results in skin excess. Excess skin can be utilised as full thickness skin grafts, local flaps, and free flaps. (a) Most common aesthetic body contouring procedures: (1) brachioplasty; (2) lateral chest skin excision; (3) different abdominoplasty techniques; (4) lower body lift; (5) medial thigh lift. (b) Their corresponding perforator flaps: (1) medial arm flap; (2) ICAP (intercostal artery perforator); TAP (thoracodorsal artery perforator) flap; (3) DIEP (deep inferior artery perforator); SIEA (superficial inferior epigastric artery) flap; (4) ALT (anterolateral thigh flap); (5) medial thigh flap.

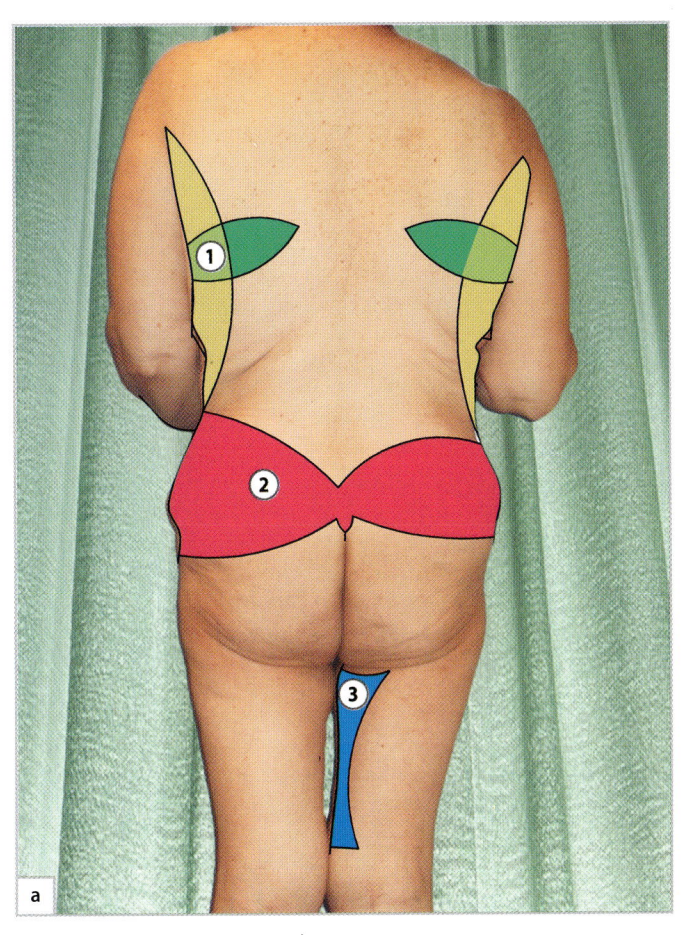

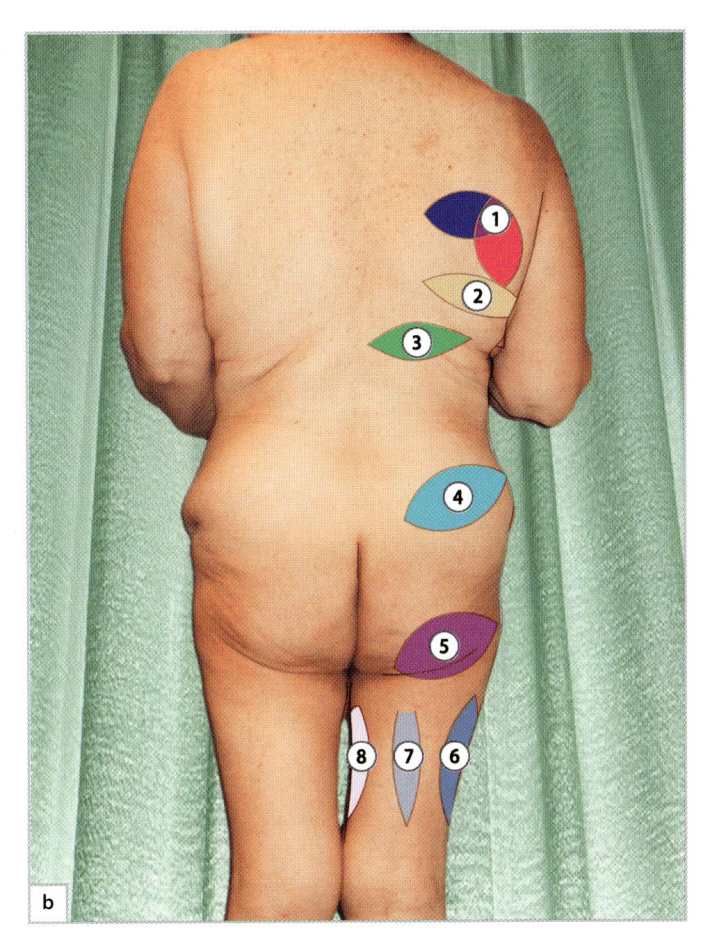

Figure 21.2 Massive weight loss results in skin excess. Excess skin can be utilised as full thickness skin grafts, local flaps, and free flaps. (a) Most common aesthetic body contouring procedures: (1) circumferential abdominal lipectomy, belt lipectomy, body lift; (2) medial thigh plasty; (3) excision of lateral chest skin excess. (b) Their corresponding perforator flaps: (1) scapular, parascapular flaps; (2) TAP (thoracodorsal artery perforator) flap; (3) lumbar artery perforator flap; (4) SGAP (superior gluteal artery perforator) flap; (5) IGAP (inferior gluteal artery perforator) flap; (6) ALT (anterolateral thigh) flap; (7) posterior thigh flap; (8) medial thigh flap.

Appropriate prophylaxis with low-molecular-weight heparin or other anticoagulant medications when needed should be administered, depending on the risk level. Sequential compression devices should be used during and after surgery. Early mobilization is necessary. Patients should be educated about signs of thromboembolism after discharge.[5]

Nutrition

Massive weight loss is variable as is the physiology, depending on the mechanism of loss. Bariatric surgery results in altered physiology when compared with diet and exercise- or cancer-related weight losses. It is emphasized that, even though less severe, patients who do not undergo bariatric surgery and have lost massive weight with diet and exercise are prone to wound-healing complications. This is due to decreased protein or micronutrient absorption.[6] Nutritional parameters should be evaluated before any surgery in the MWL patient in order to prevent and anticipate any complications. Where most relevant, the parameters are total protein, albumin, and prealbumin; a list of tests is given in **Table 21.1**.

WOUND HEALING

Wound-healing complications in the MWL patient have been reported at >40% according to a meta-analysis by Albino et al.[7] According to this study wound-healing complications related to cancer surgery were 45%. Causes are multifactorial and result in dehiscence, seroma, cellulitis, necrosis, and hematoma. Nutrition, radiation, activity, and secondary revisions all play a major role in wound healing in the MWL patient.[7-9] General complications are summarized (**Table 21.4**).

Data from body-contouring surgery are helpful in understanding the risks associated with reconstructive surgery in the MWL patient. As these patients often endure cancer treatments, including radiation and chemotherapy, risks are more likely to be increased. Some major wound-healing complications are listed in **Table 21.5**.

The following is a summary of available reconstruction options in the MWL patient:
- Musculocutaneous flaps
- Fasciocutaneous perforator flaps
- Free flaps
- Local tissue rearrangement
- Skin grafts.

Reconstruction in the MWL patient utilizing musculocutaneous flaps

The rationale of using tissues that will otherwise be discarded can be utilized for reconstruction of the defects. Most common cancers with known associations with obesity are breast and digestive tract cancers, so these reconstructions are emphasized.

Table 21.4 Most common complications of massive weight loss body contouring surgeries.[1,3]

Intraoperative concerns
Difficult airways
Blood loss
Hypothermia
Long surgical times
Early postoperative concerns
Hematoma
Thromboembolic events such as deep vein thrombosis (DVT) or pulmonary embolism (PE)
Partial or total flap necrosis
Late postoperative concerns
Minor delayed wound healing
Superficial wound dehiscence
Major wound dehiscence
Infection
Seroma requiring drainage
Minor fat necrosis
Major fat necrosis
Skin necrosis
DVT
PE
Pressure sores
Contour deformity
Skin necrosis
Infection
Seroma
Scarring

Table 21.5 Autologous augmentation with lateral intercostal perforator (LICAP) flap for massive weight loss patients.

Reference	Augmentation
Hamdi et al.[10]	Isolated LICAP and used LICAP flap for autologous breast augmentation in the massive weight loss patient
Kwei et al.[11]	Side rolls were used together with a Wise-pattern mastopexy
Rubin et al.[12]	Described a similar technique with good results
Hurwitz and Agha-Mohammadi[13]	Used a spiral flap that was extended on the lateral side of the breast
Holmstrom and Lossing[14]	Identified the perforators and used them for breast reconstruction

Technical point

It should be noted that the distance from muscle to skin will be longer and tissues much looser and lax in MWL patients than in other patients. Avulsion of the pedicle from the skin paddle is a potential risk. Care should be taken to avoid this. The quality and laxity of the skin paddle, as well as its circulation, should be checked during surgery. Skin circulation should be judged at the end of the procedure. Skin areas that appear to have poor circulation should be discarded. If necessary, it can be replaced with a full- or split-thickness graft.

Abdominal contouring techniques for body contouring after bariatric surgery are summarized in **Table 21.6**.[2]

TRAM breast reconstruction

TRAM (transverse rectus abdominis flap) has been the standard for autologous breast reconstruction for the past two decades. In the MWL patient, previous abdominal incisions such as open cholecystectomy scar or abdominoplasty scars should be considered when attempting breast reconstruction with a pedicled TRAM flap (**Fig. 21.3**).

VRAM flap for perineal reconstruction

VRAM (vertical rectus abdominis musculocutaneous) has been frequently used in perineal reconstruction. Utilizing this in the MWL patient can be advantageous. It tightens the abdominal wall and removes the excess skin in a similar pattern to a fleur-de-lis abdominoplasty (**Fig. 21.4**).

Gracilis flap

Thigh flaps such as pedicled gracilis can also be utilized in the MWL patient for the reconstruction of this area. This results in a similar pattern for a medial thigh lift (**Table 21.7**).

■ Reconstruction in the MWL patient utilizing perforator flaps

Perforator flaps have led to advancement in reconstructive surgery. Large-caliber and lengthened perforator vessels are usually associated with obesity. These large perforators maintain their sizes even after MWL. Use of these fasciocutaneous perforator flaps not only decreases morbidity associated with other muscle flaps, but also aids in aesthetic improvement.[10] The idea of using otherwise discarded tissues in MWL patients has already been described and widely utilized for autologous breast and gluteal augmentations in the MWL patient (**Tables 21.8** and **21.9**).[15]

Technical

It is important to understand that perforator flaps are a relatively new concept. The 'first do not harm' concept should remain true because there is a steep learning curve in dissection of these flaps.[16]

LICAP (lateral intercostal perforator) flap

Hamdi et al. utilized the excess tissues on the lateral thorax and 'side rolls'[10] for autologous breast augmentation. This is an example of using otherwise discarded tissues for reconstruction in the MWL patient. This concept can be translated to breast cancer mastectomy reconstruction utilizing excess sides of the breast (**Table 21.10**).

Technical

The largest or dominant perforators were found between the fifth and seventh Intercostal spaces. Perforators located between the fourth and sixth Intercostal spaces were usually chosen due to their proximity.[10] Identifying the perforator might not always be necessary if the potential arc of rotation of the flap is sufficient to perform a pedicled flap procedure.[15]

Table 21.6 Types of most commonly used abdominoplasty techniques.[2]

Type I: Full abdominoplasty
Type II: Fleur-de-lis abdominoplasty
Type III: Circumferential abdominoplasty
Type IV: Fleur-de-lis circumferential abdominoplasty
Type V: Panniculectomy
Vertical abdominoplasty

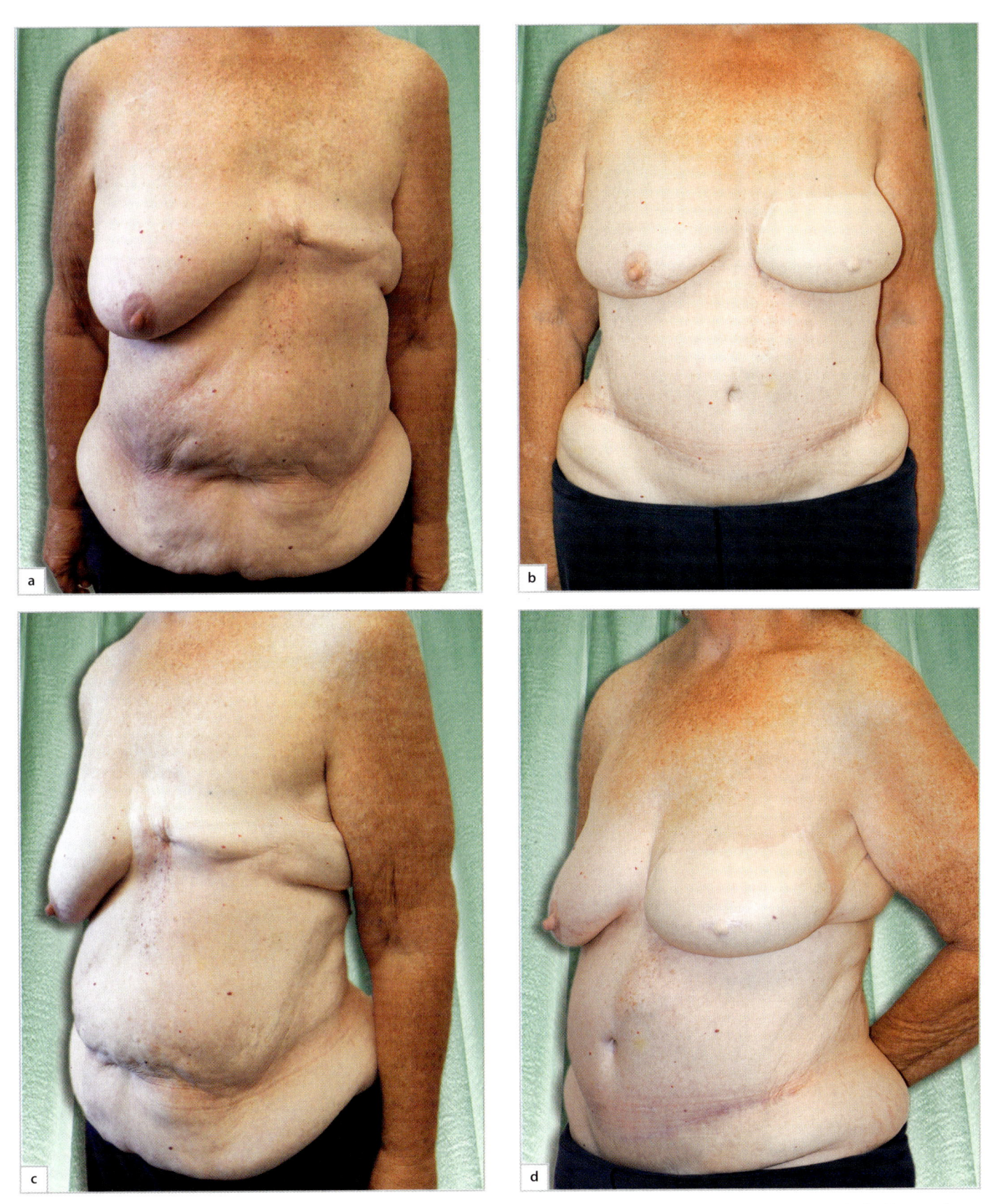

Figure 21.3 (a) A 60-year-old woman with a history of 54 kg (120 lb) massive weight loss after gastric banding and left stage 3 breast cancer who had history of chemotherapy and radiation. Six years after her original mastectomy with no recurrence, she wanted to have reconstruction. (b) She went through left breast reconstruction with a pedicled TRAM (transverse rectus abdominis flap) flap. The pedicle was tunneled laterally. Note the location of the gastric band under the abdominal skin. This should not be violated at the time of dissection. (c) Oblique preoperative view of this patient. (d) Oblique postoperative view of this patient. Note reduction of the abdominal skin.

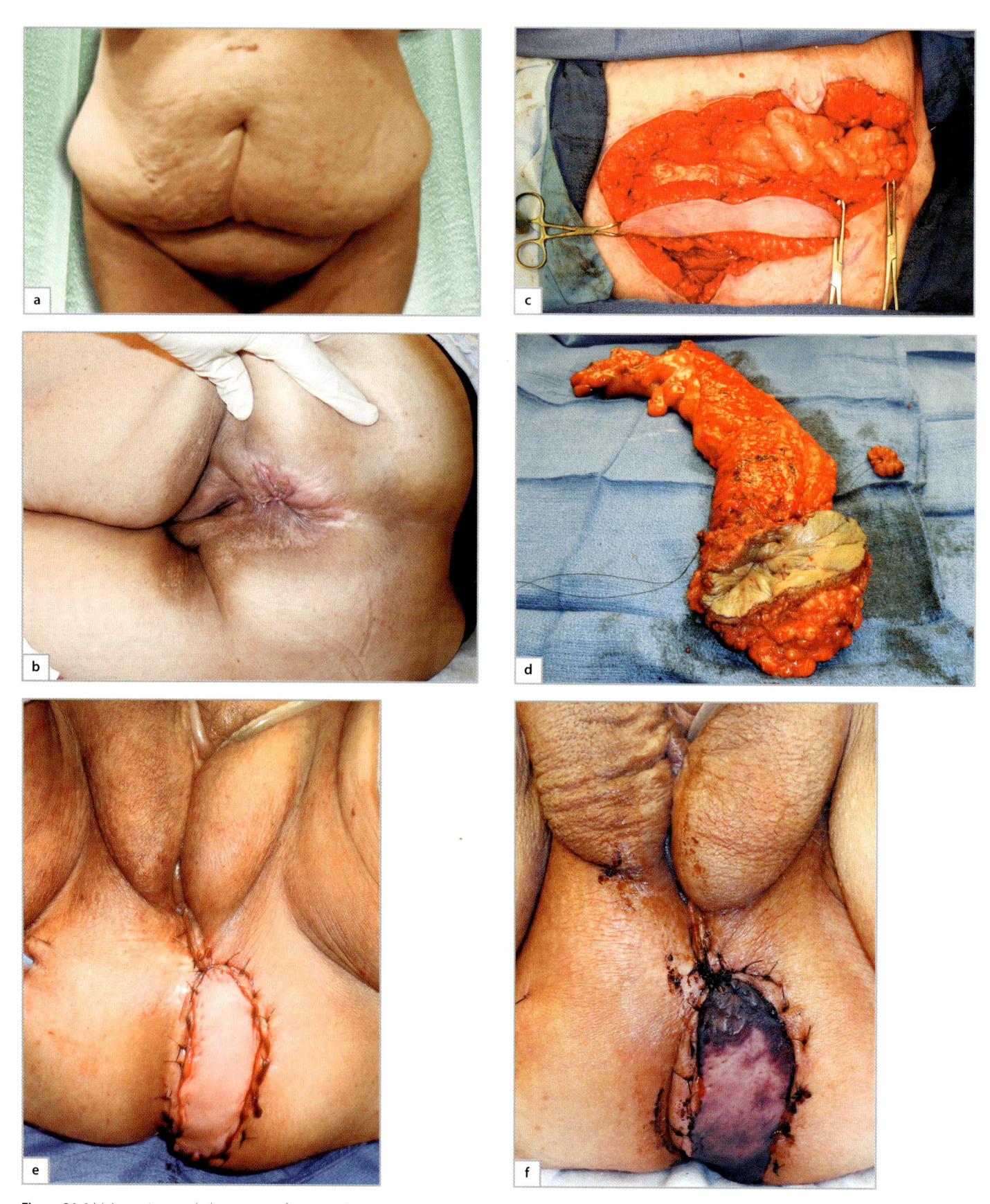

Figure 21.4 (a) A massive weight loss patient after gastric bypass had lost 60 kg (150 lb). She then had been diagnosed with anal squamous cell cancer. As a result of the history of radiation and need to fill the empty space decision was made to do vertical rectus abdominis myocutaneous (VRAM) flap. (b) She received chemotherapy and radiation. An abdominoperineal resection was planned. (c) Intraoperative view of the VRAM flap. (d) Specimen removed. Patient will receive VRAM flap to fill in the cavity. (e) Skin paddle inset in the perineum after VRAM. (f) Skin necrosis due to congestion that required total debridement of the skin paddle. Rectus muscle was healthy and was left. Skin was closed primarily. This allowed for the wound to heal without major problems and helped with her skin access on her abdomen.[15]

Table 21.7 Musculocutaneous flap examples that can result in better cosmesis after reconstructive surgery.[2]

Technique	Flap
Type I: Full abdominoplasty	TRAM
Type II: Fleur-de-lis abdominoplasty	VRAM
Medial thigh lift	Gracilis

TRAM, transverse rectus abdominis; VRAM, vertical rectus abdominis myocutaneous.

Table 21.8 Autologous breast augmentation using perforator flap options that had been already described for autologous augmentation in the massive weight loss patient after bariatric surgery.[15,18]

TAP	Thoracodorsal artery perforator flap
LICAP	Lateral intercostal perforator flap
SEAP	Superior epigastric artery perforator flap

Table 21.9 Other perforator flaps used in breast reconstruction.[10,15]

TAP (thoracodorsal artery perforator flap)
LICAP (lateral intercostal perforator flap)
DIEP (deep inferior epigastric artery)
SIEA (superficial inferior epigastric artery)
SGAP (superior gluteal artery perforator)
IGAP (inferior gluteal artery perforator)
SEAP (superior epigastric artery perforator flap)

Table 21.10 Summary of major wound healing complications data from the body-contouring literature that is relevant to reconstruction in this special population.[19]

Reference	No. of patients	Seroma complications (%)	Thromboembolic complications (%)	Wound infections (%)	Percentage of hematomas (%)
Shermak et al.[20]	138	20	2.9	Unknown	Unknown
Greco et al.[19]	222	14	Unknown	2	6

ALT (anterolateral thigh) flap
A pedicled or free ALT flap can be utilized for inguinal or perineal defects. This would produce the effect of a lateral thigh lift. In the MWL patient, it would be easier to close the donor site because of excess skin (**Fig. 21.5**).

SGAP (superior gluteal artery perforator) flap
These flaps are often de-epithelialised. They are then placed in gluteal pockets for aesthetic autologous gluteal augmentation in the MWL patient.[17] This flap could be a useful adjunct to other muscle or fasciocutaneous flaps when gluteal or sacral closure after cancer resection is necessary (see **Fig. 21.2b**).

Reconstruction in the MWL patient utilizing free flaps

DIEP free flap breast reconstruction
DIEP (deep inferior epigastric artery) free flap is an alternative to TRAM for breast reconstruction in suitable patients who want to avoid abdominal morbidity associated with TRAM. The perforators that could be used are much larger in this MWL patient population. Dissection is easier.

Due to bariatric surgery, these MWL patients might have a midline incision from an open gastric bypass or multiple incisions after laparoscopic surgery. After a midline incision, midline fascial widening and diastases might be encountered because the sutures that were used to repair the fascia tend to loosen after MWL. These patients are likely to have incisional hernias – it has been reported as frequently as in 20% of cases.[20] These hernias and dehiscence should be evaluated when planning TRAM or DIEP surgery for breast reconstruction. The abdominal anterior wall may be plicated in these cases at the time of breast reconstruction surgery.[20]

Technical
Meticulous hemostasis should be obtained due to large perforators in the abdomen (**Fig. 21.6**).

SIEA free flap breast reconstruction
The usability of the SIEA (superficial inferior epigastric artery) for free flap breast reconstruction necessitates a diameter >1.5 mm, and palpability of a pulse. Some centers utilize an algorithmic approach of exploring SIEA before DIEP dissection in order to preserve the integrity of the abdominal wall.[21] Data to use SIEA free flap breast reconstruction in the MWL population have yet to be published. However, In this study of 64 MWL patients after bariatric surgery undergoing abdominal surgery, Gusenoff et al. found that SIEA length and SIEA diameters were higher than in the normal BMI population.[21] Size was correlated with the BMI before bariatric surgery and the weight of the pannus. They suggested that this special group demonstrated a mean diameter of 1.7 mm. More conclusive data are necessary.

Free TRAM
This can be considered for patients with a BMI > 35. It is associated with more abdominal morbidity and use of mesh could be a potential hazard for infection in this sensitive population.

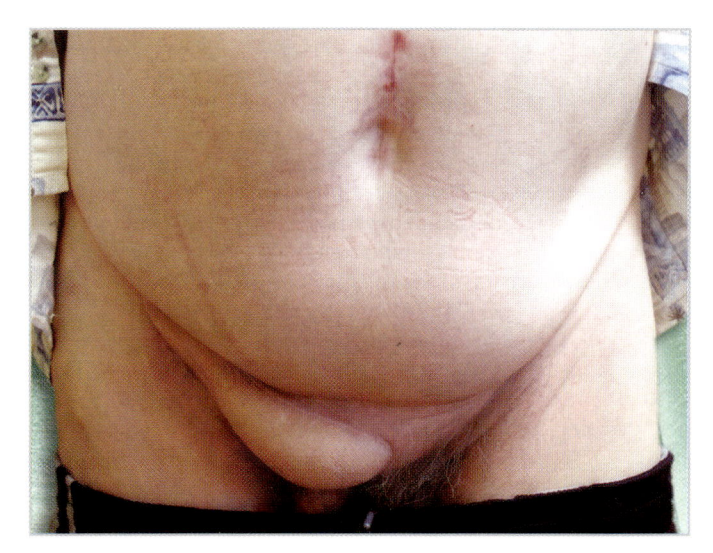

Figure 21.5 Pedicled anterolateral thigh flap for inguinal reconstruction.

■ Reconstruction in the MWL patient utilizing tissue rearrangement

Oncoplastic breast reduction

Tissue rearrangement is a viable option for lumpectomy in the suitable breast cancer patient. This approach would allow for a mastopexy effect which would result in a better aesthetic outcome in the MWL patient (**Fig. 21.7**).

■ Reconstruction in the MWL patient utilizing tissue expanders and permanent implants

Tissue expansion can be considered for this population. These patients have increased skin laxity and could have a quicker response to skin expansion. These patients carry a higher risk for infection and must be closely monitored for potential complications of tissue expanders and implant placements (**Figs 21.8** and **21.9**).

■ Reconstruction in the MWL patient utilizing skin grafts

Skin graft harvest of full and split thickness could be done in areas that will be otherwise discarded (**Table 21.11** and **Fig. 21.10**).

■ COMPLICATIONS

Common complications related to morbidly obese patients decrease after MWL. They may persist in their post-MWL state. They should be considered as risk factors when surgically treating these patients. Problems include hypertension, diabetes mellitus, sleep apnea, gastroesophageal reflux disease, thyroid problems, myocardial infarction, cardiovascular disease, hypercholesterolemia, malnutrition, stroke, thrombotic events, renal failure, seizures, and anemia.[6] Contraindications for long surgery or factors that may compromise wound healing should be corrected before reconstructive surgery.[10]

■ CONCLUSIONS

The percentage of subgroup of patients who have a cancer after bariatric surgery and before undergoing body-contouring surgery has

Table 21.11 Potential donor sites for skin graft harvest.

Full- or split-thickness skin graft donor sites
Thighplasty
Abdominoplasty
Mastopexy/Augmentation
Lower body lift
Upper body lift

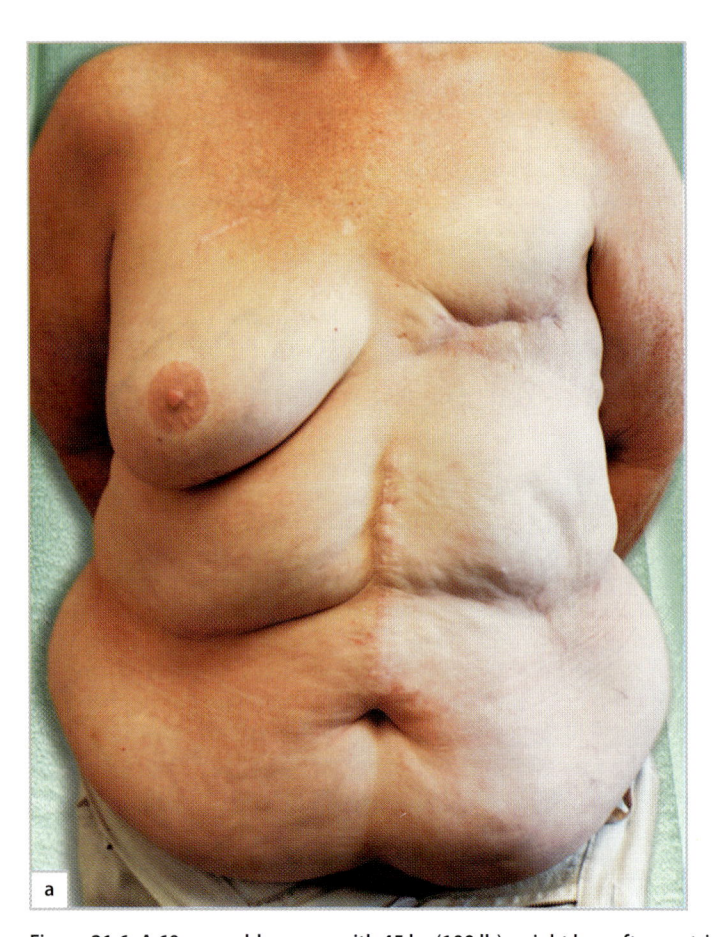

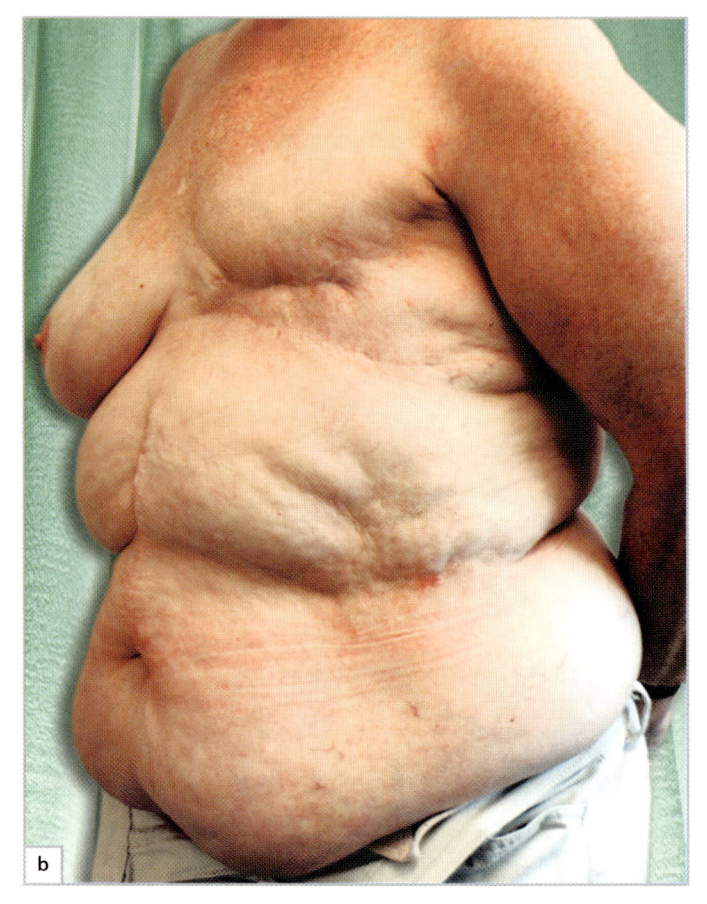

Figure 21.6 A 60-year-old woman with 45 kg (100 lb) weight loss after gastric bypass was diagnosed with breast cancer. (a, b) She had mastectomy, chemotherapy, and radiation. She was interested in using her abdominal tissues, so a unilateral DIEP (deep inferior epigastric artery perforator) free flap was performed. *Continued opposite.*

Conclusions

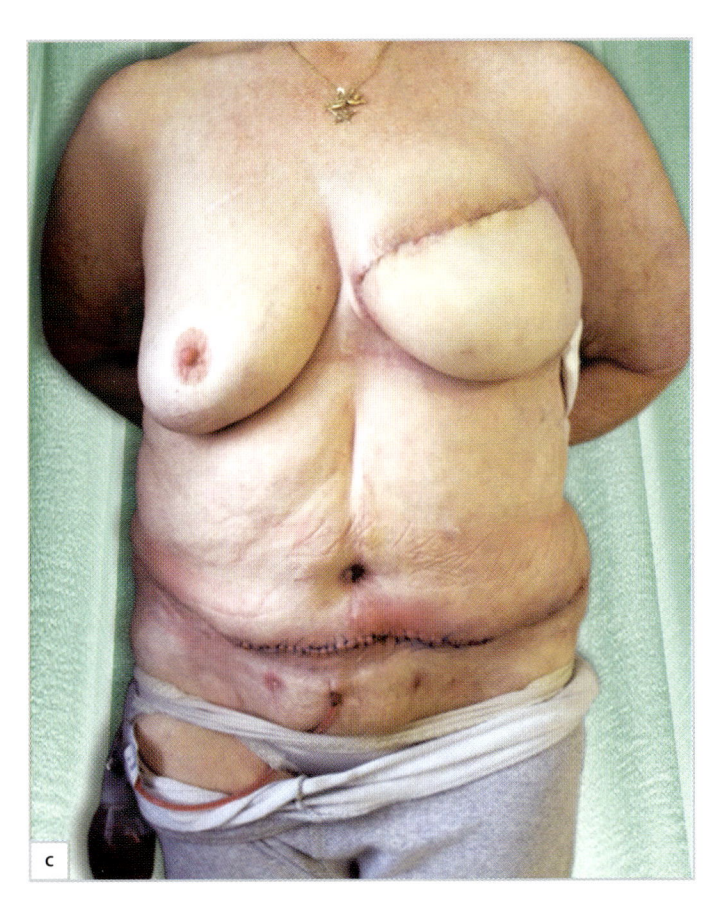

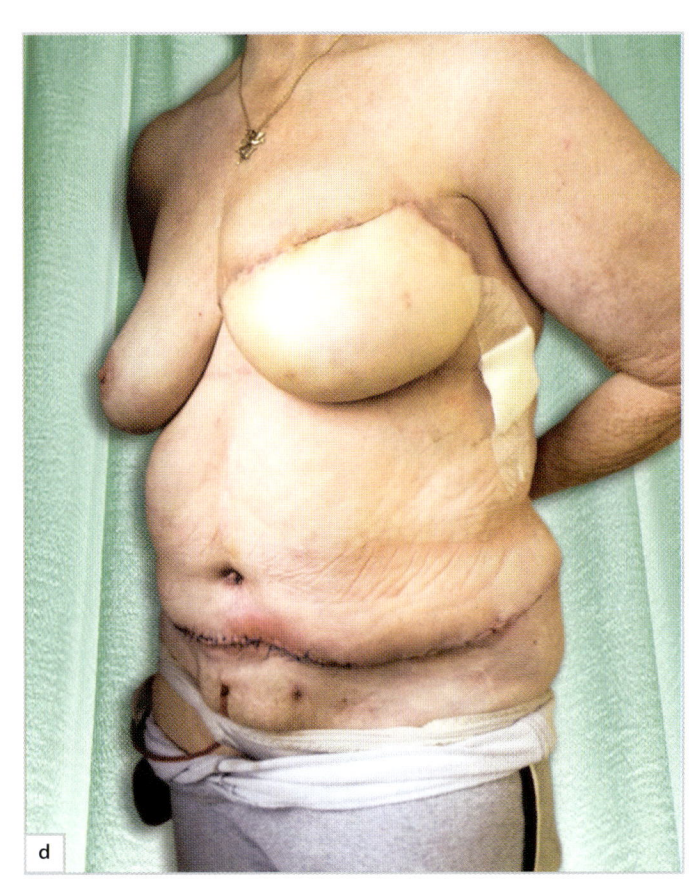

Figure 21.6 A 60-year-old woman with 45 kg (100 lb) weight loss after gastric bypass was diagnosed with breast cancer. (c, d) Early postoperative view after free DIEP reconstruction. Single perforator with remarkable diameter of 2 mm was utilized with good results of the flap. Only zone 1 was used. Incidentally a midline incisional hernia was found and repaired. Also midline plication was done. On postoperative day 3 she developed a hematoma on the abdomen that required evacuation. This might have contributed to the cellulitis and scarring of the abdomen which had to be excised and repaired later. She requested a lift on the right side, which is why the left side was designed larger and higher for now.

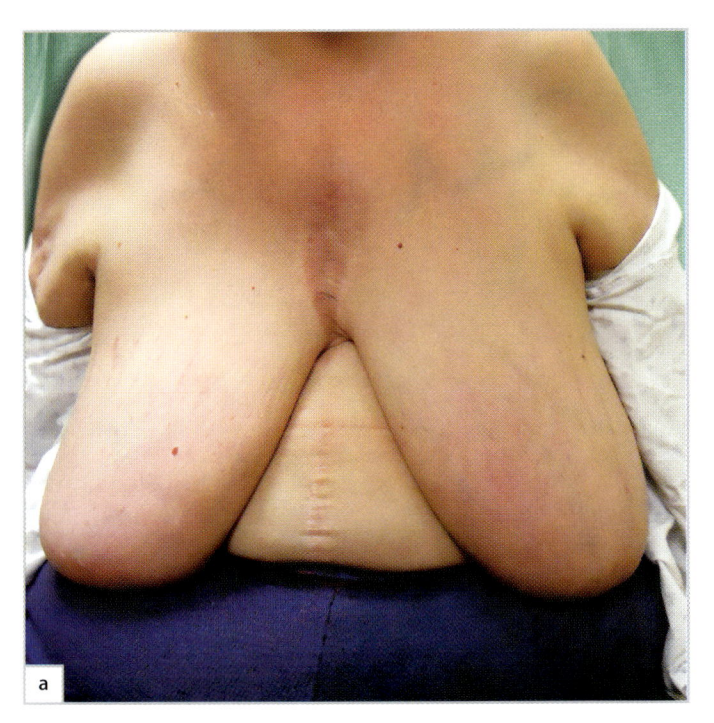

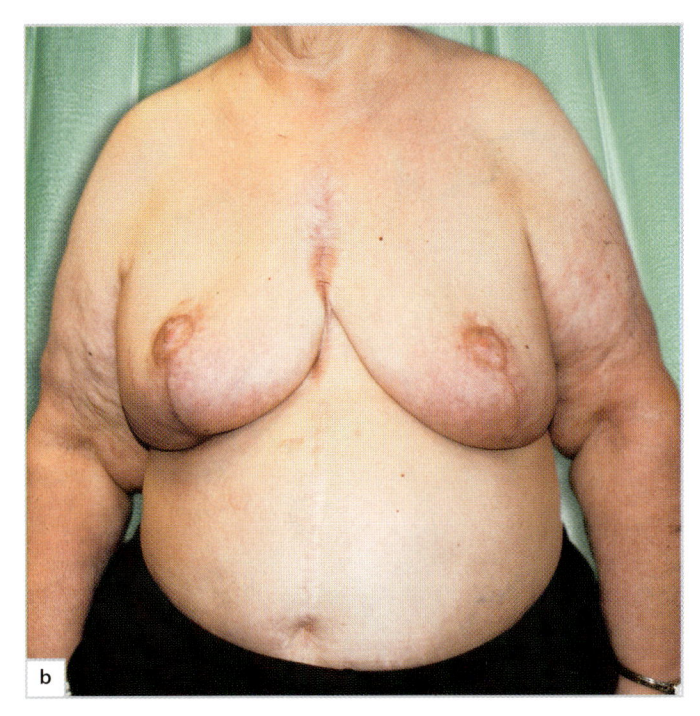

Figure 21.7 This patient had lost 50 kg (110 lb) after gastric bypass and was diagnosed with breast cancer. (a) This patient had grade 3 ptosis with excess skin and lack of fullness. Tumor was located in right side in the central area. (b) A free nipple graft and Wise-pattern reduction were used. It is of note that this patient had significant sleep apnea syndrome which is very common in the massive weight loss patient and should be taken into account.

yet to be investigated. In the MWL patient with cancer or a history of cancer, it is important to understand that the overall goal is to provide tissue coverage and reconstruction after tumor resection. It is clear that cancer reconstruction to repair a defect is not the same as an aesthetic, postbariatric, body-contouring surgery. Combining these procedures can clearly prolong the surgical or healing time as well as risk flap necrosis.[22] These factors can interfere with the reconstructive outcome in this sensitive population, already characterized by poor wound healing. Yet with careful preoperative planning that utilizes the information gathered from the postbariatric body-contouring literature, use of excess tissues that would otherwise be discarded can be a helpful adjunct for the reconstructive surgeon. The goal is to yield better functional and aesthetic results in this patient population.

ACKNOWLEDGMENTS

The author would like to thank Ceren Isil for medical drawings, and Dr Yvonne Pierpont (Division of Plastic Surgery) and Dr Michel Murr (Director of Bariatric Surgery) at the University of South Florida for their editorial input.

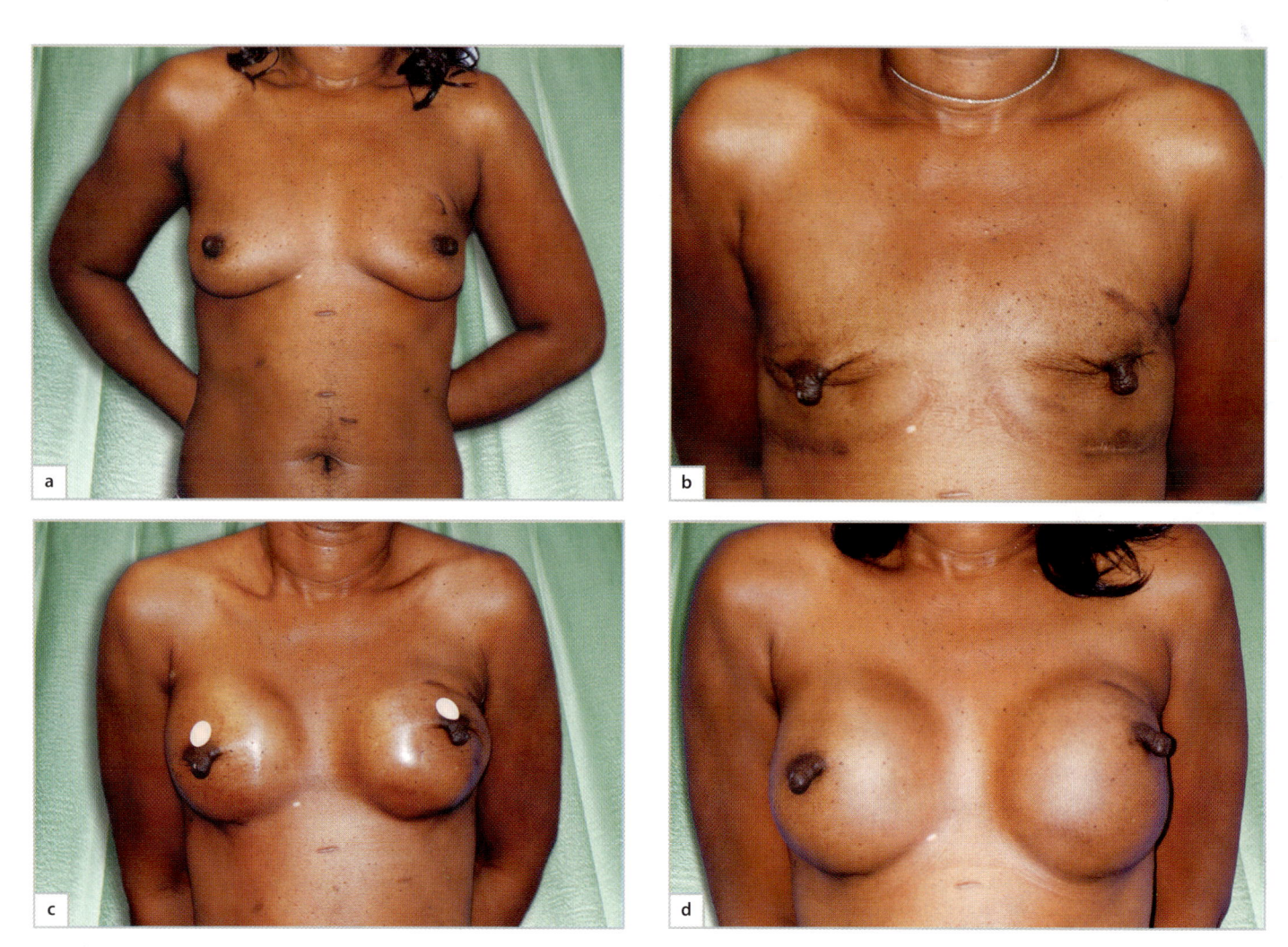

Figure 21.8 (a) A 38-year-old patient with a recently diagnosed breast cancer. She has a history of laparoscopic gastric bypass that resulted in 27 kg (60 lb) weight loss. Note the multiple incision scars on the abdomen. She was initially reconstructed with bilateral tissue expanders and acellular dermal matrix for an immediate breast reconstruction, after her bilateral nipple areola-sparing mastectomy. This patient was noncompliant for follow-up after her bariatric surgery and after reconstructive surgery, and had failed to receive nutritional support. (b) The patient had severe infection and tissue expanders had to be removed with prolonged antibiotic use. After 4 months she was operated on again, this time without complications. (c) The tissue expanders in place. (d) Implants in place.

Acknowledgments

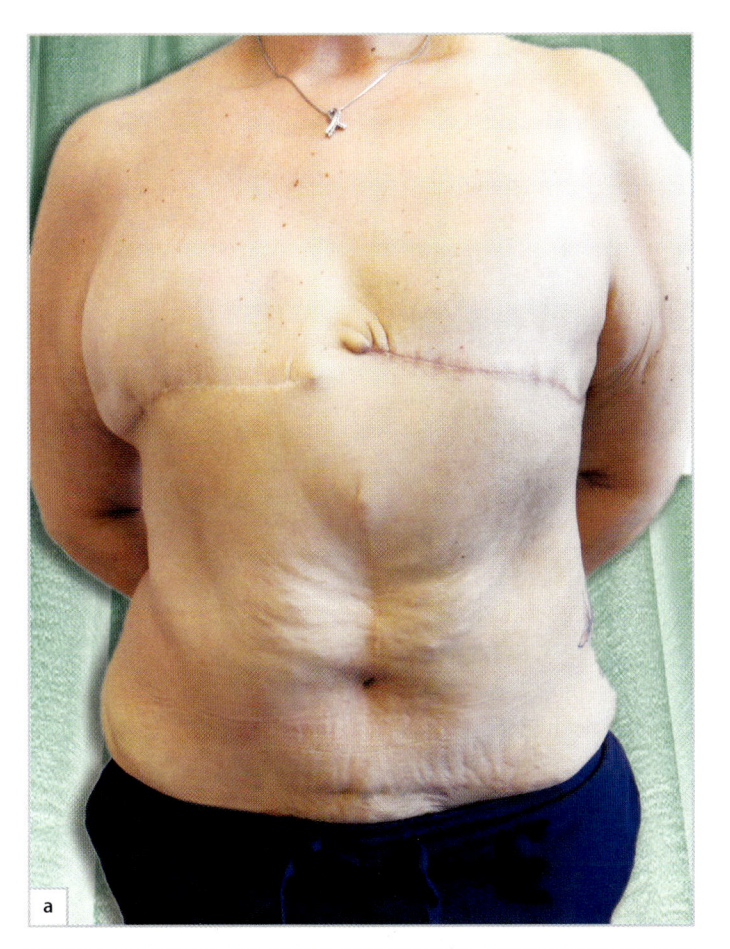

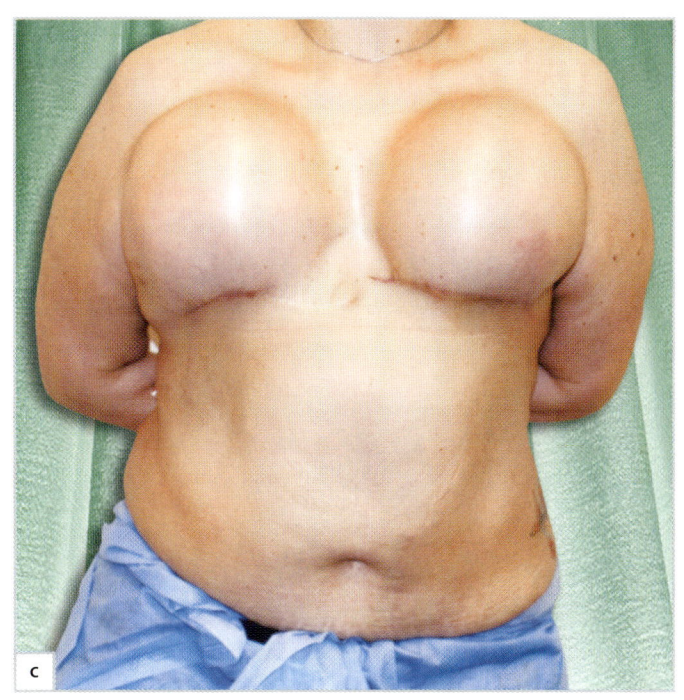

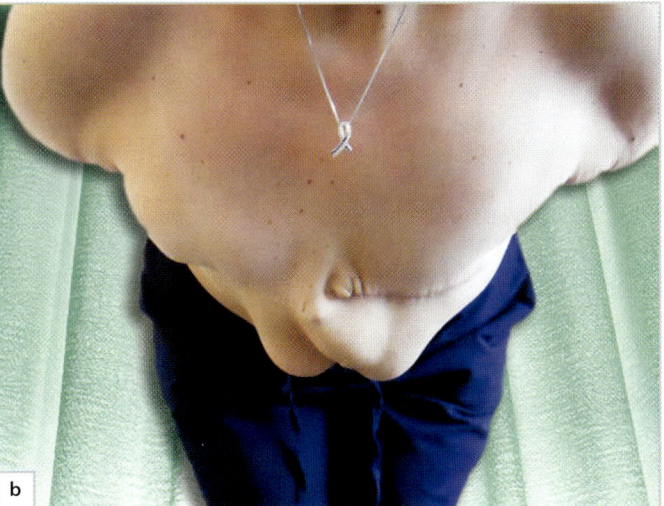

Figure 21.9 (a) A 40-year-old patient with a history of gastric by pass and having lost 45 kg (100 lb) was diagnosed with breast cancer. She had bilateral mastectomies. She wanted to be as large as possible. (b) She also had a history of fleur-de-lis abdominoplasty, but she still had excess tissues on her upper abdomen. Delayed insertion of tissue expanders was performed. She then had exchange of her tissue expanders for permanent silicone implants. Although it was initially thought to use her original tissues from her upper abdomen, later on this was presumed to be insufficient. (c) Postoperative view of silicone implants for breast reconstruction.

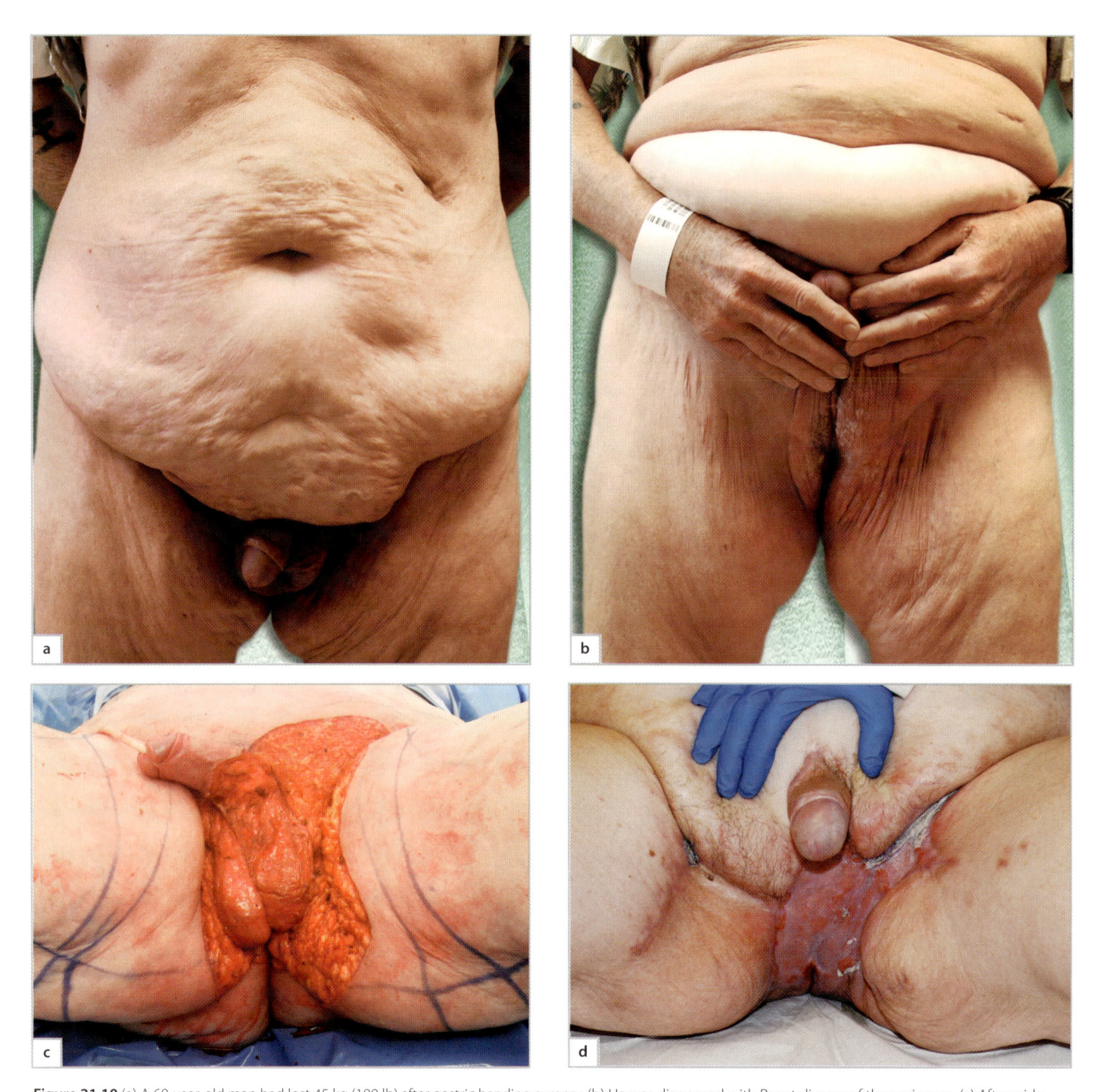

Figure 21.10 (a) A 60-year-old man had lost 45 kg (100 lb) after gastric banding surgery. (b) He was diagnosed with Paget disease of the perineum. (c) After wide local excision, the decision was made to use local flaps and skin grafts for closure. (d) Postoperative view.

■ REFERENCES

1. Centeno RF, Mendieta CG, Young VL. Gluteal contouring surgery in the massive weight loss patient. *Clin Plast Surg* 2008;**35**:73–91; discussion 93.
2. Wallach SG. Treating the abdominotorso region of the massive weight loss patient: an algorithmic approach. *Plast Reconstr Surg* 2008;**121**:1431–41.
3. Hurwitz DJ, Neavin T. L brachioplasty correction of excess tissue of the upper arm, axilla, and lateral chest. *Clin Plast Surg* 2008;**35**:131–40; discussion 149.
4. Nahai F. *Art of Aesthetic Surgery: Principles and techniques*. St Louis, MO: Quality Medical Publishing, 2005.
5. Richter DF, Stoff A, Velasco-Laguardia FJ, et al. Circumferential lower truncal dermatolipectomy. *Clin Plast Surg* 2008;**35**:53–71; discussion 93.
6. Koltz PF, Chen R, Messing S. Prospective assessment of nutrition and exercise parameters before body contouring surgery: optimizing attainability in the massive weight loss population. *Plast Reconstr Surg* 2010;**125**:1242–7.

7. Albino FP, Koltz PF, Gusenoff JA. A comparative analysis and systematic review of the wound-healing milieu: implications for body contouring after massive weight loss. *Plast Reconstr Surg* 2009;**124**:1675–82.
8. Graf RM, Mansur AE, Tenius FP, Ono MC, Romano GG, Cruz GA. Mastopexy after massive weight loss: extended chest wall-based flap associated with a loop of pectoralis muscle. *Aesthet Plast Surg* 2008;**32**:371–4.
9. Levy S, Gomes FR, Sterodimas A. Macroscopic anatomic changes of subcutaneous fat tissue in massive-weight-loss patients. *Aesthet Plast Surg* 2011;**35**:814–19.
10. Hamdi M, Van Landuyt K, Blondeel P, et al. Autologous breast augmentation with the lateral intercostal artery perforator flap in massive weight loss patients. *J Plast Reconstr Aesthet Surg* 2009;**62**:65–70.
11. Kwei S, Borud LJ, Lee BT. Mastopexy with autologous augmentation after massive weight loss: the intercostal artery perforator (ICAP) flap. *Ann Plast Surg* 2006;**57**:361–5.
12. Rubin JP, Gusenoff JA, Coon D. Dermal suspension and parenchymal reshaping mastopexy after massive weight loss: statistical analysis with concomitant procedures from a prospective registry. *Plast Reconstr Surg* 2009;**123**:782–9.
13. Hurwitz DJ, Agha-Mohammadi S. Postbariatric surgery breast reshaping: the spiral flap. *Ann Plast Surg* 2006;**56**:481–6; discussion 486.
14. Holmström H, Lossing C. The lateral thoracodorsal flap in breast reconstruction. *Plast Reconstr Surg* 1986;**77**:933–43.
15. Szychta P, Anderson WD. Islanded pedicled superior epigastric artery perforator flaps for bilateral breast augmentation with mastopexy after massive weight loss. *J Plast Reconstr Aesthet Surg* 2011;**64**:1677–81.
16. Pribaz JJ, Chan RK. Where do perforator flaps fit in our armamentarium? *Clin Plast Surg* 2010;**37**:571–9, xi.
17. Colwell AS, Borud LJ. Autologous gluteal augmentation after massive weight loss: aesthetic analysis and role of the superior gluteal artery perforator flap. *Plast Reconstr Surg* 2007;**119**:345–56.
18. Nelson RA, Butler CE. Surgical outcomes of VRAM versus thigh flaps for immediate reconstruction of pelvic and perineal cancer resection defects. *Plast Reconstr Surg* 2009;**123**:175–83.
19. Greco JA, 3rd, Castaldo ET, Nanney LB, et al. The effect of weight loss surgery and body mass index on wound complications after abdominal contouring operations. *Ann Plast Surg* 2008;**61**:235–42.
20. Shermak MA. Hernia repair and abdominoplasty in gastric bypass patients. *Plast Reconstr Surg* 2006;**117**:1145–50; discussion 1151–2.
21. Gusenoff JA, Coon D, de la Cruz C, Rubin JP, Watson JP. Superficial inferior epigastric vessels in the massive weight loss population: implications for breast reconstruction. *Plast Reconstr Surg* 2008;**122**:1621–6.
22. Rieger UM, Heider I, Bauer T, et al. Treatment algorithm for abdomino-torso body contouring in massive weight-loss patients in the presence of scars – a comprehensive review. *J Plast Reconstr Aesthet Surg* 2011;**64**:563–72.

Chapter 22 Medicolegal issues

Walter G. Sullivan

The law has a major impact on the practice of medicine, subjecting physicians to duties and obligations far beyond those experienced by other professions. This chapter covers the major areas of concern for practicing surgeons. Although cosmetic surgery after bariatric procedures is a specialized area of plastic surgery, the legal issues involve those that trouble all physicians: Medical malpractice, informed consent, record keeping, fraud and abuse concerns, and contract issues. Regarding the references to legal cases given in this chapter, it is very helpful, educational, and occasionally enjoyable to read these cases to understand the way that legal thinking is performed. It is extremely easy to find these cases using search engines.

■ MEDICAL MALPRACTICE

In an action for medical malpractice, the plaintiff must prove four things, each by a preponderance of the evidence (i.e. it is more likely than not):
1. The physicians owed a duty to the patient.
2. The physician's acts or omissions did not meet the 'standard of care.'
3. This deviation from the standard of care was the proximate cause of the patient's injury.
4. There was an injury that was the result of the physician's actions or inactions.

■ Duty

For an actionable medical malpractice to occur, the physician must have owed the patient a duty of care. In the setting of a plastic surgery practice, this is almost never a point in contention. As long as a doctor–patient relationship exists, there will be a duty. However, we frequently ask for advice from colleagues about a particular patient. Giving such advice does not create a doctor–patient relationship between the consulted physician and the patient, and therefore does not give rise to a duty. In the emergency room setting, if one is on-call and refuses to see an emergency room patient, a physician may be precluded from asserting that there was no doctor–patient relationship (*Hiser v Randolph* 1980).

However, we are still free to refuse to treat a particular patient, a situation that arises frequently in plastic surgery. If one refuses to treat a patient who is part of a legally protected class because he is a member of that class, one will open oneself to being charged with a violation of law, e.g. one could not refuse to treat a particular racial or religious group, because this would violate Civil Rights Laws. This is not a subject of malpractice law, but the issue of operating on HIV-positive patients who want cosmetic surgery is a frequent one. In the United States Supreme Court decision, (*Bragdon v Abbott*), a dentist who normally performed fillings in his office decided to treat an asymptomatic HIV-positive patient in the hospital. There was no refusal to treat, only a desire to treat differently, to perform the procedure in a hospital and avoid the possible exposure of his employees, equipment, other patients and himself to the deadly virus. Although the dentist promised not to charge any more, the patient, facing the charges from the hospital, sued under the Americans with Disability Act (ADA). It reached the US Supreme Court. Under the ADA, a disability is covered if it substantially limits a major life activity. The problem here was that the patient was asymptomatic. Her side therefore argued that she had chosen not to have children because she was HIV-positive and reproduction is a major life activity, and therefore, that she was 'disabled'. In a 5–4 decision (Rehnquist, Thomas, Scalia, and O'Connor dissenting), the court said that an HIV-positive person was disabled from the moment of initial infection and she was covered by the ADA. These learned men and women in their clean black robes, who never have to deal with such things as blood and other bodily fluids, have decided that you may not discriminate against an HIV positive patient. Though I disagree, I believe this would apply to cosmetic surgery.

■ Standard of care

Assuming a doctor–patient relationship with the resulting duty, there must be a violation of the standard of practice. This is one of the most confused issues in legal medicine, although the legal concept is clear. It is frequently misunderstood by physicians, and sometimes misused by attorneys.

First, what it is not. It is not what the average doctor would do; otherwise almost 50% of physicians would not meet the standard of care. It is not what most doctors would do. Most definitely, it is not just what you would do! Yet, this is what one sees if one looks at some experts' testimony. They criticize care because they would not have done that. Or they defend care because that is what they would have done. In other words, the standard of care is not determined by the majority; it is determined by some minimum standard of care accepted by the medical community which is needed under the circumstances. Fall below that minimum and you have violated the standard of care. Meet the minimum and, even if most physicians would not do it that way, you have not violated the standard of care. The standard is what a reasonable specialist would do in the same or similar circumstances.

Well accepted in jurisprudence is the 'respectable minority' (*Creasey v Hogan* 1981), where the law recognizes that there may be differences of opinion in the medical community with regard to proper treatment. The minority opinion needs to have some acceptance in the medical community, but certainly not widespread acceptance. In plastic surgery, where treatment is so frequently tailored to the individual patient, this becomes an important principle. Attorneys unfamiliar with plastic surgery can be at a loss when trying to decide if a treatment was within the standard of care. They turn to experts to help them decide and the unknowledgeable or unscrupulous expert may start with the usual, 'I would not have done that,' and the game begins.

■ Proximate causation

Your treatment of a patient to whom you owed a duty was below the standard of care for your profession, but did this deviation from the standard of care actually cause the injury? You did an abdominoplasty on an 'unacceptably' obese patient and the patient developed a wound infection. The plaintiff must prove by a preponderance of the evidence that the surgery on an unsuitable candidate more likely than not led to the infection. An expert says that you should not have operated on that patient and obese patients have a higher complication rate. Your expert says infection can happen after any operation and it was not related to the size of the patient. How can a jury decide this? Do they sympathize with the patient or the surgeon? Do they prefer the expert with the English accent? In some cases, it is a play where a juror roots for one character or another. This is what the surgeon and plaintiff are up against.

Injury

This is rarely disputed in plastic surgery cases. Attorneys just do not take cases where there is no injury.

THE INTERNET

Marketing on the internet is now an important component of many plastic surgeons' practices. It is very inexpensive compared with the Yellow Pages and reaches everywhere. Especially for younger generations, it is where patients find out information about plastic surgery and plastic surgeons. One must be careful about the claims made on a website. Although 'puffery' is accepted in commercial speech (e.g. 'thisssssss is the best car ever built'), professionals are held to a higher standard. Claims that cannot be supported by evidence are unacceptable both legally and ethically. If claims are made of special talents or abilities, the plastic surgeon may be held to this higher standard in court. In addition, it is now possible to recall on the internet any website's appearance on a particular date. Changing your website after the fact will not erase the record of how it appeared when the patient read it. Patients should give consent before their photographs are used on the internet. Although this consent can be oral, it is good practice to get it in writing. This permission should be included on your standard photographic consent. Patients, particularly those having facial surgery, may request that their photographs not be used on the internet and this request should be honored. When this request is made before signing the consent, draw a line through that part of the consent, and initial and date before the patient signs. When you post a photo, check the consent and make sure that the patient has given permission. Failure to do so would be a Breach of Confidentiality as well as a Breach of Fiduciary Duty. Care should be used in answering email generated by your website. Obviously, a written record of this communication will exist. If someone other than the physician answers the email, these responses should be reviewed, because the physician will be held liable for anything said. Confidentiality and privacy must be maintained. Phrase your answers in generalities to unknown patients. You cannot answer specific questions without seeing the patient.

EXPERTS

Except in cases of *res ipsa loquitor*, where 'the thing speaks for itself,' an expert is needed to define the standard of care and testify whether it has been violated. *Res ipsa* cases are frequently defined by statute, e.g. leaving an instrument in a patient, where no expert is needed to say that was wrong, but the usual case requires an expert. States define what the qualifications of the expert must be. With tort reform increasing in recent years, these qualifications have been tightened up, but generally they are still fairly lax. Nevertheless, there are board-certified plastic surgeons who will testify to almost anything. An expert could be seen as more believable if he or she testifies for both plaintiff and defendant. Personally, the author believes that this should be done in egregious cases to encourage settlement. Dragging on indefensible cases raises the costs of litigation to the insurance company, justifying premium increases for all.

An expert should obviously be well qualified and some legal experience with depositions is helpful. However, he or she should also be able to give real help to the attorney. Defense cases, in particular, are frequently handled by big law firm associates who lack experience in plastic surgery cases. The surgeon being sued should educate the attorney and provide all the assistance needed, but lawsuits take such an emotional toll that this is sometimes problematic. Experts can fill in. He or she can also help with the deposition and testimony of the opposing expert.

MALPRACTICE INSURANCE

The cost of malpractice insurance has generally escalated in recent decades, periodically leveling off and even decreasing, varying with the status of tort reform. Although, in the past, the thought of voluntarily going 'bare' was unthinkable, today it is becoming an alternative. In some communities it is not possible, because hospitals may require coverage. You may therefore be unable to operate at outpatient surgery centers or your office without having hospital admitting privileges. In other states, the legislature has responded by making it possible to practice bare rather than passing meaningful tort reform. The author does not recommend it. It is realistic enough to know that there may be circumstances where it becomes necessary. The author recommends a long talk with an attorney versed in asset protection before going bare.

Malpractice insurance comes in two varieties – claims made and occurrence. In the past, most policies were occurrence. Occurrence policies cover you for life for any patients whom you treated while you were insured. No additional coverage is required when you stop practicing to cover you when you are no longer paying premiums. Due to the long-term risks to the insurance company, these policies became prohibitively expensive or ceased all together, leaving claims-made policies to be the predominant form of insurance today. Claims made covers you for lawsuits filed while you are paying premiums. When you no longer have claims-made insurance, you no longer have coverage for the cases that you did while you were insured. Consequently, when you move and must have another company's policy, or you retire, or go bare, you will need to have a separate policy to continue to cover you after your claims-made policy is over. This separate coverage is usually called a 'tail' or 'extended reporting period' coverage. Many companies will give you a 'tail' without cost if you have been insured with them for a certain number of years and then you retire after a certain age, become disabled, or die. Everyone should check his or her policy to make sure that this protection is present. When you join another carrier, you may be able to buy a 'nose' to cover previous events.

When the author reviews a contract for a surgeon who is joining a group, I make sure that the physician understands whether the group will be paying his tail coverage if he leaves, or will be required to purchase it himself. These contracts are drawn up by the hiring group's attorney and usually can be negotiated if you are knowledgeable enough to get your own attorney familiar with health law.

LITIGATION

At some point, most surgeons will be confronted by a lawsuit. Sometimes, they come out of the blue, but, on most occasions, there are warnings that should have been heeded and not ignored.

The problem patient

We all have complications. As is said, if you do not have any complications, you are not doing surgery. We expect a certain percentage of wound complications. Patients who are ill-prepared for surgery expect that a problem would never happen to them. Informed consent is not only a legal requirement, it is also absolutely necessary to prepare patients for the possibility of an untoward event. Cosmetic and reconstructive surgery after bariatric surgery is fraught with wound risks. Abdominoplasties that might involve extensive undermining and multiple incisions can be often expected to require secondary surgery for at least minor wound problems and unsightly scars. Patients should be informed of this ahead of time, and not after the fact. Although extensive written informed consents are valuable, take the time to talk to the patient about your common experience of secondary revisions.

One can recognize the problem patient. She is the patient whose name on the appointment schedule gives the surgeon a shutter. Patients usually don't sue because of a bad result or complication. They sue because they are angry with a surgeon who did not warn them of the possibility of a bad result and then acts dismissively of the patient. It is all too common to stretch out the time between office visits for unpleasant unhappy patients. This is a significant mistake. Instead of stretching visits out, these patients should be seen even more frequently than normal. They have a problem. You wish the problem would go away. You may even know that this wound problem will in fact heal itself with minimal care, but the patient does not have your knowledge and experience. They want you to show concern. You can best show this by seeing them frequently. If you plan on going to a meeting or vacation, carefully pick the surgeon who will be seeing the patient in your absence. It is unfortunate that this covering surgeon may imagine a lawsuit coming and want to distance himself. One surgeon who covered for me did not even keep a medical record of the visits, a legal violation in itself.

Experienced surgeons have seen very significant complications and no lawsuit and also seen patients with very minor complications who filed or threatened lawsuits. The patient's complaints were waived off as being too minor to be concerned about. Remember, every bad result is severe to most patients. Treat it accordingly. All too often when I have been asked to consult on a malpractice case, the patient had a problem and the surgeon continues to note in the chart, 'Doing well.' What's the point? Is this going to prevent a lawsuit or prove to the patient once the records are obtained that you were oblivious to their concerns?

It is definitely in your interest to notify your malpractice carrier when you suspect that a patient is angry and may sue for a bad result. They will not hold this against you. They will not use this as a basis to raise your rates. They can assign you an attorney if the situation warrants, who can guide you in helping prevent a lawsuit. Sometimes the patient demands her money back. I advise not doing this unless you get a Covenant Not to Sue in exchange. This will hold up in court. It is basically like a settlement before a lawsuit. If you pay the money instead of the insurance company, it arguably need not be reported to the Malpractice Data Bank. Malpractice insurance companies encourage this and will have the document prepared for you. Refunding money only to be named in a lawsuit a month later would be adding insult to injury. Get your insurance carrier involved as soon as possible.

The lawsuit

When sued, you will get a hand-delivered complaint that can just be given to an employee at your office. Call your malpractice carrier that day. Usually, they will ask you if there is a defense attorney whom you prefer. You can ask other surgeons if they were happy with their attorney, but in no case, discuss the case with anyone except your attorney. During your deposition you will be asked with whom you have discussed the case. Anyone you talked with can then be subpoenaed and required to reveal anything that you said.

Surgeons sometimes believe that a lawsuit means that they are being accused of being an incompetent surgeon. All a lawsuit really means is that, in this particular case, you did something that was negligent, a legal word for 'careless.' Negligence is a rather low standard. It means that you did not do something wrong purposely, just carelessly. The standard of proof is a 'preponderance of the evidence,' which means it is more likely than not, or 51% instead of 49% likely. You will be assigned an attorney rather rapidly. The attorney will ask you to send all the records, the originals to his or her office. It is best to have someone from the attorney's office pick them up in person to avoid any chance of their being lost. The lawyer will file an answer to the complaint, basically denying everything. After that, discovery takes place. The plaintiff's and your deposition will be taken along with that of experts, and possibly others, e.g. nurses or assistants. It is a painful process. Understand that, generally, the plaintiff's lawyer will be inclined to settle to get the most money for the least amount of time. The defense lawyer may be inclined to spend as many billable hours as possible on the case, not necessarily in your interest. One thing to consider is whether you really committed malpractice. Malpractice does occur. Sometimes, surgeons have a bad day and the plaintiff is right. When I see a case like this, I tell the defense attorney that I would settle. That is why you have insurance. If the plaintiff is right, settle and get it over with.

If you did not commit malpractice, you can spend untold hours fighting it or settle. Most cases get settled one way or another. The civil justice system is essentially a drama where the best actors and experts have a decided advantage. Although most verdicts come in for the physician, it can be a 'crapshoot' where true justice may be absent. In a case where your liability is unlimited and your coverage may not cover the amount of the award, an independent attorney's opinion may be warranted before you get to trial. Although your defense lawyer may not mention it to you, a letter to your carrier to demand settlement under your policy limits may make your insurance carrier liable for any judgment above your policy limits. Understand that defense attorneys get their clients from the insurance company and they may have divided loyalty. A settlement where the insurance company pays does get reported to the Data Bank. However, unless you have many cases, the author has not found this to be important.

■ INFORMED CONSENT

A lawsuit based solely on an alleged lack of informed consent is quite rare. More commonly, an informed consent claim is added to the main complaint of medical negligence. In the context of plastic surgery cases, the unfavorable result is frequently the basis of the suit. Whether or not supported by the facts, the patient alleges that, had she been informed about the possibility of this unfavorable result, she never would have consented to the procedure. Thus, obtaining and documenting the informed consent becomes a valuable exercise for the plastic surgeon. Surprisingly, it was not until 1957 that the term 'informed consent' was first used by a court (*Sago v Leland Stanford, Jr., University Board of Trustees* 1957). After the 1960s, legal theories of patient autonomy expanded and the patient became a partner in the doctor–patient relationship entitled to adequate understanding of contemplated treatment plans. Physicians have a legal and ethical obligation to obtain informed consent from their patients before treatment.

■ Elements required in informed consent

It is easy to enumerate the kinds of information required to be disclosed to the patient, but it is a much more complicated task to list the details of what must be disclosed. In some cases, it will depend on in which state the surgeon practices. In other cases, it will depend on the individual nature of the particular patient. In general, five types of information are required and additional information may be required stemming from the physician's role as a fiduciary. The standard five types of information required are as follows.

Diagnosis

This is rarely an important issue in the context of plastic surgery, and it is rarely litigated.

Nature and purpose of the proposed treatment

A detailed description of the procedure is not required and, although it may be good practice, there is no case law requiring the discussion of the likelihood of success.[1]

Availability of alternative treatments

This is an extensively litigated area. The patient must be informed about any medically acceptable alternative treatment that could be used under the circumstances. This includes procedures that the informing physician could not, in fact, perform, and the patient would have to see another physician for the alternative treatment. It is not, however, necessary to inform the patient about procedures that neither the informing physician nor another specialist would recommend (*Vandi v Permanente Medical Group* 1992).

Risks, complications, and consequences

This is clearly the 'mother lode' of informed consent litigation in plastic surgery. More frequently than is justified by the facts, there is an unfavorable result, a suit for malpractice is filed, and an informed consent claim is added claiming that the patient never would have had the procedure if she had been informed of the possibility of that specific unfavorable result. A risk or complication is something that might happen as a result of the procedure, e.g. a postoperative hematoma occurs after a facelift. A consequence is something that either normally occurs after a procedure, e.g. a joint will not move after an arthrodesis, or results from the occurrence of a complication, e.g. skin loss after a post-facelift hematoma. Courts do not require that every risk be disclosed to a patient. It is generally not required that extremely unlikely risks be disclosed, but this is subject to exceptions in some states. Case law indicates that risks that are 'commonly known' need not be discussed (*Cobbs v Grant* 1972). In our present medicolegal milieu, however, reliance on this by the physician is not recommended to avoid being second guessed later. Finally, although rarely mentioned in talks and in the literature directed at physicians, what you legally need to disclose to a patient depends on the informed consent standard adopted in your particular state which is addressed shortly.

Result if no treatment

A physician is under a legal duty to inform the patient about any unfavorable results that may occur without treatment, e.g. a biopsy of a suspicious lesion may be indicated, but the patient refuses. The patient must be informed that the result of not having a biopsy may be a delay in diagnosis of a malignancy, increasing the extent of later treatment or raising the possibility of increased mortality (*Truman v Thomas* 1980).

■ THE PHYSICIAN AS FIDUCIARY

The physician–patient relationship imposes on the physician the highest standard of duty imposed by law, that of the fiduciary. A fiduciary is one who undertakes to act in the interest of another person while subordinating the fiduciary's personal interests to that of the other person.[2] This has led a court to find that a physician had a duty to disclose his alcoholism to a patient (*Hidding v Williams* 1991) and another to find a duty to disclose a physician's HIV-positive status.[1] Although not strictly an issue of informed consent, physicians are obligated to disclose a failure of treatment or the happening of a maloccurrence during a procedure (e.g. 'the nerve was accidentally cut').[3]

■ State variations in duty to disclose

There are two standards used to judge the adequacy of an informed consent, the physician-based standards (for the states AK, CA, CT, DC, GA, IA, LA, MD, MA, MN, MI, N], NM, OR, OK, PA, RI, SD, WA, WV, WI – Rosoff, Appendix 17A[1]) and the patient-based standards (for the states AK, CA, CT, DC, GA, IA, LA, MD, MA, MN, MI, NI, NM, OR, OK, PA, RI, SD, WA, WV, WI – Rosoff, Appendix 17A[1]). Some states use a hybrid rule (for the states CO, FL, HI, KY, ND, OR, TX, UT – Rosoff, Appendix 17A[1]). Although the number of physician-based states (at 22) outnumber the patient-based states (20 + DC), most of the hybrid states are more patient oriented than physician oriented, effectively making the patient-based standard the majority rule in the USA.

Initially, courts allowed the medical profession to set the standards for informed consent. What was required was what the doctors in the community thought was necessary. This evolved into the physician-based standard. Within the past few decades, some states have, instead, adopted a rule that requires disclosure of what the patient would consider material to his or her decision. This is the patient-based standard.

Physician-based standard

A plastic surgeon in a physician-based standard state needs to inform the patient what the reasonable plastic surgeon would tell the patient under similar circumstances (*Natanson v Kline* 1960). This standard is basically the same as that used for medical malpractice, where the question is whether the physician violated the standard of care as determined by the physician's specialty group. Such a standard can be determined only by an expert witness who can testify to the standards of the specialty. In an informed consent case in a physician-based standard state, the prevailing standard of informed consent in that specialty must be testified to by an expert witness.

Patient-based standard

In a patient-based standard state, the plastic surgeon must give the patient all the information 'material' to the decision that the patient must make. Rather than inform the patient about what plastic surgeons think the patient should know, the information given must be what the patient needs to know to make a decision. What the patient needs to know is what a patient would find important (i.e. material) in making the decision. Complicating matters is whether you need to tell that patient what that particular patient needs to know (subjective standard) or whether it is adequate to tell the patient what the reasonable and prudent patient would want to know under similar circumstances (objective standard). In the groundbreaking case that first elucidated the patient-based standard (*Canterbury v Spence* 1972), the court applied the 'objective' patient-based standard. The objective standard is by far the most commonly adopted standard in the states utilizing the patient-based approach. However, even using the objective approach, where you must make the patient aware of risks that the theoretical reasonable patient would want to know, the courts still insist that a physician take into account any special fears, values, or sensibilities of his particular patient. The disadvantage for the physician defendant in a patient-based standard state is that the plaintiff patient need not have an expert witness testify that the physician should have told him before surgery about a particular risk. As the standard is what the reasonable patient layman would want to know, the jury can simply put itself in the reasonable patient's position and decide if the members of the jury members themselves would have wanted to be informed.

When an informed consent is not required

There are a number of situations when an informed consent is not required.

Waiver

A competent patient may waive an informed consent. Patients have the right to refuse disclosures otherwise required for an informed consent and may not be forced to hear them.

Emergency treatment

When prompt treatment is needed and the patient is incapable of giving an informed consent, courts will generally allow consent by proxy from the patient's nearest available relation. If no such proxy is available or known, the courts presume that the patient would want such emergency care if he or she were able to consent absent evidence to the contrary (e.g. 'Living Will').

Therapeutic privilege

A physician may abstain from a complete disclosure to the patient when, in the physician's sound judgment, the disclosure itself poses a significant risk of harming the patient, e.g. a physician decided that a seriously ill patient with hypertension and a suspected thoracic aortic aneurysm should not be told the risks of thoracic aortography. The patient developed paralysis after the aortogram and contended that had he been told of the risk he would not have consented. The court held for the doctor on the basis of therapeutic privilege (*Nishi v Hartwell* 1970).

Patient's prior knowledge

Where the physician is aware that the patient has adequate prior knowledge, it is not necessary to inform the patient again.

Implied consent

A patient's conduct may legally imply consent, e.g. a patient poses for preoperative photographs in the office without objection has implied consent to be photographed.

When the procedure exceeds the consent

The extension doctrine

The extension doctrine allows the surgeon to extend the scope of the procedure when unforeseen circumstances arise that make it advisable to do so. This doctrine does not allow a surgeon carte blanche. If the extension was foreseeable and the patient was not informed about its possibility, then the doctrine does not apply. Similarly, it will not apply in situations where the extension is not so urgent that it cannot be postponed until the patient can give consent, e.g. during an authorized oophorectomy, a surgeon removed a suspicious mole from a patient's thigh without consent. The court held against the surgeon, because there was no necessity to proceed without first getting the patient's consent (*Lloyd v Kull* 1974). In another case, a surgeon harvested tensor fascia lata without consent to use in an authorized hand procedure. The court found that surgeon was unjustified (*Millard v Nagle* 1991). The additional procedure was a foreseeable possibility about which the patient should have been informed.

Documentation

Contrary to common belief, a consent need not be in writing. What a written consent may provide, however, is documentation that the informed consent actually took place. This frequently becomes an issue in litigation after an unfavorable result. Strictly speaking, a verbal disclosure meeting the legal requirements, followed by a verbal assent by the patient, are all that is required. However, the surgeon, for his own protection, should record in the patient's medical record that an informed consent was given by the patient. Listing the risks discussed may also be helpful. Another approach is to have a written consent to assure that the legal requirements are fulfilled. A very complete written consent signed by the patient is not a complete defense. Plaintiffs may contend that they were not given enough time to read it, did not understand it, and had no opportunity to ask questions, in short, that they did not know what they were doing. There is no foolproof way of preventing an informed consent claim. Some states, bowing to tort reform, have helped to make a defense easier if certain conditions are met. At least 12 states (FL, GA, ID, IA, LA, ME, NV, NC, OR, TX, UT, WA) make a signed consent form presumptively valid (see Rosoff,[1] pp 17–84). The list of required disclosures is generally short. Plastic surgeons practicing in these states should consider taking advantage of their states' laws and use a written consent. Courts have generally looked unfavorably at 'blanket' consent forms that give the surgeon virtually unlimited discretion in performing the procedure. Courts will strike down consents that include waivers of prospective liability as void against public policy. Such waivers to sue physicians for future possible malpractice are never valid.

VICARIOUS LIABILITY

Vicarious liability is liability based on some legal relationship that a party has with the person who actually commits the tort, e.g. if your employee has an accident while he or she is going to the bank for you, you are responsible in addition to the employee. As you may be the 'deep pocket,' you may be the target. Hence, it is important for incorporating or practicing as a professional corporation (PC) or limited liability company (LLC) instead of as a sole proprietorship. When a legal entity employs the employee, the legal entity is responsible (e.g. your PC's assets). When you personally employ an employee, all your personal as well as your business assets are at risk.

One area of vulnerability for plastic surgeons is their association with other plastic surgeons. A simple office-sharing arrangement with no clearly defined legal relationship can be considered a partnership. This kind of partnership is known as a 'general partnership' and there could be unlimited personal liability for each partner for the torts of any other partner or employee. One of the things that will be looked at is how the physicians present themselves to their patients, e.g. if both names are on the door without any distinction between practices, employees are shared, or the same phone number is used, the law may imply a partnership. In this case, you and/or your PC may be held liable for any acts of malpractice by the other physician. Basically, there must be a formal legal relationship between physicians who practice with each other to protect the other party. Contracts should be the foundation of any association or office sharing arrangement. A health law attorney thoroughly familiar with fraud and abuse laws, which are easy to run afoul of, is necessary.

Less serious, but potentially troublesome, is apparent authority. Apparent authority is authority that is not actual, but appears to exist, e.g. your office manager has actual authority to order supplies, schedule your surgeries, and change your Yellow Page ad. When she is fired, she no longer has any real authority. However, she is a little peeved and so orders from your magazine subscription service 'Ex-Con' magazine, cancels your ads, changes your phone number, and requests that the post office send all your mail to Sparta, Mississippi. You suffer financial damage and want to sue all these companies. Your lawyer informs you that, although she did not have actual authority, she did have apparent authority, because you had previously informed those business through your actions that she had had the authority to do those things, and you failed to notify them that she no longer had authority. Hence, from their point of view, she still had the authority, and in fact legally she did, called apparent authority. When anyone acts as your agent, and then they no longer are your agent, notify the parties that dealt with her that she no longer has authority.

ASSET PROTECTION

Briefly, there are many things that you can do to protect your assets that are perfectly legal. If you should have a financial catastrophe, you will want to limit the extent of the damage. Generally, this is done by segregating assets so that they are not all at risk. The best time to do this is when you can see no reason for doing it. After a lawsuit or even just after the bad outcome, it may be too late to avoid what is known as a fraudulent conveyance, a conveyance that is done for the sole purpose of avoiding paying a judgment. If you are incorporated, your personal assets are still at risk for any tort that you are found to have committed. Although a healthy malpractice insurance policy is a great comfort, judgments in excess of policy limits do occur and the surgeon should be prepared. Physicians usually get into financial trouble due to lawsuits resulting from business relationships and outside investments that were poorly structured and contracted rather than malpractice.

MEDICAL RECORDS

Physicians have a legal and ethical obligation to maintain adequate medical records. The importance of the patient's medical record in our litigious society cannot be overstated. Remarkably, medical evidence is thought to be involved in three-quarters of all civil cases and about a quarter of criminal cases brought to trial.[5] Medical records are vital in the communication of medical information among physicians and other healthcare entities. It allows continuity of care when the patient changes physicians, allowing future medical professionals to evaluate the patient with the benefit of knowing what came before. More narrowly, the medical record allows the physician to clearly document the progress of the patient's treatment. This will be of major importance should a legal dispute arise in the future. Medical records should be accurate and timely. A note should reflect each patient visit. Although very difficult to be consistently carried out, it is good practice to make notations for every patient contact, including telephone calls. The patient's non-compliance with treatment plans and failure to return for office visits should be documented. Patient's complaints and dissatisfactions should be noted. When dealing with children, it is the parent or guardian who will determine compliance with treatment and discussions with them should be noted. Documentation of informed consents should be reflected in the chart.

The record should be legible. Inadequate medical records could be the basis of the court finding a violation of the standard of care. There are state and federal statutes that mandate that medical records be retained for a specific number of years, usually 5–15 years and longer for children.[6] If a patient decides to see another physician, a copy of the medical record should be sent to the new physician when requested. In plastic surgery, copies of the patient's photographs are particularly useful to the new surgeon. If a surgeon moves or retires from practice, his or her records still need to be retained at least for the statutorily mandated time. Ideally, they could be transferred to the surgeon taking over the practice. Otherwise, there still needs to be some way for the patients to gain access to them.

Alteration of medical records

Errors in medical records are frequent and usually involve a spelling or transcription error. However, an error as simple as transcribing 'there is evidence of necrosis' when what was dictated was 'there is no evidence of necrosis' could make a great deal of difference in a malpractice suit for a delay in the treatment of a complication. In addition, simple but costly errors such as this are difficult to pick up without carefully reading the record. Mistakes should be corrected as soon as possible. The proper way to correct a medical record is to put a simple line through the improper entry, so that it can still be read. Then, the appropriate entry should be placed nearby with the date of the correction added, followed by the corrector's initials, which in most cases would be the physician who dictated the note. If it is not obvious from the context why the change needed to be made, then the reason should be noted. Never try to erase or obliterate an error. Never substitute an entirely new note for the old one with the intention of making the evidence of the error disappear. When the worst happens and your own words, whether or not an erroneous entry, will damn you in a malpractice case, never, never, never attempt to cover it up. You must always assume that the opposing party already has a copy of the record and would love to find an altered record on discovery. In some states, it is a criminal offense to falsify a medical record to conceal negligence or a criminal act.[4] The physician would be looking at the possible loss of his medical license and a jail term. Physicians should know that the science of documentation examination has advanced to such a point that it is very difficult to successfully falsify a medical record. Plaintiff attorneys may use experts for suspicious entries, because the effects of finding such an alteration mean a virtually guaranteed win. As an example, the ink used in pens may be labeled for the year in which it manufactured. Try explaining a 1997 entry with 1999 ink! The greatest temptation to alter a record is when the physician really is blameless and the entry was an honest mistake. Never attempt to alter the record in any way except the correct one. With electronic medical records, the information about when and who made an alteration will be in the computer in the form of 'metadata.' You will not be able to see it, but it will be there and electronic discovery of medical records is becoming a routine request. Discuss this with your attorney before making a change in a case that is or will be involved in litigation.

CONFIDENTIALITY

Flowing from the fiduciary physician–patient relationship is the duty to preserve the patient's privacy and keep his or her medical records confidential. Legally, the physical medical record belongs to the physician, but the information contained within belongs to the patient. State laws vary, but the patient largely has a right to a copy of his or her records. Exceptions usually exist for psychiatric records. Unless there is a statute providing an exception, the physician may not release the patient's medical records without the patient's permission. Even a request from the patient's attorney or the patient's insurance company cannot be released without the patient's consent. A good office policy is not to allow any medical record to leave the office without it being checked by the physician. Filing errors occur and it is possible to send someone else's note or laboratory result that was misfiled into another patient's chart. Before sending the copy of the record out, the presence of the patient's consent should be verified. Such consent should be in writing. All information about the patient is confidential. It is the patient's privilege to waive and, with rare legal exception, the physician may not reveal information about the patient without permission, e.g. in one case a plastic surgeon used a patient's pre- and postoperative photographs in a presentation at a department store and on television without permission; the court found that this was a violation of the patient's right to confidentiality (*Vassiliades v Garfinkel* 1985). Breach of confidentiality can lead to a lawsuit on multiple grounds, e.g. breach of privacy, breach of confidentiality, breach of fiduciary duty, breach of loyalty, breach of contract, negligence, infliction of emotional distress, as well as liability for violation of privacy statutes, and last but not least, HIPAA (*Doe v Roe* 1977). By statute, the patient usually waives his right to confidentiality when he puts his health in question in litigation, e.g. a malpractice action.

FRAUD AND ABUSE

There are approximately 200 000 pages of Federal rules and regulations concerning health care. This does not include the mountain of paper that will be required to enforce 'Obamacare.' Many involve fraud and abuse. We tend to think of fraud and abuse as billing for patients who were not treated. Certainly, this is a criminal offense. However, physicians are unaware of how many things are rigidly controlled and enforced with draconian laws. Upcoding, bundling, unbundling, etc. are considered serious offenses. The monetary penalties can be truly astronomical. In a representative case, the provider received from Medicare almost $25 000 over a period of years from charges that Medicare later determined were not warranted (*Mayers v Department of Health and Human Services* 1986). Hence, it was fraud. The total penalties under the law were over $5.4 million, but the government settled for only $1.79 million. As the provider could have been charged with multiple criminal offenses with a prison sentence of 5 years for each individual line item charge easily amounting to life in prison, a financial-only punishment was indeed lucky. Cases such as this are not the exception. The penalties in both monetary and prison sentence terms are truly enormous. Major healthcare providers have had settlements of over $1 billion. They settled because, if they lost in court, the financial penalty would have been much higher. Although all these laws definitely apply to any Federal Health Care program (e.g. Medicare, Medicaid, TriCare), many states apply them to private insurance as well. Physicians are usually turned in by disgruntled employees and competitors. The informing individual can file a lawsuit against the physician in the name of the government (a Qui Tam suit) and will be entitled to 15–30% of any settlement in addition to attorney fees. The Stark law, Anti-Kickback law, and the False Claims Act are the laws enforced against fraud and abuse. There are strict requirements to meet in many areas of concern to the surgeon, including any relationship with another physician where anything of value is exchanged, in the structure of ambulatory surgery centers, practice sales, and many other business relationships. All these agreements should be reviewed by a health law attorney knowledgeable in the minutiae of fraud and abuse laws. To give an example to show how detailed these laws are, if there is an ambulatory surgery center owned by physicians of different specialties, only 40% may be owned by physicians using or referring to the surgery center. Also, a minimum of 40% of their practice income must come from operating there. With the passage of the Patient Protection and Accountable Care Act ('Obamacare'), every individual charge to Medicare that involves an Anti-Kickback Violations is automatically a false claim, leading to civil and criminal prosecution with huge fines and possible imprisonment. Referral relationships with other physicians, particularly relevant when doing reconstructive procedures on patients after having the weight loss surgery by another surgeon, are also suspect and need to be evaluated. This stuff is serious. Protect yourself. Have every contract, practice arrangement, associate agreement, and lease with a hospital checked to avoid a violation.

TABLE OF CASES

Bragdon v Abbott, 524 US 624 (1998)
Canterbury v Spence, 464 F. 2d 772 (D.C. Cir. 1972)
Cobbs v Grant, 502 P. 2d 1 (1972)
Creasey v Hogan, 637 P.2d 114 (1981)
Doe v Roe, 400 N.Y.S. 2d 668 (Sup. Ct. 1977)
Helling v Carey, 519 P. 2d 981 (1974)
Hidding v Williams, 578 So. 2d 1192 (La. Ct. App. 1991)
Hiser v Randolph, 617 P.2d 774 (1980)
Lloyd v Kull, 329 F. 2d 168 (7th Cir. 1974)
Mayers v Department of Health and Human Services, 806 F. 2d 995 (11th Cir. 1986)
Millard v Nagle, 587 A. 2d 10 (1991)
Natanson v Kline, 350 P. 2d 1093 (1960)
Nishi v Hartwell, 473 P. 2d 116 (Haw. 1970)
Palsgraf v Long Island R. R. Co., 162 N.E. 99 (1928)
Sago v Leland Stanford, Jr., University Board of Trustees, 317 P.2d 170 (1957)
Schloendorff v Society of New York Hospital, 105 N.E. 92 (1914)
Toth v Community Hospital at Glen Cove, 239 N.E.2d 368 (1968)
Truman v Thomas, 611 P. 2d 902 (1980)
Vandi v Permanente Medical Group, 9 Cal. Rptr. 2d 463 (1992)
Vassiliades v Garfinckel, 492 A. 2d 580 (D.C. 1985)

REFERENCES

1. Rosoff AJ. Consent to medical treatment. In: MacDonald MG, Kaufman RM, Capron AM, Birn M (eds), *Treatise on Health Care Law*. New York: Matthew Bender & Co., 2005:17A-1, 17A-6.
2. Scott AW. *The Fiduciary Principle*. 37 Cal. L. Rev. 539 (1949),
3. LeBlang TR, King JL. *Tort Liability for Nondisclosure: The Physician's Legal Obligation to Disclose Patient Illness and Injury*. 89 Dick. L. Rev. 1 (1984).
4. Mich. Stat. Ann. 9 14.624(1) (Callaghan 1976).

Index

Note: Page numbers in **bold** or *italic* refer to tables or figures respectively.

A

Abdominal binder 107, 111, 179
Abdominal deformities 30, *30–33*, 33, 74
Abdominal wall
  anatomy 74–75, 90, 105–107, *106*
  embryology 74
  hernias 105 (*see also* Incisional hernias)
  laxity 90
Abdominal wall defect reconstruction
  abdominal lipectomy 113–114, *114*, *117*, 118, *118*, 122
  defect evaluation 115, *116*, *117*, *118*
  open wound reconstruction/panniculectomy 118–119, *120*
  patient evaluation 114–115, *115*
  technique 119, 121, *121*
  timing of procedures 116–117, *119*, *120*
  wound preparation 116
Abdominoplasty 9, 39, 192, **192**
  anesthesia considerations 77
  circumferential 83–85, *85*
  classification system 76
  complications 179–181, **180**, *180*
  contraindications 76
  fleur-de-lis 82–83, *83*
  historical perspectives 73
  incisional hernia repair 111, 112, 113
  indications and patient selection 76
  informed consent 76–77
  lipoabdominoplasty 78–79, *79*, *80*
  monsplasty *81*, 81–82
  massive weight loss (MWL) patient and 73
  nutritional assessment 75–76
  photographic documentation 76
  preoperative workup 76
  reverse abdominoplasty 79–81, *80*
  safety precautions 76
  total body lifting 85–86 (*see also* Total body lift (TBL) surgery)
Acellular dermal matrices (ADMs) 110
Adipose tissue 12, 26, 57, 60, 61, 73, 75, 147, 162, 179
Adjustable gastric band (AGB) 2, *2*, **8**, 9
Airway, assessment of 19, 21, 77
Albumin 183
American Society of Plastic Surgery (ASPS)
  body-contouring procedure 179
  brachioplasty procedures statistics 125, *125*
  venous thromboembolism (VTE) prophylaxis guide lines 162, 183
Anatomic deformities, 25
  abdomen 30, *30–33*, 33
  arms 25–26, *27*
  back 33–36, *34–36*
  face and neck 25, *26*
  female breast 27, *29*, 30
  male chest 26–27, *28*
  thigh 36, *37*

Anterior proximal extended thighlift (APEX) 181–182
Anterosuperior iliac spine (ASIS) 92
Antibiotics 82, 97, 101, 110, 122, 130, 168, 179, 181
Antidepressants 5, 14, 161
Arcuate line, abdominal wall 105
Arm *see also* Brachioplasty
  anatomy *125*, 125–126
  deformities in massive weight loss (MWL) patients 25–26, *27*
Arterial cannulation 20
Augmentation
  breast (*see also* Breast reconstruction procedures)
    implant-based 142
    with local perforator flap 140–142
    mastopexy 140
    with pedicled latissimus 142
  gluteal (*see also* Gluteal contouring)
    autologous 149, *150*, *151*
    with implants 147–149, *149*

B

Back
  blood supply 90
  deformities in massive weight loss (MWL) patients 33–36, *34–36*
Barbed sutures 132, 158
Bariatric patients 5, 20, 83, 92, 114–115, *115*
  comorbid conditions in 91
  deflated appearance 89, *89*
Bariatric surgery 1, 7, 39, 73, 105, 113
  body-contouring surgery after 5
  challenges 19–20
  complications 8, **8**
  contraindications to 1, 5
  follow up after
    medical visits 7–8, **8**
    medications 8
    nutrition 8
  malabsorptive procedures 1, 11
  mixed procedures 1, 11
  open *vs.* laparoscopic 3
  preoperative evaluation 1
  procedure options 1, *11*, 11–12, 19
    adjustable gastric band 2, *2*
    biliopancreatic diversion 1–2
    roux-en-Y technique 2–3, *3*
    sleeve gastrectomy 2, *2*
  psychological evaluation
    postbariatric patients 5–6
    preoperative 5
  restrictive procedures 11
  revisional 3
Belt lipectomy 9, 40 *see also* Outpatient lower body lift

historical perspective 89
markings for 92–93, *93*
operation 93–94
positioning 93
and total body lift 89–90, *102*, *103*
  anatomy related to 90
  complications 101
  counseling 92
  history and physical exam 90, **90**
  patient selection and timing 91
  perioperative bleeding risk 92, **92**
  postoperative care 98, 100–101
  preoperative testing 91
  procedure choice 91
  technique 92–98
Biliopancreatic diversion (BPD) 1–2, 11, 15–17
  side effects 2
Binge-eating disorder (BED) 13
Bioprosthetic materials 110
Bleeding complications 101
BMI *see* Body mass index (BMI)
Body contouring procedures 5, 8–9, 11, 19, 39, 57, 73, 179
  combined *vs.* staged procedures 9
  complications
    abdominal contouring 179–181, **180**, *180*
    breast contouring 181, **181**
    extremity contouring **181**, 181–182, *182*
    facial contouring 182
    medical comorbidities 183
    nutritional status 183
    smoking 183
    venous thromboembolism (VTE) prevention 183
  economic considerations 74
  patient expectation, managing 183–184, *184*, *185*
  preoperative evaluation 9, 11
    bariatric procedures and **11**, 11–12
    cardiac disease 12–13
    deep vein thrombosis 13
    diabetes 12
    gastroesophageal reflux disease 13
    laboratory tests 17
    macronutrients 14–15
    micronutrients 15–17
    nutritional deficiency 14, **14**
    psychiatric issues 13–14
    pulmonary disease 13
    weight loss history 12
  venous thrombosis prophylaxis use 77
Body dysmorphic disorder (BDD) 6, 14, 60
Body mass index (BMI) 1, 5, 11, 13, 19, 105, 114, *115*, *119*, 132, 138, 179
  elevated, conditions 19
  obesity 19, **19** (*see also* Obesity)

Body weight stability 12, 14, 57, 75, 85, 161
BPD see Biliopancreatic diversion (BPD)
Brachioplasty 61, 125, 166
    arm anatomy and *125*, 125–126
    complications 131
    extended technique 128, *129*, 130
    historical perspective 126
    indications 126
    liposuction in 128, 166–168, *166–171*, **172**
    minimal incision technique 126, *126*, *127*
    outcome studies 131–132
    postoperative management 128, 130–131
    preoperative preparations 126
    T-incision 126, *127*, *128–129*
Breast 9, 20, 22
    blood supply 90
    deformity from massive weight loss 27, *29*, *30*, **139**
    surgery
        female 137–143 (*see also* Breast reconstruction procedures)
        male 133–136 (*see also* Pseudogynecomastia)
    volume 138
Breast reconstruction procedures 137
    breast anatomy and 137, *137*
    patient evaluation 137
        body mass index 138
        breast volume 138
        degree of ptosis 138, *138*
        history examination 139
        inframammary fold 139
        nipple-areolar complex (NAC) assessment 138
        nicotine use 138–139
    surgical approaches 139, **139**
        dermal suspension 139–140, *140*
        implant augmentation 142
        mammoplasty 143
        parenchymal plication 140, *141*
        in ptosis with insufficient volume 140–142
        vertical mastopexy 139

C
Camper fascia 105
Cancer patients, 189, *190*
    free flaps, use of
        deep inferior epigastric artery (DIEP) free flap 195, *196–197*
        free transverse rectus abdominis (TRAM) 195
        superficial inferior epigastric artery (SIEA) free flap 195
    musculocutaneous flaps 91–192
        gracilis flap 192
        transverse rectus abdominis (TRAM) breast reconstruction 192, *193*
        vertical rectus abdominis myocutaneous (VRAM) flap 192, *194*
    perforator flaps, use of 192, **195**
        anterolateral thigh (ALT) flap 195, *195*
        lateral intercostal perforator (LICAP) flap 192
        superior epigastric artery (SGAP) flap 195
    preoperative examination and planning 189, *190*, **190,** *191*
        hernias and previous incisions 190
        history examination 189, **189**
        nutritional status 191
        patient education 190–191
        preoperative lab tests 189, **189**
        skin excess assessment 189–190, **190**

    skin graft harvest 196, **196,** *200*
    tissue expanders 196, *198*, *199*
    tissue rearrangement 196, *197*
    wound-healing complications 191, **192**
Cardiac disease, in postbariatric patient 12–13
Cautery, 179
Cellulite 160, 168
Chest
    blood supply 90
    deformities in massive weight loss (MWL) patients 26–27, *28*
Cholecalciferol 16
Circumferential abdominoplasty 83–84 *see also* Belt lipectomy
    complications 85
    surgical technique 84–85, *85*
Circumferential dermatolipectomy *see* Belt lipectomy
Circumferential lower body lift 40 *see also* Outpatient lower body lift
Coccyx 145
Component separation technique *108*, 108–109, 111, *118*, 118–119, *120*
Compression garments 101
Computed tomography (CT) 91, 101, *118*, 182
Concentric mastopexy 133–134
Copper deficiency 15

D
Deep venous thrombosis (DVT) 20, 71, 101, 110, 131, 161 *see also* Venous thromboembolism (VTE)
    in postbariatric patient 13
    prophylaxis 98, 180
Dermal bra technique 140, *140*
Dermal suspension 139–140, *140*
Diabetes, in postbariatric patient 12
Diet, after bariatric surgery 8, **8**
Digital imaging 76
Dive test 190
'Dog ear' 94, 97
Doppler ultrasonography 142
Double bubble effect 147
Dumping syndrome 15
Duodenal switch 1
DVT *see* Deep venous thrombosis (DVT)
Dysmorphophobia *see* Body dysmorphic disorder (BDD)

E
Edema 15, 60, 71, 82, 101, 130
Endermologie treatment 60, 71
Extended brachioplasty 128, *129*, *130 see also* Brachioplasty
External oblique muscles, 106, *106*
Extremity contouring procedures **181**, 181–182 *see also* Brachioplasty; Thighplasties

F
Facial contouring 161, 182
    massive weight loss (MWL) patients and 161
    postbariatric face and neck 162
    postoperative care 163
    preoperative evaluation 161
    surgical technique *162*, 162–163, *163*
Facial deformities, in massive weight loss (MWL) patients 25, *26*
Fascia lata graft 109, *109*
Fat-grafting techniques 101

Fleur-de-lis abdominoplasty 82, 119, 121
    complications 83
    surgical technique 82–83, *83*
Folate deficiency 16

G
Gastric partitioning 11
Gastroesophageal reflux disease (GERD) 13
Ghrelin 2
Gluteal contouring 145, 147 *see also* Gluteal region
    implant-based gluteal augmentation 147, *149*
        intramuscular implant 147–148
        subfascial implant 148–149
        submuscular implant 147
    multimodality approach 149
    preoperative consultation 147
Gluteal frame 146
    evaluation *147*
    types 146, *148*
Gluteal region
    anatomy *145*, 145–146
    evaluation 146–147, *147*, **148**
    landmarks 145, *145*
    ptosis 147, *149*
Gluteus maximus 146
Gracilis flap 192
Gynecomastia 27, 61, 133
    vs. pseudogynecomastia 133

H
Hematomas 17, 61, 79, 101
    abdominoplasty/panniculectomy 180–181
    breast contouring 181
    outpatient lower body lift 55
Hernias 76, 82, 84, 90, 91 *see also* Incisional hernias
Histamine H_2-receptor antagonists 20
Horizontal gastroplasty 11
Human cadavers (allogeneic) 110

I
Iliac crest 145, *145*
Implant augmentation 98, 142 *see also* Breast reconstruction procedures
Incisional hernias 3, 9, 105, 107 *see also* Abdominal wall defect reconstruction
    abdominal wall anatomy and 105–107, *106*
    development of, factors for 107
    incidence 107
    natural history 107
    repair 110, 114
        with abdominoplasty/panniculectomy 111
        complications 111–112
        component separation technique *108*, 108–109, 111
        options for *108*, 108–109, *109*
        preoperative evaluation 107–108
Informed consent 76–77, 205
    documentation 207
    elements required in 205–206
    extension doctrine 207
    non requirement of 207
    patient-based standard 206–207
    physician-based standard 206
Infragluteal fold 145, *146*
Inframammary fold (IMF) 27, *137*, 139
Intercostal artery perforator (ICAP) 142
Internal oblique muscles, abdominal wall 106, *106*
Intramuscular gluteal implant 147–148
Iron deficiency, 15

Ischemia 55
Island autologus gluteal augmentation flap 149, *150*

J
Jejunoileal bypass (JIB) 11

L
Labial spreading 160
Lamellar layer, abdominal wall 75
Laparoscopic adjustable gastric banding (LAP-BAND) 11
Legal issues 203
  asset protection 208
  confidentiality 208–209
  expert testimony 204
  fraud and abuse 209
  informed consent 205–206 (*see also* Informed consent)
  litigation 204–205
  malpractice insurance 204
  medical malpractice 203–204
  medical records 208
  vicarious liability 207–208
Lateral intercostal perforator (LICAP) flap 192
Linea alba, abdominal wall 105, *106*
Lipoabdominoplasty 78
  complications 79
  surgical technique 78–79, *79, 80*
Lipobrachioplasty 128
LMWH *see* Low-molecular-weight heparin (LMWH)
Local perforator flaps, 142
Lockwood dissector 40, *42*
Low-dose unfractionated heparin (LUDH) 162
Low-molecular-weight heparin (LMWH) 13, **21**, 22, 77, 122, 162, 183, 191
Lymphazurin blue dye injection 131
Lymphedema 36, 101, 130, 131, 159

M
Mammoplasty 143
Marsupialization 168
Massive weight loss (MWL) 11, 19, 25, 161
  anatomic deformities with 25–36 (*see also* Anatomic deformities, after bariatric weight loss)
  cancer patients 189, 190 (*see also* Cancer patients, reconstructive surgery in)
  excess skin 73
  female breast surgery after 137–143
  male breast surgery after 133–136
  pathophysiology 74
  pseudogynecomastia 133, **133**
Mastopexy 139–140, *140*
Medial antebrachial cutaneous nerve 125, *125*, 131
Medial brachial cutaneous (MBC) nerve 125, *125*, 131
Medicolegal issues *see* Legal issues
Methicillin-resistant *S. aureus* (MRSA) 180
Microcytic anemia 15
Minimal incision brachioplasty 126, *126, 127 see also* Brachioplasty
Monsplasty 9, 81
  complications 82
  surgical technique *81*, 81–82
Moustache autologus gluteal augmentation flap 149, *151*
Mutton-chop flap *see* Rectus femoris musculofascial flap
MWL *see* Massive weight loss (MWL)

N
Neuroma 131
Nicotine use 138–139
Nipple–areolar complex (NAC) 27, 30, 133–136, *136, 137*, 138
Nitrate application 167
Noninvasive positive airway pressure ventilation 20
Nutrition **7**, 8, 21, 91, 92, 131, 139, 191
Nutritional deficiencies, in weight loss patient 1, 11, **14**, 14–17, 20, 75, 183

O
Obesity 1, 7, 12, 19, 39, 73, 105, 107, 113, 146, 161
  body mass index (BMI)-based definitions 19, **19**
  control 7
  medical conditions related to **8**
  morbid 105, 107
  multidisciplinary approach for 74
  pathophysiology 74
  prevalence 74, 105
  treatment 19, 113
Obesity hypoventilation syndrome (OHS) 13
Obstructive sleep apnea (OSA) 13
Oncoplastic breast reduction 196, *197*
Outpatient lower body lift 39
  anesthesia 2–43
  complications 49–50, 54–55, **55**
    hematoma 55
    ischemia 55
    pulmonary embolus 55
    seroma/prolonged drainage 49–50, 54
    wound dehiscence 54
  patient selection 39–40, *40*
  preoperative markings 40–42, *41, 42*
  results 49, **50**, *50–54*
  surgical technique 43–49, *44–48*
    anterior closure 49
    Jackson–Pratt silicone drain placement 46
    lateral–lateral–supine position 44, *45*
    Lockwood dissection *42*, 44
    prone–supine position 44, *44*
    subdermal closure 49
    supine frog-leg positioning 44, *46*
    'V' excision technique 44
  terminology related to 40

P
Panniculectomy 9, 20, 63, 77, 111 *see also* Abdominoplasty
  complications 179–181, **180**, *180*
Pannus, abdominal 33, 61, 81, 89, 90, 95, *96*, 111
Parenchymal plication 140, *141*
Pedicled flaps, 142
Perforator flaps, 192, 195, **195**
Perforator preservation technique 111
Perineal reconstruction 192, *194*
Pinch technique 173–174, *175*
Pitanguy long skin demarcator 167, *168*
Pittsburgh rating scale 25, 33, 76, 81, 139, **139**, 181
Platypygia, of buttocks 146
Platysmaplasty, in postbariatric patient 162 *see also* Facial contouring
Postbariatric patients
  anesthetic considerations
    airway 21
    anemia screening 21
    epidural anesthesia 22
    hypothermia 21–22
    infection 21
    intraoperative 21–22
    liposuction 22
    medical comorbidities 21
    muscle relaxants 22
    NPO guidelines 20–21
    nutritional assessment 21
    positioning 22
    smoking cessation 21, **21**
    staging procedures 20
    thromboembolism prophylaxis 21
  medical management **7**, 7–8, **8**
  nutritional deficiencies in 14, **14**
    fat-soluble vitamins 16–17
    macronutrients 14–15
    micronutrients 15
    minerals 15–16
    water-soluble vitamins 16
  psychological evaluation 5–6
    body image 5–6
    eating habits 6
    quality of life 6
    social functioning 6
  surgical approach to 77–78
Posterosuperior iliac spine (PSIS) 145, *145*
Postoperative nausea and vomiting (PONV) rates, for TIVA 42
Pregnancy test 91
ProCare MD 60
Propofol 43
Protein–calorie malnutrition 14–15
Proton pump inhibitors 20
Pseudogynecomastia 26–27, 133
  classification 133, **133**
  grade 1 133–134, *134*
  grade 2 134, *134*
  grade 3 134, *135*
  surgical treatment 133–135, *134, 135*
    circumvertical technique 134, *134*
    concentric mastopexy 133–134
    midaxillary skin resection 134, *135*
    pedicled reconstruction 134, *134*
    ultrasound-assisted liposuction 133
Pseudo-saddlebag 40
Ptosis
  breast 138, 143
    grading scale 138, *138*
    with insufficient volume 140–142
  gluteal 147, *149*
  of mons pubis 9
Pulmonary embolism (PE) 13, 55, 101
Pyramidalis, abdominal wall 106
Pyridoxine (vitamin B$_6$) deficiency 16

Q
Quill barb suture device 71
Quilting sutures 179, 181

R
Rectus abdominis muscle 74, 90, 105–106, *106*, 115
Rectus diastasis 90
Rectus femoris musculofascial flap 109, *109, 110*
Reverse abdominoplasty 79–80
  complications 80–81
  surgical technique 80, *80*
Riboflavin (vitamin B$_2$) deficiency 16
Roux-en-Y- gastric bypass (RYGB) 1, 2–3, 11, 12, 15–17, 182
  complications **8**
  procedure 3

INDEX

S
Sacral triangle 145, *146*, *146–147*
Saddlebags 158–159
SAL *see* Suction-assisted lipectomy (SAL)
Scar 77, 82, 92, 130, 131, 181, *182*
　care regimen 100
　contracture 131
Scarpa fascia 105
Sciatic nerve 147
Superior epigastric artery perforator (SEAP) flap 195
Selenium deficiency 15–16
Sequential compression devices (SCDs) 13, 183
Seromas 44, 49, 101
　abdominoplasty/panniculectomy 179
　brachioplasty 167–168
　lower body lift 49–50, 54
　thighplasty 181
Superficial inferior epigastric artery (SIEA) flap 195
Silastic ring gastroplasty 11
Silicone gel sheeting 130, 131
Skin
　dehiscence
　　abdominoplasty/panniculectomy 179, *180*
　　brachioplasty 167, 181
　　breast contouring 181
　elasticity 74, 137, 138, 142
　grafts 196, **196**, *200*
　in massive weight loss (MWL) patients 73
　necrosis 111, 180, 194
Sleeve gastrectomy 2, *2*, **8**
Smoking cessation, 9, 21, 76, 179, 183
Staphylococcus aureus 180
Subfascial gluteal augmentation 148
Submuscular gluteal implant 147
Suction-assisted lipectomy (SAL) 165
　candidate for 165, *165*, *166*
　fat deposition areas and 165, *166*
　lower extremity contouring 168, *172*
　　body lift 168, *173*
　　medial thigh lift 168, 172–177, *173–177*, **177**
　upper extremity contouring 165–168 (see also Brachioplasty)
Superficial fascial system (SFS) 146
Superficial musculoaponeurotic system (SMAS) facelift, in postbariatric patient 162, *163 see also* Facial contouring
Surgical glue 158
Surgical site infection 107, 181, 183
　abdominoplasty/panniculectomy 179–180
　and incisional hernias 107

T
Tailor-tack method 158
Thiamine (vitamin B$_1$) deficiency 16
Thigh, in massive weight loss (MWL) patients 36, *37*
Thighplasties 153
　complications 159
　　cellulite 160
　　hematoma 159
　　labial spreading 160
　　lymphocele 159
　　seroma 159
　　wound dehiscence *159*, 159–160, *160*
　extended medial thigh lift 154, *156–157*, 157
　　markings for 157–158, *158*
　　patient positioning 158, *158*
　first-stage debulking 154, *154*, *155*
　history 153
　lateral thigh 158–159, *159*
　patient evaluation 153
Thoracic epidural analgesia 20
T-incision brachioplasty 126, *127*, *128–129 see also* Brachioplasty
Tissue expanders 196, *198*, *199*
Tissue inhibitor of metalloproteinase (TIMP-1) 182, 183
Total body lift (TBL) surgery 57
　anemia and malnutrition treatment 60
　dieting for weight loss 60
　documentation and assessment 57
　endermologie treatment 60
　examination 60
　　abdomen 60
　　arm deformity 61
　　breast and upper body 61
　　gynecomastia 61
　　supine abdomen 61
　groupings of operations 65–66, *65–71*
　intervals between operations 66–67
　marking for 95–97
　medical evaluation 57
　operation 97–98
　　body lift 97–98
　　breast reshaping 98
　operative combinations 61, 63, 65
　positioning 97
　postoperative view 100
　preoperative preparation 60
　preoperative view 99
　psychological assessment 60
　short-hand form for 57, *58–59*
　single-stage 67–68
　success of, 68
　　hypothermia prevention 71
　　improving efficiency 71
　　proficiency in team work 68, 71
　　reducing complications 71
　supplements intake 60
　treatment plan 61, *62–63*
Total intravenous anesthesia (TIVA) 42
Transverse rectus abdominis flap (TRAM), 192, *193*
Transversus abdominis, 106, *106*

U
Ultrasound-assisted lipectomy (UAL) 61, 133
Umbilicoplasty 84, 94
Umbilicus-to-sternal notch distance (U-SN) 135–136, *136*
Upper extremity contouring 165–168, *166*, *167*, *168*

V
Vacuum-assisted closure (VAC) therapy 116
Vascular supply, 106–107
Venous thromboembolism (VTE) 161, 180
　abdominoplasty/panniculectomy 181
　prevention 183
　prophylaxis 161–162
Vertical banded gastroplasty (VBG) 11
Vitamin A deficiency 16, 75
Vitamin B$_{12}$ (cobalamin) deficiency 16, 75
Vitamin D deficiency 16–17
Vitamin K deficiency 17
Vertical rectus abdominis musculocutaneous (VRAM) flap, for perineal reconstruction 192, *194*

W
Weight loss 1 *see also* Massive weight loss (MWL); Obesity
　after gastric bypass 196
　surgery for (see Bariatric surgery) Wernicke–Korsakoff syndrome 16
Wise-pattern incision *140*
Wise-pattern reduction mammoplasty 143
Wound dehiscence 54
　after hernia repair and lipectomy *122*
　outpatient lower body lift 54
　thighplasty *159*, 159–160, *160*

Z
Zinc deficiency, in postbariatric patients 15, 75
Z-plasty 126, 128, *130*, 131, 167